AR Signaling in Human Malignancies: Prostate Cancer and Beyond

Special Issue Editor

Emmanuel S. Antonarakis

MDPI • Basel • Beijing • Wuhan • Barcelona • Belgrade

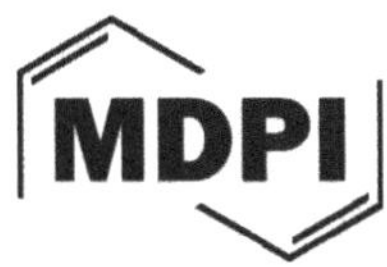

Special Issue Editor
Emmanuel S. Antonarakis
Johns Hopkins University
USA

Editorial Office
MDPI AG
St. Alban-Anlage 66
Basel, Switzerland

This edition is a reprint of the Special Issue published online in the open access journal *Cancers* (ISSN 2072-6694) from 2016–2018 (available at: http://www.mdpi.com/journal/cancers/special_issues/ar_signal).

For citation purposes, cite each article independently as indicated on the article page online and as indicated below:

Lastname, F.M.; Lastname, F.M. Article title. *Journal Name*. **Year**. *Article number*, page range.

First Edition 2018

ISBN 978-3-03842-740-7 (Pbk)
ISBN 978-3-03842-739-1 (PDF)

Table of Contents

About the Special Issue Editor

Emmanuel S. Antonarakis is an Associate Professor of Oncology and Urology at the Johns Hopkins Sidney Kimmel Comprehensive Cancer Center, and the Director of Prostate Cancer Medical Oncology Research. His work focuses on drug development and clinical trial design for patients with prostate cancer. More specifically, he is interested in developing novel androgen-directed therapies as well as immunotherapies for men with recurrent or advanced prostate cancer. He also has an interest in liquid biomarker development, specifically the clinical validation of the AR-V7 marker as well as DNA repair markers and their therapeutic implications. He is currently the PI of several phase II and III prostate cancer trials, and is an active member of the Prostate Cancer Clinical Trials Consortium (PCCTC) and the Eastern Cooperative Oncology Group (ECOG) as well as the NCI Prostate Cancer Task Force and the NCCN Prostate Cancer Panel. He is the author of over 175 peer-reviewed articles, and several book chapters.

Preface to "AR Signaling in Human Malignancies: Prostate Cancer and Beyond"

The notion that androgens and androgen receptor (AR) signaling are the hallmarks of prostate cancer oncogenesis and disease progression is generally well accepted. What is more poorly understood is the role of AR signaling in other human malignancies. This Special Issue of Cancers initially reviews the role of AR in advanced prostate cancer, and then explores the potential importance of AR signaling in other epithelial malignancies. The first few articles focus on the use of novel AR-targeting therapies in castration-resistant prostate cancer and the mechanisms of resistance to novel antiandro-gens, and they also outline the interaction between AR and other cellular pathways, including PI3 kinase signaling, transcriptional regulation, angiogenesis, stromal factors, Wnt signaling, and epige-netic regulation in prostate cancer. The next several articles review the possible role of androgens and AR signaling in breast cancer, bladder cancer, salivary gland cancer, and hepatocellular carcinoma, as well as the potential treatment implications of using antiandrogen therapies in these non-prostatic malignancies.

Emmanuel S. Antonarakis

Special Issue Editor

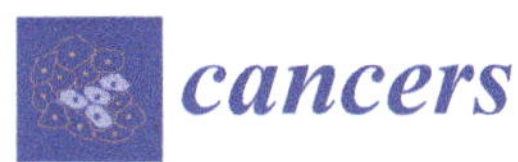

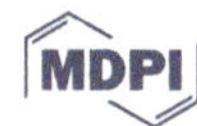

Editorial

AR Signaling in Human Malignancies: Prostate Cancer and Beyond

Emmanuel S. Antonarakis

The Sidney Kimmel Comprehensive Cancer Center at Johns Hopkins, 1650 Orleans Street, CRB1–1M45, Baltimore, MD 21287, USA; eantona1@jhmi.edu; Tel.: +1-443-287-0553

Received: 17 January 2018; Accepted: 17 January 2018; Published: 18 January 2018

Abstract: The notion that androgens and androgen receptor (AR) signaling are the hallmarks of prostate cancer oncogenesis and disease progression is generally well accepted. What is more poorly understood is the role of AR signaling in other human malignancies. This special issue of *Cancers* initially reviews the role of AR in advanced prostate cancer, and then explores the potential importance of AR signaling in other epithelial malignancies. The first few articles focus on the use of novel AR-targeting therapies in castration-resistant prostate cancer and the mechanisms of resistance to novel antiandrogens, and they also outline the interaction between AR and other cellular pathways, including PI3 kinase signaling, transcriptional regulation, angiogenesis, stromal factors, Wnt signaling, and epigenetic regulation in prostate cancer. The next several articles review the possible role of androgens and AR signaling in breast cancer, bladder cancer, salivary gland cancer, and hepatocellular carcinoma, as well as the potential treatment implications of using antiandrogen therapies in these non-prostatic malignancies.

Androgens and androgen receptor (AR) signaling are the hallmarks of prostate cancer oncogenesis and disease progression. While the medical literature is saturated by studies examining the role of androgens/AR in prostate cancer, less attention has been given to the potential importance of the AR pathway in other human malignancies. The goal of this special issue of *Cancers* is to shed more light on the clinical significance of androgen/AR signaling, not just in prostate cancer, but also in other epithelial malignancies.

This theme issue begins with a thoughtful summary by Schweizer et al. [1] introducing the AR signaling field in prostatic and other malignancies. After describing the biological and therapeutic roles of AR in prostate cancer, the authors review the evidence supporting AR-directed therapies in other tumor types including breast cancer, bladder cancer, kidney cancer, pancreatic cancer, hepatocellular cancer, ovarian and endometrial cancers, mantle cell lymphoma, and salivary gland cancers. This is followed by a review by Crumbaker et al. [2] that summarizes the interaction between AR and PI3 kinase signaling in prostate cancer, outlines the role of the PI3K pathway in prostate cancer, and reviews the potential clinical utility of dual targeting of AR and PI3K as a therapeutic strategy in prostate cancer. The next review by Obinata et al. [3] delves deeper into the interplay between AR and other collaborative transcription factors (such as FOXA1, GATA2, and OCT1), and proposes new strategies to co-target AR together with some of these transcriptional collaborators, with particular attention to pyrrole–imidazole polyamide as a candidate compound. This is followed by a review article by Eisermann et al. [4] discussing the interactions between AR, angiogenesis, and the vascular endothelial growth factor (VEGF) in prostate cancer, hormone-mediated mechanisms of VEGF regulation, and potential therapeutic strategies that take into account both AR and hypoxia as potential regulators of angiogenesis. The next article, by Leach et al. [5], reviews the important but understudied subject of AR signaling in the stromal compartment (primarily in fibroblasts and myofibroblasts) in the context of prostate cancer, suggesting that stromal AR activity strongly influences prognosis and progression of this disease. The next article, by Cucchiara et al. [6], summarizes our knowledge of epigenomic regulation of AR in prostate cancer, discusses the various types of epigenetic control (including DNA methylation, chromatin modification, and noncoding RNAs), and ends with some therapeutic implications including the use of the demethylase inhibitor SD-70. Finally, the article by Pakula et al. [7] reviews our current understanding of the interaction between AR and Wnt pathway signaling in prostate cancer, the central role of beta-catenin in this context, and possible therapeutic applications of drugs that target both AR and Wnt/beta-catenin pathways in prostate cancer.

The second series of articles begins to address the role of AR signaling in other human cancers, with a focus on potential therapeutic implications. Rahim et al. [8] begin with a thoughtful overview of the role of androgens and AR signaling in breast cancer (especially in triple-negative breast cancer), they summarize the biology and prognostic/predictive role of AR in breast cancer, and they end with some thoughts on potential therapeutic strategies. This is followed by a second review article on this topic by Narayanan et al. [9] who delve deeper into the therapeutic strategies (nonsteroidal agonists and antagonists) that target androgen/AR signaling in breast cancer. Asano et al. [10] then present an original research article investigating protein expression (by immunohistochemistry) of the AR molecule in 190 cases of triple-negative breast cancer, showing that positive AR protein expression in triple-negative breast cancer tissues is associated with a better prognosis and should perhaps be used to sub-classify cases of triple-negative disease for prognostic purposes. Next, Li et al. [11] review the current knowledge of AR signaling in urothelial carcinoma of the bladder, summarize the data linking androgens to urothelial carcinogenesis and tumor growth, and offer some chemopreventive and therapeutic options for bladder cancer management. After this, the article by Dalin et al. [12] reviews the data on AR signaling in salivary gland cancer (particularly salivary duct carcinoma), and summarizes the prevalence, biology, and therapeutic implications of AR signaling in salivary gland cancers. Finally, the last article in this special issue, by Kanda et al. [13], reviews the role of AR in hepatocellular cancer, its centrality in the development of this malignancy, the potential role of AR in regulating the innate immune response in this disease, and strategies combining sorafenib with AR inhibitors for therapeutic purposes.

We hope that the readership enjoys this this special issue of *Cancers*, that they become informed about the role of androgens and AR signaling in the context of multiple different cancer types, and that this treatise will ignite further clinical research and therapeutic trials aiming to modulate the AR pathway in various human malignancies.

Conflicts of Interest: E.S.A. is a paid consultant/advisor to Janssen, Astellas, Sanofi, Dendreon, Medivation, ESSA, AstraZeneca, Clovis, and Merck and has received research funding to his institution from Janssen, Johnson & Johnson, Sanofi, Dendreon, Genentech, Novartis, Tokai, Bristol Myers-Squibb, AstraZeneca, Clovis, and Merck; he is also the co-inventor of a biomarker technology that has been licensed to Qiagen.

References

1. Schweizer, M.T.; Yu, E.Y. AR-signaling in human malignancies: Prostate cancer and beyond. *Cancers* **2017**, *9*, 7. [CrossRef] [PubMed]
2. Crumbaker, M.; Khoja, L.; Joshua, A.M. AR signaling and the PI3K pathway in prostate cancer. *Cancers* **2017**, *9*, 34. [CrossRef] [PubMed]
3. Obinata, D.; Takayama, K.; Takahashi, S.; Inoue, S. Crosstalk of the androgen receptor with transcriptional collaborators: potential therapeutic targets for castration-resistant prostate cancer. *Cancers* **2017**, *9*, 22. [CrossRef] [PubMed]
4. Eisermann, K.; Fraizer, G. The androgen receptor and VEGF: Mechanisms of androgen-regulated angiogenesis in prostate cancer. *Cancers* **2017**, *9*, 32. [CrossRef] [PubMed]
5. Leach, D.A.; Buchanan, G. Stromal androgen receptor in prostate cancer development and progression. *Cancers* **2017**, *9*, 10. [CrossRef] [PubMed]
6. Cucchiara, V.; Yang, J.C.; Mirone, V.; Gao, A.C.; Rosenfeld, M.G.; Evans, C.P. Epigenomic regulation of androgen receptor signaling: Potential role in prostate cancer therapy. *Cancers* **2017**, *9*, 9. [CrossRef] [PubMed]

7. Pakula, H.; Xiang, D.; Li, Z. A tale of two signals: AR and WNT in development and tumorigenesis of prostate and mammary gland. *Cancers* **2017**, *9*, 14. [CrossRef] [PubMed]
8. Rahim, B.; O'Regan, R. AR signaling in breast cancer. *Cancers* **2017**, *9*, 21. [CrossRef] [PubMed]
9. Narayanan, R.; Dalton, J.T. Androgen receptor: A complex therapeutic target for breast cancer. *Cancers* **2016**, *8*, 108. [CrossRef] [PubMed]
10. Asano, Y.; Kashiwagi, S.; Goto, W.; Tanaka, S.; Morisaki, T.; Takashima, T.; Noda, S.; Onoda, N.; Ohsawa, M.; Hirakawa, K.; Ohira, M. Expression and clinical significance of androgen receptor in triple-negative breast cancer. *Cancers* **2017**, *9*, 4. [CrossRef] [PubMed]
11. Li, P.; Chen, J.; Miyamoto, H. Androgen receptor signaling in bladder cancer. *Cancers* **2017**, *9*, 20. [CrossRef] [PubMed]
12. Dalin, M.G.; Watson, P.A.; Ho, A.L.; Morris, L.G.T. Androgen Receptor signaling in salivary gland cancer. *Cancers* **2017**, *9*, 17. [CrossRef] [PubMed]
13. Kanda, T.; Takahashi, K.; Nakamura, M.; Nakamoto, S.; Wu, S.; Haga, Y.; Sasaki, R.; Jiang, X.; Yokosuka, O. Androgen receptor could be a potential therapeutic target in patients with advanced hepatocellular carcinoma. *Cancers* **2017**, *9*, 43. [CrossRef] [PubMed]

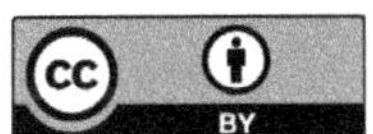

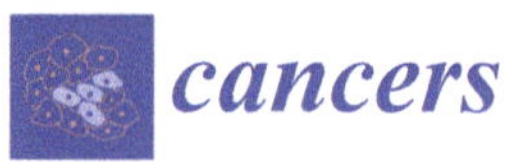

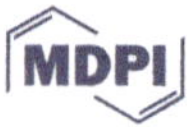

Review

AR-Signaling in Human Malignancies: Prostate Cancer and Beyond

Michael T. Schweizer [1,2,*] and Evan Y. Yu [1,2]

1 Division of Oncology, Department of Medicine, University of Washington, Seattle, WA 98109, USA; evanyu@u.washington.edu
2 Fred Hutchinson Cancer Research Center, Seattle, WA 98109, USA
* Correspondence: schweize@u.washington.edu

Academic Editor: Emmanuel S. Antonarakis
Received: 29 November 2016; Accepted: 5 January 2017; Published: 11 January 2017

Abstract: In the 1940s Charles Huggins reported remarkable palliative benefits following surgical castration in men with advanced prostate cancer, and since then the androgen receptor (AR) has remained the main therapeutic target in this disease. Over the past couple of decades, our understanding of AR-signaling biology has dramatically improved, and it has become apparent that the AR can modulate a number of other well-described oncogenic signaling pathways. Not surprisingly, mounting preclinical and epidemiologic data now supports a role for AR-signaling in promoting the growth and progression of several cancers other than prostate, and early phase clinical trials have documented preliminary signs of efficacy when AR-signaling inhibitors are used in several of these malignancies. In this article, we provide an overview of the evidence supporting the use of AR-directed therapies in prostate as well as other cancers, with an emphasis on the rationale for targeting AR-signaling across tumor types.

Keywords: prostate cancer; breast cancer; bladder cancer; renal cell carcinoma; pancreatic cancer; ovarian cancer; hepatocellular cancer; ovarian cancer; endometrial cancer; androgen receptor

---

1. Androgen Receptor Biology

Androgens, or male sex hormones, have a wide range of functions, including promoting the development of male secondary sexual characteristics, stimulating erythropoiesis, increasing metabolic rate, increasing bone density and stimulating libido [1]. In men, androgens are produced predominately by the testes, while the sole source of androgens in women are the adrenal glands. Consequently, women have considerably lower androgen levels compared to men. The normal physiologic function of androgens is a result of stimulating the androgen receptor (AR).

The AR is a member of the nuclear hormone receptor family of transcription factors, which also includes the estrogen receptor (ER), glucocorticoid receptor (GR), progesterone receptor (PR) and others [2,3]. Like the other nuclear hormone receptors, transcription of AR target genes is induced by the receptor binding androgenic ligands. Canonical AR-signaling involves a well-described series of events, including: (1) AR binding to androgens; (2) dissociating from heat-shock proteins; (3) translocating to the nucleus and the formation of AR homodimers; (4) binding to androgen response elements (AREs) within the promoter region of AR target genes; (5) recruitment of coactivators; and (6) transcription of target genes [4].

In addition to its normal physiologic role, prostatic adenocarcinomas remain dependent on AR-signaling even at later stages. Supporting the importance of AR to prostate cancer biology is the observation that AR target genes (e.g., *PSA*) are usually expressed even in men progressing on androgen deprivation therapy (ADT), with AR pathway alterations commonly observed in late stage disease [5]. This has served as the basis for ADT through medical and surgical castration, as well as the development of next generation AR-directed therapies like abiraterone and enzalutamide.

As our understanding of AR biology has improved, it has become apparent that the AR-signaling pathway can interact with a number of additional oncogenic signaling pathways, including those involved in promoting growth and resistance across a variety of tumor types (e.g., AKT/mTOR/PI3K, EGFR, HER2/Neu, Wnt) [5–12]. Interestingly, in spite of differences in consensus DNA binding motifs, AR is able to bind estrogen response elements and activate a transcriptional program similar to the ER—indicating that AR may be important mediator of breast cancer cell survival as well as other ER-dependent tumors [13,14]. The pleiotropic effects of AR-signaling raise the specter that targeting this pathway may have beneficial effects in a number of different cancers. In this review, we will outline the current evidence for testing AR-directed therapies in prostate, breast and other "non-hormonally" driven cancer like bladder, renal cell and pancreatic cancer, to name a few.

2. AR Targeting in Prostate Cancer

In 1941, Charles Huggins published his seminal paper describing the remarkable palliative effects of surgical castration in men with advanced prostate cancer [15]. We now understand that the beneficial effects of castrating therapy are a direct result of inhibiting AR-signaling, and as such targeting the AR has remained the backbone of prostate cancer therapy since the 1940s. As it stands, ADT is most often achieved through the use of luteinizing hormone releasing hormone (LHRH) agonists/antagonists as opposed to surgical castration; however, both achieve the same effect of lowering testosterone levels to the castrate range (i.e., <20–50 ng/dL) [16]. While ADT is initially highly effective, it does not represent a cure, and the vast majority of men with advanced prostate cancer will progress on ADT, developing castration-resistant prostate cancer (CRPC) [17,18].

Work over the last decade has shown that the AR remains a viable therapeutic target even in the castration-resistant setting. This was born out of the observation that AR target genes (e.g., *PSA*) are often expressed at high levels in patients with CRPC, and that expression of AR will go up in response to ADT [19,20]. It has also come to light that alternative sources of androgens, including those generated intratumorally, may also drive tumor growth in this setting [21,22]. As such, a number of next-generation AR-directed therapies have been developed to further inhibit AR-signaling, with abiraterone and enzalutamide both approved on the basis of Phase III data demonstrating improved overall survival compared to controls [23–27]. Abiraterone is a CYP17 inhibitor that targets extragonadal androgen biosynthesis in the tumor microenvironment and adrenal glands. Enzalutamide is an AR antagonist that is more effective than the first generation non-steroidal antiandrogens (e.g., bicalutamide, nilutamide). Because both of these agents target the ligand-AR interaction—abiraterone through ligand depletion and enzalutamide through antagonizing the AR-ligand binding domain—it is not surprising that numerous groups have documented evidence of cross-resistance between these drugs [28–35].

More recently, a number of studies have described mechanisms whereby AR-signaling is able to reemerge in spite of treatment with next generation AR-signaling inhibitors. Examples of these mechanisms include: AR amplification/overexpression, intratumoral androgen production, activation via feedback pathways (e.g., AKT/mTOR/Pi3K, HER2/Neu), activating AR ligand binding domain mutation, emergence of constitutively active AR splice variants and activation through other nuclear hormone transcription factors (e.g., GR) [6,7,19,21,36–48]. Several in depth reviews of these mechanisms have been published, and a detailed overview of their role in promoting resistance to AR-directed therapies is beyond the scope of this paper [3,20,49]. Suffice it to say, many ongoing drug development efforts are focused on developing more effective AR-directed therapies (e.g., drugs *not* targeting the ligand-AR interaction like EPI-506) or drugs to target key feedback pathways in selected populations (e.g., Akt inhibitors in patients with PTEN loss) [50–52].

3. Breast Cancer

3.1. AR in Breast Cancer

Like prostate cancer, breast cancer is a hormonally regulated malignancy. Indeed, shortly following the discovery that surgical castration was effective in men with advanced prostate cancer, Charles Huggins began exploring oophorectomy and adrenalectomy (with hormone replacement) as treatments for advanced breast cancer [53]. It is worth noting, however, that the German surgeon Albert Schinzinger was first credited with proposing oophorectomy as a treatment for breast cancer in the late 19th century [54]. While most hormonal-based therapies for breast cancer involve inhibiting estrogen receptor (ER)-signaling in hormone receptor positive subtypes, it has recently come to light that AR-signaling is likely an important modulator of breast cancer cell survival and may also be a viable target [55,56].

Several lines of clinical data support the biologic importance of AR-signaling in breast cancer, although AR positivity has been found to have variable prognostic impact across studies. Vera-Badillo, et al. conducted a systemic review of 19 studies that assessed AR immunohistochemistry (IHC) in 7693 patients with early stage breast cancer and found AR staining present in 60.5% of patients; interestingly, AR positivity was associated with improved overall survival (OS) [57]. The authors also found that AR positivity was more common in ER positive compared to ER negative tumors (74.8% vs. 31.8%, $p < 0.001$). However, it should be noted that AR antibodies used across studies was not consistent, nor was the cutoff defining "positivity", making it difficult to draw firm conclusion regarding the overall prevalence of AR positivity across breast cancer subtypes.

Another study analyzing AR expression from tissue microarrays (TMAs) of 931 patients reported that 58.1% stained positive for AR, and that the association of AR with improved OS was only true for patients with ER positive tumors [58]. Apocrine tumors (ER negative, AR positive) with HER2 positivity associated with poorer survival, while AR did not appear to impact OS in triple negative breast cancer (TNBC) cases. A study by Choi and colleagues focused specifically on TNBCs ($n = 559$), found that AR was expressed in 17.7% of these cases, and that AR positivity was a negative prognostic feature. Two subsequent meta-analyses found that AR expression associated with better outcomes across tumor subtypes, however (i.e., ER positive, ER negative, and TNBC) [59,60].

3.2. Targeting AR in Breast Cancer

As mentioned, AR and ER are both nuclear hormone transcription factors and share a number of similar biologic features [55]. Upon binding their respective ligands, they undergo conformational changes, dissociate from heat shock proteins, dimerize and bind to DNA response elements where they promote transcription of target genes [3,61]. A number of studies have documented mechanisms whereby crosstalk between AR and ER exists, with most evidence supporting a model in which AR inhibits ER signaling through a variety of mechanisms—providing a biological basis for why AR positivity may associate with improved outcomes in ER positive breast cancers. AR is able to compete with ER for bindings at ER response elements (EREs), and transfection of MDA-MB-231 breast cancer cells with the AR DNA binding domain has been shown to inhibit ER activity [13]. Because the transcriptional machinery of both ER and AR involves a number of shared coactivator proteins, AR also likely inhibits ER activity through competing for binding of these cofactors [62,63]. Interestingly, there is also evidence that AR and ER can directly interact, with the AR N-terminal domain binding to the ERα ligand binding domain leading to decreased ERα transactivation [64].

The biologic action of AR in ER-negative breast cancers may differ significantly. AR is expressed in 12% to 36% of TNBCs, and in contrast to ER-positive breast cancers, data suggests that AR may be able to drive progression in some ER-negative cell lines [65–71]. Supporting the biologic importance of AR, and its viability as a therapeutic target, preclinical data has shown that AR antagonists (e.g., bicalutamide, enzalutamide) exert an anti-tumor effect in a number of ER-negative breast cancer models [65,67,72].

AR positive TNBCs are generally referred to as molecular apocrine tumors; however, more recent work has defined TNBCs on the basis of their molecular phenotype [73,74]. Work by Lehmann and colleagues have defined six subtypes of TNBC on the basis of their gene expression profiles: basal-like 1 and 2, immunomodulatory, mesenchymal, mesenchymal stem-like, and luminal androgen receptor (LAR) [74]. Interestingly, in spite of being ER-negative, the LAR subtype shares a gene expression signature similar to the luminal, ER-positive breast cancers. Chromatin immunoprecipitation (ChIP)-sequencing studies demonstrate that AR-binding events are similar to those of ERα in ER-positive breast cancer cell lines, indicating that AR may be able to substitute for ER in this context [14].

It should be noted that in addition to LAR tumors, other ER-negative, AR-positive breast cancer subtypes are sensitive to the effects of androgens [65,67]. Ni and colleagues have shown that in HER2-positive, ER-negative cell lines, AR mediates activation of Wnt and HER2 signaling in a ligand-dependent manner [67]. Further speaking to the importance of AR across breast cancer subtypes, Barton and colleagues reported that the next-generation AR antagonist enzalutamide is effective in several non-LAR TNBC subtypes. Interestingly, it has been shown that constitutively active AR splice variants (AR-Vs)—a well-described resistance mechanism in prostate cancer—are present in a large subset of breast cancer tumors, and that treatment of MDA-MB-453 cells (ER/PR-negative, HER2-negative, AR-positive) with enzalutamide can lead to the induction of AR-Vs [75]. The fact that a well-known resistance mechanism to AR-directed therapy appears relevant to breast cancer provides further support for the importance of AR-signaling in breast cancer.

3.3. *Clinical Trials Targeting AR-Signaling in Breast Cancer*

Early clinical data reported by Gucalp and colleagues supported AR as a therapeutic target in AR-positive, ER-negative/PR-negative breast cancers [76]. They conducted a single-arm, Phase II study testing bicalutamide 150 mg daily in patients with >10% nuclear AR staining. The primary endpoint was clinical benefit rate (CBR) defined as complete response (CR), partial response (PR) or stable disease >6 months. Overall, 51 of 424 (12%) screened patients were AR-positive as defined by the study. Twenty-eight patients were treated per protocol, with only 26 being evaluable for the primary endpoint. The study reported a clinical benefit in five patients (all with stable disease), which exceeded the predefined threshold (CBR = 4/28 patients) needed to justify further study.

A single-arm Phase II study testing enzalutamide in AR-positive TNBCs was more recently reported [77]. The primary endpoint was the CBR in "evaluable" patients which were defined as those with $\geq$10% AR staining and a response assessment. After testing 404 patient samples, 55% were found to have AR staining in $\geq$10% of cells. 118 patients were treated with enzalutamide, and 75 were "evaluable". Of the evaluable patients, the CBR at 16 and 24 weeks was 35% and 29% respectively. The median progression free survival (PFS) in this group was 14 weeks. In patients with an AR gene signature (n = 56), clinical outcomes were numerically improved compared to the overall "evaluable" group and those lacking the gene signature (N = 62)—suggesting that further refinement of predictive biomarkers beyond AR IHC is necessary.

Table 1. Ongoing studies testing AR-directed therapies in breast cancer. Abi, abiraterone; Enza, enzalutamide; AR, androgen receptor; AE, adverse event; MTD, maximum tolerated dose; CR, complete response; PR, partial response; and SD, stable disease.

Indication	Therapeutic Agent(s)	Disease State	Study Phase	Sample Size	Primary Endpoint	NCT Number
Breast cancer	Enza, enza + anastrozole, enza + exemestane, enza + fulvestrant	Advanced	Phase I	101	Safety	NCT01597193
Breast cancer	Enza + exemestane	Advanced	Phase II	247	Progression free survival	NCT02007512
Triple-negative breast cancer	Enza + paclitaxel vs. placebo + paclitaxel	Advanced	Phase III	780	Progression free survival	NCT02929576
AR positive, triple-negative breast cancer	Enza + taselisib	Advanced	Phase I/II	73	MTD	NCT02457910
AR positive, triple-negative breast cancer	Enza + paclitaxel	Localized (neoadjuvant)	Phase II	37	Pathologic complete response and minimal residual disease	NCT02689427
HER2 positive and AR positive breast cancer	Enza + trastuzumab	Advanced	Phase II	80	Clinical benefit rate: combined CR, PR and SD	NCT02091960
AR positive, triple-negative breast cancer	Enza	Localized (adjuvant)	Phase II	200	Treatment discontinuation rate	NCT02750358
AR positive, triple-negative breast cancer	Enza	Advanced	Phase II	118	Clinical benefit rate: combined CR, PR and SD	NCT01889238
Breast cancer	VT-464	Advanced	Phase I/II	110	MTD	NCT02580448
Breast cancer	Abi	Advanced	Phase I/II	74	MTD, causality of AEs, and clinical benefit rate: combined CR, PR and SD	NCT00755885
ER positive HER2 negative breast cancer	Abi	Advanced	Phase II	299	Progression free survival	NCT01381874
HER2 negative breast cancer	Abi	Advanced	Phase II	31	Clinical benefit rate: combined CR, PR and SD	NCT01842321
ER positive HER2 negative breast cancer	Abi vs. anastrozole	Localized (neoadjuvant)	Phase II	–	Gene expression differences	NCT01814865
AR positive breast cancer	Orteronel	Advanced	Phase II	86	Response rate: complete and partial responses	NCT01990209
Breast cancer	Orteronel	Advanced	Phase I	8	Safety, recommended Phase II dose, and decrease in estradiol levels	NCT01808040

Abiraterone, an inhibitor of extragonadal androgen biosynthesis, has also been tested in breast cancer [78]. In a randomized Phase II trial, abiraterone was compared to the aromatase inhibitor exemestane or the combination. In contrast to the aforementioned studies, this study focused on ER-positive patients and did not require positive AR staining in order to enroll. The authors cited two reasons for not mandating AR-positivity: (1) upwards of 80% of ER-positive breast cancers are also positive for AR; and (2) inhibition of CYP17 will also decrease estrogen levels. The primary endpoint was PFS. A total of 297 patients were randomized between treatment arms, with 102 receiving exemestane, 106 receiving exemestane plus abiraterone and 89 receiving abiraterone. Of note, enrollment to the abiraterone monotherapy arm was discontinued early after a pre-specified analysis determined that futility conditions had been met. After a median follow up of 11.4 months, there was no difference in median PFS between when abiraterone was compared to exemestane (3.7 vs. 3.7 months, $p = 0.437$), or when abiraterone plus exemestane was compared to exemestane (4.5 vs. 3.7 months, $p = 0.794$). Of note, there was also no difference in PFS in the subset of patients with AR-positive disease.

Given that some studies have shown signs of activity for AR-signaling inhibitors, a number of additional trials are either planned or underway testing AR-directed therapies in breast cancer patients (Table 1). However, it seems likely that these agents will only be effective in a subset of patients, and as such, the development of predictive biomarkers will be critical. Whether the AR will prove to be a clinically important target in breast cancer remains to be seen, but evidence to date does support further testing of drugs designed to inhibit this oncogenic pathway.

4. Other Tumor Types

In addition to prostate and breast cancer, there are a number of other malignancies in which AR-signaling appears to play a role in driving tumor growth. As such, there are several ongoing clinical trials testing AR-directed therapies across an array of cancer types (Table 2). A brief overview of the rationale for targeting AR in these malignancies is provided below.

4.1. Bladder Cancer

In 2016, it is estimated that 58,950 American men will be diagnosed with bladder cancer compared to only 18,010 women [79]. Even after controlling for environmental risk factors (e.g., tobacco exposure) men still have a 3–4-fold increased risk of developing bladder cancer [80–82]. The observed epidemiologic differences in bladder cancer risk between the sexes points to the potential for sex steroid pathways to play a role in the pathogenesis of this disease [83]. Women have also been found to have a worse prognosis compared to men after adjusting for stage at presentation, further bolstering the case that underlying biologic differences between the sexes influencing outcomes [84].

Androgen receptor has been found to be variably expressed in urothelial carcinoma specimens, with AR staining present in 12% to 77% of patients [85–89]. In general, AR expression appears comparable in men and women [85,86]. There is no clear relationship between AR expression and clinical outcomes, and gene expression profiling studies do not demonstrate a clear relationship between AR expression levels and The Cancer Genome Atlas (TCGA) subtype [86,90,91].

Preclinical studies evaluating the effect of androgens and AR-signaling on urothelial carcinoma tumorigenesis have found that AR-signaling may promote tumor formation. In vitro siRNA studies have found that AR knockdown can lead to decreased tumor cell proliferation and increased apoptosis, possibly mediated through AR's effect on *cyclin D1*, *Bcl-x(L)* and *MMP-9* gene expression [92]. In a separate set of experiments, mice engineered to not express AR in urothelial cells were found to have a lower incidence of bladder cancer following exposure to the carcinogen BBN [*N*-butyl-*N*-(4-hydroxybutyl)-nitrosamine] [93]. In vitro experiments found that this effect may be due to modulation of p53 and DNA damage repair. Studies have also implicated AR in modulating various other oncogenic signaling pathways (e.g., EGFR, ERBB2, β-catenin), offering more evidence for the importance of AR-signaling as it pertains to bladder cancer biology [94,95].

Table 2. Ongoing studies testing AR-directed therapies in cancers other than breast or prostate cancer. Enza, enzalutamide; AR, androgen receptor; and MTD, maximum tolerated dose.

Indication	Therapeutic Agent(s)	Disease State	Study Phase	Sample Size	Primary Endpoint	NCT Number
Endometrial cancer	Enza + carboplatin + paclitaxel	Advanced	Phase II	69	Safety/objective tumor response	NCT02684227
Hepatocellular carcinoma	Enza vs. placebo	Advanced	Phase II	144	Overall survival	NCT02528643
Hepatocellular carcinoma	Enza vs. Enza + sorafenib	Advanced	Phase I/II	73	Safety	NCT02642913
Non-muscle invasive bladder cancer	Enza	Localized (chemoprevention)	Phase II	50	Recurrence rate	NCT02605863
Bladder cancer	Enza + cisplatin + gemcitabine	Advanced	Phase I	24	MTD	NCT02300610
AR positive ovarian cancer	Enza	Advanced	Phase II	58	Response rate: complete and partial responses	NCT01974765
Pancreatic cancer	Enza + gemcitabine + nab-paclitaxel	Advanced	Phase I	38	MTD	NCT02138383
Renal cell carcinoma	Enza	Localized (neoadjuvant)	Pilot/Phase 0	20	Cell proliferation and tumor apoptosis	NCT02885649
Mantle cell lymphoma	Enza	Advanced	Pilot/Phase 0	20	Response rate: complete and partial responses	NCT02489123
AR positive salivary cancer	Enza	Advanced	Phase II	45	Response rate: complete and partial responses	NCT02749903

Kawahara and colleagues recently published a paper describing a series of in vitro and in vivo experiments in AR-positive and AR-null bladder cancer models [96]. They found that DHT increased AR-positive bladder cancer cell line viability and migration in culture, while AR antagonists (i.e., hydroxyflutamide, bicalutamide and enzalutamide) inhibited viability and migration. Similarly, apoptosis was decreased following exposure to DHT, and anti-androgens had the opposite effect. Importantly, enzalutamide was found to inhibit AR-positive bladder cancer xenograft growth in vivo. On the basis of these findings, two clinical trials have opened to test enzalutamide in patients with bladder cancer. One is testing enzalutamide monotherapy as a chemoprevention strategy in patients with non-muscle invasive bladder cancer [clinicaltrials.gov: NCT02605863], and the other is testing it in patients with advanced bladder cancer in combination with gemcitabine plus cisplatin [clinicaltrials.gov: NCT02300610].

4.2. Renal Cell Carcinoma

Androgen receptor is expressed in the distal and proximal tubules of normal kidneys and is expressed in approximately 15% to 42% of renal cell carcinomas (RCC) [97–99]. IHC studies correlating AR expression with clinical outcomes have not been consistent, with some reporting an association with decreased survival, while others have found that AR expression was correlated with a favorable pathologic stage and an overall favorable prognosis [97,100,101].

In a study evaluating AR transcript levels using real-time PCR, it was found that AR mRNA expression levels correlated with pathologic T stage and cancer specific survival. Multivariate regression analysis found AR transcript levels were independently associated with cancer specific survival. Of note, AR mRNA levels did not differ between sexes.

A more recent analysis of the TCGA data revealed that high AR protein and transcript levels was associated with improved overall survival in patients with clear cell RCC (the most common pathologic subtype), but not other histologic subtypes of RCC (i.e., papillary or chromophobe) [102]. Interestingly, in clear cell RCC cases they found that AR mRNA expression did not differ between men and women, but that AR protein expression was significantly higher in men. The authors concluded that AR might function as a tumor suppressor in this context.

In vitro experiments have reported that exposure to DHT causes proliferation in AR-positive RCC cells, while enzalutamide can reduce cell viability [103]. Other groups have found that AR may mediate tumor growth through activating HIF-2α/VEGF-signaling [104]. Preclinical studies have shown that enzalutamide can inhibit RCC cell migration and invasion by modulating HIF-2α/VEGF expression at the mRNA and protein levels. A neoadjuvant Pilot study testing enzalutamide in RCC patients is currently underway, with the primary goal to determine the effects of enzalutamide on RCC apoptosis and cellular proliferation [clinicaltrials.gov: NCT02885649].

4.3. Pancreatic Cancer

Although the incidence of AR expression is not well defined in pancreatic cancer, AR does appear to be expressed [105]. A number of in vitro/in vivo studies have tested the effects of antiandrogens and/or androgen deprivation in pancreatic cancer models, and have, for the most part, shown that inhibiting AR-signaling exerts anti-tumor effect [106–113]. Preclinical work has demonstrated that this effect may be mediated through IL-6, with a model whereby IL-6 activates AR-signaling via STAT3 and MAPK. Importantly, IL-6 has been shown to enhance pancreatic cell migration, an effect that is blocked through AR knockdown with an AR siRNA [114].

Greenway reported the results of a randomized trial comparing flutamide (a non-steroidal antiandrogen) vs. placebo ($n = 49$) in patients with both localized and metastatic pancreatic cancer [115]. It should be noted that histologic confirmation of pancreatic cancer was not required, and 32 included subjects were diagnosed on the basis of clinical presentation/imaging studies. This trial reported a median survival of 226 vs. 120 days in the flutamide and placebo groups, respectively ($p = 0.079$,

Wilcoxon; $p = 0.01$, log-rank). Several other studies in patients with pancreatic cancer have not shown hormonal therapies to be beneficial, however [116–121].

Preliminary results from an ongoing Phase I study testing enzalutamide in combination with gemcitabine and nab-paclitaxel in patients with metastatic pancreatic cancer have recently been reported [122]. They have treated 19 patients, and report that 37% had tumor tissue positive for AR. Among 15 evaluable patients, two had a partial response and 13 had stable disease. Pharmacokinetic (PK) analyses did not find any evidence that enzalutamide altered the PK of either chemotherapeutic agent. Whether enzalutamide will prove to be an effective treatment for pancreatic cancer remains to be seen.

4.4. *Hepatocellular Carcinoma*

Androgen receptor appears to be expressed in subset of hepatocellular carcinomas (HCC), although, like pancreatic cancer, the incidence has not been well defined [123–126]. The majority of studies show that AR-positivity is associated with worse outcomes, including decreased progression free and overall survival as well as increased tumor size [126–129]. Studies have also linked AR-signaling with increased risk of developing hepatitis B and C related HCC [130–133]. AR has been found to promote HCC growth, migration and invasion in several preclinical studies, possibly through increasing oxidative stress and DNA damage, as well as suppressing p53 [134–136]. In vitro and in vivo studies targeting AR with either AR-siRNA or ASC-J9 (an AR protein degrader) resulted in decreased tumor growth [134]. A randomized Phase II study testing enzalutamide vs. placebo in HCC is currently underway [clinicaltrials.gov: NCT02528643].

4.5. *Ovarian Cancer*

In 1998, Risch hypothesized that epithelial ovarian cancers may develop as a result of androgens stimulating epithelial cell proliferation, and as it stands, a number of lines of evidence support the role for AR-signaling in the pathogenesis of the disease [137,138]. AR is highly expressed in ovarian cancers, with approximately 44% to 82% of tumors staining positive for AR [139–141]. Polycystic ovarian syndrome (PCOS), and its resultant hyperandrogenic state, are associated with hyperplastic and metaplastic changes in the surface epithelium of the ovaries, and women with ovarian cancer are more likely to have a history of PCOS compared to control cases [142,143]. The use of exogenous androgens (i.e., danazol, testosterone) has been associated with a >3-fold increased risk of developing ovarian cancer [144]. Preclinical models also support the hypothesis that androgens play a role in the development of epithelial ovarian cancers, with a number of oncogenic signaling pathways implicated in this process (e.g., TGF-β, IL-6/IL-8, EGFR) [138,145–147]. However, as it stand, the prognostic impact of AR expression in epithelial ovarian cancers is not clear [138].

A handful of clinical trials testing AR-signaling inhibitors in women with ovarian cancer have been completed, with no clear signs of activity. A single-arm Phase II study testing flutamide in ovarian cancer patients progressing on platinum chemotherapy has previously been reported [148]. Out of 68 women enrolled, only two objective responses (one complete and one partial response) were observed. In a second single-arm Phase II study, flutamide was given to 24 ovarian cancer patients who failed chemotherapy and only one partial response was observed [149]. Finally, in a single-arm Phase II study, Levine and colleagues treated 35 women with ovarian cancer who were in second or greater complete remission with bicalutamide and goserelin (LHRH agonist) [150]. This trial failed to meet the pre-specified metric to justify further studies testing this regimen, which was arbitrarily set at median PFS >13.5 months. More recent preclinical work has shown that enzalutamide is able to significantly inhibit the growth of ovarian cancer xenografts [151]. On this basis, a Phase II study has been launched to test enzalutamide in women with AR-positive, advanced ovarian cancer [clinicaltrials.gov: NCT01974765].

4.6. Endometrial Cancer

Similar to prostate and breast cancer, endometrial cancers are hormonally dependent, and hormonal agents targeting ER-/PR-signaling are options for select patients [152]. Given the similarities to breast and prostate cancer, Tangen and colleagues sought to explore the potential for targeting AR-signaling in advanced endometrial cancer [153]. They found that the majority of hyperplastic endometrial specimens evaluated (93%) had evidence of AR expression. This number decreased in primary tumors, and high-grade tumors (i.e., grade 3) were found to express less AR than low-grade tumors (i.e., grade 1) (53% vs. 74%). Metastatic specimens from 142 patients revealed AR expression in 48% of samples. On multivariate analyses, AR status did not provide additional prognostic value, however. Short-term cell culture experiments demonstrated that cell proliferation was inhibited by enzalutamide, and stimulated by the synthetic androgen R1881, providing justification for a Phase II study testing enzalutamide in combination with carboplatin and paclitaxel [clinicaltrials.gov: NCT02684227].

4.7. Mantle Cell Lymphoma

Mantle cell lymphoma shows a male predominance, and interestingly, male sex appears to associate with higher mortality based on a retrospective SEER analysis [154]. While it is not clear what underlies the poor outcomes in men with mantle cell lymphoma, AR is expressed across an array of hematopoietic cells, and may account for gender differences in the function of platelets and the immune system [155–157]. Furthermore, in contrast to other lymphomas, *AR* appears to be hypomethylated in mantle cell lymphoma—indicating that epigenetic silencing of *AR* gene expression may not be present in mantle cell lymphoma [158,159]. To our knowledge, large studies examining AR protein expression in mantle cell lymphoma samples have not been conducted. On the basis of these observations a pilot study was recently launched to assess the clinical effects of enzalutamide in patients with mantle cell lymphoma [clinicaltrials.gov: NCT02489123].

4.8. Salivary Gland Cancer

AR is expressed in the majority of lacrimal gland ductal carcinomas, and as a result AR staining is often used as part of the workup to confirm the diagnosis [160–166]. To date, there have been a handful of case reports/series documenting favorable outcomes in patients with salivary gland cancers treated with AR-directed therapies. A small case series ($n = 10$) reported a clinical benefit when ADT—most often single agent bicalutamide—was given to patients with salivary ductal carcinoma, with 50% of patients experiencing clinical benefit (i.e., stable disease, $n = 3$; partial response, $n = 2$) [167]. A case report has also reported favorable outcomes when ADT was combined with radiation therapy in a patient with AR-positive salivary gland cancer [168]. A single arm Phase II study testing enzalutamide in AR-positive salivary gland cancers is ongoing [clinicaltrials.gov: NCT02749903].

5. Conclusions

AR signaling is involved in a number of normal physiologic processes, and there is varying levels of evidence for its role in promoting cancer growth and progression across an array of malignancies. To date, prostate cancer remains the only malignancy with Level 1 evidence supporting the use of AR-directed therapies as an integral part of its treatment paradigm. However, mounting preclinical, epidemiologic and early phase clinical trial data support the further exploration of these drugs in diseases as varied as breast and salivary gland cancers, and it is likely that in the ensuing decade next generation AR-directed drugs will extend their reach beyond prostate cancer.

Acknowledgments: M.T.S. has received funding through a Prostate Cancer Foundation Young Investigator Award and DOD award W81XWH-16-1-0484.

Conflicts of Interest: The authors declare no conflict of interest.

References

1. Heemers, H.V.; Tindall, D.J. Androgen receptor (AR) coregulators: A diversity of functions converging on and regulating the ar transcriptional complex. *Endocr. Rev.* **2007**, *28*, 778–808. [CrossRef] [PubMed]
2. Robinson-Rechavi, M.; Escriva Garcia, H.; Laudet, V. The nuclear receptor superfamily. *J. Cell Sci.* **2003**, *116*, 585–586. [CrossRef] [PubMed]
3. Schweizer, M.T.; Yu, E.Y. Persistent androgen receptor addiction in castration-resistant prostate cancer. *J. Hematol. Oncol.* **2015**, *8*, 128. [CrossRef] [PubMed]
4. Koryakina, Y.; Ta, H.Q.; Gioeli, D. Androgen receptor phosphorylation: Biological context and functional consequences. *Endocr. Relat. Cancer* **2014**, *21*, T131–T145. [CrossRef] [PubMed]
5. Robinson, D.; van Allen, E.M.; Wu, Y.M.; Schultz, N.; Lonigro, R.J.; Mosquera, J.M.; Montgomery, B.; Taplin, M.E.; Pritchard, C.C.; Attard, G.; et al. Integrative clinical genomics of advanced prostate cancer. *Cell* **2015**, *161*, 1215–1228. [CrossRef] [PubMed]
6. Yeh, S.; Lin, H.K.; Kang, H.Y.; Thin, T.H.; Lin, M.F.; Chang, C. From HER2/Neu signal cascade to androgen receptor and its coactivators: A novel pathway by induction of androgen target genes through map kinase in prostate cancer cells. *Proc. Natl. Acad. Sci. USA* **1999**, *96*, 5458–5463. [CrossRef] [PubMed]
7. Drake, J.M.; Graham, N.A.; Lee, J.K.; Stoyanova, T.; Faltermeier, C.M.; Sud, S.; Titz, B.; Huang, J.; Pienta, K.J.; Graeber, T.G.; et al. Metastatic castration-resistant prostate cancer reveals intrapatient similarity and interpatient heterogeneity of therapeutic kinase targets. *Proc. Natl. Acad. Sci. USA* **2013**, *110*, E4762–E4769. [CrossRef] [PubMed]
8. Hsieh, A.C.; Liu, Y.; Edlind, M.P.; Ingolia, N.T.; Janes, M.R.; Sher, A.; Shi, E.Y.; Stumpf, C.R.; Christensen, C.; Bonham, M.J.; et al. The translational landscape of mtor signalling steers cancer initiation and metastasis. *Nature* **2012**, *485*, 55–61. [CrossRef] [PubMed]
9. Mulholland, D.J.; Cheng, H.; Reid, K.; Rennie, P.S.; Nelson, C.C. The androgen receptor can promote beta-catenin nuclear translocation independently of adenomatous polyposis coli. *J. Biol. Chem.* **2002**, *277*, 17933–17943. [CrossRef] [PubMed]
10. Chesire, D.R.; Isaacs, W.B. Beta-catenin signaling in prostate cancer: An early perspective. *Endocr. Relat. Cancer* **2003**, *10*, 537–560. [CrossRef] [PubMed]
11. Yang, F.; Li, X.; Sharma, M.; Sasaki, C.Y.; Longo, D.L.; Lim, B.; Sun, Z. Linking beta-catenin to androgen-signaling pathway. *J. Biol. Chem.* **2002**, *277*, 11336–11344. [CrossRef] [PubMed]
12. Traish, A.M.; Morgentaler, A. Epidermal growth factor receptor expression escapes androgen regulation in prostate cancer: A potential molecular switch for tumour growth. *Br. J. Cancer* **2009**, *101*, 1949–1956. [CrossRef] [PubMed]
13. Peters, A.A.; Buchanan, G.; Ricciardelli, C.; Bianco-Miotto, T.; Centenera, M.M.; Harris, J.M.; Jindal, S.; Segara, D.; Jia, L.; Moore, N.L.; et al. Androgen receptor inhibits estrogen receptor-alpha activity and is prognostic in breast cancer. *Cancer Res.* **2009**, *69*, 6131–6140. [CrossRef]
14. Robinson, J.L.; Macarthur, S.; Ross-Innes, C.S.; Tilley, W.D.; Neal, D.E.; Mills, I.G.; Carroll, J.S. Androgen receptor driven transcription in molecular apocrine breast cancer is mediated by foxa1. *EMBO J.* **2011**, *30*, 3019–3027. [CrossRef] [PubMed]
15. Huggins, C.; Hodges, C.V. Studies on prostatic cancer. I. The effect of castration, of estrogen and of androgen injection on serum phosphatases in metastatic carcinoma of the prostate. 1941. *J. Urol.* **2002**, *168*, 948–952. [CrossRef]
16. Nishiyama, T. Serum testosterone levels after medical or surgical androgen deprivation: A comprehensive review of the literature. *Urol. Oncol.* **2014**, *32*, 38.e17–38.e28. [CrossRef]
17. Scher, H.I.; Halabi, S.; Tannock, I.; Morris, M.; Sternberg, C.N.; Carducci, M.A.; Eisenberger, M.A.; Higano, C.; Bubley, G.J.; Dreicer, R.; et al. Design and end points of clinical trials for patients with progressive prostate cancer and castrate levels of testosterone: Recommendations of the prostate cancer clinical trials working group. *J. Clin. Oncol.* **2008**, *26*, 1148–1159. [CrossRef] [PubMed]
18. Scher, H.I.; Morris, M.J.; Stadler, W.M.; Higano, C.S.; Halabi, S.; Smith, M.R.; Basch, E.M.; Fizazi, K.; Ryan, C.J.; Antonarakis, E.S.; et al. The prostate cancer working group 3 (PCWG3) consensus for trials in castration-resistant prostate cancer (CRPC). In Proceedings of the American Society of Clinical Oncology Annual Meeting, Chicago, IL, USA, 29 May–2 June 2015.

19. Chen, C.D.; Welsbie, D.S.; Tran, C.; Baek, S.H.; Chen, R.; Vessella, R.; Rosenfeld, M.G.; Sawyers, C.L. Molecular determinants of resistance to antiandrogen therapy. *Nat. Med.* **2004**, *10*, 33–39. [CrossRef] [PubMed]
20. Scher, H.I.; Sawyers, C.L. Biology of progressive, castration-resistant prostate cancer: Directed therapies targeting the androgen-receptor signaling axis. *J. Clin. Oncol.* **2005**, *23*, 8253–8261. [CrossRef] [PubMed]
21. Montgomery, R.B.; Mostaghel, E.A.; Vessella, R.; Hess, D.L.; Kalhorn, T.F.; Higano, C.S.; True, L.D.; Nelson, P.S. Maintenance of intratumoral androgens in metastatic prostate cancer: A mechanism for castration-resistant tumor growth. *Cancer Res.* **2008**, *68*, 4447–4454. [CrossRef] [PubMed]
22. Mohler, J.L.; Titus, M.A.; Bai, S.; Kennerley, B.J.; Lih, F.B.; Tomer, K.B.; Wilson, E.M. Activation of the androgen receptor by intratumoral bioconversion of androstanediol to dihydrotestosterone in prostate cancer. *Cancer Res.* **2011**, *71*, 1486–1496. [CrossRef] [PubMed]
23. Scher, H.I.; Fizazi, K.; Saad, F.; Taplin, M.E.; Sternberg, C.N.; Miller, K.; de Wit, R.; Mulders, P.; Chi, K.N.; Shore, N.D.; et al. Increased survival with enzalutamide in prostate cancer after chemotherapy. *N. Engl. J. Med.* **2012**, *367*, 1187–1197. [PubMed]
24. Beer, T.M.; Armstrong, A.J.; Rathkopf, D.E.; Loriot, Y.; Sternberg, C.N.; Higano, C.S.; Iversen, P.; Bhattacharya, S.; Carles, J.; Chowdhury, S.; et al. Enzalutamide in metastatic prostate cancer before chemotherapy. *N. Engl. J. Med.* **2014**, *371*, 424–433. [CrossRef] [PubMed]
25. De Bono, J.S.; Logothetis, C.J.; Molina, A.; Fizazi, K.; North, S.; Chu, L.; Chi, K.N.; Jones, R.J.; Goodman, O.B., Jr.; Saad, F.; et al. Abiraterone and increased survival in metastatic prostate cancer. *N. Engl. J. Med.* **2011**, *364*, 1995–2005. [CrossRef]
26. Ryan, C.J.; Smith, M.R.; de Bono, J.S.; Molina, A.; Logothetis, C.J.; de Souza, P.; Fizazi, K.; Mainwaring, P.; Piulats, J.M.; Ng, S.; et al. Abiraterone in metastatic prostate cancer without previous chemotherapy. *N. Engl. J. Med.* **2013**, *368*, 138–148. [CrossRef] [PubMed]
27. Ryan, C.J.; Smith, M.R.; Fizazi, K.; Saad, F.; Mulders, P.F.; Sternberg, C.N.; Miller, K.; Logothetis, C.J.; Shore, N.D.; Small, E.J.; et al. Abiraterone acetate plus prednisone versus placebo plus prednisone in chemotherapy-naive men with metastatic castration-resistant prostate cancer (cou-aa-302): Final overall survival analysis of a randomised, double-blind, placebo-controlled phase 3 study. *Lancet Oncol.* **2015**, *16*, 152–160. [CrossRef]
28. Loriot, Y.; Bianchini, D.; Ileana, E.; Sandhu, S.; Patrikidou, A.; Pezaro, C.; Albiges, L.; Attard, G.; Fizazi, K.; de Bono, J.S.; et al. Antitumour activity of abiraterone acetate against metastatic castration-resistant prostate cancer progressing after docetaxel and enzalutamide (MDV3100). *Ann. Oncol.* **2013**, *24*, 1807–1812. [CrossRef] [PubMed]
29. Noonan, K.L.; North, S.; Bitting, R.L.; Armstrong, A.J.; Ellard, S.L.; Chi, K.N. Clinical activity of abiraterone acetate in patients with metastatic castration-resistant prostate cancer progressing after enzalutamide. *Ann. Oncol.* **2013**, *24*, 1802–1807. [CrossRef] [PubMed]
30. Schrader, A.J.; Boegemann, M.; Ohlmann, C.H.; Schnoeller, T.J.; Krabbe, L.M.; Hajili, T.; Jentzmik, F.; Stoeckle, M.; Schrader, M.; Herrmann, E.; et al. Enzalutamide in castration-resistant prostate cancer patients progressing after docetaxel and abiraterone. *Eur. Urol.* **2014**, *65*, 30–36. [CrossRef] [PubMed]
31. Bianchini, D.; Lorente, D.; Rodriguez-Vida, A.; Omlin, A.; Pezaro, C.; Ferraldeschi, R.; Zivi, A.; Attard, G.; Chowdhury, S.; de Bono, J.S. Antitumour activity of enzalutamide (MDV3100) in patients with metastatic castration-resistant prostate cancer (CRPC) pre-treated with docetaxel and abiraterone. *Eur. J. Cancer* **2014**, *50*, 78–84. [CrossRef] [PubMed]
32. Suzman, D.L.; Luber, B.; Schweizer, M.T.; Nadal, R.; Antonarakis, E.S. Clinical activity of enzalutamide versus docetaxel in men with castration-resistant prostate cancer progressing after abiraterone. *Prostate* **2014**, *74*, 1278–1285. [CrossRef] [PubMed]
33. Badrising, S.; van der Noort, V.; van Oort, I.M.; van den Berg, H.P.; Los, M.; Hamberg, P.; Coenen, J.L.; van den Eertwegh, A.J.; de Jong, I.J.; Kerver, E.D.; et al. Clinical activity and tolerability of enzalutamide (MDV3100) in patients with metastatic, castration-resistant prostate cancer who progress after docetaxel and abiraterone treatment. *Cancer* **2014**, *120*, 968–975. [CrossRef] [PubMed]
34. Cheng, H.H.; Gulati, R.; Azad, A.; Nadal, R.; Twardowski, P.; Vaishampayan, U.N.; Agarwal, N.; Heath, E.I.; Pal, S.K.; Rehman, H.T.; et al. Activity of enzalutamide in men with metastatic castration-resistant prostate cancer is affected by prior treatment with abiraterone and/or docetaxel. *Prostate Cancer Prostatic Dis.* **2015**, *18*, 122–127. [CrossRef]

35. Azad, A.A.; Eigl, B.J.; Murray, R.N.; Kollmannsberger, C.; Chi, K.N. Efficacy of enzalutamide following abiraterone acetate in chemotherapy-naive metastatic castration-resistant prostate cancer patients. *Eur. Urol.* **2015**, *67*, 23–29. [CrossRef]
36. Antonarakis, E.S.; Lu, C.; Wang, H.; Luber, B.; Nakazawa, M.; Roeser, J.C.; Chen, Y.; Mohammad, T.A.; Chen, Y.; Fedor, H.L.; et al. Ar-v7 and resistance to enzalutamide and abiraterone in prostate cancer. *N. Engl. J. Med.* **2014**, *371*, 1028–1038. [CrossRef] [PubMed]
37. Asangani, I.A.; Dommeti, V.L.; Wang, X.; Malik, R.; Cieslik, M.; Yang, R.; Escara-Wilke, J.; Wilder-Romans, K.; Dhanireddy, S.; Engelke, C.; et al. Therapeutic targeting of bet bromodomain proteins in castration-resistant prostate cancer. *Nature* **2014**, *510*, 278–282. [CrossRef] [PubMed]
38. Carreira, S.; Romanel, A.; Goodall, J.; Grist, E.; Ferraldeschi, R.; Miranda, S.; Prandi, D.; Lorente, D.; Frenel, J.S.; Pezaro, C.; et al. Tumor clone dynamics in lethal prostate cancer. *Science Transl. Med.* **2014**, *6*, 254ra125. [CrossRef]
39. Chang, K.H.; Li, R.; Kuri, B.; Lotan, Y.; Roehrborn, C.G.; Liu, J.; Vessella, R.; Nelson, P.S.; Kapur, P.; Guo, X.; et al. A gain-of-function mutation in dht synthesis in castration-resistant prostate cancer. *Cell* **2013**, *154*, 1074–1084. [CrossRef] [PubMed]
40. Cho, E.; Montgomery, R.B.; Mostaghel, E.A. Minireview: Slco and abc transporters: A role for steroid transport in prostate cancer progression. *Endocrinology* **2014**, *155*, 4124–4132. [CrossRef] [PubMed]
41. Evaul, K.; Li, R.; Papari-Zareei, M.; Auchus, R.J.; Sharifi, N. 3beta-hydroxysteroid dehydrogenase is a possible pharmacological target in the treatment of castration-resistant prostate cancer. *Endocrinology* **2010**, *151*, 3514–3520. [CrossRef] [PubMed]
42. Li, Z.; Bishop, A.C.; Alyamani, M.; Garcia, J.A.; Dreicer, R.; Bunch, D.; Liu, J.; Upadhyay, S.K.; Auchus, R.J.; Sharifi, N. Conversion of abiraterone to d4a drives anti-tumour activity in prostate cancer. *Nature* **2015**, *523*, 347–351. [CrossRef] [PubMed]
43. Malik, R.; Khan, A.P.; Asangani, I.A.; Cieslik, M.; Prensner, J.R.; Wang, X.; Iyer, M.K.; Jiang, X.; Borkin, D.; Escara-Wilke, J.; et al. Targeting the mll complex in castration-resistant prostate cancer. *Nat. Med.* **2015**, *21*, 344–352. [CrossRef] [PubMed]
44. Mostaghel, E.A.; Marck, B.T.; Plymate, S.R.; Vessella, R.L.; Balk, S.; Matsumoto, A.M.; Nelson, P.S.; Montgomery, R.B. Resistance to CYP17A1 inhibition with abiraterone in castration-resistant prostate cancer: Induction of steroidogenesis and androgen receptor splice variants. *Clin. Cancer Res.* **2011**, *17*, 5913–5925. [CrossRef]
45. Mostaghel, E.A.; Solomon, K.R.; Pelton, K.; Freeman, M.R.; Montgomery, R.B. Impact of circulating cholesterol levels on growth and intratumoral androgen concentration of prostate tumors. *PLoS ONE* **2012**, *7*, e30062. [CrossRef] [PubMed]
46. Wright, J.L.; Kwon, E.M.; Ostrander, E.A.; Montgomery, R.B.; Lin, D.W.; Vessella, R.; Stanford, J.L.; Mostaghel, E.A. Expression of slco transport genes in castration-resistant prostate cancer and impact of genetic variation in SLCO1B3 and SLCO2B1 on prostate cancer outcomes. *Cancer Epidemiol. Biomark. Prev.* **2011**, *20*, 619–627. [CrossRef] [PubMed]
47. Yang, M.; Xie, W.; Mostaghel, E.; Nakabayashi, M.; Werner, L.; Sun, T.; Pomerantz, M.; Freedman, M.; Ross, R.; Regan, M.; et al. SLCO2B1 and SLCO1B3 may determine time to progression for patients receiving androgen deprivation therapy for prostate cancer. *J. Clin. Oncol.* **2011**, *29*, 2565–2573. [CrossRef] [PubMed]
48. Yu, Z.; Chen, S.; Sowalsky, A.G.; Voznesensky, O.S.; Mostaghel, E.A.; Nelson, P.S.; Cai, C.; Balk, S.P. Rapid induction of androgen receptor splice variants by androgen deprivation in prostate cancer. *Clin. Cancer Res.* **2014**, *20*, 1590–1600. [CrossRef] [PubMed]
49. Boudadi, K.; Antonarakis, E.S. Resistance to novel antiandrogen therapies in metastatic castration-resistant prostate cancer. *Clin. Med. Insights Oncol.* **2016**, *10*, 1–9. [PubMed]
50. De Bono, J.; De Giorgi, U.; Massard, C.; Bracarda, S.; Rodrigues, D.; Kocak, I.; Font, A.; Arija, J.; Shih, K.; Radavoi, G.; et al. Pten loss as a predictive biomarker for the akt inhibitor ipatasertib combined with abiraterone acetate in patients with metastatic castration-resistant prostate cancer (MCRPC). *Ann. Oncol.* **2016**, *27*, vi243–vi265.
51. Montgomery, R.B.; Antonarakis, E.S.; Hussain, M.; Fizazi, K.; Joshua, A.M.; Attard, G.; Sadar, M.; Perabo, F.; Chi, K.N. A phase 1/2 open-label study of safety and antitumor activity of epi-506, a novel ar n-terminal domain inhibitor, in men with metastatic castration-resistant prostate cancer (MCRPC) with progression after enzalutamide or abiraterone. In Proceedings of the American Society of Clinical Oncology Annual Meeting, Chicago, IL, USA, 29 May–2 June 2015.

52. Dehm, S.M.; Tindall, D.J. Androgen receptor structural and functional elements: Role and regulation in prostate cancer. *Mol. Endocrinol.* **2007**, *21*, 2855–2863. [CrossRef] [PubMed]
53. Huggins, C.; Dao, T.L. Adrenalectomy and oophorectomy in treatment of advanced carcinoma of the breast. *J. Am. Med. Assoc.* **1953**, *151*, 1388–1394. [PubMed]
54. Love, R.R.; Philips, J. Oophorectomy for breast cancer: History revisited. *J. Natl. Cancer Inst.* **2002**, *94*, 1433–1434. [CrossRef] [PubMed]
55. Fioretti, F.M.; Sita-Lumsden, A.; Bevan, C.L.; Brooke, G.N. Revising the role of the androgen receptor in breast cancer. *J. Mol. Endocrinol.* **2014**, *52*, R257–R265. [CrossRef] [PubMed]
56. Pietri, E.; Conteduca, V.; Andreis, D.; Massa, I.; Melegari, E.; Sarti, S.; Cecconetto, L.; Schirone, A.; Bravaccini, S.; Serra, P.; et al. Androgen receptor signaling pathways as a target for breast cancer treatment. *Endocr. Relat. Cancer* **2016**, *23*, R485–R498. [CrossRef] [PubMed]
57. Vera-Badillo, F.E.; Templeton, A.J.; de Gouveia, P.; Diaz-Padilla, I.; Bedard, P.L.; Al-Mubarak, M.; Seruga, B.; Tannock, I.F.; Ocana, A.; Amir, E. Androgen receptor expression and outcomes in early breast cancer: A systematic review and meta-analysis. *J. Natl. Cancer Inst.* **2014**, *106*, djt319. [CrossRef] [PubMed]
58. Park, S.; Koo, J.S.; Kim, M.S.; Park, H.S.; Lee, J.S.; Lee, J.S.; Kim, S.I.; Park, B.W.; Lee, K.S. Androgen receptor expression is significantly associated with better outcomes in estrogen receptor-positive breast cancers. *Ann. Oncol.* **2011**, *22*, 1755–1762. [CrossRef] [PubMed]
59. Qu, Q.; Mao, Y.; Fei, X.C.; Shen, K.W. The impact of androgen receptor expression on breast cancer survival: A retrospective study and meta-analysis. *PLoS ONE* **2013**, *8*, e82650. [CrossRef] [PubMed]
60. Kim, Y.; Jae, E.; Yoon, M. Influence of androgen receptor expression on the survival outcomes in breast cancer: A meta-analysis. *J. Breast Cancer* **2015**, *18*, 134–142. [CrossRef] [PubMed]
61. Le Romancer, M.; Poulard, C.; Cohen, P.; Sentis, S.; Renoir, J.M.; Corbo, L. Cracking the estrogen receptor's posttranslational code in breast tumors. *Endocr. Rev.* **2011**, *32*, 597–622. [CrossRef] [PubMed]
62. Risbridger, G.P.; Davis, I.D.; Birrell, S.N.; Tilley, W.D. Breast and prostate cancer: More similar than different. *Nat. Rev. Cancer* **2010**, *10*, 205–212. [CrossRef] [PubMed]
63. Lanzino, M.; De Amicis, F.; McPhaul, M.J.; Marsico, S.; Panno, M.L.; Ando, S. Endogenous coactivator ara70 interacts with estrogen receptor alpha (eralpha) and modulates the functional eralpha/androgen receptor interplay in MCF-7 cells. *J. Biol. Chem.* **2005**, *280*, 20421–20430. [CrossRef] [PubMed]
64. Panet-Raymond, V.; Gottlieb, B.; Beitel, L.K.; Pinsky, L.; Trifiro, M.A. Interactions between androgen and estrogen receptors and the effects on their transactivational properties. *Mol. Cell. Endocrinol.* **2000**, *167*, 139–150. [CrossRef]
65. Barton, V.N.; D'Amato, N.C.; Gordon, M.A.; Lind, H.T.; Spoelstra, N.S.; Babbs, B.L.; Heinz, R.E.; Elias, A.; Jedlicka, P.; Jacobsen, B.M.; et al. Multiple molecular subtypes of triple-negative breast cancer critically rely on androgen receptor and respond to enzalutamide in vivo. *Mol. Cancer Ther.* **2015**, *14*, 769–778. [CrossRef] [PubMed]
66. Bianchini, G.; Balko, J.M.; Mayer, I.A.; Sanders, M.E.; Gianni, L. Triple-negative breast cancer: Challenges and opportunities of a heterogeneous disease. *Nature Rev. Clin. Oncol.* **2016**, *13*, 674–690. [CrossRef] [PubMed]
67. Ni, M.; Chen, Y.; Lim, E.; Wimberly, H.; Bailey, S.T.; Imai, Y.; Rimm, D.L.; Liu, X.S.; Brown, M. Targeting androgen receptor in estrogen receptor-negative breast cancer. *Cancer Cell* **2011**, *20*, 119–131. [CrossRef] [PubMed]
68. Collins, L.C.; Cole, K.S.; Marotti, J.D.; Hu, R.; Schnitt, S.J.; Tamimi, R.M. Androgen receptor expression in breast cancer in relation to molecular phenotype: Results from the nurses' health study. *Mod. Pathol.* **2011**, *24*, 924–931. [CrossRef] [PubMed]
69. Mrklic, I.; Pogorelic, Z.; Capkun, V.; Tomic, S. Expression of androgen receptors in triple negative breast carcinomas. *Acta Histochem.* **2013**, *115*, 344–348. [CrossRef] [PubMed]
70. Thike, A.A.; Yong-Zheng Chong, L.; Cheok, P.Y.; Li, H.H.; Wai-Cheong Yip, G.; Huat Bay, B.; Tse, G.M.; Iqbal, J.; Tan, P.H. Loss of androgen receptor expression predicts early recurrence in triple-negative and basal-like breast cancer. *Mod. Pathol.* **2014**, *27*, 352–360. [CrossRef] [PubMed]
71. Safarpour, D.; Pakneshan, S.; Tavassoli, F.A. Androgen receptor (AR) expression in 400 breast carcinomas: Is routine ar assessment justified? *Am. J. Cancer Res.* **2014**, *4*, 353–368. [PubMed]
72. Cochrane, D.R.; Bernales, S.; Jacobsen, B.M.; Cittelly, D.M.; Howe, E.N.; D'Amato, N.C.; Spoelstra, N.S.; Edgerton, S.M.; Jean, A.; Guerrero, J.; et al. Role of the androgen receptor in breast cancer and preclinical analysis of enzalutamide. *Breast Cancer Res.* **2014**, *16*, R7. [CrossRef] [PubMed]

73. Farmer, P.; Bonnefoi, H.; Becette, V.; Tubiana-Hulin, M.; Fumoleau, P.; Larsimont, D.; Macgrogan, G.; Bergh, J.; Cameron, D.; Goldstein, D.; et al. Identification of molecular apocrine breast tumours by microarray analysis. *Oncogene* **2005**, *24*, 4660–4671. [CrossRef] [PubMed]
74. Lehmann, B.D.; Bauer, J.A.; Chen, X.; Sanders, M.E.; Chakravarthy, A.B.; Shyr, Y.; Pietenpol, J.A. Identification of human triple-negative breast cancer subtypes and preclinical models for selection of targeted therapies. *J. Clin. Investig.* **2011**, *121*, 2750–2767. [CrossRef] [PubMed]
75. Hickey, T.E.; Irvine, C.M.; Dvinge, H.; Tarulli, G.A.; Hanson, A.R.; Ryan, N.K.; Pickering, M.A.; Birrell, S.N.; Hu, D.G.; Mackenzie, P.I.; et al. Expression of androgen receptor splice variants in clinical breast cancers. *Oncotarget* **2015**, *6*, 44728–44744. [PubMed]
76. Gucalp, A.; Tolaney, S.; Isakoff, S.J.; Ingle, J.N.; Liu, M.C.; Carey, L.A.; Blackwell, K.; Rugo, H.; Nabell, L.; Forero, A.; et al. Phase II trial of bicalutamide in patients with androgen receptor-positive, estrogen receptor-negative metastatic breast cancer. *Clin. Cancer Res.* **2013**, *19*, 5505–5512. [CrossRef] [PubMed]
77. Traina, T.; Miller, K.; Yardley, D.; O'Shaughnessy, J.; Cortes, J.; Awada, A.; Kelly, C.; Trudeau, M.; Schmid, P.; Gianni, L.; et al. Results from a phase 2 study of enzalutamide (ENZA), an androgen receptor (AR) inhibitor, in advanced AR+ triple-negative breast cancer (TNBC). In Proceedings of the ASCO Annual Meeting, Chicago, IL, USA, 29 May–2 June 2015.
78. O'Shaughnessy, J.; Campone, M.; Brain, E.; Neven, P.; Hayes, D.; Bondarenko, I.; Griffin, T.W.; Martin, J.; De Porre, P.; Kheoh, T.; et al. Abiraterone acetate, exemestane or the combination in postmenopausal patients with estrogen receptor-positive metastatic breast cancer. *Ann. Oncol.* **2016**, *27*, 106–113. [CrossRef] [PubMed]
79. Siegel, R.L.; Miller, K.D.; Jemal, A. Cancer statistics, 2016. *CA Cancer J. Clin.* **2016**, *66*, 7–30. [CrossRef] [PubMed]
80. Scosyrev, E.; Noyes, K.; Feng, C.; Messing, E. Sex and racial differences in bladder cancer presentation and mortality in the us. *Cancer* **2009**, *115*, 68–74. [CrossRef] [PubMed]
81. Castelao, J.E.; Yuan, J.M.; Skipper, P.L.; Tannenbaum, S.R.; Gago-Dominguez, M.; Crowder, J.S.; Ross, R.K.; Yu, M.C. Gender- and smoking-related bladder cancer risk. *J. Natl. Cancer Inst.* **2001**, *93*, 538–545. [CrossRef] [PubMed]
82. Hartge, P.; Harvey, E.B.; Linehan, W.M.; Silverman, D.T.; Sullivan, J.W.; Hoover, R.N.; Fraumeni, J.F., Jr. Unexplained excess risk of bladder cancer in men. *J. Natl. Cancer Inst.* **1990**, *82*, 1636–1640. [CrossRef] [PubMed]
83. Godoy, G.; Gakis, G.; Smith, C.L.; Fahmy, O. Effects of androgen and estrogen receptor signaling pathways on bladder cancer initiation and progression. *Bladder Cancer* **2016**, *2*, 127–137. [CrossRef] [PubMed]
84. Mungan, N.A.; Aben, K.K.; Schoenberg, M.P.; Visser, O.; Coebergh, J.W.; Witjes, J.A.; Kiemeney, L.A. Gender differences in stage-adjusted bladder cancer survival. *Urology* **2000**, *55*, 876–880. [CrossRef]
85. Boorjian, S.; Ugras, S.; Mongan, N.P.; Gudas, L.J.; You, X.; Tickoo, S.K.; Scherr, D.S. Androgen receptor expression is inversely correlated with pathologic tumor stage in bladder cancer. *Urology* **2004**, *64*, 383–388. [CrossRef] [PubMed]
86. Mir, C.; Shariat, S.F.; van der Kwast, T.H.; Ashfaq, R.; Lotan, Y.; Evans, A.; Skeldon, S.; Hanna, S.; Vajpeyi, R.; Kuk, C.; et al. Loss of androgen receptor expression is not associated with pathological stage, grade, gender or outcome in bladder cancer: A large multi-institutional study. *BJU Int.* **2011**, *108*, 24–30. [CrossRef] [PubMed]
87. Nam, J.K.; Park, S.W.; Lee, S.D.; Chung, M.K. Prognostic value of sex-hormone receptor expression in non-muscle-invasive bladder cancer. *Yonsei Med. J.* **2014**, *55*, 1214–1221. [CrossRef] [PubMed]
88. Williams, E.M.; Higgins, J.P.; Sangoi, A.R.; McKenney, J.K.; Troxell, M.L. Androgen receptor immunohistochemistry in genitourinary neoplasms. *Int. Urol. Nephrol.* **2015**, *47*, 81–85. [CrossRef]
89. Zhuang, Y.H.; Blauer, M.; Tammela, T.; Tuohimaa, P. Immunodetection of androgen receptor in human urinary bladder cancer. *Histopathology* **1997**, *30*, 556–562. [CrossRef] [PubMed]
90. Cancer Genome Atlas Research Network. Comprehensive molecular characterization of urothelial bladder carcinoma. *Nature* **2014**, *507*, 315–322.
91. Choi, W.; Porten, S.; Kim, S.; Willis, D.; Plimack, E.R.; Hoffman-Censits, J.; Roth, B.; Cheng, T.; Tran, M.; Lee, I.L.; et al. Identification of distinct basal and luminal subtypes of muscle-invasive bladder cancer with different sensitivities to frontline chemotherapy. *Cancer Cell* **2014**, *25*, 152–165. [CrossRef] [PubMed]
92. Wu, J.T.; Han, B.M.; Yu, S.Q.; Wang, H.P.; Xia, S.J. Androgen receptor is a potential therapeutic target for bladder cancer. *Urology* **2010**, *75*, 820–827. [CrossRef] [PubMed]

93. Hsu, J.W.; Hsu, I.; Xu, D.; Miyamoto, H.; Liang, L.; Wu, X.R.; Shyr, C.R.; Chang, C. Decreased tumorigenesis and mortality from bladder cancer in mice lacking urothelial androgen receptor. *Am. J. Pathol.* **2013**, *182*, 1811–1820. [CrossRef] [PubMed]
94. Li, Y.; Zheng, Y.; Izumi, K.; Ishiguro, H.; Ye, B.; Li, F.; Miyamoto, H. Androgen activates beta-catenin signaling in bladder cancer cells. *Endocr. Relat. Cancer* **2013**, *20*, 293–304. [CrossRef] [PubMed]
95. Zheng, Y.; Izumi, K.; Yao, J.L.; Miyamoto, H. Dihydrotestosterone upregulates the expression of epidermal growth factor receptor and erbb2 in androgen receptor-positive bladder cancer cells. *Endocr. Relat. Cancer* **2011**, *18*, 451–464. [CrossRef]
96. Kawahara, T.; Ide, H.; Kashiwagi, E.; El-Shishtawy, K.A.; Li, Y.; Reis, L.O.; Zheng, Y.; Miyamoto, H. Enzalutamide inhibits androgen receptor-positive bladder cancer cell growth. *Urol. Oncol.* **2016**, *34*, 432.e15–432.e23. [CrossRef] [PubMed]
97. Langner, C.; Ratschek, M.; Rehak, P.; Schips, L.; Zigeuner, R. Steroid hormone receptor expression in renal cell carcinoma: An immunohistochemical analysis of 182 tumors. *J. Urol.* **2004**, *171*, 611–614. [CrossRef] [PubMed]
98. Brown, D.F.; Dababo, M.A.; Hladik, C.L.; Eagan, K.P.; White, C.L., 3rd; Rushing, E.J. Hormone receptor immunoreactivity in hemangioblastomas and clear cell renal cell carcinomas. *Mod. Pathol.* **1998**, *11*, 55–59. [PubMed]
99. Quinkler, M.; Bujalska, I.J.; Kaur, K.; Onyimba, C.U.; Buhner, S.; Allolio, B.; Hughes, S.V.; Hewison, M.; Stewart, P.M. Androgen receptor-mediated regulation of the alpha-subunit of the epithelial sodium channel in human kidney. *Hypertension* **2005**, *46*, 787–798. [CrossRef] [PubMed]
100. Noh, S.J.; Kang, M.J.; Kim, K.M.; Bae, J.S.; Park, H.S.; Moon, W.S.; Chung, M.J.; Lee, H.; Lee, D.G.; Jang, K.Y. Acetylation status of p53 and the expression of DBC1, SIRT1, and androgen receptor are associated with survival in clear cell renal cell carcinoma patients. *Pathology* **2013**, *45*, 574–580. [CrossRef] [PubMed]
101. Zhu, G.; Liang, L.; Li, L.; Dang, Q.; Song, W.; Yeh, S.; He, D.; Chang, C. The expression and evaluation of androgen receptor in human renal cell carcinoma. *Urology* **2014**, *83*, 510.e519–510.e524. [CrossRef] [PubMed]
102. Zhao, H.; Leppert, J.T.; Peehl, D.M. A protective role for androgen receptor in clear cell renal cell carcinoma based on mining tcga data. *PLoS ONE* **2016**, *11*, e0146505. [CrossRef]
103. Ha, Y.S.; Lee, G.T.; Modi, P.; Kwon, Y.S.; Ahn, H.; Kim, W.J.; Kim, I.Y. Increased expression of androgen receptor mrna in human renal cell carcinoma cells is associated with poor prognosis in patients with localized renal cell carcinoma. *J. Urol.* **2015**, *194*, 1441–1448. [CrossRef] [PubMed]
104. He, D.; Li, L.; Zhu, G.; Liang, L.; Guan, Z.; Chang, L.; Chen, Y.; Yeh, S.; Chang, C. Asc-j9 suppresses renal cell carcinoma progression by targeting an androgen receptor-dependent HIF2ALPHA/vegf signaling pathway. *Cancer Res.* **2014**, *74*, 4420–4430. [CrossRef] [PubMed]
105. Corbishley, T.P.; Iqbal, M.J.; Wilkinson, M.L.; Williams, R. Androgen receptor in human normal and malignant pancreatic tissue and cell lines. *Cancer* **1986**, *57*, 1992–1995. [CrossRef]
106. Konduri, S.; Schwarz, M.A.; Cafasso, D.; Schwarz, R.E. Androgen receptor blockade in experimental combination therapy of pancreatic cancer. *J. Surg. Res.* **2007**, *142*, 378–386. [CrossRef] [PubMed]
107. Sumi, C.; Brinck-Johnsen, T.; Longnecker, D.S. Inhibition of a transplantable pancreatic carcinoma by castration and estradiol administration in rats. *Cancer Res.* **1989**, *49*, 6687–6692. [PubMed]
108. Lhoste, E.F.; Roebuck, B.D.; Stern, J.E.; Longnecker, D.S. Effect of orchiectomy and testosterone on the early stages of azaserine-induced pancreatic carcinogenesis in the rat. *Pancreas* **1987**, *2*, 38–43. [CrossRef] [PubMed]
109. Sumi, C.; Longnecker, D.S.; Roebuck, B.D.; Brinck-Johnsen, T. Inhibitory effects of estrogen and castration on the early stage of pancreatic carcinogenesis in fischer rats treated with azaserine. *Cancer Res.* **1989**, *49*, 2332–2336. [PubMed]
110. Lhoste, E.F.; Roebuck, B.D.; Brinck-Johnsen, T.; Longnecker, D.S. Effect of castration and hormone replacement on azaserine-induced pancreatic carcinogenesis in male and female fischer rats. *Carcinogenesis* **1987**, *8*, 699–703. [CrossRef] [PubMed]
111. Meijers, M.; Visser, C.J.; Klijn, J.G.; Lamberts, S.W.; van Garderen-Hoetmer, A.; de Jong, F.H.; Foekens, J.A.; Woutersen, R.A. Effects of orchiectomy, alone or in combination with testosterone, and cyproterone acetate on exocrine pancreatic carcinogenesis in rats and hamsters. *Int. J. Pancreatol.* **1992**, *11*, 137–146. [CrossRef] [PubMed]
112. Siu, T.O.; Kwan, W.B. Hormones in chemotherapy for pancreatic cancer, chemoagents or carriers? *In Vivo* **1989**, *3*, 255–258. [PubMed]

113. Selvan, R.S.; Metzgar, R.S.; Petrow, V. Growth modulatory effects of some 6-methylenic steroids on human and hamster pancreatic adenocarcinoma cells in vitro. *Drug Des. Discov.* **1992**, *9*, 119–133. [PubMed]
114. Okitsu, K.; Kanda, T.; Imazeki, F.; Yonemitsu, Y.; Ray, R.B.; Chang, C.; Yokosuka, O. Involvement of interleukin-6 and androgen receptor signaling in pancreatic cancer. *Genes Cancer* **2010**, *1*, 859–867. [CrossRef] [PubMed]
115. Greenway, B.A. Effect of flutamide on survival in patients with pancreatic cancer: Results of a prospective, randomised, double blind, placebo controlled trial. *BMJ* **1998**, *316*, 1935–1938. [CrossRef] [PubMed]
116. Sharma, J.J.; Razvillas, B.; Stephens, C.D.; Hilsenbeck, S.G.; Sharma, A.; Rothenberg, M.L. Phase II study of flutamide as second line chemotherapy in patients with advanced pancreatic cancer. *Investig. New Drugs* **1997**, *15*, 361–364. [CrossRef]
117. Negi, S.S.; Agarwal, A.; Chaudhary, A. Flutamide in unresectable pancreatic adenocarcinoma: A randomized, double-blind, placebo-controlled trial. *Investig. New Drugs* **2006**, *24*, 189–194. [CrossRef] [PubMed]
118. Corrie, P.; Mayer, A.; Shaw, J.; D'Ath, S.; Blagden, S.; Blesing, C.; Price, P.; Warner, N. Phase II study to evaluate combining gemcitabine with flutamide in advanced pancreatic cancer patients. *Br. J. Cancer* **2002**, *87*, 716–719. [CrossRef] [PubMed]
119. Keating, J.J.; Johnson, P.J.; Cochrane, A.M.; Gazzard, B.G.; Krasner, N.; Smith, P.M.; Trewby, P.N.; Wheeler, P.; Wilkinson, S.P.; Williams, R. A prospective randomised controlled trial of tamoxifen and cyproterone acetate in pancreatic carcinoma. *Br. J. Cancer* **1989**, *60*, 789–792. [CrossRef] [PubMed]
120. Philip, P.A.; Carmichael, J.; Tonkin, K.; Buamah, P.K.; Britton, J.; Dowsett, M.; Harris, A.L. Hormonal treatment of pancreatic carcinoma: A phase II study of lhrh agonist goserelin plus hydrocortisone. *Br. J. Cancer* **1993**, *67*, 379–382. [CrossRef] [PubMed]
121. Swarovsky, B.; Wolf, M.; Havemann, K.; Arnold, R. Tamoxifen or cyproterone acetate in combination with buserelin are ineffective in patients with pancreatic adenocarcinoma. *Oncology* **1993**, *50*, 226–229. [CrossRef] [PubMed]
122. Mahipal, A.; Springett, G.; Burke, N.; Neuger, A.; Copolla, D.; Kim, R. Phase I trial of gemcitabine, nab-paclitaxel and enzalutamide for treatment of advanced pancreatic cancer. In Proceedings of the AACR-NCI-EORTC International Conference: Molecular Targets and Cancer, Boston, MA, USA, 5–9 November 2015.
123. Vizoso, F.J.; Rodriguez, M.; Altadill, A.; Gonzalez-Dieguez, M.L.; Linares, A.; Gonzalez, L.O.; Junquera, S.; Fresno-Forcelledo, F.; Corte, M.D.; Rodrigo, L. Liver expression of steroid hormones and apolipoprotein d receptors in hepatocellular carcinoma. *World J. Gastroenterol.* **2007**, *13*, 3221–3227. [CrossRef]
124. Nagasue, N.; Ito, A.; Yukaya, H.; Ogawa, Y. Androgen receptors in hepatocellular carcinoma and surrounding parenchyma. *Gastroenterology* **1985**, *89*, 643–647. [CrossRef]
125. Negro, F.; Papotti, M.; Pacchioni, D.; Galimi, F.; Bonino, F.; Bussolati, G. Detection of human androgen receptor mrna in hepatocellular carcinoma by in situ hybridisation. *Liver* **1994**, *14*, 213–219. [CrossRef] [PubMed]
126. Kalra, M.; Mayes, J.; Assefa, S.; Kaul, A.K.; Kaul, R. Role of sex steroid receptors in pathobiology of hepatocellular carcinoma. *World J. Gastroenterol.* **2008**, *14*, 5945–5961. [CrossRef] [PubMed]
127. Nagasue, N.; Yu, L.; Yukaya, H.; Kohno, H.; Nakamura, T. Androgen and oestrogen receptors in hepatocellular carcinoma and surrounding liver parenchyma: Impact on intrahepatic recurrence after hepatic resection. *Br. J. Surg.* **1995**, *82*, 542–547. [CrossRef] [PubMed]
128. Boix, L.; Castells, A.; Bruix, J.; Sole, M.; Bru, C.; Fuster, J.; Rivera, F.; Rodes, J. Androgen receptors in hepatocellular carcinoma and surrounding liver: Relationship with tumor size and recurrence rate after surgical resection. *J. Hepatol.* **1995**, *22*, 616–622. [CrossRef]
129. Zhang, X.; He, L.; Lu, Y.; Liu, M.; Huang, X. Androgen receptor in primary hepatocellular carcinoma and its clinical significance. *Chin. Med. J.* **1998**, *111*, 1083–1086. [PubMed]
130. Yu, M.W.; Yang, Y.C.; Yang, S.Y.; Cheng, S.W.; Liaw, Y.F.; Lin, S.M.; Chen, C.J. Hormonal markers and hepatitis b virus-related hepatocellular carcinoma risk: A nested case-control study among men. *J. Natl. Cancer Inst.* **2001**, *93*, 1644–1651. [CrossRef] [PubMed]
131. Kanda, T.; Steele, R.; Ray, R.; Ray, R.B. Hepatitis c virus core protein augments androgen receptor-mediated signaling. *J. Virol.* **2008**, *82*, 11066–11072. [CrossRef] [PubMed]
132. White, D.L.; Tavakoli-Tabasi, S.; Kuzniarek, J.; Pascua, R.; Ramsey, D.J.; El-Serag, H.B. Higher serum testosterone is associated with increased risk of advanced hepatitis c-related liver disease in males. *Hepatology* **2012**, *55*, 759–768. [CrossRef] [PubMed]

133. Kanda, T.; Jiang, X.; Yokosuka, O. Androgen receptor signaling in hepatocellular carcinoma and pancreatic cancers. *World J. Gastroenterol.* **2014**, *20*, 9229–9236. [PubMed]
134. Ma, W.L.; Hsu, C.L.; Wu, M.H.; Wu, C.T.; Wu, C.C.; Lai, J.J.; Jou, Y.S.; Chen, C.W.; Yeh, S.; Chang, C. Androgen receptor is a new potential therapeutic target for the treatment of hepatocellular carcinoma. *Gastroenterology* **2008**, *135*, 947–955.e5. [CrossRef] [PubMed]
135. Ma, W.L.; Hsu, C.L.; Yeh, C.C.; Wu, M.H.; Huang, C.K.; Jeng, L.B.; Hung, Y.C.; Lin, T.Y.; Yeh, S.; Chang, C. Hepatic androgen receptor suppresses hepatocellular carcinoma metastasis through modulation of cell migration and anoikis. *Hepatology* **2012**, *56*, 176–185. [CrossRef]
136. Ao, J.; Meng, J.; Zhu, L.; Nie, H.; Yang, C.; Li, J.; Gu, J.; Lin, Q.; Long, W.; Dong, X.; et al. Activation of androgen receptor induces id1 and promotes hepatocellular carcinoma cell migration and invasion. *Mol. Oncol.* **2012**, *6*, 507–515. [CrossRef] [PubMed]
137. Risch, H.A. Hormonal etiology of epithelial ovarian cancer, with a hypothesis concerning the role of androgens and progesterone. *J. Natl. Cancer Inst.* **1998**, *90*, 1774–1786. [CrossRef] [PubMed]
138. Zhu, H.; Zhu, X.; Zheng, L.; Hu, X.; Sun, L.; Zhu, X. The role of the androgen receptor in ovarian cancer carcinogenesis and its clinical implications. *Oncotarget* **2016**. [CrossRef]
139. Lee, P.; Rosen, D.G.; Zhu, C.; Silva, E.G.; Liu, J. Expression of progesterone receptor is a favorable prognostic marker in ovarian cancer. *Gynecol. Oncol.* **2005**, *96*, 671–677. [CrossRef] [PubMed]
140. Cardillo, M.R.; Petrangeli, E.; Aliotta, N.; Salvatori, L.; Ravenna, L.; Chang, C.; Castagna, G. Androgen receptors in ovarian tumors: Correlation with oestrogen and progesterone receptors in an immunohistochemical and semiquantitative image analysis study. *J. Exp. Clin. Cancer Res. CR* **1998**, *17*, 231–237. [PubMed]
141. Chadha, S.; Rao, B.R.; Slotman, B.J.; van Vroonhoven, C.C.; van der Kwast, T.H. An immunohistochemical evaluation of androgen and progesterone receptors in ovarian tumors. *Hum. Pathol.* **1993**, *24*, 90–95. [CrossRef]
142. Schildkraut, J.M.; Schwingl, P.J.; Bastos, E.; Evanoff, A.; Hughes, C. Epithelial ovarian cancer risk among women with polycystic ovary syndrome. *Obstet. Gynecol.* **1996**, *88*, 554–559. [CrossRef]
143. Resta, L.; Russo, S.; Colucci, G.A.; Prat, J. Morphologic precursors of ovarian epithelial tumors. *Obstet. Gynecol.* **1993**, *82*, 181–186. [PubMed]
144. Cottreau, C.M.; Ness, R.B.; Modugno, F.; Allen, G.O.; Goodman, M.T. Endometriosis and its treatment with danazol or lupron in relation to ovarian cancer. *Clin. Cancer Res.* **2003**, *9*, 5142–5144. [PubMed]
145. Edmondson, R.J.; Monaghan, J.M.; Davies, B.R. The human ovarian surface epithelium is an androgen responsive tissue. *Br. J. Cancer* **2002**, *86*, 879–885. [CrossRef] [PubMed]
146. Elattar, A.; Warburton, K.G.; Mukhopadhyay, A.; Freer, R.M.; Shaheen, F.; Cross, P.; Plummer, E.R.; Robson, C.N.; Edmondson, R.J. Androgen receptor expression is a biological marker for androgen sensitivity in high grade serous epithelial ovarian cancer. *Gynecol. Oncol.* **2012**, *124*, 142–147. [CrossRef] [PubMed]
147. Gruessner, C.; Gruessner, A.; Glaser, K.; AbuShahin, N.; Zhou, Y.; Laughren, C.; Wright, H.; Pinkerton, S.; Yi, X.; Stoffer, J.; et al. Flutamide and biomarkers in women at high risk for ovarian cancer: Preclinical and clinical evidence. *Cancer Prev. Res.* **2014**, *7*, 896–905. [CrossRef] [PubMed]
148. Tumolo, S.; Rao, B.R.; van der Burg, M.E.; Guastalla, J.P.; Renard, J.; Vermorken, J.B. Phase II trial of flutamide in advanced ovarian cancer: An eortc gynaecological cancer cooperative group study. *Eur. J. Cancer* **1994**, *30A*, 911–914. [CrossRef]
149. Vassilomanolakis, M.; Koumakis, G.; Barbounis, V.; Hajichristou, H.; Tsousis, S.; Efremidis, A. A phase II study of flutamide in ovarian cancer. *Oncology* **1997**, *54*, 199–202. [CrossRef] [PubMed]
150. Levine, D.; Park, K.; Juretzka, M.; Esch, J.; Hensley, M.; Aghajanian, C.; Lewin, S.; Konner, J.; Derosa, F.; Spriggs, D.; et al. A phase II evaluation of goserelin and bicalutamide in patients with ovarian cancer in second or higher complete clinical disease remission. *Cancer* **2007**, *110*, 2448–2456. [CrossRef] [PubMed]
151. Park, B.Y.; Grisham, R.N.; den Hollander, B.; Thapi, D.; Berman, T.; de Stanchina, E.; Zhou, Q.; Iyer, G.; Aghajanian, C.; Spriggs, D.R. Tumor inhibition by enzalutamide in a xenograft model of ovarian cancer. *Cancer Investig.* **2016**, *34*, 517–520. [CrossRef] [PubMed]
152. Fleming, G.F. Second-line therapy for endometrial cancer: The need for better options. *J. Clin. Oncol.* **2015**, *33*, 3535–3540. [CrossRef] [PubMed]
153. Tangen, I.L.; Onyango, T.B.; Kopperud, R.; Berg, A.; Halle, M.K.; Oyan, A.M.; Werner, H.M.; Trovik, J.; Kalland, K.H.; Salvesen, H.B.; et al. Androgen receptor as potential therapeutic target in metastatic endometrial cancer. *Oncotarget* **2016**, *7*, 49289–49298. [CrossRef] [PubMed]

154. Chandran, R.; Gardiner, S.K.; Simon, M.; Spurgeon, S.E. Survival trends in mantle cell lymphoma in the united states over 16 years 1992–2007. *Leuk. Lymphoma* **2012**, *53*, 1488–1493. [CrossRef] [PubMed]
155. Danel, L.; Menouni, M.; Cohen, J.H.; Magaud, J.P.; Lenoir, G.; Revillard, J.P.; Saez, S. Distribution of androgen and estrogen receptors among lymphoid and haemopoietic cell lines. *Leuk. Res.* **1985**, *9*, 1373–1378. [CrossRef]
156. Khetawat, G.; Faraday, N.; Nealen, M.L.; Vijayan, K.V.; Bolton, E.; Noga, S.J.; Bray, P.F. Human megakaryocytes and platelets contain the estrogen receptor beta and androgen receptor (AR): Testosterone regulates ar expression. *Blood* **2000**, *95*, 2289–2296. [PubMed]
157. Klein, S.L. Immune cells have sex and so should journal articles. *Endocrinology* **2012**, *153*, 2544–2550. [CrossRef] [PubMed]
158. Yang, H.; Chen, C.M.; Yan, P.; Huang, T.H.; Shi, H.; Burger, M.; Nimmrich, I.; Maier, S.; Berlin, K.; Caldwell, C.W. The androgen receptor gene is preferentially hypermethylated in follicular non-hodgkin's lymphomas. *Clin. Cancer Res.* **2003**, *9*, 4034–4042.
159. Shi, H.; Maier, S.; Nimmrich, I.; Yan, P.S.; Caldwell, C.W.; Olek, A.; Huang, T.H. Oligonucleotide-based microarray for DNA methylation analysis: Principles and applications. *J. Cell. Biochem.* **2003**, *88*, 138–143. [CrossRef] [PubMed]
160. Andreasen, S.; Grauslund, M.; Heegaard, S. Lacrimal gland ductal carcinomas: Clinical, morphological and genetic characterization and implications for targeted treatment. *Acta Ophthalmol.* **2016**. [CrossRef] [PubMed]
161. Rahimi, S.; Lambiase, A.; Brennan, P.A.; Abdolrahimzadeh, S. An androgen receptor-positive carcinoma of the lacrimal drainage system resembling salivary duct carcinoma: Case report and review of the literature. *Appl. Immunohistochem. Mol. Morphol.* **2016**, *24*, e69–e71. [CrossRef] [PubMed]
162. Simpson, R.H. Salivary duct carcinoma: New developments–morphological variants including pure in situ high grade lesions; proposed molecular classification. *Head Neck Pathol.* **2013**, *7*, S48–S58. [CrossRef] [PubMed]
163. Kapadia, S.B.; Barnes, L. Expression of androgen receptor, gross cystic disease fluid protein, and CD44 in salivary duct carcinoma. *Mod. Pathol.* **1998**, *11*, 1033–1038. [PubMed]
164. Di Palma, S.; Simpson, R.H.; Marchio, C.; Skalova, A.; Ungari, M.; Sandison, A.; Whitaker, S.; Parry, S.; Reis-Filho, J.S. Salivary duct carcinomas can be classified into luminal androgen receptor-positive, her2 and basal-like phenotypes. *Histopathology* **2012**, *61*, 629–643. [CrossRef] [PubMed]
165. Williams, M.D.; Roberts, D.; Blumenschein, G.R., Jr.; Temam, S.; Kies, M.S.; Rosenthal, D.I.; Weber, R.S.; El-Naggar, A.K. Differential expression of hormonal and growth factor receptors in salivary duct carcinomas: Biologic significance and potential role in therapeutic stratification of patients. *Am. J. Surg. Pathol.* **2007**, *31*, 1645–1652. [CrossRef] [PubMed]
166. Fan, C.Y.; Wang, J.; Barnes, E.L. Expression of androgen receptor and prostatic specific markers in salivary duct carcinoma: An immunohistochemical analysis of 13 cases and review of the literature. *Am. J. Surg. Pathol.* **2000**, *24*, 579–586. [CrossRef] [PubMed]
167. Jaspers, H.C.; Verbist, B.M.; Schoffelen, R.; Mattijssen, V.; Slootweg, P.J.; van der Graaf, W.T.; van Herpen, C.M. Androgen receptor-positive salivary duct carcinoma: A disease entity with promising new treatment options. *J. Clin. Oncol.* **2011**, *29*, e473–e476. [CrossRef] [PubMed]
168. Soper, M.S.; Iganej, S.; Thompson, L.D. Definitive treatment of androgen receptor-positive salivary duct carcinoma with androgen deprivation therapy and external beam radiotherapy. *Head Neck* **2014**, *36*, E4–E7. [CrossRef]

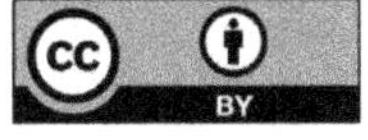

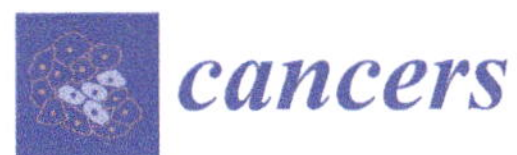

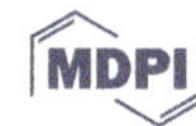

Review

AR Signaling and the PI3K Pathway in Prostate Cancer

Megan Crumbaker [1,2], Leila Khoja [3,4] and Anthony M. Joshua [1,2,5,*]

1. Kinghorn Cancer Centre, St Vincent's Hospital, 370 Victoria Street, Darlinghurst, Sydney, NSW 2010, Australia; m.crumbaker@garvan.org.au
2. Garvan Institute of Medical Research, St Vincent's Clinical School, University of New South Wales, Sydney, 384 Victoria St, Darlinghurst, Sydney, NSW 2010, Australia
3. AstraZeneca UK, Clinical Discovery Unit, Early Clinical Development Innovative Medicines, da Vinci Building, Melbourn Science Park, Melbourn, Hertfordshire SG8 6HB, UK; lkhoja@yahoo.com
4. Addenbrookes Hospital, Cambridge University Hospitals NHS Foundation Trust Cambridge Biomedical Campus, Hills Rd, Cambridge CB2 0QQ, UK
5. Princess Margaret Cancer Centre, University Health Network, University of Toronto, University Avenue, Toronto, ON M5G 2M9, Canada

* Correspondence: anthony.joshua@svha.org.au; Tel.: +61-(02)-9355-5655

Academic Editor: Emmanuel S. Antonarakis
Received: 27 February 2017; Accepted: 11 April 2017; Published: 15 April 2017

Abstract: Prostate cancer is a leading cause of cancer-related death in men worldwide. Aberrant signaling in the androgen pathway is critical in the development and progression of prostate cancer. Despite ongoing reliance on androgen receptor (AR) signaling in castrate resistant disease, in addition to the development of potent androgen targeting drugs, patients invariably develop treatment resistance. Interactions between the AR and PI3K pathways may be a mechanism of treatment resistance and inhibitors of this pathway have been developed with variable success. Herein we outline the role of the PI3K pathway in prostate cancer and, in particular, its association with androgen receptor signaling in the pathogenesis and evolution of prostate cancer, as well as a review of the clinical utility of PI3K targeting.

Keywords: PI3K; prostate cancer; AR signaling; castrate resistant prostate cancer

---

1. Introduction

Prostate cancer is the second most common non-cutaneous cancer in men and the fifth cause of cancer death in men worldwide [1]. The understanding that androgen receptor signaling continues to influence the evolution and development of metastatic castrate-resistant prostate cancer (mCRPC) has prompted the development of novel androgen pathway targeting agents such as enzalutamide and abiraterone acetate. These drugs have yielded practice-changing results with improvements in overall survival as well as a number of meaningful surrogate endpoints. Both enzalutamide and abiraterone are now licensed for the treatment of mCRPC pre- or post-chemotherapy [2–5].

However, resistance to these agents invariably develops via multi-factorial mechanisms [6,7]. It is generally believed that strategies to target inherent and or acquired resistance will lead to more efficacious therapeutic combinations. Activation of the phosphatidylinositol 3-kinase (PI3K) pathway is seen commonly in castrate-resistant disease, and this pathway may represent a therapeutic target with which to overcome treatment resistance. Herein we outline the role of the PI3K pathway in prostate cancer and, in particular, its association with androgen receptor signaling in the pathogenesis and evolution of prostate cancer as well as a review of the clinical utility of PI3K targeting.

2. The Androgen Receptor Pathway

The AR is a ligand-dependent nuclear transcription factor expressed in a variety of tissues which, in the absence of ligand, remains in the cytosol bound to heat shock proteins (Hsps). Though numerous ligands interact with the AR, its predominant native ligands are the androgens, 5α-dihydrotestosterone (DHT) and testosterone. The binding of these ligands to the AR initiates male sexual development and pubertal changes in addition to maintaining libido, spermatogenesis, muscle mass, erythropoiesis and bone mineral density in adult males [8].

Once the AR is engaged its effects manifest via three mechanisms. Firstly, classical AR signaling occurs when androgen binds to the ligand binding domain (LBD) to displace the Hsps triggering AR dimerization, phosphorylation and conformational change leading to exposure of the nuclear localization sequence (NLS). The AR then translocates to the nucleus and the DNA binding domain (DBD) binds to androgen responsive elements (AREs) to induce transcription of specific AR-responsive genes that recruit transcription co-activators and co-suppressors [9,10]. Alternatively, the androgen/AR complex can also trigger second messenger pathways leading to activation of several signaling cascades including MAPK/ERK and AKT [10,11]. This occurs in the cytosol through non-nuclear signaling and is rapid in onset as compared to classical signaling [10,12]. Thirdly ligand-independent activation of the AR is possible via growth factors (such as cytokines e.g., IL-6 [13,14]) and subsequent protein kinase and MAPK pathway activation, phosphorylation of the AR or co-activator stimulation such as insulin-like growth factor (IGF) activation of the AR [15,16]. Such alternative activation can stimulate distinct genes compared to classical AR signaling and may be particularly important in mCRPC [6].

In the normal prostate gland, AR is expressed in the stromal and epithelial compartments [12,17]; postnatal development of the gland is dependent on reciprocal signaling between these two compartments [18]. AR is expressed in both basal and luminal cells of the prostatic epithelium where its primary role is to promote expression of genes involved in terminal differentiation, secretion and suppression of proliferation to maintain homeostasis [12,19–24].

3. AR Signaling in Prostate Cancer

Aberrant AR signaling is critical to the evolution of prostatic carcinogenesis. The AR has been shown to be necessary for cell proliferation, survival and invasion in early and late prostate cancer [25–27]. Rates of cell proliferation and programmed cell death are balanced in the normal prostatic epithelium but this balance is lost in prostate cancer cells [28]. The mechanism for the switch from homeostatic to proliferative AR signaling in prostate cancer is unknown [12]. AR-regulated cancer-specific gene fusions are relatively common and may play a role. Fusion of the ARE-containing promoter from the AR target gene TMPRSS2 to the coding sequence of several members of the Ets family has been well-described [29,30]. These fusions result in AR-driven production of Ets transcription factors potentially leading to proliferation and promotion of cell survival. These fusions however are not present in all tumors. Alternatively, studies mapping genomic binding sites of the AR using ChIP technology have revealed that direct AR binding to aberrant targets may drive prostate pathogenesis [31].

The reliance of prostate cancer on AR signaling has led to the development of potent androgen pathway targeted treatments. Despite initial responses in many however, resistance to these agents is inevitable and remains an intractable problem. Resistance to these therapies may occur broadly through at least three mechanisms [6,10,12,15,24,32–35]: (1) AR-independent activation of AR-dependent pathways via bypass mechanisms, such as through up-regulation of glucocorticoid receptor expression [32]; (2) De-differentiation such as BRN2-mediated trans-differentiation to neuroendocrine prostate carcinoma [36]; and (3) The most commonly targeted mechanism, direct reactivation of the AR and its signaling despite castrate levels of androgens. The third mechanism can occur via AR gene amplification or AR protein overexpression. It may be ligand-dependent, such as intra-tumoral androgen synthesis activating classical signaling and AR LBD mutations leading to increased sensitivity to agonists or alternate non-androgen ligands [37,38]. Conversely,

AR reactivation may also be ligand-independent; examples include AR splice variants resulting in constitutive activation [39–42] (reviewed by Sprenger and Plymate [43]) or AR activation through other proliferation pathways. The PI3K pathway may be involved in more than one of the above mechanisms through non-nuclear interactions between ligand-activated AR and PI3K [10,12] and direct stimulatory feedback from the PI3K pathway [44].

4. The PI3K Signaling Pathway

PI3Ks are a family of lipid kinases that regulate anabolic and catabolic activities in the cell through phosphorylation of the 3′-hydroxyl group of phosphoinositides and phosphatidylinositol. PI3Ks are divided into three classes according to their preferred substrate and sequence homology with class IA thought to be most relevant to human cancers [45].

Class IA PI3Ks are heterodimers made up of a regulatory subunit (p85α, p55α, p50α, p85β or p85γ) and a catalytic subunit (p110α, β or δ) that can be activated by receptor tyrosine kinases, G-protein coupled receptors or oncogenes [46,47]. Following stimulation, the catalytic subunit of PI3K phosphorylates phosphatidylinositol-4,5-biphosphate (PIP2) to phosphatidylinositol-3,4,5-triphosphate (PIP3), a reaction negatively regulated by the phosphatase and tensin homolog chromosome 10 (PTEN) and INPP4B. PIP3 acts as a second messenger to propagate intracellular signaling by binding pleckstrin homology domains. This signaling cascade eventually leads to AKT activation through phosphorylation by PDK1 and the mTORC 1/2 complexes. AKT, in turn, phosphorylates several cellular proteins which regulate cellular processes including cell growth, survival, proliferation, metabolism and angiogenesis through effectors such as p27, BAD, glycogen synthetase kinase 3 (GSK3) and forkhead box O (FOXO) transcription factors [46].

PIK3CA, PIK3CB and PIK3CD genes encode the p110α, β and δ isoforms respectively. The p110α and 110β isoforms are both widely expressed but p110δ is generally only found in leucocytes. Both the alpha and beta isoforms generate PIP3 but have differing roles: p110α is mainly found in the cytoplasm and is crucial in insulin signaling, glucose metabolism and G1 cell cycle entry while p110β is found in the nucleus and is important in DNA synthesis and replication and cell mitosis [48]. Both isoforms have been implicated in human cancer. Oncogenicity of the p110α isoform is well established [49–52] and mutations of PIK3CA play a causative role in the development of many cancer types (reviewed by Samuels [53]). PIK3CB and PIK3CD genes are rarely mutated in cancers but are often amplified or over-expressed [54]. Aberrant PI3K signaling in cancer can also occur via PTEN abnormalities including mutations, promotor hypermethylation or loss of heterozygosity; AKT isoform mutations or amplifications can occur as well (reviewed by Sadeghi and Gerber [55]).

5. PI3K Pathway Activation in Prostate Cancer

Aberrations in PI3K/AKT/mTOR signaling have been identified in approximately 40% of early prostate cancer cases and 70–100% in advanced disease [56,57]. In particular, loss of PTEN leading to constitutive activation of the PI3K pathway has been documented in 30% of primary and 60% of castrate-resistant prostate cancers [58]. Activation of the PI3K pathway is associated with resistance to androgen deprivation therapy, disease progression and poor outcomes in prostate cancer [59–62]. Over-activation via PTEN loss has been shown to initiate prostate cancer development. Varying rates of prostatic hyperplasia and cancer are seen in mouse models with heterozygous loss of PTEN [63–66] and combined deletion of a second tumor suppressor gene can induce prostate cancer with complete penetrance in some models [67]; heterozygous models failed to develop metastatic disease however. Conditional PTEN knockout mice though can mimic the course of human prostate cancer with progression from hyperplasia to invasive cancer to metastatic disease [68]. Moreover, pre-clinical data demonstrate that some PTEN-deficient neoplasms, including prostate cancer, particularly activate the PI3K pathway through the p110β isoform of the PI3K catalytic subunit [69–71]. Ablation of p110β but not p110α inhibits downstream AKT signaling resulting in reduced tumorogenesis in these models. Importantly however, selective p110β inhibition only temporarily inhibits signaling in PTEN deficient models because it removes feedback inhibition on receptors which in turn up-regulate signaling via p110α [72]. Combined inhibition of p110α and p110β results in more sustained suppression of signaling with improved tumor shrinkage in PTEN null models of prostate cancer as compared to p110β inhibition alone.

The association of PI3K pathway activation with castrate-refractory disease suggests that a critical component of the poor prognostic value of PI3K aberrations may be its interaction with androgen signaling. Additionally, responses to AR inhibitors in prostate cancers with PTEN loss may depend on the level of PI3K pathway activation.

6. Interaction of PI3K and AR Signaling

Despite the association outlined above, the effect of PI3K activation on prostate cancer growth pre-clinically is not dichotomous as some cell lines with PTEN loss (e.g., LNCaP) retain sensitivity to castration, while the robust response to castration in de novo disease suggests that most PTEN null tumors retain some sensitivity to androgen deprivation. The mechanism of the interaction between these two pathways remained unclear until relatively recently.

Two landmark papers defined the interplay between PTEN loss/PI3K activation and AR signaling in the development of prostate cancer [56,73]. Carver et al. first demonstrated in a series of studies on PTEN deficient murine and human cell lines that pharmacological PI3K inhibition increased AR protein thereby activating AR-related gene expression through a HER3 dependent mechanism (HER2 and Her3 promote AR activity and stability); similar effects were seen with AKT inhibition. They cross-validated this data in human samples indirectly demonstrating that a gene set enrichment score (GESA) of AR activity was significantly repressed in PTEN null human samples, as well as being associated with decreased HER2 expression [74,75]. Thereafter, they also demonstrated the inverse relationship with AR inhibition being associated with upregulated AKT signaling as a result of increased phosphorylation of AKT target genes such as GSK-alpha and PRAS40. The mechanism was determined to be through AR inhibition causing downregulation of the androgen dependent immunophilin FKBP5 that in turn is a chaperone for the AKT phosphatase PHLPP [8,76]. Finally, to confirm their finding of cross-regulation between the AR and PI3K pathways, they tested the effect of single pathway and combined pathway inhibition on PTEN deficient models. While single pathway inhibition with either enzalutamide or BEZ235 (a PI3K inhibitor) only had modest cytostatic effects, the combination of AR and PI3K pathway inhibition (in particular PI3K and/or mTORC 1/2) or PI3K inhibition and HER2/3 inhibition led to significant tumor reductions.

Utilizing a PTEN conditional murine prostate cancer model, Mulholland et al. demonstrated that PTEN loss suppresses AR transcriptional output and generally drives gene expression towards a castrate-like phenotype. To determine how PTEN loss causes suppression of AR transcriptional output, they used a doxycycline-dependent PTEN loss murine model. They found PTEN re-expression did not affect AR expression but did lead to reduced expression of EGR1 and c-JUN transcription factors, factors that are known to be up-regulated particularly in CRPC and to promote cancer growth in an androgen-depleted environment through direct interaction with and downregulation of the AR [77,78]. Through Network Component Analysis, they showed that PTEN re-expression was associated with reduced transcription factor activities (TFAs) of EGR1 and c-JUN followed by increased AR TFA. Reduced AR TFA seen in PTEN null models can be reversed by mTOR inhibition, suggesting involvement of the PI3K/AKT/mTOR pathway as seen by Carver et al. Additionally, Mulholland et al. found that downregulation of FKBP5/PHLPP by AR inhibition/loss may release the negative feedback on the AKT pathway to promote AKT-dependent, AR-independent cell growth. They showed more significant tumor regressions with dual pathway inhibition via Enzalutamide and rapamycin rather than single pathway inhibition in both PTEN null/AR+ prostate cancer cell lines and PTEN null mice.

Given the complexity of the AR and PI3K pathways, they likely interact at numerous levels. AR-induced PI3K stimulation may also occur through Src-mediated non-nuclear signaling, particularly in the context of ADT [79,80]. Androgen-bound AR can form a complex with Src to induce cell proliferation pathways. Aberrant Src signaling is present in prostate cancer cells. In low passage, androgen sensitive LNCaP prostate cancer cell lines, Src signaling is androgen-dependent. High passage cell lines however demonstrate constitutively activated AR/Src-induced proliferation in the absence of androgen [81]. AR and PI3K cross talk may occur through interactions of AR/Src and the p85α subunit of PI3K may trigger downstream pathway activation to promote cell survival in androgen-deplete conditions [10]. These interactions may be particularly important in patients treated with enzalutamide which prevents translocation of the AR into the nucleus promoting more cytosolic interactions which stimulate non-nuclear signaling.

Though Mulholland and Carver proposed somewhat different mechanisms, they independently demonstrated with both pharmacologic and genetic approaches PI3K/AKT activation via PTEN loss promotes prostate cancer growth in the absence of AR signaling; as a result, they hypothesize that strong suppression of AR-signaling with potent anti-androgen therapy may select for tumors with PI3K pathway activation and repressed AR activity leading to CRPC. They showed that dual pathway inhibition with androgen deprivation and a PI3K, AKT or mTOR inhibitor could lead to significant tumor regression as compared to single pathway inhibition.

Subsequent studies have supported the presence of AR-PI3K pathway interactions. Zhu et al. showed that conditional expression of human AR transgene in transgenic mice prostates not only induced malignancy but also resulted in decreased AKT activation in the tumor cells [82]. They further investigated the interaction between the PI3K/AKT and AR pathways in a series of in vitro and in vivo experiments [83] which confirmed a functional interaction between the pathways. They showed that depletion of androgens by various means results in increased expression of phosphorylated AKT and castration of conditional PTEN knockout mice increases AKT expression in prostate cancer cells. Furthermore, they demonstrated decreased endogenous AR expression in PTEN-null prostatic cells.

7. Therapeutic Implications

Recognition of the role the PI3K pathway plays in the development and propagation of cancer has led to the development of several PI3K inhibitors. Classes of drugs targeting the PI3K pathway and its downstream targets include pan-class I PI3K inhibitors, isoform-selective PI3K inhibitors, rapamycin analogues, active-site mTOR inhibitors, pan-PI3K/mTOR inhibitors and AKT inhibitors (Figure 1). Though some studies have yet to be reported, early studies in both pan-PI3K class I inhibitors and isoform-specific PI3K inhibitors have shown limited activity due to a combination of dose limiting toxicities, inadequate target inhibition and likely up-regulation of compensatory pathways [84–86]. For example, Hotte et al. presented data at ASCO 2013 on the use of PX-866, an irreversible pan-isoform inhibitor of class I PI3K, in men with mCRPC [87]. In this single-arm phase II study, 43 docetaxel-naïve men with mCRPC were treated with PX-866 with a primary endpoint of lack of progression at 12 weeks. Overall, PX-866 was well tolerated, but only 12 patients (28.4%) were progression-free at 12 weeks with one confirmed prostate-specific antigen (PSA) response. This agent did not meet the a priori benchmarks for further development as a single agent in unselected patients. Trials of monotherapy with AKT or mTOR inhibitors have also failed to progress. Burris et al., reported at ASCO 2011 the safety, pharmacokinetics and pharmacodynamics of the pan-AKT inhibitor GSK2141795 in nine prostate cancer patients of whom five were documented to have had PTEN loss [88]. In this cohort, seven patients had measurable responses, and six had stable disease with two having treatment durations in excess of 180 days; based on the phase I study results, development of this agent as monotherapy was not pursued, however. A recent systematic review of mTOR inhibition for mCRPC similarly found limited efficacy [89].

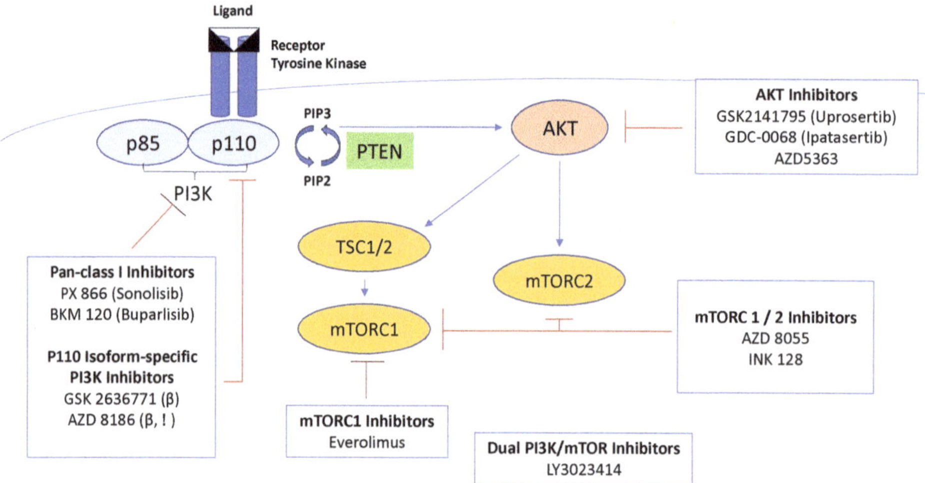

Figure 1. PI3K pathway targeting agents in development for the treatment of prostate cancer.

There are a number of explanations for the lack of efficacy seen in these trials of single pathway inhibition. Clinical correlation of the pre-clinical data on AR and PI3K pathway crosstalk was suggested in a phase I/II trial of everolimus, an mTOR inhibitor, in combination with gefitinib in patients with metastatic CRPC [90]. Rapid PSA rises occurred which often declined upon treatment discontinuation. In light of Carver and Mulholland's work, these transient PSA rises may represent a surrogate marker of AR reactivation and AR-dependent transcription as a result of mTOR inhibition.

8. Combined Therapeutic Targeting of AR and PI3K Signaling

If the mutual inhibition of both pathways is required, and from the results above it seems that PI3K activation is not the sole route of standard androgen resistance, then the combination of AR targeting and PI3K targeting would appear to be intuitive. Studies currently underway in prostate cancer are particularly focused on using PI3K inhibitors to overcome castrate-resistance. Thus, PI3K inhibitors are largely being tested in combinations in patients who have progressed on either enzalutamide or abiraterone to test the hypothesis of emerging resistance to these agents via the PI3K pathway.

Hotte et al. presented the second part of their phase 2 study of PX-866 at ASCO GU 2015; 25 patients with progressive CRPC on abiraterone/prednisone were treated with a combination of PX-866 and continued abiraterone/prednisone [91]. Six patients (24%) were progression-free at 12 weeks, but no objective or PSA responses (PCWG2) were seen. Similarly, in another phase 2 study presented at the same meeting, PI3K inhibition with BKM120 with or without AR inhibition with enzalutamide failed to improve progression-free survival (PFS) in men with progressive CRPC on enzalutamide [92]. However, AKT inhibition with ipatasertib in combination with abiraterone improved radiographic PFS and overall survival (OS) in men with CRPC previously treated with docetaxel [93]. Unlike the two previous studies, only a small portion (23/253) of these patients had received treatment with a novel anti-androgen prior to enrolment. Two other phase 2 studies have been published exploring the combination of the mTOR inhibitor, everolimus and bicalutamide. Nakabayashi et al. reported a study of bicalutamide in combination with everolimus in which only two of 36 patients (6%) treated with bicalutamide in combination with everolimus achieved a PSA fall ≥50% [94]. Thirty-one (86%) of the men had been treated with bicalutamide previously. Chow et al. however, reported on 24 bicalutamide naïve men with CRPC treated with this combination based on a historic PSA response rate of 25% for bicalutamide alone in CRPC [95]. Though they achieved a PSA response (50% PSA fall) rate of 62.5%, this level of activity was abrogated by a high rate (54%) of grade 3 or 4 adverse events attributable to treatment.

These studies raise the question of whether earlier PI3K pathway inhibition, prior to development of castrate resistance or significant pre-treatment with androgen-targeted treatments, would be more efficacious. Some pre-clinical models have shown more durable responses to dual AR and PI3K pathway inhibition in castrate sensitive-cell lines as compared to castrate-resistant [96–98]. Another issue may be patient selection as most of the data are in unselected, heavily pre-treated patients.

9. Biomarkers for PI3K Inhibition

The prolonged responses seen in two of the patients presented by Burris et al. raise the question of whether patient selection may be another contributing factor to the lack of overall efficacy seen in many of these trials. Attempts to identify subpopulations that will yield maximum benefit from PI3K inhibitors are underway with testing for PIK3CA or AKT alterations and PTEN loss. Pre-clinical data indicate that tumors with PIK3CA mutations or PTEN loss are more sensitive to PIK3CA and AKT inhibition but the value of these markers in clinical practice is uncertain due to the complexity of the pathway and unknown effects of these agents on the tumor microenvironment [99]. Some PIK3CA mutations result in minimal activation of AKT as compared to PTEN loss suggesting that AKT inhibitors may be more efficacious in cancers with AKT alterations and PTEN loss [99,100]. One patient with mCRPC harboring a PIK3CA mutation treated with PX-866 on the phase I study achieved a prolonged clinical response to the PI3K inhibitor [84]. However, the predictive value of PIK3CA mutations has not been confirmed in other studies [85,101].

Most recently, de Bono, et al. presented data supporting PTEN loss as a predictor of response to treatment with ipatasertib in combination with abiraterone acetate in men with mCRPC [102]. PTEN expression was assessed by immunohistochemistry (IHC) in archival or fresh tumor samples and genomic loss was detected by fluorescence in situ hybridization (FISH) and next generation sequencing (NGS). Of the 253 patients randomized, PTEN IHC was evaluable in 165 with PTEN loss detected in 71 (41%). There was good concordance between IHC, FISH and NGS results. Median radiographic progression-free survival (rPFS) was 5.6 months vs. 7.5 months in the non-PTEN loss abiraterone plus placebo arm and abiraterone plus ipatasertib arms respectively. PTEN loss was associated with a shorter rPFS in the placebo plus abiraterone arm and a greater treatment effect in the 400 mg ipatasertib plus abiraterone arm (4.6 months and 11.5 months). Based on these results, this combination is planned to proceed to a phase III trial.

10. Current Clinical Trials of PI3K Pathway Inhibitors in Prostate Cancer

Table 1 details the different agents in development and the trials currently being conducted with these agents. Three of the five trials actively recruiting involve PI3K/AKT/mTOR agents in combination with anti-androgen therapy while another is examining combination with docetaxel. GSK2636771 is a p110β isoform-specific inhibitor with preliminary signs of activity in PTEN-deficient tumors [103]. AZD8186 inhibits both p110β and -δ isoforms and has demonstrated anti-tumor effects in vitro as monotherapy and in combination with docetaxel in prostate cancer models [104]. Interestingly, AZD8186 showed activity in both PTEN null and PTEN wildtype models. LY3023414 is a dual class I PI3K and mTOR inhibitor with phase I monotherapy data in advanced solid tumors [105]. AZD5363, on the other hand, is an inhibitor of AKT isoforms 1, 2 and 3 which has synergy with enzalutamide in preclinical models of enzalutamide-resistant prostate cancer and docetaxel in CRPC [106]. AZD5363 in combination with docetaxel is proceeding to a phase II study following determination of the recommended dose in the recently published ProCaid study in men with mCRPC [107]. In this study, 10 patients were treated, of whom seven (70%) had a >50% reduction of PSA from baseline to 12 weeks. The most common toxicities were rash and diarrhea with self-limiting hyperglycemia seen in all patients.

Table 1. PI3K and AKT inhibitor agents in clinical development.

Agent	Pharmaceutical Company	Sponsor	Trial	Endpoint	Patient Population	Status	Biomarkers
BKM120 (PI3K)	Novartis	Duke University	Phase II, BKM120 in mCRPC (NCT01385293)	PFS	Post chemo; prior sipuleucel-T, abiraterone (Abi), or enzalutamide (enza) allowed. $n = 66$	Study accrued, results awaited	Circulating tumor cells (CTCs), Tissue PI3K signature, PTEN status, PI3K activation, PSA levels
		University of California	Phase II, neoadjuvant BKM120 for high-risk prostate cancer pre radical prostatectomy (RP) (NCT01695473)	PI3K inhibition in tumor measured by IHC	Candidates for RP; high risk defined by trial Target $n = 24$	Study accrued, results awaited	IHC for phosphorylation of: S6, 4EBP1, or AKT
GSK2636771 (PI3K)	GlaxoSmithKline	GSK	Phase I, GSK2636771 in combination with Enza for mCRPC (NCT02215096)	Safety and tolerability	PTEN deficient tumors post progression on Enza $n = 44$	Recruiting	PTEN status PSA levels
AZD8186 (PI3K)	AstraZeneca	AZ	Phase I, AZD8186 +/− Abi or AZD2014 in TNBC/NSCLC or CRPC or known PTEN-deficient/PI3 mutated disease (NCT01884285)	Safety and tolerability	mCRPC (Total) Target $n = 180$	Recruiting	PSA levels
LY3023414 (PI3K + mTOR)	Eli Lilly	Eli Lilly	Phase II Study of Enzalutamide +/− LY3023414 in mCRPC (NCT02407054)	PFS	mCRPC post progression on Abi; no prior chemo in castrate-refractory setting, immunotherapy, or Ra223 Target $n = 144$	Recruiting	PSA levels
AZD5363 (AKT)	AstraZenica	Institute of Cancer Research, UK	Phase I/II, Enza +/− AZD5363 in mCRPC	Phase II: Best overall tumor response	mCRPC with tissue for PTEN testing Target $n = 136$	Recruiting	PTEN PSA levels
		University Hospital Southampton NHS Foundation Trust	Randomised Phase II, Docetaxel +/− AZD 5363 in mCRPC	PFS	Chemotherapy-naïve mCRPC	Recruiting	PSA levels
MK2206 (AKT)	Merck	National Cancer Institute	Phase II, bicalutamide +/− MK2206 in men with HSPC	Proportion undetectable PSA	Biochemically relapsed hormone-sensitive PC following definitive treatment $n = 104$	Study accrued, results awaited	PSA levels

11. Conclusions

The androgen receptor and PI3K pathways are the two most commonly deregulated pathways in prostate cancer. There is evidence that PI3K signaling is involved in the evolution to castrate-resistant disease, a form of prostate cancer that remains lethal despite recent advances. This understanding has led to the development of several drugs targeting the PI3K pathway and its downstream targets but, unfortunately, early results overall have been disappointing. Adding complexity to early trials is the issue of interpreting a rising PSA, the most commonly measured marker of response in prostate cancer, in the context of potential activation of AR transcription with resultant PSA rises following PI3K pathway inhibition. Pre-clinical data supporting combined pathway inhibition coupled with the lack of substantial single-agent activity have prompted studies of PI3K pathway inhibition in combination with androgen pathway inhibition and/or additional downstream AKT/mTOR inhibition; the results continue to be mixed with efficacy often compromised by toxicity. There is a suggestion that earlier treatment with these agents, to prevent rather than overcome castrate-resistance, may be a useful strategy.

Ongoing studies to address the optimal timing, sequence and combinations of these treatments in addition to potential predictive biomarkers are underway. Given the reciprocal activation of p110α upon p110β inhibition in PTEN null tumors, it will be interesting to see the outcomes with the isoform-specific PI3K inhibitors in combination with enzalutamide. It is unclear whether the preferred agent should target multiple nodes of the pathway, such as with LY3023414, or induce pan-isoform inhibition of a single node, such as with AZD 5363. Despite their promise, it is yet to be seen whether these strategies can successfully overcome endocrine resistance to yield a significant improvement in outcomes for patients.

Author Contributions: All of the authors contributed to the design and development of this manuscript.

Conflicts of Interest: The authors declare no conflict of interest. Anthony Joshua holds a research grant from Astellas.

References

1. Globocan. Prostate Cancer Incidence, Mortality and Prevalence Worldwide. Available online: http://globocan.iarc.fr/Pages/online.aspx (accessed on 15 January 2017).
2. Beer, T.M.; Armstrong, A.J.; Rathkopf, D.E.; Loriot, Y.; Sternberg, C.N.; Higano, C.S.; Iversen, P.; Bhattacharya, S.; Carles, J.; Chowdhury, S.; et al. Enzalutamide in metastatic prostate cancer before chemotherapy. *N. Engl. J. Med.* **2014**, *371*, 424–433. [CrossRef] [PubMed]
3. De Bono, J.S.; Logothetis, C.J.; Molina, A.; Fizazi, K.; North, S.; Chu, L.; Chi, K.N.; Jones, R.J.; Goodman, O.B., Jr.; Saad, F.; et al. Abiraterone and increased survival in metastatic prostate cancer. *N. Engl. J. Med.* **2011**, *364*, 1995–2005. [CrossRef] [PubMed]
4. Ryan, C.J.; Smith, M.R.; Fizazi, K.; Saad, F.; Mulders, P.F.; Sternberg, C.N.; Miller, K.; Logothetis, C.J.; Shore, N.D.; Small, E.J.; et al. Abiraterone acetate plus prednisone versus placebo plus prednisone in chemotherapy-naive men with metastatic castration-resistant prostate cancer (COU-AA-302): Final overall survival analysis of a randomised, double-blind, placebo-controlled phase 3 study. *Lancet Oncol.* **2015**, *16*, 152–160. [CrossRef]
5. Scher, H.I.; Fizazi, K.; Saad, F.; Taplin, M.E.; Sternberg, C.N.; Miller, K.; de Wit, R.; Mulders, P.; Chi, K.N.; Shore, N.D.; et al. Increased survival with enzalutamide in prostate cancer after chemotherapy. *N. Engl. J. Med.* **2012**, *367*, 1187–1197. [PubMed]
6. Chandrasekar, T.; Yang, J.C.; Gao, A.C.; Evans, C.P. Mechanisms of resistance in castration-resistant prostate cancer (CRPC). *Transl. Androl. Urol.* **2015**, *4*, 365–380. [PubMed]
7. Watson, P.A.; Arora, V.K.; Sawyers, C.L. Emerging mechanisms of resistance to androgen receptor inhibitors in prostate cancer. *Nat. Rev. Cancer* **2015**, *15*, 701–711. [CrossRef] [PubMed]
8. Gao, T.; Furnari, F.; Newton, A.C. Phlpp: A phosphatase that directly dephosphorylates AKT, promotes apoptosis, and suppresses tumor growth. *Mol. Cells* **2005**, *18*, 13–24. [CrossRef] [PubMed]

9. Eder, I.E.; Culig, Z.; Putz, T.; Nessler-Menardi, C.; Bartsch, G.; Klocker, H. Molecular biology of the androgen receptor: From molecular understanding to the clinic. *Eur. Urol.* **2001**, *40*, 241–251. [CrossRef] [PubMed]
10. Leung, J.K.; Sadar, M.D. Non-genomic actions of the androgen receptor in prostate cancer. *Front. Endocrinol.* **2017**, *8*, 2. [CrossRef] [PubMed]
11. Davey, R.A.; Grossmann, M. Androgen receptor structure, function and biology: From bench to bedside. *Clin. Biochem. Rev.* **2016**, *37*, 3–15. [PubMed]
12. Zarif, J.C.; Miranti, C.K. The importance of non-nuclear AR signaling in prostate cancer progression and therapeutic resistance. *Cell Signal.* **2016**, *28*, 348–356. [CrossRef] [PubMed]
13. Hobisch, A.; Eder, I.E.; Putz, T.; Horninger, W.; Bartsch, G.; Klocker, H.; Culig, Z. Interleukin-6 regulates prostate-specific protein expression in prostate carcinoma cells by activation of the androgen receptor. *Cancer Res.* **1998**, *58*, 4640–4645. [PubMed]
14. Ueda, T.; Mawji, N.R.; Bruchovsky, N.; Sadar, M.D. Ligand-independent activation of the androgen receptor by interleukin-6 and the role of steroid receptor coactivator-1 in prostate cancer cells. *J. Biol. Chem.* **2002**, *277*, 38087–38094. [CrossRef] [PubMed]
15. Kim, H.J.; Lee, W.J. Ligand-independent activation of the androgen receptor by insulin-like growth factor-I and the role of the MAPK pathway in skeletal muscle cells. *Mol. Cells* **2009**, *28*, 589–593. [CrossRef] [PubMed]
16. Kim, H.J.; Lee, W.J. Insulin-like growth factor-I induces androgen receptor activation in differentiating C2C12 skeletal muscle cells. *Mol. Cells* **2009**, *28*, 189–194. [CrossRef] [PubMed]
17. Planz, B.; Aretz, H.T.; Wang, Q.; Tabatabaei, S.; Kirley, S.D.; Lin, C.W.; McDougal, W.S. Immunolocalization of the keratinocyte growth factor in benign and neoplastic human prostate and its relation to androgen receptor. *Prostate* **1999**, *41*, 233–242. [CrossRef]
18. Hayward, S.W.; Haughney, P.C.; Rosen, M.A.; Greulich, K.M.; Weier, H.U.; Dahiya, R.; Cunha, G.R. Interactions between adult human prostatic epithelium and rat urogenital sinus mesenchyme in a tissue recombination model. *Differentiation* **1998**, *63*, 131–140. [CrossRef] [PubMed]
19. Berger, R.; Febbo, P.G.; Majumder, P.K.; Zhao, J.J.; Mukherjee, S.; Signoretti, S.; Campbell, K.T.; Sellers, W.R.; Roberts, T.M.; Loda, M.; et al. Androgen-induced differentiation and tumorigenicity of human prostate epithelial cells. *Cancer Res.* **2004**, *64*, 8867–8875. [CrossRef] [PubMed]
20. Niu, Y.; Altuwaijri, S.; Lai, K.P.; Wu, C.T.; Ricke, W.A.; Messing, E.M.; Yao, J.; Yeh, S.; Chang, C. Androgen receptor is a tumor suppressor and proliferator in prostate cancer. *Proc. Natl. Acad. Sci. USA* **2008**, *105*, 12182–12187. [CrossRef] [PubMed]
21. Sensibar, J.A. Analysis of cell death and cell proliferation in embryonic stages, normal adult, and aging prostates in human and animals. *Microsc. Res. Tech.* **1995**, *30*, 342–350. [CrossRef] [PubMed]
22. Whitacre, D.C.; Chauhan, S.; Davis, T.; Gordon, D.; Cress, A.E.; Miesfeld, R.L. Androgen induction of in vitro prostate cell differentiation. *Cell Growth Differ.* **2002**, *13*, 1–11. [PubMed]
23. Yadav, N.; Heemers, H.V. Androgen action in the prostate gland. *Minerva Urol. Nefrol.* **2012**, *64*, 35–49. [PubMed]
24. Zhou, Y.; Bolton, E.C.; Jones, J.O. Androgens and androgen receptor signaling in prostate tumorigenesis. *J. Mol. Endocrinol.* **2015**, *54*, R15–R29. [CrossRef] [PubMed]
25. Haag, P.; Bektic, J.; Bartsch, G.; Klocker, H.; Eder, I.E. Androgen receptor down regulation by small interference rna induces cell growth inhibition in androgen sensitive as well as in androgen independent prostate cancer cells. *J. Steroid Biochem. Mol. Biol.* **2005**, *96*, 251–258. [CrossRef] [PubMed]
26. Hara, T.; Miyazaki, H.; Lee, A.; Tran, C.P.; Reiter, R.E. Androgen receptor and invasion in prostate cancer. *Cancer Res.* **2008**, *68*, 1128–1135. [CrossRef] [PubMed]
27. Snoek, R.; Cheng, H.; Margiotti, K.; Wafa, L.A.; Wong, C.A.; Wong, E.C.; Fazli, L.; Nelson, C.C.; Gleave, M.E.; Rennie, P.S. In vivo knockdown of the androgen receptor results in growth inhibition and regression of well-established, castration-resistant prostate tumors. *Clin. Cancer Res.* **2009**, *15*, 39–47. [CrossRef] [PubMed]
28. Denmeade, S.R.; Lin, X.S.; Isaacs, J.T. Role of programmed (apoptotic) cell death during the progression and therapy for prostate cancer. *Prostate* **1996**, *28*, 251–265. [CrossRef]
29. Tomlins, S.A.; Rhodes, D.R.; Perner, S.; Dhanasekaran, S.M.; Mehra, R.; Sun, X.W.; Varambally, S.; Cao, X.; Tchinda, J.; Kuefer, R.; et al. Recurrent fusion of TMPRSS2 and ets transcription factor genes in prostate cancer. *Science* **2005**, *310*, 644–648. [CrossRef] [PubMed]

30. Tu, J.J.; Rohan, S.; Kao, J.; Kitabayashi, N.; Mathew, S.; Chen, Y.-T. Gene fusions between TMPRSS2 and ETS family genes in prostate cancer: Frequency and transcript variant analysis by RT-PCR and fish on paraffin-embedded tissues. *Mod. Pathol.* **2007**, *20*, 921–928. [CrossRef] [PubMed]
31. Massie, C.E.; Lynch, A.; Ramos-Montoya, A.; Boren, J.; Stark, R.; Fazli, L.; Warren, A.; Scott, H.; Madhu, B.; Sharma, N.; et al. The androgen receptor fuels prostate cancer by regulating central metabolism and biosynthesis. *EMBO J.* **2011**, *30*, 2719–2733. [CrossRef] [PubMed]
32. Arora, V.K.; Schenkein, E.; Murali, R.; Subudhi, S.K.; Wongvipat, J.; Balbas, M.D.; Shah, N.; Cai, L.; Efstathiou, E.; Logothetis, C.; et al. Glucocorticoid receptor confers resistance to antiandrogens by bypassing androgen receptor blockade. *Cell* **2013**, *155*, 1309–1322. [CrossRef] [PubMed]
33. Gao, H.; Ouyang, X.; Banach-Petrosky, W.A.; Shen, M.M.; Abate-Shen, C. Emergence of androgen independence at early stages of prostate cancer progression in Nkx3.1; pten mice. *Cancer Res.* **2006**, *66*, 7929–7933. [CrossRef] [PubMed]
34. Isaacs, J.T.; Coffey, D.S. Adaptation versus selection as the mechanism responsible for the relapse of prostatic cancer to androgen ablation therapy as studied in the dunning R-3327-H adenocarcinoma. *Cancer Res.* **1981**, *41*, 5070–5075. [PubMed]
35. Montgomery, R.B.; Mostaghel, E.A.; Vessella, R.; Hess, D.L.; Kalhorn, T.F.; Higano, C.S.; True, L.D.; Nelson, P.S. Maintenance of intratumoral androgens in metastatic prostate cancer: A mechanism for castration-resistant tumor growth. *Cancer Res.* **2008**, *68*, 4447–4454. [CrossRef] [PubMed]
36. Bishop, J.L.; Thaper, D.; Vahid, S.; Davies, A.; Ketola, K.; Kuruma, H.; Jama, R.; Nip, K.M.; Angeles, A.; Johnson, F.; et al. The master neural transcription factor BRN2 is an androgen receptor-suppressed driver of neuroendocrine differentiation in prostate cancer. *Cancer Discov.* **2017**, *7*, 54–71. [CrossRef] [PubMed]
37. Suzuki, H.; Akakura, K.; Komiya, A.; Aida, S.; Akimoto, S.; Shimazaki, J. Codon 877 mutation in the androgen receptor gene in advanced prostate cancer: Relation to antiandrogen withdrawal syndrome. *Prostate* **1996**, *29*, 153–158. [CrossRef]
38. Suzuki, H.; Sato, N.; Watabe, Y.; Masai, M.; Seino, S.; Shimazaki, J. Androgen receptor gene mutations in human prostate cancer. *J. Steroid Biochem. Mol. Biol.* **1993**, *46*, 759–765. [CrossRef]
39. Guo, Z.; Yang, X.; Sun, F.; Jiang, R.; Linn, D.E.; Chen, H.; Chen, H.; Kong, X.; Melamed, J.; Tepper, C.G.; et al. A novel androgen receptor splice variant is up-regulated during prostate cancer progression and promotes androgen depletion-resistant growth. *Cancer Res.* **2009**, *69*, 2305–2313. [CrossRef] [PubMed]
40. Hu, R.; Dunn, T.A.; Wei, S.; Isharwal, S.; Veltri, R.W.; Humphreys, E.; Han, M.; Partin, A.W.; Vessella, R.L.; Isaacs, W.B.; et al. Ligand-independent androgen receptor variants derived from splicing of cryptic exons signify hormone-refractory prostate cancer. *Cancer Res.* **2009**, *69*, 16–22. [CrossRef] [PubMed]
41. Nakazawa, M.; Antonarakis, E.S.; Luo, J. Androgen receptor splice variants in the era of enzalutamide and abiraterone. *Horm. Cancer* **2014**, *5*, 265–273. [CrossRef] [PubMed]
42. Ware, K.E.; Garcia-Blanco, M.A.; Armstrong, A.J.; Dehm, S.M. Biologic and clinical significance of androgen receptor variants in castration resistant prostate cancer. *Endocr. Relat. Cancer* **2014**, *21*, T87–T103. [CrossRef] [PubMed]
43. Sprenger, C.C.T.; Plymate, S.R. The link between androgen receptor splice variants and castration resistant prostate cancer. *Horm. Cancer* **2014**, *5*, 207–217. [CrossRef] [PubMed]
44. Tan, M.H.; Li, J.; Xu, H.E.; Melcher, K.; Yong, E.L. Androgen receptor: Structure, role in prostate cancer and drug discovery. *Acta Pharmacol. Sin.* **2015**, *36*, 3–23. [CrossRef] [PubMed]
45. Yuan, T.L.; Cantley, L.C. PI3K pathway alterations in cancer: Variations on a theme. *Oncogene* **2008**, *27*, 5497–5510. [CrossRef] [PubMed]
46. Edlind, M.P.; Hsieh, A.C. PI3K-AKT-mtor signaling in prostate cancer progression and androgen deprivation therapy resistance. *Asian J. Androl.* **2014**, *16*, 378–386. [PubMed]
47. LoRusso, P.M. Inhibition of the PI3K/AKT/mTOR pathway in solid tumors. *J. Clin. Oncol.* **2016**. [CrossRef] [PubMed]
48. Li, B.; Sun, A.; Jiang, W.; Thrasher, J.B.; Terranova, P. PI-3 kinase p110β: A therapeutic target in advanced prostate cancers. *Am. J. Clin. Exp. Urol.* **2014**, *2*, 188–198. [PubMed]
49. Chang, H.W.; Aoki, M.; Fruman, D.; Auger, K.R.; Bellacosa, A.; Tsichlis, P.N.; Cantley, L.C.; Roberts, T.M.; Vogt, P.K. Transformation of chicken cells by the gene encoding the catalytic subunit of PI 3-kinase. *Science* **1997**, *276*, 1848–1850. [CrossRef] [PubMed]

50. Klippel, A.; Escobedo, J.A.; Hu, Q.; Williams, L.T. A region of the 85-kilodalton (kda) subunit of phosphatidylinositol 3-kinase binds the 110-kda catalytic subunit in vivo. *Mol. Cell. Biol.* **1993**, *13*, 5560–5566. [CrossRef] [PubMed]
51. Zhao, J.J.; Gjoerup, O.V.; Subramanian, R.R.; Cheng, Y.; Chen, W.; Roberts, T.M.; Hahn, W.C. Human mammary epithelial cell transformation through the activation of phosphatidylinositol 3-kinase. *Cancer Cell* **2003**, *3*, 483–495. [CrossRef]
52. Zhao, J.J.; Liu, Z.; Wang, L.; Shin, E.; Loda, M.F.; Roberts, T.M. The oncogenic properties of mutant p110α and p110β phosphatidylinositol 3-kinases in human mammary epithelial cells. *Proc. Natl. Acad. Sci. USA* **2005**, *102*, 18443–18448. [CrossRef] [PubMed]
53. Samuels, Y.; Waldman, T. Oncogenic mutations of pik3ca in human cancers. *Curr. Top. Microbiol. Immunol.* **2010**, *347*, 21–41. [PubMed]
54. Thorpe, L.M.; Yuzugullu, H.; Zhao, J.J. PI3k in cancer: Divergent roles of isoforms, modes of activation and therapeutic targeting. *Nat. Rev. Cancer* **2015**, *15*, 7–24. [CrossRef] [PubMed]
55. Sadeghi, N.; Gerber, D.E. Targeting the PI3k pathway for cancer therapy. *Futur. Med. Chem.* **2012**, *4*, 1153–1169. [CrossRef] [PubMed]
56. Carver, B.S.; Chapinski, C.; Wongvipat, J.; Hieronymus, H.; Chen, Y.; Chandarlapaty, S.; Arora, V.K.; Le, C.; Koutcher, J.; Scher, H.; et al. Reciprocal feedback regulation of PI3k and androgen receptor signaling in PTEN-deficient prostate cancer. *Cancer Cell* **2011**, *19*, 575–586. [CrossRef] [PubMed]
57. Taylor, B.S.; Schultz, N.; Hieronymus, H.; Gopalan, A.; Xiao, Y.; Carver, B.S.; Arora, V.K.; Kaushik, P.; Cerami, E.; Reva, B.; et al. Integrative genomic profiling of human prostate cancer. *Cancer Cell* **2010**, *18*, 11–22. [CrossRef] [PubMed]
58. Vivanco, I.; Sawyers, C.L. The phosphatidylinositol 3-kinase-AKT pathway in human cancer. *Nat. Rev. Cancer* **2002**, *2*, 489–501. [CrossRef] [PubMed]
59. Bitting, R.L.; Armstrong, A.J. Targeting the PI3K/AKT/mTOR pathway in castration-resistant prostate cancer. *Endocr. Relat. Cancer* **2013**, *20*, R83–R99. [CrossRef] [PubMed]
60. Jiao, J.; Wang, S.; Qiao, R.; Vivanco, I.; Watson, P.A.; Sawyers, C.L.; Wu, H. Murine cell lines derived from PTEN null prostate cancer show the critical role of pten in hormone refractory prostate cancer development. *Cancer Res.* **2007**, *67*, 6083–6091. [CrossRef] [PubMed]
61. Liu, L.; Dong, X. Complex impacts of PI3K/AKT inhibitors to androgen receptor gene expression in prostate cancer cells. *PLoS ONE* **2014**, *9*, e108780. [CrossRef] [PubMed]
62. Reid, A.H.; Attard, G.; Ambroisine, L.; Fisher, G.; Kovacs, G.; Brewer, D.; Clark, J.; Flohr, P.; Edwards, S.; Berney, D.M.; et al. Molecular characterisation of ERG, ETV1 and PTEN gene loci identifies patients at low and high risk of death from prostate cancer. *Br. J. Cancer* **2010**, *102*, 678–684. [CrossRef] [PubMed]
63. Di Cristofano, A.; Pesce, B.; Cordon-Cardo, C.; Pandolfi, P.P. PTEN is essential for embryonic development and tumour suppression. *Nat. Genet.* **1998**, *19*, 348–355. [PubMed]
64. Podsypanina, K.; Ellenson, L.H.; Nemes, A.; Gu, J.; Tamura, M.; Yamada, K.M.; Cordon-Cardo, C.; Catoretti, G.; Fisher, P.E.; Parsons, R. Mutation of Pten/Mmac1 in mice causes neoplasia in multiple organ systems. *Proc. Natl. Acad. Sci. USA* **1999**, *96*, 1563–1568. [CrossRef] [PubMed]
65. Stambolic, V.; Suzuki, A.; de la Pompa, J.L.; Brothers, G.M.; Mirtsos, C.; Sasaki, T.; Ruland, J.; Penninger, J.M.; Siderovski, D.P.; Mak, T.W. Negative regulation of PKB/Akt-dependent cell survival by the tumor suppressor pten. *Cell* **1998**, *95*, 29–39. [CrossRef]
66. Suzuki, A.; de la Pompa, J.L.; Stambolic, V.; Elia, A.J.; Sasaki, T.; del Barco Barrantes, I.; Ho, A.; Wakeham, A.; Itie, A.; Khoo, W.; et al. High cancer susceptibility and embryonic lethality associated with mutation of the PTEN tumor suppressor gene in mice. *Curr. Biol.* **1998**, *8*, 1169–1178. [CrossRef]
67. Di Cristofano, A.; De Acetis, M.; Koff, A.; Cordon-Cardo, C.; Pandolfi, P.P. Pten and p27KIP1 cooperate in prostate cancer tumor suppression in the mouse. *Nat. Genet.* **2001**, *27*, 222–224. [CrossRef] [PubMed]
68. Wang, S.; Gao, J.; Lei, Q.; Rozengurt, N.; Pritchard, C.; Jiao, J.; Thomas, G.V.; Li, G.; Roy-Burman, P.; Nelson, P.S.; et al. Prostate-specific deletion of the murine Pten tumor suppressor gene leads to metastatic prostate cancer. *Cancer Cell* **2003**, *4*, 209–221. [CrossRef]
69. Jia, S.; Liu, Z.; Zhang, S.; Liu, P.; Zhang, L.; Lee, S.H.; Zhang, J.; Signoretti, S.; Loda, M.; Roberts, T.M.; et al. Essential roles of PI(3)K-p110beta in cell growth, metabolism and tumorigenesis. *Nature* **2008**, *454*, 776–779. [PubMed]

70. Ni, J.; Liu, Q.; Xie, S.; Carlson, C.B.; Von, T.; Vogel, K.W.; Riddle, S.M.; Benes, C.H.; Eck, M.J.; Roberts, T.M.; et al. Functional characterization of an isoform-selective inhibitor of PI3K-p110β as a potential anti-cancer agent. *Cancer Discov.* **2012**, *2*, 425–433. [CrossRef] [PubMed]
71. Wee, S.; Wiederschain, D.; Maira, S.-M.; Loo, A.; Miller, C.; deBeaumont, R.; Stegmeier, F.; Yao, Y.-M.; Lengauer, C. PTEN-deficient cancers depend on PIK3CB. *Proc. Natl. Acad. Sci. USA* **2008**, *105*, 13057–13062. [CrossRef] [PubMed]
72. Schwartz, S.; Wongvipat, J.; Trigwell, C.B.; Hancox, U.; Carver, B.S.; Rodrik-Outmezguine, V.; Will, M.; Yellen, P.; de Stanchina, E.; Baselga, J.; et al. Feedback suppression of PI3Kalpha signaling in PTEN-mutated tumors is relieved by selective inhibition of PI3Kbeta. *Cancer Cell* **2015**, *27*, 109–122. [CrossRef] [PubMed]
73. Mulholland, D.J.; Tran, L.M.; Li, Y.; Cai, H.; Morim, A.; Wang, S.; Plaisier, S.; Garraway, I.P.; Huang, J.; Graeber, T.G.; et al. Cell autonomous role of PTEN in regulating castration-resistant prostate cancer growth. *Cancer Cell* **2011**, *19*, 792–804. [CrossRef] [PubMed]
74. Mahajan, N.P.; Liu, Y.; Majumder, S.; Warren, M.R.; Parker, C.E.; Mohler, J.L.; Earp, H.S.; Whang, Y.E. Activated Cdc42-associated kinase Ack1 promotes prostate cancer progression via androgen receptor tyrosine phosphorylation. *Proc. Natl. Acad. Sci. USA* **2007**, *104*, 8438–8443. [CrossRef] [PubMed]
75. Mellinghoff, I.K.; Vivanco, I.; Kwon, A.; Tran, C.; Wongvipat, J.; Sawyers, C.L. HER2/neu kinase-dependent modulation of androgen receptor function through effects on DNA binding and stability. *Cancer Cell* **2004**, *6*, 517–527. [CrossRef] [PubMed]
76. Pei, H.; Li, L.; Fridley, B.L.; Jenkins, G.D.; Kalari, K.R.; Lingle, W.; Petersen, G.; Lou, Z.; Wang, L. FKBP51 affects cancer cell response to chemotherapy by negatively regulating Akt. *Cancer Cell* **2009**, *16*, 259–266. [CrossRef] [PubMed]
77. Gitenay, D.; Baron, V.T. Is EGR1 a potential target for prostate cancer therapy? *Futur. Oncol.* **2009**, *5*, 993–1003. [CrossRef] [PubMed]
78. Yuan, H.; Young, C.Y.; Tian, Y.; Liu, Z.; Zhang, M.; Lou, H. Suppression of the androgen receptor function by quercetin through protein-protein interactions of Sp1, c-Jun, and the androgen receptor in human prostate cancer cells. *Mol. Cell. Biochem.* **2010**, *339*, 253–262. [CrossRef] [PubMed]
79. Castoria, G.; Lombardi, M.; Barone, M.V.; Bilancio, A.; Di Domenico, M.; Bottero, D.; Vitale, F.; Migliaccio, A.; Auricchio, F. Androgen-stimulated DNA synthesis and cytoskeletal changes in fibroblasts by a nontranscriptional receptor action. *J. Cell Biol.* **2003**, *161*, 547–556. [CrossRef] [PubMed]
80. Gelman, I.H. Androgen receptor activation in castration-recurrent prostate cancer: The role of Src-family and Ack1 tyrosine kinases. *Int. J. Biol. Sci.* **2014**, *10*, 620–626. [CrossRef] [PubMed]
81. Unni, E.; Sun, S.; Nan, B.; McPhaul, M.J.; Cheskis, B.; Mancini, M.A.; Marcelli, M. Changes in androgen receptor nongenotropic signaling correlate with transition of LNCaP cells to androgen independence. *Cancer Res.* **2004**, *64*, 7156–7168. [CrossRef] [PubMed]
82. Zhu, C.; Luong, R.; Zhuo, M.; Johnson, D.T.; McKenney, J.K.; Cunha, G.R.; Sun, Z. Conditional expression of the androgen receptor induces oncogenic transformation of the mouse prostate. *J. Biol. Chem.* **2011**, *286*, 33478–33488. [CrossRef] [PubMed]
83. Lee, S.H.; Johnson, D.; Luong, R.; Sun, Z. Crosstalking between androgen and PI3k/AKT signaling pathways in prostate cancer cells. *J. Biol. Chem.* **2015**, *290*, 2759–2768. [CrossRef] [PubMed]
84. Hotte, S.J. Ncic ctg, ind-205: A phase ii study of px-866 in patients with recurrent or metastatic castration-resistant prostate cancer (crpc). In Proceedings of the ASCO Annual Meeting, Chicago, IL USA, 2–6 June 2013.
85. Fruman, D.A.; Rommel, C. PI3K and cancer: Lessons, challenges and opportunities. *Nat. Rev. Drug Discov.* **2014**, *13*, 140–156. [CrossRef] [PubMed]
86. Hong, D.S.; Bowles, D.W.; Falchook, G.S.; Messersmith, W.A.; George, G.C.; O'Bryant, C.L.; Vo, A.C.; Klucher, K.; Herbst, R.S.; Eckhardt, S.G.; et al. A multicenter phase I trial of PX-866, an oral irreversible phosphatidylinositol 3-kinase inhibitor, in patients with advanced solid tumors. *Clin. Cancer Res.* **2012**, *18*, 4173–4182. [CrossRef] [PubMed]
87. Burris, H.A. Safety, pharmacokinetics (pk), pharmacodynamics (pd), and clinical activity of the oral AKT inhibitor GSK2141795 (GSK795) in a phase I first-in-human study. *J. Clin. Oncol.* **2011**, *29*, 3003. [CrossRef]
88. Statz, C.M.; Patterson, S.E.; Mockus, S.M. Mtor inhibitors in castration-resistant prostate cancer: A systematic review. *Target. Oncol.* **2017**, *12*, 47–59. [CrossRef] [PubMed]

89. Rathkopf, D.E.; Larson, S.M.; Anand, A.; Morris, M.J.; Slovin, S.F.; Shaffer, D.R.; Heller, G.; Carver, B.; Rosen, N.; Scher, H.I. Everolimus combined with gefitinib in patients with metastatic castration-resistant prostate cancer: Phase 1/2 results and signaling pathway implications. *Cancer* **2015**, *121*, 3853–3861. [CrossRef] [PubMed]
90. Bendell, J.C.; Rodon, J.; Burris, H.A.; de Jonge, M.; Verweij, J.; Birle, D.; Demanse, D.; De Buck, S.S.; Ru, Q.C.; Peters, M.; et al. Phase I, dose-escalation study of BKM120, an oral pan-class I pi3k inhibitor, in patients with advanced solid tumors. *J. Clin. Oncol.* **2012**, *30*, 282–290. [CrossRef] [PubMed]
91. Hotte, S.J.; Joshua, A.M.; Torri, V.; Macfarlane, R.J.; Basappa, N.S.; Powers, J.; Winquist, E.; Mukherjee, S.; Gregg, R.W.; Kollmannsberger, C.K.; et al. IND 205b: A phase II study of the PI3k inhibitor PX-866 and continued abiraterone/prednisone in patients with recurrent or metastatic castration resistant prostate cancer (CRPC) with PSA progression on abiraterone/prednisone. *J. Clin. Oncol.* **2015**, *33*, 279. [CrossRef]
92. Armstrong, A.J.; Halabi, S.; Healy, P.; Alumkal, J.J.; Yu, E.Y.; Winters, C.; Hobbs, C.; Soleau, C.; Slottke, R.; Mundy, K.; et al. Phase II trial of the PI3 kinase inhibitor BKM120 with or without enzalutamide in men with metastatic castration resistant prostate cancer (mCRPC). *J. Clin. Oncol.* **2015**, *33*, 5025.
93. De Bono, J.S. Randomized phase II study of AKT blockade with ipatasertib (GDC-0068) and abiraterone (abi) vs. Abi alone in patients with metastatic castration-resistant prostate cancer (mCRPC) after docetaxel chemotherapy. *J. Clin. Oncol.* **2016**, *34*. Abstrct 5017.
94. Nakabayashi, M.; Werner, L.; Courtney, K.D.; Buckle, G.; Oh, W.K.; Bubley, G.J.; Hayes, J.H.; Weckstein, D.; Elfiky, A.; Sims, D.M.; et al. Phase II trial of RAD001 and bicalutamide for castration-resistant prostate cancer. *BJU Int.* **2012**, *110*, 1729–1735. [CrossRef] [PubMed]
95. Chow, H.; Ghosh, P.M.; deVere White, R.; Evans, C.P.; Dall'Era, M.A.; Yap, S.A.; Li, Y.; Beckett, L.A.; Lara, P.N., Jr.; Pan, C.X. A phase 2 clinical trial of everolimus plus bicalutamide for castration-resistant prostate cancer. *Cancer* **2016**, *122*, 1897–1904. [CrossRef] [PubMed]
96. Qi, W.; Morales, C.; Cooke, L.S.; Johnson, B.; Somer, B.; Mahadevan, D. Reciprocal feedback inhibition of the androgen receptor and PI3K as a novel therapy for castrate-sensitive and -resistant prostate cancer. *Oncotarget* **2015**, *6*, 41976–41987. [PubMed]
97. Thomas, C.; Lamoureux, F.; Crafter, C.; Davies, B.R.; Beraldi, E.; Fazli, L.; Kim, S.; Thaper, D.; Gleave, M.E.; Zoubeidi, A. Synergistic targeting of PI3K/aAKT pathway and androgen receptor axis significantly delays castration-resistant prostate cancer progression in vivo. *Mol. Cancer Ther.* **2013**, *12*, 2342–2355. [CrossRef] [PubMed]
98. Toren, P.; Kim, S.; Cordonnier, T.; Crafter, C.; Davies, B.R.; Fazli, L.; Gleave, M.E.; Zoubeidi, A. Combination AZD5363 with enzalutamide significantly delays enzalutamide-resistant prostate cancer in preclinical models. *Eur. Urol.* **2015**, *67*, 986–990. [CrossRef] [PubMed]
99. Josephs, D.H.; Sarker, D. Pharmacodynamic biomarker development for PI3K pathway therapeutics. *Transl. Oncogenom.* **2015**, *7*, 33–49.
100. Vasudevan, K.M.; Barbie, D.A.; Davies, M.A.; Rabinovsky, R.; McNear, C.J.; Kim, J.J.; Hennessy, B.T.; Tseng, H.; Pochanard, P.; Kim, S.Y.; et al. Akt-independent signaling downstream of oncogenic PIK3CA mutations in human cancer. *Cancer Cell* **2009**, *16*, 21–32. [CrossRef] [PubMed]
101. Bowles, D.W.; Ma, W.W.; Senzer, N.; Brahmer, J.R.; Adjei, A.A.; Davies, M.; Lazar, A.J.; Vo, A.; Peterson, S.; Walker, L.; et al. A multicenter phase 1 study of PX-866 in combination with docetaxel in patients with advanced solid tumours. *Br. J. Cancer* **2013**, *109*, 1085–1092. [CrossRef] [PubMed]
102. De Bono, J.S.; De Giorgi, U.; Massard, C.; Bracarda, S.; Nava Rodrigues, D.; Kocak, I.; Font, A.; Arija, J.A.; Shih, K.; Radavoi, G.D.; et al. Pten loss as a predictive biomarker for the Akt inhibitor ipatasertib combined with abiraterone acetate in patients with metastatic castration-resistant prostate cancer (mCRPC). *Ann. Oncol.* **2016**, *27*, 718O. [CrossRef]
103. Arkenau, H.-T. A phase I/II, first-in-human dose-escalation study of GSK2636771 in patients (pts) with PTEN-deficient advanced tumors. *J. Clin. Oncol.* **2014**, *32*, 2514.
104. Hancox, U.; Cosulich, S.; Hanson, L.; Trigwell, C.; Lenaghan, C.; Ellston, R.; Dry, H.; Crafter, C.; Barlaam, B.; Fitzek, M.; et al. Inhibition of PI3Kbeta signaling with AZD8186 inhibits growth of PTEN-deficient breast and prostate tumors alone and in combination with docetaxel. *Mol. Cancer Ther.* **2015**, *14*, 48–58. [CrossRef] [PubMed]

105. Moore, K.N.; Varghese, A.M.; Hyman, D.M.; Callies, S.; Lin, J.; Wacheck, V.; Pant, S.; Bauer, T.M.; Bendell, J.C. A phase I, first-in-human dose study of the dual PI3K/mTOR inhibitor LY3023414 (LY) in patients (pts) with advanced cancer. *J. Clin. Oncol.* **2015**, *33*, 11075.
106. Davies, B.R.; Greenwood, H.; Dudley, P.; Crafter, C.; Yu, D.H.; Zhang, J.; Li, J.; Gao, B.; Ji, Q.; Maynard, J.; et al. Preclinical pharmacology of AZD5363, an inhibitor of akt: Pharmacodynamics, antitumor activity, and correlation of monotherapy activity with genetic background. *Mol. Cancer Ther.* **2012**, *11*, 873–887. [CrossRef] [PubMed]
107. Crabb, S.J.; Birtle, A.J.; Martin, K.; Downs, N.; Ratcliffe, I.; Maishman, T.; Ellis, M.; Griffiths, G.; Thompson, S.; Ksiazek, L.; et al. ProCAID: A phase I clinical trial to combine the AKT inhibitor AZD5363 with docetaxel and prednisolone chemotherapy for metastatic castration resistant prostate cancer. *Investig. New Drugs* **2017**. [CrossRef] [PubMed]

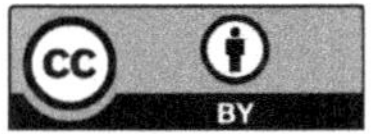

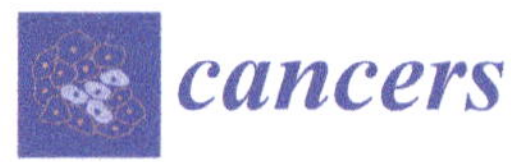

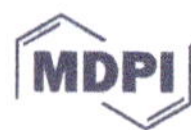

Review

Crosstalk of the Androgen Receptor with Transcriptional Collaborators: Potential Therapeutic Targets for Castration-Resistant Prostate Cancer

Daisuke Obinata [1,2], Kenichi Takayama [2], Satoru Takahashi [1] and Satoshi Inoue [2,3,*]

1. Department of Urology, Nihon University School of Medicine, Tokyo 173-8610, Japan; obinata.daisuke@nihon-u.ac.jp (D.O.); takahashi.satoru@nihon-u.ac.jp (S.T.)
2. Department of Functional Biogerontology, Tokyo Metropolitan Institute of Gerontology, Tokyo 173-0015, Japan; ktakayama-tky@umin.ac.jp
3. Division of Gene Regulation and Signal Transduction, Research Center for Genomic Medicine, Saitama Medical University, Saitama 350-1241, Japan

* Correspondence: sinoue@tmig.or.jp; Tel.: +81-3-5800-8834

Academic Editor: Emmanuel S. Antonarakis
Received: 28 November 2016; Accepted: 21 February 2017; Published: 28 February 2017

Abstract: Prostate cancer is the second leading cause of death from cancer among males in Western countries. It is also the most commonly diagnosed male cancer in Japan. The progression of prostate cancer is mainly influenced by androgens and the androgen receptor (AR). Androgen deprivation therapy is an established therapy for advanced prostate cancer; however, prostate cancers frequently develop resistance to low testosterone levels and progress to the fatal stage called castration-resistant prostate cancer (CRPC). Surprisingly, AR and the AR signaling pathway are still activated in most CRPC cases. To overcome this problem, abiraterone acetate and enzalutamide were introduced for the treatment of CRPC. Despite the impact of these drugs on prolonged survival, CRPC acquires further resistance to keep the AR pathway activated. Functional molecular studies have shown that some of the AR collaborative transcription factors (TFs), including octamer transcription factor (OCT1), GATA binding protein 2 (GATA2) and forkhead box A1 (FOXA1), still stimulate AR activity in the castration-resistant state. Therefore, elucidating the crosstalk between the AR and collaborative TFs on the AR pathway is critical for developing new strategies for the treatment of CRPC. Recently, many compounds targeting this pathway have been developed for treating CRPC. In this review, we summarize the AR signaling pathway in terms of AR collaborators and focus on pyrrole-imidazole (PI) polyamide as a candidate compound for the treatment of prostate cancer.

Keywords: androgen receptor; androgen receptor signaling pathway; coregulator; octamer transcription factor 1; pyrrole-imidazole polyamide

1. Introduction

Prostate cancer is the major cause of death from cancer among males in Western countries. For example, the American Cancer Society has estimated 180,890 new cases of prostate cancer and 26,120 deaths from the disease in the United States in 2016. The Australian Institute of Health and Welfare estimated 18,138 new diagnoses and 3398 deaths from prostate cancer in 2016. This amounts to 21.4% and 12.8% of all male deaths from cancer in each country in 2016. In Japan, although prostate cancer is the seventh-leading cause of cancer death, recently both the number of cases and the mortality rate due to prostate cancer have increased significantly. The increased population of older males is presumed to be one of the contributors in Japan.

The androgen receptor (AR) signaling pathway plays an integral role in the progression of prostate cancer. The AR is a member of the steroid hormone receptor superfamily. The AR is activated by ligands, such as dihydrotestosterone (DHT), and then functions as a transcription factor to modulate the expression of its target genes. Approximately 80%–90% of prostate cancers are androgen-dependent at the time of diagnosis [1–5]. Since the finding in the 1940s that castration inhibits the progression of prostate cancer [6,7], androgen deprivation therapy (ADT), or castration, has become the most effective and widely used treatment for unresectable prostate cancer, which includes metastasis and recurrence after local therapies [8–11]. Through the combination of luteinizing hormone-releasing hormone (LH-RH) analogs and anti-androgens, ADT decreases the production of androgens and inhibits androgen binding to the AR. ADT can inhibit the progression of prostate cancer for up to 3 years, however, prostate cancer cells eventually adapt to low testosterone levels and progress to castration-resistant prostate cancer (CRPC). Surprisingly, even in a low testosterone environment, AR and its target genes, including prostate-specific antigen (PSA), are still highly expressed in the majority of CRPC lesions [10–12]. Indeed, the rise in serum PSA levels in patients that no longer respond to ADT shows that CRPC is not hormone-insensitive. In addition, anti-androgen drugs can work as AR agonists in CRPC [13]. Some tumours acquire genomic amplifications of the AR gene, which increases their sensitivity to androgens and maintains AR signaling under the low testosterone environment of ADT [14,15]. About 30% of CRPC cases have amplifications of the AR locus [16]. Using AR-overexpressing cells, an in vitro study showed that first generation anti-androgen drugs promote AR nuclear translocation, DNA binding and co-activator recruitment [17]. AR stability also relates to AR hypersensitivity. Under physiological androgen levels, the AR is involved in a negative feedback where it suppresses the expression of genes that promote its translation. In ADT, the testosterone level is too low for the AR to inhibit these genes, but is still sufficient to stimulate AR signaling in CRPC [18]. Furthermore, deregulation of the interplay of AR with AR collaborating factors commonly occurs in CRPC cells [19].

The extragonadal androgens synthesized in adrenal or CRPC cells are one of the key mechanisms for sustaining AR signaling in CRPC. They activate the cytochrome P450 (CYP) family, which facilitates the unusual conversion of cholesterol to androgen under low testosterone conditions. Thus, the expression of androgen-dependent genes is induced by a very small amount of androgens under castration [20]. Abiraterone acetate and enzalutamide strongly target the AR pathway and improve cancer specific survival in the case with CRPC [21–23]. Abiraterone is a dual inhibitor of the 17α-hydroxylase and 17,20-lyase, which belong to the CYP17 family and play a key role in the novel androgen synthesis pathway in CRPC cells [24]. Enzalutamide is a novel AR antagonist that binds directly to AR with a higher affinity than bicalutamide or flutamide and targets multiple steps including AR nuclear translocation, DNA binding, and co-activator recruitment [21]. Despite the development of these notable drugs in the last decade, CRPC still evolves to acquire further resistance to these drugs. Aberrant AR function and cross-talk with factors that activate the AR pathway are assumed to be involved in this cancer evolution. Thus, the study of AR signaling pathways and their collaborative factors will facilitate greater understanding of the mechanisms underlying the progression of advanced prostate cancer as well as the development of novel drugs.

This article reviews the AR signaling pathway in CRPC as well as the development of novel therapeutic medicines targeting AR collaborators, especially collaborative DNA binding transcription factors (TFs).

2. AR Structure and Collaborating Factors in AR Signaling Pathway

The AR contains an N-terminal domain (NTD; 555 amino acids encoded by exon 1), a DNA-binding domain (DBD; 68 amino acids encoded by exons 2 and 3), a hinge region, and a ligand binding domain (LBD; 295 amino acids encoded by exons 4–8) [25]. The NTD includes the activation function (AF) 1 element, which enables the transactivation of the AR [26]. The LBD is located in the C-terminal region where androgens, such as DHT, bind in the first step of the androgen signaling pathway. After activation by ligands, the AR translocates into the nucleus and then binds to specific

DNA sequences, called androgen response elements (AREs). The DBD plays an important role at this stage involving AR nuclear localization, homodimer formation, and specific DNA binding.

The increased frequency of functional AR mutations in CRPC enhances resistance to ADT. In addition, ADT drugs mediate a conformational change in the AR [27,28]. The proportions of AR mutations in prostate cancer are 40% in the NTD, 49% in the LBD, and 7% in the DBD [29]. Important mutations cause gain-of-function in the LBD [30], one of the most common of which is T878A. Because this mutation broadens ligand specificity, the anti-androgen flutamide, as well as other steroids, become partial agonists [31,32]. This mutation can be found in approximately one-third of CRPC [33,34], whilst the other mutations appear to be rare [35].

Previous reports have shown that constitutively active AR isoforms (splice variants: ARVs) were detected in CRPC cell lines and patient tissues [36]. These ARVs have common structural characteristics of the NTD, encoded by exons 1 and 2 or exons 1 to 3, followed by a truncated C-terminal domain (CTD) originating from introns 2 or 3. Among these ARVs, AR-V7, encoded by exons 1 to 3 with the cryptic exons, is the most abundantly detected variant in prostate cancer [37]. Lacking the LBD in the CTD, it is expected that: (1) enzalutamide is unable to bind to AR-V7; and (2) AR-V7 is activated independently, despite the low androgen levels due to abiraterone acetate. A recent report showed that positive AR-V7 expression in circulating prostate cancer cells was associated with the resistance to enzalutamide and abiraterone acetate [38].

The regulation of AR-targeted gene expression requires the recruitment of coregulators to regulatory regions of the AR protein. Coregulators promote (named coactivators), or inhibit (named corepressors) AR transactivation. Although coregulators do not need to bind DNA, they recruit general TFs associated with RNA polymerase II (Rpol II) to gene promoters [39]. The actions of AR coactivators have been well characterized for *PSA*, a classical AR-regulated gene. The AR and coactivator complex first occupies the *PSA* enhancer region and then bridges to the promoter, which allows Rpol II to track to this region [40]. Since the discovery of steroid receptor coactivator-1 (SRC-1), more than 200 nuclear receptor coregulators have been identified [39,41–43]. The elevated expression of SRC-1, 2 and 3 is related to poor prognosis of patients with localized prostate cancer as well as CRPC [44].

In addition to AR coregulators, TFs that collaborate with AR are also important for androgen responsive gene expression. Generally, most genes are packed and condensed into nucleosomes by being wound around the four core histones [45]. Thus, nucleosomes prevent the AR from binding to AREs. Some TFs make histone modifications to support AR binding to target regions. Wang et al. identified 90 functional AR binding regions in chromosomes 21 and 22 using high-throughput technologies [46]. Interestingly, they reported that the canonical ARE (AGAACAnnnTGTTCT) [47] existed in only 10% of these AR binding regions, whilst 68% of the AR binding regions harbored non-canonical, but functional AREs where motifs for three TFs, GATA binding protein 2 (GATA2), forkhead box A1 (FOXA1), and octamer transcription factor (OCT1), were significantly enriched [46].

GATA and FoxA family members are known to play important roles in liver and gut development in mouse embryos [48]. In vivo footprinting analysis revealed both families commonly bind to their target gene elements first in nascent liver buds and gut endoderm to induce development [48,49]. Zaret et al. [48] proposed these factors as pioneer factors, which are able to bind DNA, even in condensed chromatin, and facilitate DNA binding of other factors by opening the chromatin [50,51].

Consistent with the results of liver developmental studies, one member of the FoxA family, FOXA1, works as a pioneer factor in the AR and estrogen receptor (ER) pathways in prostate cancer and breast cancer cells [52–54]. Interestingly, although overexpression of FOXA1 is associated with poor prognosis in prostate cancer [55], ERα-positive breast cancer with high FOXA1 expression shows favorable sensitivity to endocrine therapy [56]. Lupien et al. [57] reported that FOXA1 is recruited into target DNA regions according to the methylation of histone H3 lysine 4 (H3K4), which differs between cell types. These data indicate that the pioneer factor FOXA1 is first recruited to a specific DNA binding region, then facilitates the recruitment of other collaborating factors, and finally induces cell type specific gene expression.

GATA family proteins are also recruited to compact chromatin [54]. GATA2 and 3 are pioneer factors for prostate cancer and breast cancer [48]. GATA2 is required for AR binding in prostate cancer cells, whereas GATA3 is necessary for ER mediated gene expression in breast cancer [46,58]. High expression of GATA2 is related to high risk of prostate cancer [59]. Recent ChIP combined with genome-wide studies have shown that GATA2 promotes the AR pathway by (1) binding to enhancer regions before androgen stimulation; (2) modifying the histone code to allow the AR easy access; and (3) establishing chromatin loop formation [60]. In addition, GATA2 cooperates with FOXA1 to perform these actions regardless of the hormone status [60]. This means that GATA2 is functionally similar to FOXA1 in the AR pathway. Like FOXA1, which induces chromatin looping for AR target gene expression in CRPC cells, GATA2 establishes the loop via the recruitment of loop formation factor mediator complex subunit 1 (MED1) [60–62]. These data indicate that GATA2 and FOXA1 correlate with abundant AR hypersensitivity in CRPC cells.

OCT1 acts downstream of these pioneer factors. For prostate cancer cells, GATA2 and OCT1 work in a hierarchical network as GATA2 is recruited with AR, followed by OCT1 binding to its motifs [46]. OCT1 is comprised of two DNA-binding domains that are connected to each other by a flexible linker [63]. Previous reports showed that OCT1 is weakly recruited to some AR binding regions, and OCT1 reduced *TGM2* and *C20orf77* expression by inhibiting AR activity [64,65]. These data suggest that OCT1 recruitment is limited to specific AR regulated regions where it plays an OCT1 specialized function. Interestingly, some reports indicate that OCT1 is related to the cellular stress response [66,67]. Tantin et al. [67] reported that fibroblasts deficient in OCT1 showed hypersensitivity to radiation, doxorubicin, and hydrogen peroxide and harbored elevated levels of reactive oxygen species. Kang et al. [66] showed that a large number of stress response-related genes were regulated by OCT1. These stress response genes included DNA repair genes, such as poly(ADP-ribose) polymerase 1 (*PARP1*), and metabolic genes [68]. PARP1 plays an integral role in DNA repair, in addition, a recent report showed that PARP1 was recruited to AR binding regions and promoted AR function in advanced prostate cancer [69]. These data indicate that OCT1 might correlate with drug resistance in prostate cancer by enhancement of the AR and DNA repair pathways. Consistent with these reports, we previously reported that high OCT1 expression in prostate cancer tissues is related to poor prognosis and high AR expression [70]. These data raise the hypothesis that the major downstream target genes of the OCT1 and AR complex play an important role for prostate cancer progression. Using chromatin immunoprecipitation sequencing (ChIP-Seq) and microarray techniques, we identified acyl-CoA synthetase long-chain family member 3 (*ACSL3*) [71] as the most highly expressed gene regulated by AR and OCT1 in LNCaP cells [72]. In addition, we also revealed that high *ACSL3* expression in prostate cancer tissues was associated with poor patient prognosis [72].

In addition to these primary factors, several groups have subsequently identified ETS proto-oncogene 1, transcription factor (ETS1), ERG, ETS transcription factor (ERG), CCAAT/enhancer binding proteins (C/EBPs), nuclear factor I (NFI), NK3 homeobox 1 (NKX3-1), runt related transcription factor 1 (RUNX1), and forkhead box P1 (FOXP1) as other AR collaborative TFs [65,73–78]. The roles of C/EBPs and NFI in the AR signaling pathway are still unknown. Both factors have various subtypes (e.g., C/EBPα, β, NFIA, and NFIB), and each has different effects depending on AR response genes [65,79,80].

ETS1 is a member of the ETS (v-ets erythroblastosis virus E26 oncogene) family. Massie et al. [73] reported the enrichment of ETS consensus binding motifs and non-canonical AREs in about 70% of AR binding promoter regions. ETS1 was known to activate AR, as well as multiple cancer-associated pathways, which resulted in enhanced energy metabolism, cancer cell growth and survival [81,82]. Consistent with these data, Smith et al. [83] reported that increased *ETS1* expression is related to high-grade prostate cancer and the resistance to flutamide in prostate cancer cell lines. In addition, ETS1 directly interacts with AR and stimulates *NKX3-1* expression [73,84].

The NKX family belongs to the homeodomain class of TFs, which are critical regulators of whole organ development [85]. The role of NKX3-1 in tumor progression is still controversial. Since the *NKX3-1* gene region is frequently lost in prostate cancer and this leads to increase vascular endothelial growth factor-C (*VEGF-C*) expression, *NKX3-1* is known as a tumor suppressor gene [86,87]. On the other hand, a previous study showed that *NKX3-1* is an AR response gene as well as an AR collaborating TF [75]. This study suggested that NKX3-1 forms a positive autoregulatory loop with AR and FOXA1, and mediates cancer cell survival via induction of *RAB3B*, a member of the RAS oncogene family [75].

Similar to ETS1, ERG belongs to the class I ETS family (ERG, ETS1 and 2, ETS variant: ETV1–5, ELK1, ELK3, ELK4, ETS2 repressor factor: ERF, FEV, Fli-1 proto-oncogene: FLI1 and GA binding protein transcription factor alpha subunit: GABPα) and possesses oncogenic properties, which activate the phosphoinositide 3-kinase (PI3K) pathway to promote prostate cancer progression [88,89]. On the other hand, chromosomal rearrangements between TMPRSS2 and ERG (TMPRSS2:ERG), made by AR binding to the "breakpoint ARE" in this region, occur in around 50% of prostate cancers [90–93]. Interestingly, Bowen et al. [94] recently reported that NKX3-1 bound to the region adjacent to the "break point ARE" to prevent the TMPRSS2:ERG rearrangement and its expression.

Unlike ETS1, ERG has a unique role in the AR signaling pathway. Yu et al. [76] showed that approximately 44% of AR binding sites overlap with ERG binding sites where ERG repressed AR activity. Indeed, ERG represses a number of prostate epithelium-specific genes (*PSA*, solute carrier family 45 member 3: *SLC45A3*, microseminoprotein beta: *MSMB*, and secretoglobin family 1D member 2: *SCGB1D2*). In other words, these genes are prostate epithelial differentiation markers [95]. Yu et al. [76] suggest that TMPRSS2:ERG activates a malignant regulatory switch that inhibits physiological AR signaling by induction of enhancer of zeste 2 polycomb repressive complex 2 subunit (*EZH2*). TMPRSS2:ERG expression decreases during ADT, but is reactivated in the castration resistant state [96]. EZH2, which is a member of polycomb repressive complex 2 (PRC2), mediates the trimethylation of H3K27 [97]. This means that EZH2 represses target gene expression, and facilitates cellular dedifferentiation. For example, the tumor suppressive gene, DAB2 interacting protein (*DAB2IP*) was inhibited by EZH2/PRC2 [98]. *EZH2* is also overexpressed in hormone-refractory metastatic prostate cancer, suggesting EZH2 promotes AR independent growth [97]. Furthermore, Xu et al. [99] has shown that EZH2 works not only as a methyltransferase, but also as an activator of target genes that cooperate with AR. Unlike ERG, we have reported that the AR response gene *RUNX1* functions as an AR collaborative factor to maintain AR activity. In addition, EZH2 is recruited to the *RUNX1* promoter to repress its expression [77]. The *RUNX1* expression level in clinical prostate cancer tissues is negatively associated with *EZH2* expression, and decreased *RUNX1* expression is correlated with poor prognosis [77]. These data indicate that long-term ADT and high *EZH2* expression in androgen-independent prostate cancer inhibits *RUNX1* and the negative effect of *RUNX1* on prostate cancer progression. In addition to EZH2, Ma et al. [100] showed that the TMPRSS2:ERG activates SRY-box 9 (SOX9), which stimulates WNT signaling and tumor progression in a subset of prostate cancer.

Interestingly, previous reports have shown that high dose testosterone supplementation of castrate-resistant cells inhibits their proliferation [101,102]. This negative feedback mechanism of the AR signaling pathway might maintain prostate cancer in a well differentiated type of adenocarcinoma.

3. The Unique Features of Transcription Factors in Castration-Resistant Prostate Cancer

AR binding regions might keep changing with prostate cancer progression under a low testosterone environment. Recently, Sharma et al. [103] elucidated the differences in AR binding regions between ADT naïve prostate cancer and CRPC. Notably, 44% of genes with AR binding sites unique to CRPC showed no response to androgen in prostate cancer cell lines [103]. These AR binding sites are enriched in promoter regions and predominantly included E2F transcription factor (E2F), v-myc avian myelocytomatosis viral oncogene homolog (*MYC*), and signal transducer and activator of transcription (STAT) motifs compared to those in ADT naïve and prostate cancer cell lines [103].

E2F-1 activates genes related to G_1–S transition and DNA synthesis and induces cell cycle progression [104]. The expression of *E2F-1* is regulated by the tumor suppressor gene RB transcriptional corepressor 1 (*RB1*). RB1 inhibits G_1–S transition related gene expression by directly obstructing the transactivation domain of E2F and the promoter activity of these genes [105]. Since *RB1* loss is frequently observed in CRPC, the RB1/E2F-1 complex could play a significant role in tumor progression. A previous report suggested that loss of *RB1* enhances AR activity via *E2F-1* activation to induce resistance to ADT [106].

c-MYC is known as an oncogenic transcription factor that regulates ribosomal RNA expression, glutamine metabolism, and energy and reactive oxygen species [107–109]. Bernard et al. [110] reported that c-MYC was regulated by the AR and was required for AR-dependent and AR-independent growth in AR positive prostate cancer cell lines. Previous fluorescence in situ hybridization data showed the specific amplification of the *c-MYC* gene in 72% of CRPC [111,112]. Some c-MYC repressed genes, *Bin1* and *MXI1*, were inactivated in advanced prostate cancer [113,114]. Consistent with the report by Yu et al. [76] about the TMPRSS2:ERG/EZH pathway, Sun et al. [115] also reported that TMPRSS2:ERG activates *c-MYC* and represses prostate epithelial differentiation genes.

STAT3 is regulated by the Janus kinase (Jak) family/interleukin 6 (IL-6) and is also oncogenic, promoting cytosolic dimerization, nuclear translocation and DNA binding [116–118]. STAT3 activation is observed in 82% of prostate cancer tissues compared to matched adjacent non-cancer tissues, and elevated STAT3 activity was correlated with a malignant phenotype [119]. Interestingly, Culig et al. [120] reported that IL-6 activates AR in androgen depleted conditions to promote the growth of almost all prostate cancer cell lines. However, IL-6 stimulation inhibited LNCaP cell proliferation regardless of STAT3 activation. In addition, a recent report showed that inhibition of IL-6/STAT3 signaling in a phosphatase and tensin homolog (PTEN)-deficient prostate cancer model promotes cancer progression [121]. These data indicate that the effect of STAT3 on prostate cancer progression is still controversial. Reinforcing the report by Sharma et al. [103], a recent study shows that the pluripotency transcription factor Nanog homeobox (NANOG) alters FOXA1 and AR target genes during reprogramming of androgen-dependent prostate cancer cells to CRPC [122].

Collectively, these studies suggest that the role of the AR signaling pathway in prostate cancer progression is more complicated than expected, because AR collaborating TFs are entangled with each other and have differing effects on AR activity depending on testosterone levels and the duration of anti-androgen drug treatment.

4. Development of Novel Drugs

4.1. *Pyrrole-Imidazole Polyamide*

Different classes of drugs are under investigation to inhibit AR collaborative TFs. In this section, we review the development of one new class of compounds, pyrrole-imidazole (PI) polyamides, before discussing specific examples of compounds that target AR collaborative TFs in the following section. PI polyamides are small synthetic molecules made up of *N*-methylimidazole (Im) and *N*-methylpyrrole (Py) amino acids, the side by side pairings of which recognize and attach to the minor groove of DNA with high affinity and sequence specificity [123–125]. Im/Py pairs recognise G/C nucleotides and Py/Py pairs bind to A/T and T/A nucleotides (Figure 1) [126,127].

In addition, the C-terminal β-alanine residue next to dimethylpropylamine (Dp) and the γ-aminobutyric acid turns a unit, which enforces an antiparallel hairpin configuration and enhances both DNA binding affinity and specificity [124,128,129]. Vector-assisted delivery systems are not necessary for PI polyamide translocation to the nucleus. Following PI polyamide binding to DNA, the minor groove is widened and the major groove is bent and compressed to block TFs binding [130]. Unlike most DNA targeted therapies, PI polyamides bind to DNA non-covalently without a drug delivery system [131]. In addition, PI polyamides are fully resistant to biological degradation by nucleases and do not induce unnecessary normal cell damage and carcinogenesis [132]. These are advantages of PI polyamides compared to other chemical drugs.

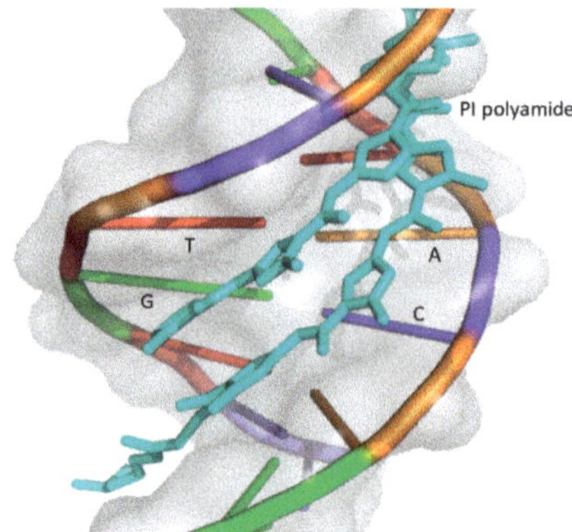

Figure 1. A schematic view of pyrrole-imidazole (PI) polyamide binding to a target DNA sequence. Image of 1CVY [124] created with Open-Source PyMOL Molecular Graphics System, Version 1.7, Schrödinger, LLC.

The pharmacokinetics of PI polyamides provide promise for future clinical applications. Previous reports have shown that PI polyamides are not absorbed from the intestine [133]. After transvenous distribution in rat organs, PI polyamides were excreted into urine and bile without any metabolism [133,134]. Matsuda et al. showed that PI polyamides accumulated in nuclei of kidney cells in rats and were maintained for about two weeks without any drug delivery system [135,136]. Recently, Igarashi et al. [137] studied the possible clinical applications of PI polyamides using a primate model. They developed an ointment including a PI polyamide targeting human transforming growth factor beta (TGF-β) 1 and tested for hypertrophic scars in marmosets. The PI polyamide bound to keratinocyte nuclei in marmosets and suppressed hypertrophic scarring without any side effects [137]. These reports are fundamental evidence for the clinical application of PI polyamides and increasing interest in their use for AR and some AR collaborative TFs, such as OCT1 and ETS family genes.

4.2. Novel Drugs Targeting TFs Related to the AR Pathway

4.2.1. The Pioneer Factors (FOXA1 and GATA2)

Targeting the pioneer factor FOXA1 showed contradictory results for AR activity and prostate cancer prognosis [138]. Increasing FOXA1 activity causes indiscriminate opening of closed chromatin, attracting the AR to ARE half sites at the expense of genes with canonical ARE that promote prostate cancer progression. Conversely, inhibition of FOXA1 reprogrammed the arrangement of the AR and led to overexpression some androgen-responsive genes to promote CRPC cell growth [139]. We also reported that the AR/FOXA1 response gene *FOXP1* acts as a negative AR collaborative transcriptional factor, and represses tumor activity by binding to adjacent regions to AREs [78,140]. Interestingly, the EZH2 methyltransferase inhibitor, GSK126, promotes *FOXA1* expression and inhibits breast cancer growth via cooperation with *BRCA1* [141]. Recently, Zhao et al. [142] elucidated the dichotomous functions of FOXA1 in the AR signaling pathway. They indicated that FOXA1 reprograms the AR and GATA2 cistromes as a pioneer factor [142]. Whilst FOXA1 represses AR binding to DNA, GATA2 positively collaborates with the AR in androgen-mediated gene expression in prostate cancer [142]. Previous reports showed that GATA2 specific inhibition using the low-molecular-weight compound K-7174 [143] suppressed AR expression and the proliferation of CRPC cells [144]. Although it is not known whether this compound is suitable for clinical applications, it is ingestible and possesses beneficial effects for haematological diseases [145–147].

4.2.2. OCT1

Whilst many studies have focused on FOXA1 and GATA2, OCT1 is often overlooked, so we have developed a novel drug targeting Oct1/AR using PI polyamides. A previous report showed that a PI polyamide targeting AREs suppressed androgen-responsive gene expression in LNCaP cells [148]. This sophisticated report showed that targeting canonical AREs was clearly effective; however, it is possible that PI polyamides that also cover non-canonical AREs might block the proliferation of CRPC even further. We identified the ACSL3 enhancer region, where AR and OCT1 regulate transcriptional activity, and developed a PI polyamide targeting OCT1 binding elements in this region [72]. This PI polyamide suppressed ACSL3 expression and CRPC cell growth. In addition, it specifically repressed global OCT1 chromatin association and AR signaling in prostate cancer cells [72]. These data reinforce the evidence that OCT1 is also important for AR recruitment to mediate global AR-response gene expression. Our study supports a novel therapeutic strategy using PI polyamides in patients with CRPC.

4.2.3. ETS Family Genes

There is one report of an ETS-1 inhibitor using double-strand oligodeoxynucleotides (ODNs) that represses gastric cancer cell proliferation [149]. ODNs mimic transcription factor binding sites and act as decoys that compete with the original DNA binding sites in promoter regions [150]. Unlike PI polyamides, ODNs require improvements to the drug delivery systems to target cells and greater in vivo stability before they are suitable for clinical applications.

Since ERG was shown to be an oncogenic protein, ERG target drugs became attractive agents for prostate cancer. PARP inhibitors, a direct ERG binding small molecule (YK-4-279), a DNA-binding inhibitor targeting ETS consensus sites (DB1255), and a drug that enhances ERG ubiquitination (WP1130) are all promising compounds for prostate cancer [151–154]. In terms of TMPRSS2:ERG, we previously developed a PI polyamide targeting a common sequence in AR-related DNA break points among *TMPRSS2* and *ERG* gene loci to repress TMPRSS2:ERG expression and prostate cancer cell growth [155]. Furthermore, a recent report showed that targeting AREs downregulated TMPRSS2:ERG expression in VCaP cells and inhibited the growth of VCaP cells in vivo [156].

4.2.4. NKX3-1

Ren et al. [157] developed NKX3-1 targeting compounds using RNA activation (RNAa). RNAa is system that uses small double-stranded RNA (dsRNA) that target selected gene promoter regions [158]. Transfecting the synthesized dsRNA into human cell lines causes induction of target gene expression. Ren et al. showed that increased *NKX3-1* expression by RNAa formulated in lipid nanoparticles significantly inhibited prostate tumor growth both in vitro and in vivo [157].

4.2.5. C/EBP Family

Although the role of the C/EBP family in prostate cancer is still unknown, a recent report showed that RNAa targeting *C/EBPα* repressed the proliferation of pancreatic ductal adenocarcinoma cells [159]. In addition, a phase I clinical study of RNAa targeting *C/EBPα* is underway for severe liver cancer (NCT02716012).

4.2.6. E2F-1

Several studies of E2F-1 inhibitors have been reported. Kaseb et al. [160] studied the efficacy of a herbal product, thymoquinone, extracted from *Nigella sativa* seeds for prostate cancer. Interestingly, thymoquinone inhibited the tumor growth of CRPC xenografts and repressed E2F-1 and AR expression [160]. Xie et al. [161] also developed a peptide binding to the *E2F-1* consensus sequence. Treatment of mice with this peptide encapsulated in PEGylated liposomes inhibited the growth of an AR negative prostate cancer cell line without toxicity [162].

4.2.7. c-MYC

Like ERG, there are several agents targeting c-MYC [163–166]. Recently, Rebello et al. [167] reported the efficacy of a combination of RNA polymerase I (Rpol I) and proto-oncogene serine/threonine-protein (PIM) kinase inhibitors (CX-5461 and CX-6258) for MYC-driven prostate cancer. They showed that c-MYC is related to both Rpol I and PIM kinase activation, which were significantly inhibited by both drugs in Hi-MYC mice [167].

4.2.8. STAT3

Leong et al. [168] showed that inhibiting *STAT3* using ODNs repressed head and neck cancer cell growth. In addition, Hedvat et al. showed favorable results in prostate cancer for a STAT3 inhibitor, AZD1480, which is a potent ATP competitive inhibitor of Jak2 kinase [169]. However, Fizazi et al. [170] reported an anti-IL-6 monoclonal antibody, siltuximab, inhibited *STAT3* expression, but did not find a survival improvement in patients with advanced prostate cancer.

The information about AR collaborative TFs and related drugs discussed in this section is summarized in Table 1.

Table 1. AR collaborative TFs.

Factor	Functions for AR	Efficacy for Cancer Progression	FOXA1 Interaction	Related Drugs	Reference
FOXA1	Pioneer factor	Controversial		GSK126	[141]
GATA2	Pioneer factor/ Activator	Promote	+	K-7174	[143,145–147]
OCT1	Activator	Promote	+	PI polyamide	[72]
ETS1	Activator	Promote	−	ODNs	[149,150]
ERG	Repressor	Promote	−	PI polyamide/ YK-4-279/ DB1255/WP1130	[151,153–155]
NKX3-1	Activator	Controversial	+	RNAa	[157]
C/EBPs	Repressor	Unknown	−	RNAa	[159]
NFI	Diverse effects on gene regulation	Unknown	+	-	
RUNX1	Activator	Inhibit	−	-	
FOXP1	Repressor	Inhibit	+	-	
E2F	Activator (CRPC)	Promote	−	Thymoquinone/Peptide	[160–162]
MYC	Controversial (CRPC)	Promote	−	CX5461/CX6258	[167]
STAT3	Activator (CRPC)	Controversial	−	ODNs/AZD1480/ Siltuximab	[168–170]

FOXA1: forkhead box A1; GATA2: GATA binding protein 2; OCT1: octamer transcription factor; ETS1: ETS proto-oncogene 1, transcription factor; ERG: ETS transcription factor; NKX3-1: NK3 homeobox 1; C/EBPs: CCAAT/enhancer binding proteins: NFI: nuclear factor I; RUNX1: runt related transcription factor 1; FOXP1: forkhead box P1; E2F: E2F transcription factor; MYC: v-myc avian myelocytomatosis viral oncogene homolog; STAT3: signal transducer and activator of transcription; CRPC: castration resistant prostate cancer; ODN: oligodeoxynucleotides; PI: pyrrole-imidazole; RNAa: RNA activation.

5. Conclusions

AR collaborators, such as collaborative TFs, are important in the extraordinary hypersensitivity of the AR in CRPC. In addition, activation of AR-regulated genes promotes prostate cancer progression. Over the last decade, sophisticated technologies for investigating transcriptional networks have broadened our understanding of AR signaling in prostate cancer. Various functional studies, including our own work, have elucidated the complicated influence that AR collaborators have on prostate cancer progression. These reports provide fundamental evidence to support the premise that developing novel drugs against AR collaborators could provide promising strategies to treat CRPC. Thus, further studies of these novel candidate compounds with pre-clinical drug screening models will be crucial for developing new strategies to treat CRPC [24,171–174].

Acknowledgments: This work was supported by grants from the P-CREATE and P-DIRECT (Satoshi Inoue) and Cell Innovation Program (Satoshi Inoue) from the MEXT, Japan; JSPS, Japan (Daisuke Obinata, Kenichi Takayama, Satoru Takahashi, Satoshi Inoue; number 24791675, 26861302, 15K15581, 15K10610, and 15K15353); the 60th Anniversary Memorial Fund from Nihon University Medical Alumni Association (2010 Research Grant, Daisuke Obinata); the Nihon University School of Medicine 50th Anniversary Fund (Daisuke Obinata); the Japanese Urological Association (Young Researcher Promotion Grant, Daisuke Obinata); Uehara Memorial Foundation (Satoshi Inoue); and the Program for Promotion of Fundamental Studies in Health Sciences (Satoshi Inoue), NIBIO, Japan.

Author Contributions: Conceived the concepts: Daisuke Obinata, Kenichi Takayama, Satoru Takahashi, and Sathoshi Inoue. Wrote the first draft of the manuscript: Daisuke Obinata. Agreed with manuscript results and conclusions: Daisuke Obinata, Kenichi Takayama, Satoru Takahashi, and Sathoshi Inoue. All authors reviewed and approved of the final manuscript.

Conflicts of Interest: The authors declare no conflicts of interest.

References

1. Hobisch, A.; Culig, Z.; Radmayr, C.; Bartsch, G.; Klocker, H.; Hittmair, A. Distant metastases from prostatic carcinoma express androgen receptor protein. *Cancer Res.* **1995**, *55*, 3068–3072. [PubMed]
2. Hobisch, A.; Culig, Z.; Radmayr, C.; Bartsch, G.; Klocker, H.; Hittmair, A. Androgen receptor status of lymph node metastases from prostate cancer. *Prostate* **1996**, *28*, 129–135. [CrossRef]
3. Sadi, M.V.; Walsh, P.C.; Barrack, E.R. Immunohistochemical study of androgen receptors in metastatic prostate cancer. Comparison of receptor content and response to hormonal therapy. *Cancer* **1991**, *67*, 3057–3064. [CrossRef]
4. Tilley, W.D.; Lim-Tio, S.S.; Horsfall, D.J.; Aspinall, J.O.; Marshall, V.R.; Skinner, J.M. Detection of discrete androgen receptor epitopes in prostate cancer by immunostaining: Measurement by color video image analysis. *Cancer Res.* **1994**, *54*, 4096–4102. [PubMed]
5. Van der Kwast, T.H.; Tetu, B. Androgen receptors in untreated and treated prostatic intraepithelial neoplasia. *Eur. Urol.* **1996**, *30*, 265–268. [PubMed]
6. Huggins, C. Effect of Orchiectomy and Irradiation on Cancer of the Prostate. *Ann. Surg.* **1942**, *115*, 1192–1200. [CrossRef] [PubMed]
7. Huggins, C.; Hodges, C.V. The effect of castration, of estrogen and of androgen injection on serum phosphatases in metastatic carcinoma of the prostate. *Cancer Res.* **1941**, *1*, 293–297.
8. Trapman, J.; Brinkmann, A.O. The androgen receptor in prostate cancer. *Pathol. Res. Pract.* **1996**, *192*, 752–760. [CrossRef]
9. Taplin, M.E.; Balk, S.P. Androgen receptor: A key molecule in the progression of prostate cancer to hormone independence. *J. Cell. Biochem.* **2004**, *91*, 483–490. [CrossRef] [PubMed]
10. Feldman, B.J.; Feldman, D. The development of androgen-independent prostate cancer. *Nat. Rev. Cancer* **2001**, *1*, 34–45. [CrossRef] [PubMed]
11. Denmeade, S.R.; Isaacs, J.T. A history of prostate cancer treatment. *Nat. Rev. Cancer* **2002**, *2*, 389–396. [CrossRef] [PubMed]
12. Arnold, J.T.; Isaacs, J.T. Mechanisms involved in the progression of androgen-independent prostate cancers: It is not only the cancer cell's fault. *Endocr. Relat. Cancer* **2002**, *9*, 61–73. [CrossRef] [PubMed]
13. Culig, Z.; Hoffmann, J.; Erdel, M.; Eder, I.E.; Hobisch, A.; Hittmair, A.; Bartsch, G.; Utermann, G.; Schneider, M.R.; Parczyk, K.; et al. Switch from antagonist to agonist of the androgen receptor bicalutamide is associated with prostate tumour progression in a new model system. *Br. J. Cancer* **1999**, *81*, 242–251. [CrossRef] [PubMed]
14. Liu, W.; Xie, C.C.; Zhu, Y.; Li, T.; Sun, J.; Cheng, Y.; Ewing, C.M.; Dalrymple, S.; Turner, A.R.; Sun, J.; et al. Homozygous deletions and recurrent amplifications implicate new genes involved in prostate cancer. *Neoplasia* **2008**, *10*, 897–907. [CrossRef] [PubMed]

15. Heemers, H.V.; Regan, K.M.; Schmidt, L.J.; Anderson, S.K.; Ballman, K.V.; Tindall, D.J. Androgen modulation of coregulator expression in prostate cancer cells. *Mol. Endocrinol.* **2009**, *23*, 572–583. [CrossRef] [PubMed]
16. Ford, O.H., 3rd; Gregory, C.W.; Kim, D.; Smitherman, A.B.; Mohler, J.L. Androgen receptor gene amplification and protein expression in recurrent prostate cancer. *J. Urol.* **2003**, *170*, 1817–1821. [CrossRef] [PubMed]
17. Chen, C.D.; Welsbie, D.S.; Tran, C.; Baek, S.H.; Chen, R.; Vessella, R.; Rosenfeld, M.G.; Sawyers, C.L. Molecular determinants of resistance to antiandrogen therapy. *Nat. Med.* **2004**, *10*, 33–39. [CrossRef] [PubMed]
18. Cai, C.; He, H.H.; Chen, S.; Coleman, I.; Wang, H.; Fang, Z.; Chen, S.; Nelson, P.S.; Liu, X.S.; Brown, M.; et al. Androgen receptor gene expression in prostate cancer is directly suppressed by the androgen receptor through recruitment of lysine-specific demethylase 1. *Cancer Cell* **2011**, *20*, 457–471. [CrossRef] [PubMed]
19. Coutinho, I.; Day, T.K.; Tilley, W.D.; Selth, L.A. Androgen receptor signaling in castration-resistant prostate cancer: A lesson in persistence. *Endocr. Relat. Cancer* **2016**, *23*, T179–T197. [CrossRef] [PubMed]
20. Yamaoka, M.; Hara, T.; Kusaka, M. Overcoming persistent dependency on androgen signaling after progression to castration-resistant prostate cancer. *Clin. Cancer Res.* **2010**, *16*, 4319–4324. [CrossRef] [PubMed]
21. Scher, H.I.; Fizazi, K.; Saad, F.; Taplin, M.E.; Sternberg, C.N.; Miller, K.; de Wit, R.; Mulders, P.; Chi, K.N.; Shore, N.D.; et al. Increased survival with enzalutamide in prostate cancer after chemotherapy. *N. Engl. J. Med.* **2012**, *367*, 1187–1197. [PubMed]
22. Beer, T.M.; Armstrong, A.J.; Rathkopf, D.E.; Loriot, Y.; Sternberg, C.N.; Higano, C.S.; Iversen, P.; Bhattacharya, S.; Carles, J.; Chowdhury, S.; et al. Enzalutamide in Metastatic Prostate Cancer before Chemotherapy. *N. Engl. J. Med.* **2014**, *371*, 424–433. [CrossRef] [PubMed]
23. De Bono, J.S.; Logothetis, C.J.; Molina, A.; Fizazi, K.; North, S.; Chu, L.; Chi, K.N.; Jones, R.J.; Goodman, O.B., Jr.; Saad, F.; et al. Abiraterone and increased survival in metastatic prostate cancer. *N. Engl. J. Med.* **2011**, *364*, 1995–2005. [CrossRef] [PubMed]
24. Schweizer, M.T.; Antonarakis, E.S. Abiraterone and other novel androgen-directed strategies for the treatment of prostate cancer: A new era of hormonal therapies is born. *Ther. Adv. Urol.* **2012**, *4*, 167–178. [CrossRef] [PubMed]
25. Tsai, M.J.; O'Malley, B.W. Molecular mechanisms of action of steroid/thyroid receptor superfamily members. *Annu. Rev. Biochem.* **1994**, *63*, 451–486. [CrossRef] [PubMed]
26. Jenster, G.; van der Korput, H.A.; Trapman, J.; Brinkmann, A.O. Identification of two transcription activation units in the N-terminal domain of the human androgen receptor. *J. Biol. Chem.* **1995**, *270*, 7341–7346. [PubMed]
27. Beltran, H.; Yelensky, R.; Frampton, G.M.; Park, K.; Downing, S.R.; MacDonald, T.Y.; Jarosz, M.; Lipson, D.; Tagawa, S.T.; Nanus, D.M.; et al. Targeted next-generation sequencing of advanced prostate cancer identifies potential therapeutic targets and disease heterogeneity. *Eur. Urol.* **2013**, *63*, 920–926. [CrossRef] [PubMed]
28. Steinkamp, M.P.; O'Mahony, O.A.; Brogley, M.; Rehman, H.; Lapensee, E.W.; Dhanasekaran, S.; Hofer, M.D.; Kuefer, R.; Chinnaiyan, A.; Rubin, M.A.; et al. Treatment-dependent androgen receptor mutations in prostate cancer exploit multiple mechanisms to evade therapy. *Cancer Res.* **2009**, *69*, 4434–4442. [CrossRef] [PubMed]
29. Egan, A.; Dong, Y.; Zhang, H.; Qi, Y.; Balk, S.P.; Sartor, O. Castration-resistant prostate cancer: Adaptive responses in the androgen axis. *Cancer Treat. Rev.* **2014**, *40*, 426–433. [CrossRef] [PubMed]
30. Schrecengost, R.; Knudsen, K.E. Molecular pathogenesis and progression of prostate cancer. *Semin. Oncol.* **2013**, *40*, 244–258. [CrossRef] [PubMed]
31. Middleman, M.N.; Lush, R.M.; Figg, W.D. The mutated androgen receptor and its implications for the treatment of metastatic carcinoma of the prostate. *Pharmacotherapy* **1996**, *16*, 376–381. [PubMed]
32. Knudsen, K.E.; Penning, T.M. Partners in crime: Deregulation of AR activity and androgen synthesis in prostate cancer. *Trends Endocrinol. Metab.* **2010**, *21*, 315–324. [CrossRef] [PubMed]
33. Gaddipati, J.P.; McLeod, D.G.; Heidenberg, H.B.; Sesterhenn, I.A.; Finger, M.J.; Moul, J.W.; Srivastava, S. Frequent detection of codon 877 mutation in the androgen receptor gene in advanced prostate cancers. *Cancer Res.* **1994**, *54*, 2861–2864. [PubMed]
34. Taplin, M.E.; Bubley, G.J.; Ko, Y.J.; Small, E.J.; Upton, M.; Rajeshkumar, B.; Balk, S.P. Selection for androgen receptor mutations in prostate cancers treated with androgen antagonist. *Cancer Res.* **1999**, *59*, 2511–2515. [PubMed]

35. Gottlieb, B.; Beitel, L.K.; Wu, J.H.; Trifiro, M. The androgen receptor gene mutations database (ARDB): 2004 update. *Hum. Mutat.* **2004**, *23*, 527–533. [CrossRef] [PubMed]
36. Dehm, S.M.; Schmidt, L.J.; Heemers, H.V.; Vessella, R.L.; Tindall, D.J. Splicing of a novel androgen receptor exon generates a constitutively active androgen receptor that mediates prostate cancer therapy resistance. *Cancer Res.* **2008**, *68*, 5469–5477. [CrossRef] [PubMed]
37. Hu, R.; Dunn, T.A.; Wei, S.; Isharwal, S.; Veltri, R.W.; Humphreys, E.; Han, M.; Partin, A.W.; Vessella, R.L.; Isaacs, W.B.; et al. Ligand-independent androgen receptor variants derived from splicing of cryptic exons signify hormone-refractory prostate cancer. *Cancer Res.* **2009**, *69*, 16–22. [CrossRef] [PubMed]
38. Antonarakis, E.S.; Lu, C.; Wang, H.; Luber, B.; Nakazawa, M.; Roeser, J.C.; Chen, Y.; Mohammad, T.A.; Chen, Y.; Fedor, H.L.; et al. AR-V7 and resistance to enzalutamide and abiraterone in prostate cancer. *N. Engl. J. Med.* **2014**, *371*, 1028–1038. [CrossRef] [PubMed]
39. Heemers, H.V.; Tindall, D.J. Androgen receptor (AR) coregulators: A diversity of functions converging on and regulating the AR transcriptional complex. *Endocr. Rev.* **2007**, *28*, 778–808. [CrossRef] [PubMed]
40. Wang, Q.; Carroll, J.S.; Brown, M. Spatial and temporal recruitment of androgen receptor and its coactivators involves chromosomal looping and polymerase tracking. *Mol. Cell* **2005**, *19*, 631–642. [CrossRef] [PubMed]
41. Onate, S.A.; Tsai, S.Y.; Tsai, M.J.; O'Malley, B.W. Sequence and characterization of a coactivator for the steroid hormone receptor superfamily. *Science* **1995**, *270*, 1354–1357. [PubMed]
42. Takayama, K.; Horie-Inoue, K.; Katayama, S.; Suzuki, T.; Tsutsumi, S.; Ikeda, K.; Urano, T.; Fujimura, T.; Takagi, K.; Takahashi, S.; et al. Androgen-responsive long noncoding RNA CTBP1-AS promotes prostate cancer. *EMBO J.* **2013**, *32*, 1665–1680. [CrossRef] [PubMed]
43. Takayama, K.; Suzuki, T.; Fujimura, T.; Urano, T.; Takahashi, S.; Homma, Y.; Inoue, S. CtBP2 modulates the androgen receptor to promote prostate cancer progression. *Cancer Res.* **2014**, *74*, 6452–6453. [CrossRef] [PubMed]
44. Taylor, B.S.; Schultz, N.; Hieronymus, H.; Gopalan, A.; Xiao, Y.; Carver, B.S.; Arora, V.K.; Kaushik, P.; Cerami, E.; Reva, B.; et al. Integrative genomic profiling of human prostate cancer. *Cancer Cell* **2010**, *18*, 11–22. [CrossRef] [PubMed]
45. Kornberg, R.D. Structure of chromatin. *Annu. Rev. Biochem.* **1977**, *46*, 931–954. [CrossRef] [PubMed]
46. Wang, Q.; Li, W.; Liu, X.S.; Carroll, J.S.; Janne, O.A.; Keeton, E.K.; Chinnaiyan, A.M.; Pienta, K.J.; Brown, M. A hierarchical network of transcription factors governs androgen receptor-dependent prostate cancer growth. *Mol. Cell* **2007**, *27*, 380–392. [CrossRef] [PubMed]
47. Mangelsdorf, D.J.; Thummel, C.; Beato, M.; Herrlich, P.; Schutz, G.; Umesono, K.; Blumberg, B.; Kastner, P.; Mark, M.; Chambon, P.; et al. The nuclear receptor superfamily: The second decade. *Cell* **1995**, *83*, 835–839. [CrossRef]
48. Zaret, K.S.; Carroll, J.S. Pioneer transcription factors: Establishing competence for gene expression. *Genes Dev.* **2011**, *25*, 2227–2241. [CrossRef] [PubMed]
49. Bossard, P.; Zaret, K.S. GATA transcription factors as potentiators of gut endoderm differentiation. *Development* **1998**, *125*, 4909–4917. [PubMed]
50. Cuesta, I.; Zaret, K.S.; Santisteban, P. The forkhead factor FoxE1 binds to the thyroperoxidase promoter during thyroid cell differentiation and modifies compacted chromatin structure. *Mol. Cell. Biol.* **2007**, *27*, 7302–7314. [CrossRef] [PubMed]
51. Cirillo, L.A.; Zaret, K.S. Specific interactions of the wing domains of FOXA1 transcription factor with DNA. *J. Mol. Biol.* **2007**, *366*, 720–724. [CrossRef] [PubMed]
52. Carroll, J.S.; Liu, X.S.; Brodsky, A.S.; Li, W.; Meyer, C.A.; Szary, A.J.; Eeckhoute, J.; Shao, W.; Hestermann, E.V.; Geistlinger, T.R.; et al. Chromosome-wide mapping of estrogen receptor binding reveals long-range regulation requiring the forkhead protein FoxA1. *Cell* **2005**, *122*, 33–43. [CrossRef] [PubMed]
53. Gao, N.; Zhang, J.; Rao, M.A.; Case, T.C.; Mirosevich, J.; Wang, Y.; Jin, R.; Gupta, A.; Rennie, P.S.; Matusik, R.J. The role of hepatocyte nuclear factor-3 alpha (Forkhead Box A1) and androgen receptor in transcriptional regulation of prostatic genes. *Mol. Endocrinol.* **2003**, *17*, 1484–1507. [CrossRef] [PubMed]
54. Cirillo, L.A.; Lin, F.R.; Cuesta, I.; Friedman, D.; Jarnik, M.; Zaret, K.S. Opening of compacted chromatin by early developmental transcription factors HNF3 (FoxA) and GATA-4. *Mol. Cell* **2002**, *9*, 279–289. [CrossRef]
55. Gerhardt, J.; Montani, M.; Wild, P.; Beer, M.; Huber, F.; Hermanns, T.; Muntener, M.; Kristiansen, G. FOXA1 promotes tumor progression in prostate cancer and represents a novel hallmark of castration-resistant prostate cancer. *Am. J. Pathol.* **2012**, *180*, 848–861. [CrossRef] [PubMed]

56. Badve, S.; Turbin, D.; Thorat, M.A.; Morimiya, A.; Nielsen, T.O.; Perou, C.M.; Dunn, S.; Huntsman, D.G.; Nakshatri, H. FOXA1 expression in breast cancer—Correlation with luminal subtype A and survival. *Clin. Cancer Res.* **2007**, *13*, 4415–4421. [CrossRef] [PubMed]
57. Lupien, M.; Eeckhoute, J.; Meyer, C.A.; Wang, Q.; Zhang, Y.; Li, W.; Carroll, J.S.; Liu, X.S.; Brown, M. FoxA1 translates epigenetic signatures into enhancer-driven lineage-specific transcription. *Cell* **2008**, *132*, 958–970. [CrossRef] [PubMed]
58. Eeckhoute, J.; Keeton, E.K.; Lupien, M.; Krum, S.A.; Carroll, J.S.; Brown, M. Positive cross-regulatory loop ties GATA-3 to estrogen receptor alpha expression in breast cancer. *Cancer Res.* **2007**, *67*, 6477–6483. [CrossRef] [PubMed]
59. Bohm, M.; Locke, W.J.; Sutherland, R.L.; Kench, J.G.; Henshall, S.M. A role for GATA-2 in transition to an aggressive phenotype in prostate cancer through modulation of key androgen-regulated genes. *Oncogene* **2009**, *28*, 3847–3856. [CrossRef] [PubMed]
60. Wu, D.; Sunkel, B.; Chen, Z.; Liu, X.; Ye, Z.; Li, Q.; Grenade, C.; Ke, J.; Zhang, C.; Chen, H.; et al. Three-tiered role of the pioneer factor GATA2 in promoting androgen-dependent gene expression in prostate cancer. *Nucleic Acids Res.* **2014**, *42*, 3607–3622. [CrossRef] [PubMed]
61. Chen, Z.; Zhang, C.; Wu, D.; Chen, H.; Rorick, A.; Zhang, X.; Wang, Q. Phospho-MED1-enhanced UBE2C locus looping drives castration-resistant prostate cancer growth. *EMBO J.* **2011**, *30*, 2405–2419. [CrossRef] [PubMed]
62. Hagege, H.; Klous, P.; Braem, C.; Splinter, E.; Dekker, J.; Cathala, G.; de Laat, W.; Forne, T. Quantitative analysis of chromosome conformation capture assays (3C-qPCR). *Nat. Protoc.* **2007**, *2*, 1722–1733. [CrossRef] [PubMed]
63. Klemm, J.D.; Rould, M.A.; Aurora, R.; Herr, W.; Pabo, C.O. Crystal structure of the Oct-1 POU domain bound to an octamer site: DNA recognition with tethered DNA-binding modules. *Cell* **1994**, *77*, 21–32. [CrossRef]
64. Jariwala, U.; Cogan, J.P.; Jia, L.; Frenkel, B.; Coetzee, G.A. Inhibition of AR-mediated transcription by binding of Oct1 to a motif enriched in AR-occupied regions. *Prostate* **2009**, *69*, 392–400. [CrossRef] [PubMed]
65. Jia, L.; Berman, B.P.; Jariwala, U.; Yan, X.; Cogan, J.P.; Walters, A.; Chen, T.; Buchanan, G.; Frenkel, B.; Coetzee, G.A. Genomic androgen receptor-occupied regions with different functions, defined by histone acetylation, coregulators and transcriptional capacity. *PLoS ONE* **2008**, *3*, e3645. [CrossRef] [PubMed]
66. Kang, J.; Gemberling, M.; Nakamura, M.; Whitby, F.G.; Handa, H.; Fairbrother, W.G.; Tantin, D. A general mechanism for transcription regulation by Oct1 and Oct4 in response to genotoxic and oxidative stress. *Genes Dev.* **2009**, *23*, 208–222. [CrossRef] [PubMed]
67. Tantin, D.; Schild-Poulter, C.; Wang, V.; Hache, R.J.; Sharp, P.A. The octamer binding transcription factor Oct-1 is a stress sensor. *Cancer Res.* **2005**, *65*, 10750–10758. [CrossRef] [PubMed]
68. Nie, J.; Sakamoto, S.; Song, D.; Qu, Z.; Ota, K.; Taniguchi, T. Interaction of Oct-1 and automodification domain of poly(ADP-ribose) synthetase. *FEBS Lett.* **1998**, *424*, 27–32. [CrossRef]
69. Schiewer, M.J.; Goodwin, J.F.; Han, S.; Brenner, J.C.; Augello, M.A.; Dean, J.L.; Liu, F.; Planck, J.L.; Ravindranathan, P.; Chinnaiyan, A.M.; et al. Dual roles of PARP-1 promote cancer growth and progression. *Cancer Discov.* **2012**, *2*, 1134–1149. [CrossRef] [PubMed]
70. Obinata, D.; Takayama, K.; Urano, T.; Murata, T.; Kumagai, J.; Fujimura, T.; Ikeda, K.; Horie-Inoue, K.; Homma, Y.; Ouchi, Y.; et al. Oct1 regulates cell growth of LNCaP cells and is a prognostic factor for prostate cancer. *Int. J. Cancer* **2012**, *130*, 1021–1028. [CrossRef] [PubMed]
71. Minekura, H.; Kang, M.J.; Inagaki, Y.; Suzuki, H.; Sato, H.; Fujino, T.; Yamamoto, T.T. Genomic organization and transcription units of the human acyl-CoA synthetase 3 gene. *Gene* **2001**, *278*, 185–192. [CrossRef]
72. Obinata, D.; Takayama, K.; Fujiwara, K.; Suzuki, T.; Tsutsumi, S.; Fukuda, N.; Nagase, H.; Fujimura, T.; Urano, T.; Homma, Y.; et al. Targeting Oct1 genomic function inhibits androgen receptor signaling and castration-resistant prostate cancer growth. *Oncogene* **2016**, *35*, 6350–6358. [CrossRef] [PubMed]
73. Massie, C.E.; Adryan, B.; Barbosa-Morais, N.L.; Lynch, A.G.; Tran, M.G.; Neal, D.E.; Mills, I.G. New androgen receptor genomic targets show an interaction with the ETS1 transcription factor. *EMBO Rep.* **2007**, *8*, 871–878. [CrossRef] [PubMed]
74. Rickman, D.S.; Chen, Y.B.; Banerjee, S.; Pan, Y.; Yu, J.; Vuong, T.; Perner, S.; Lafargue, C.J.; Mertz, K.D.; Setlur, S.R.; et al. ERG cooperates with androgen receptor in regulating trefoil factor 3 in prostate cancer disease progression. *Neoplasia* **2010**, *12*, 1031–1040. [CrossRef] [PubMed]

75. Tan, P.Y.; Chang, C.W.; Chng, K.R.; Wansa, K.D.; Sung, W.K.; Cheung, E. Integration of regulatory networks by NKX3–1 promotes androgen-dependent prostate cancer survival. *Mol. Cell. Biol.* **2012**, *32*, 399–414. [CrossRef] [PubMed]
76. Yu, J.; Mani, R.S.; Cao, Q.; Brenner, C.J.; Cao, X.; Wang, X.; Wu, L.; Li, J.; Hu, M.; Gong, Y.; et al. An integrated network of androgen receptor, polycomb, and TMPRSS2-ERG gene fusions in prostate cancer progression. *Cancer Cell* **2010**, *17*, 443–454. [CrossRef] [PubMed]
77. Takayama, K.; Suzuki, T.; Tsutsumi, S.; Fujimura, T.; Urano, T.; Takahashi, S.; Homma, Y.; Aburatani, H.; Inoue, S. *RUNX1*, an androgen- and EZH2-regulated gene, has differential roles in AR-dependent and -independent prostate cancer. *Oncotarget* **2015**, *6*, 2263–2276. [CrossRef] [PubMed]
78. Takayama, K.; Suzuki, T.; Tsutsumi, S.; Fujimura, T.; Takahashi, S.; Homma, Y.; Urano, T.; Aburatani, H.; Inoue, S. Integrative analysis of FOXP1 function reveals a tumor-suppressive effect in prostate cancer. *Mol. Endocrinol.* **2014**, *28*, 2012–2024. [CrossRef] [PubMed]
79. Grabowska, M.M.; Elliott, A.D.; DeGraff, D.J.; Anderson, P.D.; Anumanthan, G.; Yamashita, H.; Sun, Q.; Friedman, D.B.; Hachey, D.L.; Yu, X.; et al. NFI transcription factors interact with FOXA1 to regulate prostate-specific gene expression. *Mol. Endocrinol.* **2014**, *28*, 949–964. [CrossRef] [PubMed]
80. Zhang, J.; Gonit, M.; Salazar, M.D.; Shatnawi, A.; Shemshedini, L.; Trumbly, R.; Ratnam, M. C/EBPα redirects androgen receptor signaling through a unique bimodal interaction. *Oncogene* **2010**, *29*, 723–738. [CrossRef] [PubMed]
81. Turner, D.P.; Watson, D.K. ETS transcription factors: Oncogenes and tumor suppressor genes as therapeutic targets for prostate cancer. *Expert Rev. Anticancer Ther.* **2008**, *8*, 33–42. [CrossRef] [PubMed]
82. Verschoor, M.L.; Wilson, L.A.; Verschoor, C.P.; Singh, G. Ets-1 regulates energy metabolism in cancer cells. *PLoS ONE* **2010**, *5*, e13565. [CrossRef] [PubMed]
83. Smith, A.M.; Findlay, V.J.; Bandurraga, S.G.; Kistner-Griffin, E.; Spruill, L.S.; Liu, A.; Golshayan, A.R.; Turner, D.P. ETS1 transcriptional activity is increased in advanced prostate cancer and promotes the castrate-resistant phenotype. *Carcinogenesis* **2012**, *33*, 572–580. [CrossRef] [PubMed]
84. Preece, D.M.; Harvey, J.M.; Bentel, J.M.; Thomas, M.A. ETS1 regulates NKX3.1 5′ promoter activity and expression in prostate cancer cells. *Prostate* **2011**, *71*, 403–414. [CrossRef] [PubMed]
85. Wotton, K.R.; Weierud, F.K.; Juarez-Morales, J.L.; Alvares, L.E.; Dietrich, S.; Lewis, K.E. Conservation of gene linkage in dispersed vertebrate NK homeobox clusters. *Dev. Genes Evol.* **2009**, *219*, 481–496. [CrossRef] [PubMed]
86. He, W.W.; Sciavolino, P.J.; Wing, J.; Augustus, M.; Hudson, P.; Meissner, P.S.; Curtis, R.T.; Shell, B.K.; Bostwick, D.G.; Tindall, D.J.; et al. A novel human prostate-specific, androgen-regulated homeobox gene (*NKX3.1*) that maps to 8p21, a region frequently deleted in prostate cancer. *Genomics* **1997**, *43*, 69–77. [CrossRef] [PubMed]
87. Zhang, H.; Muders, M.H.; Li, J.; Rinaldo, F.; Tindall, D.J.; Datta, K. Loss of NKX3.1 favors vascular endothelial growth factor-C expression in prostate cancer. *Cancer Res.* **2008**, *68*, 8770–8778. [CrossRef] [PubMed]
88. King, J.C.; Xu, J.; Wongvipat, J.; Hieronymus, H.; Carver, B.S.; Leung, D.H.; Taylor, B.S.; Sander, C.; Cardiff, R.D.; Couto, S.S.; et al. Cooperativity of TMPRSS2-ERG with PI3-kinase pathway activation in prostate oncogenesis. *Nat. Genet.* **2009**, *41*, 524–526. [CrossRef] [PubMed]
89. King, J.C.; Xu, J.; Wongvipat, J.; Hieronymus, H.; Carver, B.S.; Leung, D.H.; Taylor, B.S.; Sander, C.; Cardiff, R.D.; Couto, S.S.; et al. Role of the *TMPRSS2-ERG* gene fusion in prostate cancer. *Neoplasia* **2008**, *10*, 177–188.
90. Perner, S.; Demichelis, F.; Beroukhim, R.; Schmidt, F.H.; Mosquera, J.M.; Setlur, S.; Tchinda, J.; Tomlins, S.A.; Hofer, M.D.; Pienta, K.G.; et al. *TMPRSS2:ERG* fusion-associated deletions provide insight into the heterogeneity of prostate cancer. *Cancer Res.* **2006**, *66*, 8337–8341. [CrossRef] [PubMed]
91. Tomlins, S.A.; Laxman, B.; Dhanasekaran, S.M.; Helgeson, B.E.; Cao, X.; Morris, D.S.; Menon, A.; Jing, X.; Cao, Q.; Han, B.; et al. Distinct classes of chromosomal rearrangements create oncogenic *ETS* gene fusions in prostate cancer. *Nature* **2007**, *448*, 595–599. [CrossRef] [PubMed]
92. Lin, C.; Yang, L.; Tanasa, B.; Hutt, K.; Ju, B.G.; Ohgi, K.; Zhang, J.; Rose, D.W.; Fu, X.D.; Glass, C.K.; et al. Nuclear receptor-induced chromosomal proximity and DNA breaks underlie specific translocations in cancer. *Cell* **2009**, *139*, 1069–1083. [CrossRef] [PubMed]

93. Hermans, K.G.; van Marion, R.; van Dekken, H.; Jenster, G.; van Weerden, W.M.; Trapman, J. *TMPRSS2:ERG* fusion by translocation or interstitial deletion is highly relevant in androgen-dependent prostate cancer, but is bypassed in late-stage androgen receptor-negative prostate cancer. *Cancer Res.* **2006**, *66*, 10658–10663. [CrossRef] [PubMed]
94. Bowen, C.; Zheng, T.; Gelmann, E.P. NKX3.1 Suppresses *TMPRSS2-ERG* Gene Rearrangement and Mediates Repair of Androgen Receptor-Induced DNA Damage. *Cancer Res.* **2015**, *75*, 2686–2698. [CrossRef] [PubMed]
95. Adamo, P.; Ladomery, M.R. The oncogene *ERG*: A key factor in prostate cancer. *Oncogene* **2016**, *35*, 403–414. [CrossRef] [PubMed]
96. Cai, C.; Wang, H.; Xu, Y.; Chen, S.; Balk, S.P. Reactivation of androgen receptor-regulated *TMPRSS2:ERG* gene expression in castration-resistant prostate cancer. *Cancer Res.* **2009**, *69*, 6027–6032. [CrossRef] [PubMed]
97. Varambally, S.; Dhanasekaran, S.M.; Zhou, M.; Barrette, T.R.; Kumar-Sinha, C.; Sanda, M.G.; Ghosh, D.; Pienta, K.J.; Sewalt, R.G.; Otte, A.P.; et al. The polycomb group protein EZH2 is involved in progression of prostate cancer. *Nature* **2002**, *419*, 624–629. [CrossRef] [PubMed]
98. Chen, H.; Tu, S.W.; Hsieh, J.T. Down-regulation of human *DAB2IP* gene expression mediated by polycomb Ezh2 complex and histone deacetylase in prostate cancer. *J. Biol. Chem.* **2005**, *280*, 22437–22444. [CrossRef] [PubMed]
99. Xu, K.; Wu, Z.J.; Groner, A.C.; He, H.H.; Cai, C.; Lis, R.T.; Wu, X.; Stack, E.C.; Loda, M.; Liu, T.; et al. EZH2 oncogenic activity in castration-resistant prostate cancer cells is Polycomb-independent. *Science* **2012**, *338*, 1465–1469. [CrossRef] [PubMed]
100. Ma, F.; Ye, H.; He, H.H.; Gerrin, S.J.; Chen, S.; Tanenbaum, B.A.; Cai, C.; Sowalsky, A.G.; He, L.; Wang, H.; et al. SOX9 drives WNT pathway activation in prostate cancer. *J. Clin. Investig.* **2016**, *126*, 1745–1758. [CrossRef] [PubMed]
101. Kokontis, J.M.; Hay, N.; Liao, S. Progression of LNCaP prostate tumor cells during androgen deprivation: Hormone-independent growth, repression of proliferation by androgen, and role for p27Kip1 in androgen-induced cell cycle arrest. *Mol. Endocrinol.* **1998**, *12*, 941–953. [CrossRef] [PubMed]
102. Morris, M.J.; Huang, D.; Kelly, W.K.; Slovin, S.F.; Stephenson, R.D.; Eicher, C.; Delacruz, A.; Curley, T.; Schwartz, L.H.; Scher, H.I. Phase 1 trial of high-dose exogenous testosterone in patients with castration-resistant metastatic prostate cancer. *Eur. Urol.* **2009**, *56*, 237–244. [CrossRef] [PubMed]
103. Sharma, N.L.; Massie, C.E.; Ramos-Montoya, A.; Zecchini, V.; Scott, H.E.; Lamb, A.D.; MacArthur, S.; Stark, R.; Warren, A.Y.; Mills, I.G.; et al. The androgen receptor induces a distinct transcriptional program in castration-resistant prostate cancer in man. *Cancer Cell* **2013**, *23*, 35–47. [CrossRef] [PubMed]
104. DeGregori, J.; Kowalik, T.; Nevins, J.R. Cellular targets for activation by the E2F1 transcription factor include DNA synthesis- and G_1/S-regulatory genes. *Mol. Cell. Biol.* **1995**, *15*, 4215–4224. [CrossRef] [PubMed]
105. Giacinti, C.; Giordano, A. RB and cell cycle progression. *Oncogene* **2006**, *25*, 5220–5227. [CrossRef] [PubMed]
106. Sharma, N.L.; Massie, C.E.; Ramos-Montoya, A.; Zecchini, V.; Scott, H.E.; Lamb, A.D.; MacArthur, S.; Stark, R.; Warren, A.Y.; Mills, I.G.; et al. The retinoblastoma tumor suppressor controls androgen signaling and human prostate cancer progression. *J. Clin. Investig.* **2010**, *120*, 4478–4492. [CrossRef] [PubMed]
107. Gao, P.; Tchernyshyov, I.; Chang, T.C.; Lee, Y.S.; Kita, K.; Ochi, T.; Zeller, K.I.; De Marzo, A.M.; Van Eyk, J.E.; Mendell, J.T.; et al. c-Myc suppression of miR-23a/b enhances mitochondrial glutaminase expression and glutamine metabolism. *Nature* **2009**, *458*, 762–765. [CrossRef] [PubMed]
108. Grandori, C.; Gomez-Roman, N.; Felton-Edkins, Z.A.; Ngouenet, C.; Galloway, D.A.; Eisenman, R.N.; White, R.J. c-Myc binds to human ribosomal DNA and stimulates transcription of rRNA genes by RNA polymerase I. *Nat. Cell. Biol.* **2005**, *7*, 311–318. [CrossRef] [PubMed]
109. Koh, C.M.; Bieberich, C.J.; Dang, C.V.; Nelson, W.G.; Yegnasubramanian, S.; De Marzo, A.M. *MYC* and Prostate Cancer. *Genes Cancer* **2010**, *1*, 617–628. [CrossRef] [PubMed]
110. Bernard, D.; Pourtier-Manzanedo, A.; Gil, J.; Beach, D.H. Myc confers androgen-independent prostate cancer cell growth. *J. Clin. Investig.* **2003**, *112*, 1724–1731. [CrossRef] [PubMed]
111. Kaltz-Wittmer, C.; Klenk, U.; Glaessgen, A.; Aust, D.E.; Diebold, J.; Lohrs, U.; Baretton, G.B. FISH analysis of gene aberrations (*MYC, CCND1, ERBB2, RB,* and *AR*) in advanced prostatic carcinomas before and after androgen deprivation therapy. *Lab. Investig.* **2000**, *80*, 1455–1464. [CrossRef] [PubMed]
112. Nupponen, N.N.; Kakkola, L.; Koivisto, P.; Visakorpi, T. Genetic alterations in hormone-refractory recurrent prostate carcinomas. *Am. J. Pathol.* **1998**, *153*, 141–148. [CrossRef]

113. Eagle, L.R.; Yin, X.; Brothman, A.R.; Williams, B.J.; Atkin, N.B.; Prochownik, E.V. Mutation of the *MXI1* gene in prostate cancer. *Nat. Genet.* **1995**, *9*, 249–255. [CrossRef] [PubMed]
114. Ge, K.; Minhas, F.; Duhadaway, J.; Mao, N.C.; Wilson, D.; Buccafusca, R.; Sakamuro, D.; Nelson, P.; Malkowicz, S.B.; Tomaszewski, J.; et al. Loss of heterozygosity and tumor suppressor activity of Bin1 in prostate carcinoma. *Int. J. Cancer* **2000**, *86*, 155–161. [CrossRef]
115. Sun, C.; Dobi, A.; Mohamed, A.; Li, H.; Thangapazham, R.L.; Furusato, B.; Shaheduzzaman, S.; Tan, S.H.; Vaidyanathan, G.; Whitman, E.; et al. *TMPRSS2-ERG* fusion, a common genomic alteration in prostate cancer activates C-MYC and abrogates prostate epithelial differentiation. *Oncogene* **2008**, *27*, 5348–5353. [CrossRef] [PubMed]
116. Darnell, J.E., Jr.; Kerr, I.M.; Stark, G.R. Jak-STAT pathways and transcriptional activation in response to IFNs and other extracellular signaling proteins. *Science* **1994**, *264*, 1415–1421. [CrossRef] [PubMed]
117. Schindler, C.; Darnell, J.E., Jr. Transcriptional responses to polypeptide ligands: The JAK–STAT pathway. *Annu. Rev. Biochem.* **1995**, *64*, 621–651. [CrossRef] [PubMed]
118. Yu, H.; Jove, R. The STATs of cancer—new molecular targets come of age. *Nat. Rev. Cancer* **2004**, *4*, 97–105. [CrossRef] [PubMed]
119. Mora, L.B.; Buettner, R.; Seigne, J.; Diaz, J.; Ahmad, N.; Garcia, R.; Bowman, T.; Falcone, R.; Fairclough, R.; Cantor, A.; et al. Constitutive activation of STAT3 in human prostate tumors and cell lines: Direct inhibition of STAT3 signaling induces apoptosis of prostate cancer cells. *Cancer Res.* **2002**, *62*, 6659–6666. [PubMed]
120. Culig, Z.; Steiner, H.; Bartsch, G.; Hobisch, A. Interleukin-6 regulation of prostate cancer cell growth. *J. Cell. Biochem.* **2005**, *95*, 497–505. [CrossRef] [PubMed]
121. Pencik, J.; Schlederer, M.; Gruber, W.; Unger, C.; Walker, S.M.; Chalaris, A.; Marie, I.J.; Hassler, M.R.; Javaheri, T.; Aksoy, O.; et al. STAT3 regulated *ARF* expression suppresses prostate cancer metastasis. *Nat. Commun.* **2015**, *6*, 7736. [CrossRef] [PubMed]
122. Jeter, C.R.; Liu, B.; Lu, Y.; Chao, H.P.; Zhang, D.; Liu, X.; Chen, X.; Li, Q.; Rycaj, K.; Calhoun-Davis, T.; et al. NANOG reprograms prostate cancer cells to castration resistance via dynamically repressing and engaging the AR/FOXA1 signaling axis. *Cell Discov.* **2016**, *2*, 16041. [CrossRef] [PubMed]
123. Trauger, J.W.; Baird, E.E.; Dervan, P.B. Recognition of DNA by designed ligands at subnanomolar concentrations. *Nature* **1996**, *382*, 559–561. [CrossRef] [PubMed]
124. Kielkopf, C.L.; Bremer, R.E.; White, S.; Szewczyk, J.W.; Turner, J.M.; Baird, E.E.; Dervan, P.B.; Rees, D.C. Structural effects of DNA sequence on T·A recognition by hydroxypyrrole/pyrrole pairs in the minor groove. *J. Mol. Biol.* **2000**, *295*, 557–567. [CrossRef] [PubMed]
125. Dervan, P.B.; Edelson, B.S. Recognition of the DNA minor groove by pyrrole-imidazole polyamides. *Curr. Opin. Struct. Biol.* **2003**, *13*, 284–299. [CrossRef]
126. Kielkopf, C.L.; Baird, E.E.; Dervan, P.B.; Rees, D.C. Structural basis for G.C recognition in the DNA minor groove. *Nat. Struct. Biol.* **1998**, *5*, 104–109. [CrossRef] [PubMed]
127. White, S.; Szewczyk, J.W.; Turner, J.M.; Baird, E.E.; Dervan, P.B. Recognition of the four Watson–Crick base pairs in the DNA minor groove by synthetic ligands. *Nature* **1998**, *391*, 468–471. [CrossRef] [PubMed]
128. Meier, J.L.; Montgomery, D.C.; Dervan, P.B. Enhancing the cellular uptake of Py-Im polyamides through next-generation aryl turns. *Nucleic Acids Res.* **2012**, *40*, 2345–2356. [CrossRef] [PubMed]
129. Zhang, W.; Bando, T.; Sugiyama, H. Discrimination of hairpin polyamides with an alpha-substituted-gamma-aminobutyric acid as a 5′-TG-3′ reader in DNA minor groove. *J. Am. Chem. Soc.* **2006**, *128*, 8766–8776. [CrossRef] [PubMed]
130. Chenoweth, D.M.; Dervan, P.B. Allosteric modulation of DNA by small molecules. *Proc. Natl. Acad. Sci. USA* **2009**, *106*, 13175–13179. [CrossRef] [PubMed]
131. Kielkopf, C.L.; White, S.; Szewczyk, J.W.; Turner, J.M.; Baird, E.E.; Dervan, P.B.; Rees, D.C. A structural basis for recognition of A·T and T·A base pairs in the minor groove of B-DNA. *Science* **1998**, *282*, 111–115. [CrossRef] [PubMed]
132. Enoch, S.J.; Cronin, M.T. A review of the electrophilic reaction chemistry involved in covalent DNA binding. *Crit. Rev. Toxicol.* **2010**, *40*, 728–748. [CrossRef] [PubMed]
133. Nagashima, T.; Aoyama, T.; Yokoe, T.; Fukasawa, A.; Fukuda, N.; Ueno, T.; Sugiyama, H.; Nagase, H.; Matsumoto, Y. Pharmacokinetic modeling and prediction of plasma pyrrole-imidazole polyamide concentration in rats using simultaneous urinary and biliary excretion data. *Biol. Pharm. Bull.* **2009**, *32*, 921–927. [CrossRef] [PubMed]

134. Fukasawa, A.; Aoyama, T.; Nagashima, T.; Fukuda, N.; Ueno, T.; Sugiyama, H.; Nagase, H.; Matsumoto, Y. Pharmacokinetics of pyrrole-imidazole polyamides after intravenous administration in rat. *Biopharm. Drug Dispos.* **2009**, *30*, 81–89. [CrossRef] [PubMed]
135. Matsuda, H.; Fukuda, N.; Ueno, T.; Tahira, Y.; Ayame, H.; Zhang, W.; Bando, T.; Sugiyama, H.; Saito, S.; Matsumoto, K.; et al. Development of gene silencing pyrrole-imidazole polyamide targeting the TGF-β1 promoter for treatment of progressive renal diseases. *J. Am. Soc. Nephrol.* **2006**, *17*, 422–432. [CrossRef] [PubMed]
136. Matsuda, H.; Fukuda, N.; Ueno, T.; Katakawa, M.; Wang, X.; Watanabe, T.; Matsui, S.; Aoyama, T.; Saito, K.; Bando, T.; et al. Transcriptional inhibition of progressive renal disease by gene silencing pyrrole-imidazole polyamide targeting of the transforming growth factor-β1 promoter. *Kidney Int.* **2011**, *79*, 46–56. [CrossRef] [PubMed]
137. Igarashi, J.; Fukuda, N.; Inoue, T.; Nakai, S.; Saito, K.; Fujiwara, K.; Matsuda, H.; Ueno, T.; Matsumoto, Y.; Watanabe, T.; et al. Preclinical Study of Novel Gene Silencer Pyrrole-Imidazole Polyamide Targeting Human TGF-β1 Promoter for Hypertrophic Scars in a Common Marmoset Primate Model. *PLoS ONE* **2015**, *10*, e0125295. [CrossRef] [PubMed]
138. Foley, C.; Mitsiades, N. Moving Beyond the Androgen Receptor (AR): Targeting AR-Interacting Proteins to Treat Prostate Cancer. *Horm. Cancer* **2016**, *7*, 84–103. [CrossRef] [PubMed]
139. Jin, H.J.; Zhao, J.C.; Wu, L.; Kim, J.; Yu, J. Cooperativity and equilibrium with FOXA1 define the androgen receptor transcriptional program. *Nat. Commun.* **2014**, *5*, 3972. [CrossRef] [PubMed]
140. Takayama, K.; Horie-Inoue, K.; Ikeda, K.; Urano, T.; Murakami, K.; Hayashizaki, Y.; Ouchi, Y.; Inoue, S. FOXP1 is an androgen-responsive transcription factor that negatively regulates androgen receptor signaling in prostate cancer cells. *Biochem. Biophys. Res. Commun.* **2008**, *374*, 388–393. [CrossRef] [PubMed]
141. Gong, C.; Fujino, K.; Monteiro, L.J.; Gomes, A.R.; Drost, R.; Davidson-Smith, H.; Takeda, S.; Khoo, U.S.; Jonkers, J.; Sproul, D.; et al. FOXA1 repression is associated with loss of *BRCA1* and increased promoter methylation and chromatin silencing in breast cancer. *Oncogene* **2015**, *34*, 5012–5024. [CrossRef] [PubMed]
142. Zhao, J.C.; Fong, K.W.; Jin, H.J.; Yang, Y.A.; Kim, J.; Yu, J. FOXA1 acts upstream of *GATA2* and *AR* in hormonal regulation of gene expression. *Oncogene* **2016**, *35*, 4335–4344. [CrossRef] [PubMed]
143. Umetani, M.; Nakao, H.; Doi, T.; Iwasaki, A.; Ohtaka, M.; Nagoya, T.; Mataki, C.; Hamakubo, T.; Kodama, T. A novel cell adhesion inhibitor, K-7174, reduces the endothelial VCAM-1 induction by inflammatory cytokines, acting through the regulation of GATA. *Biochem. Biophys. Res. Commun.* **2000**, *272*, 370–374. [CrossRef] [PubMed]
144. He, B.; Lanz, R.B.; Fiskus, W.; Geng, C.; Yi, P.; Hartig, S.M.; Rajapakshe, K.; Shou, J.; Wei, L.; Shah, S.S.; et al. GATA2 facilitates steroid receptor coactivator recruitment to the androgen receptor complex. *Proc. Natl. Acad. Sci. USA* **2014**, *111*, 18261–18266. [CrossRef] [PubMed]
145. Imagawa, S.; Nakano, Y.; Obara, N.; Suzuki, N.; Doi, T.; Kodama, T.; Nagasawa, T.; Yamamoto, M. A GATA-specific inhibitor (K-7174) rescues anemia induced by IL-1β, TNF-α, or L-NMMA. *FASEB J.* **2003**, *17*, 1742–1744. [PubMed]
146. Kikuchi, J.; Yamada, S.; Koyama, D.; Wada, T.; Nobuyoshi, M.; Izumi, T.; Akutsu, M.; Kano, Y.; Furukawa, Y. The novel orally active proteasome inhibitor K-7174 exerts anti-myeloma activity in vitro and in vivo by down-regulating the expression of class I histone deacetylases. *J. Biol. Chem.* **2013**, *288*, 25593–25602. [CrossRef] [PubMed]
147. Takano, Y.; Hiramatsu, N.; Okamura, M.; Hayakawa, K.; Shimada, T.; Kasai, A.; Yokouchi, M.; Shitamura, A.; Yao, J.; Paton, A.W.; et al. Suppression of cytokine response by GATA inhibitor K-7174 via unfolded protein response. *Biochem. Biophys. Res. Commun.* **2007**, *360*, 470–475. [CrossRef] [PubMed]
148. Nickols, N.G.; Dervan, P.B. Suppression of androgen receptor-mediated gene expression by a sequence-specific DNA-binding polyamide. *Proc. Natl. Acad. Sci. USA* **2007**, *104*, 10418–10423. [CrossRef] [PubMed]
149. Taniguchi, H.; Fujiwara, Y.; Doki, Y.; Sugita, Y.; Sohma, I.; Miyata, H.; Takiguchi, S.; Yasuda, T.; Tomita, N.; Morishita, R.; et al. Gene therapy using ETS-1 transcription factor decoy for peritoneal dissemination of gastric cancer. *Int. J. Cancer* **2007**, *121*, 1609–1617. [CrossRef] [PubMed]
150. Mann, M.J. Transcription factor decoys: A new model for disease intervention. *Ann. N. Y. Acad. Sci.* **2005**, *1058*, 128–139. [CrossRef] [PubMed]

151. Wang, S.; Kollipara, R.K.; Srivastava, N.; Li, R.; Ravindranathan, P.; Hernandez, E.; Freeman, E.; Humphries, C.G.; Kapur, P.; Lotan, Y.; et al. Ablation of the oncogenic transcription factor ERG by deubiquitinase inhibition in prostate cancer. *Proc. Natl. Acad. Sci. USA* **2014**, *111*, 4251–4256. [CrossRef] [PubMed]
152. Brenner, J.C.; Ateeq, B.; Li, Y.; Yocum, A.K.; Cao, Q.; Asangani, I.A.; Patel, S.; Wang, X.; Liang, H.; Yu, J.; et al. Mechanistic rationale for inhibition of poly(ADP-ribose) polymerase in *ETS* gene fusion-positive prostate cancer. *Cancer Cell* **2011**, *19*, 664–678. [CrossRef] [PubMed]
153. Nhili, R.; Peixoto, P.; Depauw, S.; Flajollet, S.; Dezitter, X.; Munde, M.M.; Ismail, M.A.; Kumar, A.; Farahat, A.A.; Stephens, C.E.; et al. Targeting the DNA-binding activity of the human ERG transcription factor using new heterocyclic dithiophene diamidines. *Nucleic Acids Res.* **2013**, *41*, 125–138. [CrossRef] [PubMed]
154. Rahim, S.; Beauchamp, E.M.; Kong, Y.; Brown, M.L.; Toretsky, J.A.; Uren, A. YK-4-279 inhibits ERG and ETV1 mediated prostate cancer cell invasion. *PLoS ONE* **2011**, *6*, e19343. [CrossRef] [PubMed]
155. Obinata, D.; Ito, A.; Fujiwara, K.; Takayama, K.; Ashikari, D.; Murata, Y.; Yamaguchi, K.; Urano, T.; Fujimura, T.; Fukuda, N.; et al. Pyrrole-imidazole polyamide targeted to break fusion sites in *TMPRSS2* and *ERG* gene fusion represses prostate tumor growth. *Cancer Sci.* **2014**, *105*, 1272–1278. [CrossRef] [PubMed]
156. Hargrove, A.E.; Martinez, T.F.; Hare, A.A.; Kurmis, A.A.; Phillips, J.W.; Sud, S.; Pienta, K.J.; Dervan, P.B. Tumor Repression of VCaP Xenografts by a Pyrrole-Imidazole Polyamide. *PLoS ONE* **2015**, *10*, e0143161. [CrossRef] [PubMed]
157. Ren, S.; Kang, M.R.; Wang, J.; Huang, V.; Place, R.F.; Sun, Y.; Li, L.C. Targeted induction of endogenous NKX3-1 by small activating RNA inhibits prostate tumor growth. *Prostate* **2013**, *73*, 1591–1601. [CrossRef] [PubMed]
158. Li, L.C.; Okino, S.T.; Zhao, H.; Pookot, D.; Place, R.F.; Urakami, S.; Enokida, H.; Dahiya, R. Small dsRNAs induce transcriptional activation in human cells. *Proc. Natl. Acad. Sci. USA* **2006**, *103*, 17337–17342. [CrossRef] [PubMed]
159. Yoon, S.; Huang, K.W.; Reebye, V.; Mintz, P.; Tien, Y.W.; Lai, H.S.; Saetrom, P.; Reccia, I.; Swiderski, P.; Armstrong, B.; et al. Targeted Delivery of C/EBPα -saRNA by Pancreatic Ductal Adenocarcinoma-specific RNA Aptamers Inhibits Tumor Growth In Vivo. *Mol. Ther.* **2016**, *24*, 1106–1116. [CrossRef] [PubMed]
160. Kaseb, A.O.; Chinnakannu, K.; Chen, D.; Sivanandam, A.; Tejwani, S.; Menon, M.; Dou, Q.P.; Reddy, G.P. Androgen receptor and E2F-1 targeted thymoquinone therapy for hormone-refractory prostate cancer. *Cancer Res.* **2007**, *67*, 7782–7788. [CrossRef] [PubMed]
161. Xie, X.; Kerrigan, J.E.; Minko, T.; Garbuzenko, O.; Lee, K.C.; Scarborough, A.; Abali, E.E.; Budak-Alpdogan, T.; Johnson-Farley, N.; Banerjee, D.; et al. Antitumor and modeling studies of a penetratin-peptide that targets E2F-1 in small cell lung cancer. *Cancer Biol. Ther.* **2013**, *14*, 742–751. [CrossRef] [PubMed]
162. Xie, X.; Bansal, N.; Shaik, T.; Kerrigan, J.E.; Minko, T.; Garbuzenko, O.; Abali, E.E.; Johnson-Farley, N.; Banerjee, D.; Scotto, K.W.; et al. A novel peptide that inhibits *E2F* transcription and regresses prostate tumor xenografts. *Oncotarget* **2014**, *5*, 901–907. [CrossRef] [PubMed]
163. Leonetti, C.; D'Agnano, I.; Lozupone, F.; Valentini, A.; Geiser, T.; Zon, G.; Calabretta, B.; Citro, G.C.; Zupi, G. Antitumor effect of c-myc antisense phosphorothioate oligodeoxynucleotides on human melanoma cells in vitro and and in mice. *J. Natl. Cancer Inst.* **1996**, *88*, 419–429. [CrossRef] [PubMed]
164. McGuffie, E.M.; Catapano, C.V. Design of a novel triple helix-forming oligodeoxyribonucleotide directed to the major promoter of the *c-myc* gene. *Nucleic Acids Res.* **2002**, *30*, 2701–2709. [PubMed]
165. Wang, H.; Hammoudeh, D.I.; Follis, A.V.; Reese, B.E.; Lazo, J.S.; Metallo, S.J.; Prochownik, E.V. Improved low molecular weight Myc-Max inhibitors. *Mol. Cancer Ther.* **2007**, *6*, 2399–2408. [CrossRef] [PubMed]
166. Mishra, R.; Watanabe, T.; Kimura, M.T.; Koshikawa, N.; Ikeda, M.; Uekusa, S.; Kawashima, H.; Wang, X.; Igarashi, J.; Choudhury, D.; et al. Identification of a novel E-box binding pyrrole-imidazole polyamide inhibiting MYC-driven cell proliferation. *Cancer Sci.* **2015**, *106*, 421–429. [CrossRef] [PubMed]
167. Rebello, R.J.; Kusnadi, E.; Cameron, D.P.; Pearson, H.B.; Lesmana, A.; Devlin, J.R.; Drygin, D.; Clark, A.K.; Porter, L.; Pedersen, J.; et al. The dual inhibition of RNA Pol I transcription and PIM kinase as a new therapeutic approach to treat advanced prostate cancer. *Clin. Cancer Res.* **2016**, *22*, 5539–5552. [CrossRef] [PubMed]

168. Leong, P.L.; Andrews, G.A.; Johnson, D.E.; Dyer, K.F.; Xi, S.; Mai, J.C.; Robbins, P.D.; Gadiparthi, S.; Burke, N.A.; Watkins, S.F.; et al. Targeted inhibition of STAT3 with a decoy oligonucleotide abrogates head and neck cancer cell growth. *Proc. Natl. Acad. Sci. USA* **2003**, *100*, 4138–4143. [CrossRef] [PubMed]
169. Leong, P.L.; Andrews, G.A.; Johnson, D.E.; Dyer, K.F.; Xi, S.; Mai, J.C.; Robbins, P.D.; Gadiparthi, S.; Burke, N.A.; Watkins, S.F.; et al. The JAK2 inhibitor AZD1480 potently blocks STAT3 signaling and oncogenesis in solid tumors. *Cancer Cell* **2009**, *16*, 487–497.
170. Fizazi, K.; De Bono, J.S.; Flechon, A.; Heidenreich, A.; Voog, E.; Davis, N.B.; Qi, M.; Bandekar, R.; Vermeulen, J.T.; Cornfeld, M.; et al. Randomised phase II study of siltuximab (CNTO 328), an anti-IL-6 monoclonal antibody, in combination with mitoxantrone/prednisone versus mitoxantrone/prednisone alone in metastatic castration-resistant prostate cancer. *Eur. J. Cancer* **2012**, *48*, 85–93. [CrossRef] [PubMed]
171. Montgomery, B.; Eisenberger, M.A.; Rettig, M.B.; Chu, F.; Pili, R.; Stephenson, J.J.; Vogelzang, N.J.; Koletsky, A.J.; Nordquist, L.T.; Edenfield, W.J.; et al. Androgen Receptor Modulation Optimized for Response (ARMOR) Phase I and II Studies: Galeterone for the Treatment of Castration-Resistant Prostate Cancer. *Clin. Cancer Res.* **2016**, *22*, 1356–1363. [CrossRef] [PubMed]
172. Asangani, I.A.; Wilder-Romans, K.; Dommeti, V.L.; Krishnamurthy, P.M.; Apel, I.J.; Escara-Wilke, J.; Plymate, S.R.; Navone, N.M.; Wang, S.; Feng, F.Y.; et al. BET Bromodomain Inhibitors Enhance Efficacy and Disrupt Resistance to AR Antagonists in the Treatment of Prostate Cancer. *Mol. Cancer Res.* **2016**, *14*, 324–331. [CrossRef] [PubMed]
173. Centenera, M.M.; Gillis, J.L.; Hanson, A.R.; Jindal, S.; Taylor, R.A.; Risbridger, G.P.; Sutherland, P.D.; Scher, H.I.; Raj, G.V.; Knudsen, K.E.; et al. Evidence for Efficacy of New Hsp90 Inhibitors Revealed by Ex Vivo Culture of Human Prostate Tumors. *Clin. Cancer Res.* **2012**, *18*, 3562–3570. [CrossRef] [PubMed]
174. Lawrence, M.G.; Taylor, R.A.; Toivanen, R.; Pedersen, J.; Norden, S.; Pook, D.W.; Frydenberg, M.; Australian Prostate Cancer, B.; Papargiris, M.M.; Niranjan, B.; et al. A preclinical xenograft model of prostate cancer using human tumors. *Nat. Protoc.* **2013**, *8*, 836–848. [CrossRef] [PubMed]

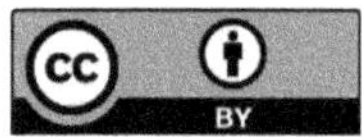

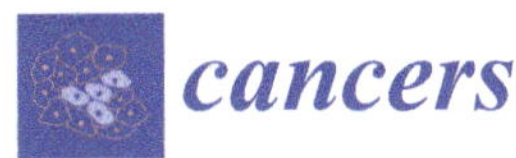
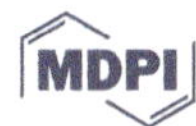

Review

The Androgen Receptor and VEGF: Mechanisms of Androgen-Regulated Angiogenesis in Prostate Cancer

Kurtis Eisermann [1] and Gail Fraizer [2,*]

[1] School of Biomedical Sciences, Kent State University, Kent, OH 44242, USA; keiserma@kent.edu
[2] Department of Biological Sciences, Kent State University, Kent, OH 44242, USA
* Correspondence: gfraizer@kent.edu; Tel.: +1-330-672-1398

Academic Editor: Emmanuel S. Antonarakis
Received: 31 January 2017; Accepted: 4 April 2017; Published: 10 April 2017

Abstract: Prostate cancer progression is controlled by the androgen receptor and new blood vessel formation, or angiogenesis, which promotes metastatic prostate cancer growth. Angiogenesis is induced by elevated expression of vascular endothelial growth factor (VEGF). VEGF is regulated by many factors in the tumor microenvironment including lowered oxygen levels and elevated androgens. Here we review evidence delineating hormone mediated mechanisms of VEGF regulation, including novel interactions between the androgen receptor (AR), epigenetic and zinc-finger transcription factors, AR variants and the hypoxia factor, HIF-1. The relevance of describing the impact of both hormones and hypoxia on VEGF expression and angiogenesis is revealed in recent reports of clinical therapies targeting both VEGF and AR signaling pathways. A better understanding of the complexities of VEGF expression could lead to improved targeting and increased survival time for a subset of patients with metastatic castration-resistant prostate cancer.

Keywords: androgen receptor; AR; VEGF; angiogenesis; hypoxia; prostate cancer; CRPC

---

1. Introduction

Androgen Signaling and Angiogenesis

Hormones are known to regulate many genes involved in prostate cancer (PC) and prostate cancer progression to castration-resistant prostate cancer (CRPC). Classical androgen signaling requires the androgen receptor (AR) to bind to Dihydrotestosterone (DHT) or testosterone (T) and dissociate from heat shock proteins. AR is then phosphorylated and translocated to the nucleus where it binds DNA and other protein co-factors at dimeric AR recognition elements (ARE) and activates transcription of androgen responsive genes such as PSA, TMPRSS2, Nkx3.1, and FKBP5 [1–6]. Many co-factors that regulate AR signaling have been identified [7–10] including co-factors with chromatin remodeling functions such as histone acetyltransferases, methyltransferases, and demethylases recruited by the AR to regulate its signaling pathways.

Identification of hormone-activated targets of the AR has been fueled by the need for useful markers of prostate cancer progression. While PSA remains the most widely used test for the presence of cancer of the prostate, it provides a large percentage of false positive results [11]. Thus, evidence of hormone responsive genes important in prostate cancer progression has been sought. One such androgen mediated gene is vascular endothelial growth factor (VEGF), a mitogen secreted by tumor cells that is essential for tumor angiogenesis and is necessary for tumor growth beyond 1–3 mm^3 in volume [12]. Patients with metastatic prostate cancer have greater VEGF plasma levels than those with localized disease, as over-expression of VEGF contributes to tumor growth and metastasis [13]. VEGF is regulated by multiple transcription factors (TFs), that respond to changes in the micro-environment such as, HIF-1 (responsive to hypoxic conditions) [14], AR (responsive to hormone levels) [15–17], and other zinc-finger TFs that bind GC-rich promoter regions, e.g., Sp1 and WT1 [16,18]. This review will outline what is known about mechanisms of androgen regulation of VEGF and the importance of VEGF in angiogenesis in prostate cancer and prostate cancer progression. The relevance of delineating the androgen and VEGF pathways in PC is demonstrated in recent clinical trials targeting both AR and VEGF pathways (including HIF1-α) [19,20].

VEGF regulation is complex and occurs at both transcriptional and post-transcriptional levels [21–23]. While the VEGF promoter lacks a TATA-binding site, it contains a GC-rich core promoter region and additional distal enhancer sites including hypoxia response elements that bind HIF1-α [24] (Figure 1A). Transcriptional and post-transcriptional regulation of VEGF has been well studied and both genetic and epigenetic mechanisms have been identified. For nearly 20 years it has been known that androgen up-regulates VEGF expression [17,25,26]. However, the mechanism of activation, whether via classical or non-classical pathways, is not yet entirely understood. The VEGF promoter lacks canonical androgen receptor (AR) DNA binding sites (ARE) either dimeric inverted or direct repeats. Whether androgens may instead be activating VEGF through non-classical pathways via src/MAPK is also unclear [27]. However, VEGF is activated via multiple pathways both in normoxia and hypoxia conditions. Below we discuss the roles of epigenetic and transcription factors AR, Sp1 (specificity protein 1), WT1 (Wilms tumor gene 1) and HIF1-α Hypoxia inducible factor 1-α) in regulating VEGF expression in conjunction with hormone.

2. Androgen and Epigenetic Regulation of VEGF

2.1. VEGF Regulation by Histone Modifiers

AR co-factors either co-activate or co-repress AR target gene expression, and several of the AR co-factors do so by modifying histone proteins. One well studied epigenetic modifier of AR target gene expression is Lysine specific demethylase 1 (LSD1/KDM1A) which has been identified in complexes with ligand bound AR [28]. LSD1 demethylates repressive histone marks and thereby can increase AR dependent transcription [28,29]. However, since AR autoregulates its own expression, it is noteworthy that AR recruitment of LSD1 to the AR promoter itself leads to a negative feedback loop repression of AR transcription [30]. Thus, LSD1, like traditional transcription factors, acts to regulate transcription, but the repressive or enhancing consequences are gene promoter context specific. Nonetheless, LSD1 up-regulates VEGF-A expression in both hormone responsive PC cells such as LNCaP, or non-responsive PC3 cells [29].

Recently, protein arginine methyltransferase 5 (PRMT5) has been shown to activate AR expression and promote PC cell growth [31]. PRMT5 binds the proximal promoter of the AR gene in a complex with Sp1 and the chromatin remodeling enzyme Brg1. Since VEGF is transcriptionally activated by androgens, PRMT5 can be expected to indirectly up-regulate VEGF and angiogenesis as well. This would be consistent with elevated PRMT expression observed in PC compared to BPH, and suggestive of an oncogenic function [31]. Although epigenetic regulators of AR and VEGF have been identified, evidence of their direct interaction with the AR on the VEGF promoter has been limited to that described for LSD1 [29].

2.2. Post-Transcriptional Regulation of VEGF by mRNA Stabilizers

VEGF mRNA is typically short-lived with a half-life of 15–40 min [32], but VEGF mRNA message stability is enhanced by low oxygen levels (hypoxia) through the binding of stabilizing proteins to the 3′untranslated regions (3′UTR). Members of the ELAV family of RNA binding proteins, like HuR, and heterogeneous nuclear ribonucleoprotein L (hnRNPL) bind to the AU-rich elements of the 3′UTR [33,34]. One potential mechanism for VEGF mRNA stabilization by HuR binding is that these stabilizing proteins block binding by the de-stabilizing micro RNAs also known to bind the 3′UTR. Indeed the binding sites for HuR and miR-200b overlap and miR-200b can compete with HuR binding to suppress VEGF mRNA expression [35]. Similarly, competition for 3′UTR binding between the hnRNPL and the γ-IFN-activated inhibitor of translation complex (GAIT) has been referred to as a riboswitch [36]. Hypoxia elevates hnRNPL protein levels and they bind and stabilize VEGF mRNA which acquires a secondary structure that blocks binding by the repressive GAIT complex [36].

As an example of the complexity of VEGF regulation, the riboswitch region is also a binding area for several microRNAs that also compete with hnRNPL for binding at the VEGF 3′UTR [37]. Of note, this is not an AU-rich but rather a CA-rich region (CARE). Overall, multiple miRNAs that bind to the 3′UTR of VEGF have been identified (reviewed in [38]) but their sensitivity to androgen is not known. Interestingly, the AR primarily up-regulates mi-RNAs considered to be oncogenic (oncomirs) and but none of these have been reported to up-regulate VEGF. Recently, androgen has been shown to suppress a miRNA cluster (miR-99a/let7c/miR-125b2), but this suppression still enhances PC cell proliferation [39].

2.3. Translational Regulation of VEGF

The relative importance of the 3′UTR region of VEGF for post-transcriptional regulation of VEGF is not greater than that of the 5′ UTR where two internal ribosome entry sites (IRES) permit cap independent translation of two separate translation start sites (AUG and upstream CUG sites) (reviewed in [38]). Of note, a sequence within the IRES-A promotes G-Quadruplex formation, conferring a suppressive structure on the VEGF 5′UTR [40]. Importantly, the 5′UTR is a critical regulatory area and in response to stress such as hypoxia, the IRES-B upstream of the CUG start sites will promote cap independent translation of the L-VEGF form encoding a longer isoform, that after proteolysis provides both an internal and the secreted VEGF peptide [41]. The clinical significance of the IRES-B was suggested when a single nucleotide polymorphism (SNP) was identified that suppressed the IRES-B function, reducing CUG translation initiation, and thereby decreasing L-VEGF protein levels. This SNP was associated with an elevated risk of prostate cancer [42].

Although this review will not cover the diversity of alternative VEGF isoforms, clearly the several alternative start codons, alternative splicing and the post translational proteolysis lead to a large number of variant VEGF protein isoforms with alternative functions (Reviewed in [38]). Use of the AUG translation initiation site is dependent upon specific exonic sequences that may be deleted in some alternatively spliced transcripts. For example, the alternatively spliced transcript encoding VEGF 121 (the diffusible form of VEGF lacking exons 6 and 7 encoding the heparin binding domains) cannot be translated from the AUG initiation site, but rather its translation initiates from an upstream CUG site [43]. The wide variety of VEGF isoforms have a variety of functions differentially affecting angiogenesis, varying from distal activity (EGF 121), to locally restricted activity (VEGF 189), to antiangiogenic activity (VEGF 165b). The role of androgen in altering VEGF isoform ratios is not yet understood but can be expected to be of clinical significance.

3. Transcription Factors that Regulate Androgen Induction of VEGF Expression

3.1. Sp1

Androgen treatment of prostatic fibroblasts and LNCaP cells significantly increases VEGF mRNA expression levels [15,16,44,45]. Additionally, VEGF protein levels have been demonstrated to be up-regulated after treatment of LNCaP cells with hormone [17], and the androgen antagonist flutamide blocks this up-regulation [46]. The mechanism of androgen-mediated regulation of VEGF expression, however, is less well understood. Three potential monomeric ARE half-sites were predicted by in silico analyses within the VEGF promoter, (Figure 1A) similar to sites reported in other gene promoters [47–49]. Furthermore, the androgen analog R1881 was shown to up-regulate both the proximal and distal VEGF promoter activity in 22Rv1 and LNCaP cells [18,24]. Taken together these results indicate the VEGF promoter is hormone responsive.

Interestingly, regions in the VEGF promoter near predicted ARE half-sites contain G-rich binding sites for other zinc finger transcription factors (ZFTF) such as Sp1, EGR1 (early growth response 1) or WT1 that could potentially interact with the AR. Non-classical AR half-sites were also identified adjacent to G-rich WT1/EGR1/Sp1 sites in 8 of 11 promoters analyzed, including VEGF [50]. Co-transfection of WT1 expression plasmids enhances VEGF promoter activity [18,24], with addition of the androgen analog R1881 increasing WT1 effectiveness, and mutation of a WT1 site reducing VEGF promoter activity [18]. These results were consistent with chromatin immunoprecipitation of WT1, Sp1 and AR at the VEGF promoter and co-immunoprecipitation of AR with Sp1 or WT1 [18,50].

Surprisingly, the ARE half-sites identified in the VEGF promoter are not required for hormone induction of VEGF expression, as site directed mutagenesis failed to eliminate hormone response [16]. Rather a single GC-box in the core promoter is essential for hormone responsiveness of the VEGF promoter [16]. This indicates that the AR is not bound to an ARE binding site, but rather is tethered via a ZFTF, which is bound to the GC boxes (Sp1/Sp3 binding sites) (Figure 1B). This GC-rich VEGF core promoter lacking ARE half-sites is responsive to androgen stimulation of PC cells, inhibited by the anti-androgen casodex [16], and is also the region of estrogen responsiveness in breast cancer cells [51,52]. In addition to lacking canonical dimeric ARE sites, the VEGF promoter also lacks canonical estrogen receptor (ER) binding sites [51,52]. Similarly, VEGF regulation by estrogen in endometrial and breast cancer cells involves interactions of ER-α and Sp1 (or Sp3) with GC boxes in the core promoter region of VEGF [51,52]. VEGF mRNA levels are significantly induced in ZR-75 breast cancer cells treated with estradiol, and the intact GC-rich core VEGF promoter region is required for such activation. The relevance of Sp1 and Sp3 in estradiol regulation of VEGF in breast cancer was demonstrated by binding assays in vitro (by EMSA) and in vivo (by ChIP) [51,52]. The VEGF core promoter contains four Sp1 binding sites and mutation of only the Sp1 site closest to the transcription start site inhibited androgen activation of VEGF in PC cells, while other adjacent sites were not required for hormone response [16]. Together, these results indicate a mechanism of androgen-mediated induction of VEGF expression in PC cells involving interaction of the AR with a specific, critical Sp1 binding site in the VEGF core promoter region [16] (Figure 1B).

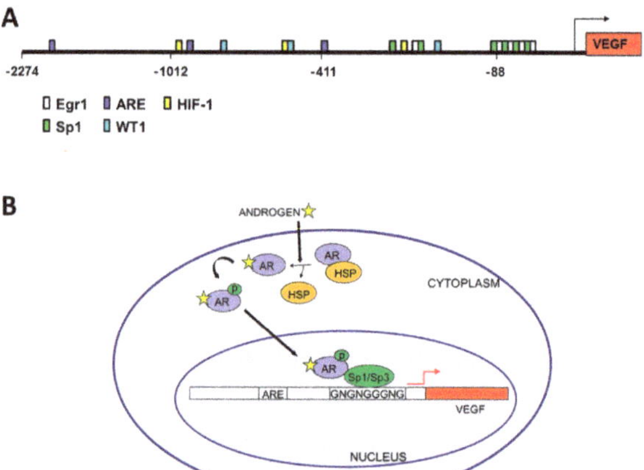

Figure 1. Androgen mediated regulation of vascular endothelial cell growth factor (VEGF) transcription. (**A**) Promoter analysis of VEGF. The VEGF promoter (VEGFA accession number AB021221) was downloaded from Ensembl and binding sites were predicted by MatInspector and located on the VEGF promoter sequence [50]. Potential androgen receptor binding sites (ARE), HIF1α binding sites (HIF-1) and zinc finger transcription factor binding sites (Sp1, Egr1, and WT1) thought to play a role in VEGF regulation are color coded according to the legend; (**B**) Model of androgen regulation of VEGF in prostate cancer showing the AR in a complex with Sp1 and bound to the GC-rich region of the VEGF core promoter. Note that ligand binding replaces HSP binding in the cytoplasm, but within the nucleus Sp1 binding recruits the AR to the core promoter region of the VEGF gene.

3.2. *Hypoxia (HIF-1α)*

VEGF expression is up-regulated in response to hypoxia and this is mediated by the stabilization of the transcription factor hypoxia-inducible factor 1 (HIF-1α) that up-regulates transcription of VEGF via binding at HIF-Responsive elements. Importantly, HIF-1α itself is up-regulated by DHT both via transcript stabilization [53] and via an autocrine loop involving EGF-R and AKT [46]. The clinical importance of HIF-1α expression in prostate cancer has been demonstrated and HIF-1α has been examined as a potential prognostic marker, being elevated in high grade PIN and not BPH [54]. Response to androgen deprivation therapy in mice with CWR22RV1 xenografts, suggests that AR may regulate HIF-1α levels, as expression of both AR and HIF-1α target genes were affected even outside of hypoxic tumor areas [55].

Conversely, substantial evidence exists for the effect of HIF-1α (and hypoxia) on AR signaling. Combined hypoxia and hormone treatment synergistically increased PSA levels [56]. Hypoxia increases transcriptional activity of ARE-luciferase reporters in low or high DHT conditions, but has no effect in the absence of DHT [57]. Thus, androgen signaling is influenced by hypoxia, which itself up-regulates VEGF expression. Overall, this suggests that VEGF response to hypoxia may be mediated in part by HIF-1α but in the case of endocrine tumors, also by hormone effects on HIF-1α [53].

4. AR Variants

Currently, a family of AR splice variants are being identified that lack the LBD, but arise in patients undergoing androgen deprivation therapy [58]. These splice forms lacking the LBD region have been seen in BPH and localized prostate cancers, but are up-regulated in castration resistant prostate cancer [59–61]. The presence of these variants is significant, as patients with a high level of AR-V7 and ARv567es expression have a shorter survival expectancy than CRPC patients lacking these AR variants [59]. Additionally, AR-V7 (the AR-V most commonly expressed in clinical specimens) has been shown to be involved in resistance to both enzalutamide and abiraterone in clinical studies [62,63]. Importantly in CWR22Rv1 cells, which contain AR splice variants (including AR-V7) [61,64,65], we have shown that Sp1 and the AR interact to activate the VEGF promoter [16]. If AR variants interact with Sp1 (either directly or through complex formation with full-length AR) they could influence VEGF expression in response to hormone. Additionally, these AR variants can recruit and form complexes with co-factors that have chromatin remodeling functions discussed above, such as histone acetyltransferases, methyltransferases, and demethylases, potentially impacting the epigenetic regulation of the AR and VEGF [29]. Thus, it will be important to determine if these novel splice variants of the AR are involved in VEGF regulation in CRPC, particularly if improved response is observed in clinical trials with CRPC patients being treated with both anti-androgens and VEGF inhibitors.

5. Relevance of Dual Targeting of Hormone Signaling and VEGF in PC Tumor Angiogenesis

Metastatic PC is associated with higher VEGF levels than localized disease [66–68]. Thus, anti-VEGF therapies have been the target of multiple clinical trials for treatment of men with CRPC. Bevacizumab is a monoclonal antibody to VEGF-A which has been shown to decrease tumor volume in many cancers. However, in clinical trials for treatment of CRPC, it has not improved the overall survival time of patients getting chemotherapy (docetaxol) along with the immunosuppressant prednisone [69]. Therefore, it is thought that angiogenesis may play a smaller role in CRPC than other cancers and current studies are investigating dual targeting of both androgen signaling and VEGF.

Studies targeting both the androgen signaling pathway (with bicalutamide or enzalutamide) and VEGF (either directly with a VEGF inhibitor or indirectly through HIF1-α inhibition) have recently been performed [19,20]. Figure 2 illustrates the steps at which dual drug targeting could impact both (1) the androgen signaling pathway (through abiraterone blocking androgen synthesis, enzalutamide binding to AR, or docetaxel inhibiting microtubule driven transport of AR-androgen complex) and

(2) the angiogenic pathway (through bevacizumab blocking VEGF binding). The effects of targeting both the AR signaling pathway and HIF-1α pathway have also been investigated and the authors found that combinatorial targeting both of these pathways lead to greater inhibition of prostate cancer cell growth than either one alone in both LNCaP and CWR22Rv1 cells [20]. Also, this study determined that VEGF protein levels were significantly reduced in the presence of both enzalutamide and siHIF-1α, suggesting that VEGF could be a biomarker for enzalutamide response [20].

A new phase II clinical trial of patients with recurring prostate cancer treated with or without the VEGF inhibitor Bevacizumab after ADT revealed that ADT combined with Bevacizumab resulted in an increased relapse free survival rate, although modestly, compared to ADT alone [19]. These results suggested that combining ADT with Bevacizumab could prolong the off-ADT-cycle during intermittent ADT and thus benefit a subset of patients that have hormone sensitive prostate cancer. These studies demonstrate the need for understanding mechanistically the relationship between AR and VEGF and how they interact in CRPC patients.

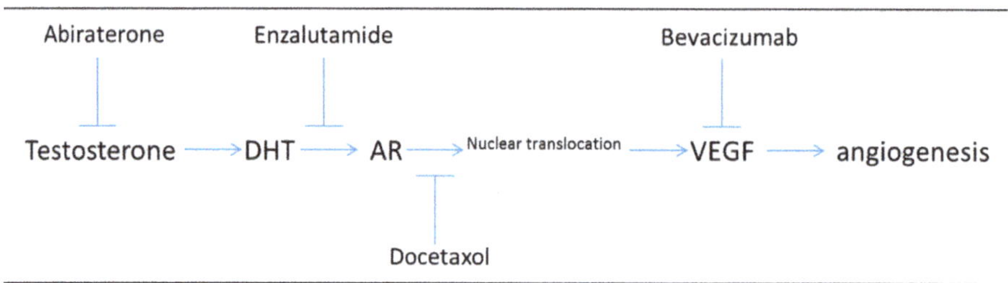

Figure 2. Targeting both VEGF induction of angiogenesis and androgen synthesis or AR signaling inhibits two critical signaling pathways in prostate cancer (PC) progression. Note that hypoxia induced VEGF can also be suppressed by targeting HIF1α with HIF1 inhibitors (not shown).

6. Conclusions

Treatment of CRPC involves targeting many factors and signaling pathways which are still being uncovered, but dual targeting of both AR and VEGF signaling should result in better efficacy for patients than either one alone. Mechanistically, it appears that androgen induction of VEGF is regulated through AR complex formation with Sp1 in the core promoter region in prostate cancer cells and not via ARE binding sites in the distal VEGF promoter. Therefore, addition of Sp1 or HIF-1α inhibitors could further add to the significant effect seen by targeting AR signaling with enzalutamide and VEGF with Bevacizumab. Further delineation of the mechanism(s) involved in the progression of CRPC and the pathways utilized will help to produce even better treatment plans for this subset of patients.

Acknowledgments: This work was funded in part by: NIH 1CA33160(GF).

Conflicts of Interest: The authors declare no conflict of interest.

References

1. Heinlein, C.A.; Chang, C. Androgen receptor in prostate cancer. *Endocr. Rev.* **2004**, *25*, 276. [CrossRef] [PubMed]
2. Cleutjens, K.B.J.M.; van der Korput, H.A.G.M.; van Eekelen, C.C.E.M.; van Rooij, H.C.J.; Faber, P.W.; Trapman, J. An androgen response element in a far upstream enhancer region is essential for high, androgen-regulated activity of the prostate-specific antigen promoter. *Mol. Endocrinol.* **1997**, *11*, 148. [CrossRef] [PubMed]
3. Tomlins, S.A.; Rhodes, D.R.; Perner, S.; Dhanasekaran, S.M.; Mehra, R.; Sun, X.W.; Varambally, S.; Cao, X.; Tchinda, J.; Kuefer, R.; et al. Recurrent fusion of TMPRSS2 and ETS transcription factor genes in prostate cancer. *Science* **2005**, *310*, 644–648. [CrossRef] [PubMed]

4. Lin, B.; Ferguson, C.; White, J.T.; Wang, S.; Vessella, R.; True, L.D.; Hood, L.; Nelson, P.S. Prostate-localized and androgen-regulated expression of the membrane-bound serine protease TMPRSS2. *Cancer Res.* **1999**, *59*, 4180–4184. [PubMed]
5. He, W.W.; Sciavolino, P.J.; Wing, J.; Augustus, M.; Hudson, P.; Meissner, P.S.; Curtis, R.T.; Shell, B.K.; Bostwick, D.G.; Tindall, D.J. A novel human prostate-specific, androgen-regulated homeobox gene (NKX3. 1) that maps to 8p21, a region frequently deleted in prostate cancer. *Genomics* **1997**, *43*, 69–77. [CrossRef] [PubMed]
6. Magee, J.A.; Chang, L.; Stormo, G.D.; Milbrandt, J. Direct, androgen receptor-mediated regulation of the FKBP5 gene via a distal enhancer element. *Endocrinology* **2006**, *147*, 590–598. [CrossRef] [PubMed]
7. O'Malley, B.W.; Kumar, R. Nuclear receptor coregulators in cancer biology. *Cancer Res.* **2009**, *69*, 8217–8222. [CrossRef] [PubMed]
8. Heemers, H.V.; Tindall, D.J. Androgen receptor (AR) coregulators: A diversity of functions converging on and regulating the AR transcriptional complex. *Endocr. Rev.* **2007**, *28*, 778–808. [CrossRef] [PubMed]
9. Agoulnik, I.U.; Weigel, N.L. Androgen Receptor Coactivators and Prostate Cancer. In *Hormonal Carcinogenesis V*; Springer: New York, NY, USA, 2008.
10. Wang, L.; Hsu, C.; Chang, C. Androgen receptor corepressors: An overview. *Prostate* **2005**, *63*, 117–130. [CrossRef] [PubMed]
11. Moyer, V.A. Screening for prostate cancer: US Preventive Services Task Force recommendation statement. *Ann. Intern. Med.* **2012**, *157*, 120–134. [CrossRef] [PubMed]
12. Fox, W.D.; Higgins, B.; Maiese, K.M.; Drobnjak, M.; Cordon-Cardo, C.; Scher, H.I.; Agus, D.B. Antibody to vascular endothelial growth factor slows growth of an androgen-independent xenograft model of prostate cancer. *Clin. Cancer Res.* **2002**, *8*, 3226–3231. [PubMed]
13. Delongchamps, N.B.; Peyromaure, M.; Dinh-Xuan, A.T. Role of vascular endothelial growth factor in prostate cancer. *Urology* **2006**, *68*, 244–248. [CrossRef] [PubMed]
14. Forsythe, J.A.; Jiang, B.H.; Iyer, N.V.; Agani, F.; Leung, S.W.; Koos, R.D.; Semenza, G.L. Activation of vascular endothelial growth factor gene transcription by hypoxia-inducible factor 1. *Mol. Cell Biol.* **1996**, *16*, 4604–4613. [CrossRef] [PubMed]
15. Stewart, R.J.; Panigrahy, D.; Flynn, E.; Folkman, J. Vascular endothelial growth factor expression and tumor angiogenesis are regulated by androgens in hormone responsive human prostate carcinoma: evidence for androgen dependent destabilization of vascular endothelial growth factor transcripts. *J. Urol.* **2001**, *165*, 688–693. [CrossRef] [PubMed]
16. Eisermann, K.; Broderick, C.J.; Bazarov, A.; Moazam, M.M.; Fraizer, G.C. Androgen up-regulates vascular endothelial growth factor expression in prostate cancer cells via an Sp1 binding site. *Mol. Cancer* **2013**, *12*, 7. [CrossRef] [PubMed]
17. Joseph, I.B.; Nelson, J.B.; Denmeade, S.R.; Isaacs, J.T. Androgens regulate vascular endothelial growth factor content in normal and malignant prostatic tissue. *Clin. Cancer Res.* **1997**, *3*, 2507–2511. [PubMed]
18. Fraizer, G.C.; Eisermann, K.; Pandey, S.; Brett-Morris, A.; Bazarov, A.; Nock, S.; Ghimirey, N.; Kuerbitz, S.J. Functional Role of WT1 in Prostate Cancer. In *Wilms Tumor*; Codon Publications: Brisbane, Australia, 2016.
19. McKay, R.R.; Zurita, A.J.; Werner, L.; Bruce, J.Y.; Carducci, M.A.; Stein, M.N.; Heath, E.I.; Hussain, A.; Tran, H.T.; Sweeney, C.J.; et al. A randomized phase II trial of short-course androgen deprivation therapy with or without bevacizumab for patients with recurrent prostate cancer after Definitive local therapy. *J. Clin. Oncol.* **2016**, *34*, 1913–1920. [CrossRef] [PubMed]
20. Fernandez, E.V.; Reece, K.M.; Ley, A.M.; Troutman, S.M.; Sissung, T.M.; Price, D.K.; Chau, C.H.; Figg, W.D. Dual targeting of the androgen receptor and hypoxia-inducible factor 1alpha pathways synergistically inhibits castration-resistant prostate cancer cells. *Mol. Pharmacol.* **2015**, *87*, 1006–1012. [CrossRef] [PubMed]
21. Loureiro, R.M.; D'Amore, P.A. Transcriptional regulation of vascular endothelial growth factor in cancer. *Cytokine Growth Factor Rev.* **2005**, *16*, 77–89. [CrossRef] [PubMed]
22. de Brot, S.; Ntekim, A.; Cardenas, R.; James, V.; Allegrucci, C.; Heery, D.M.; Bates, D.O.; Odum, N.; Persson, J.L.; Mongan, N.P. Regulation of vascular endothelial growth factor in prostate cancer. *Endocr. Relat. Cancer* **2015**, *22*, R107–123. [CrossRef] [PubMed]
23. Wagner, K.D.; Wagner, N.; Vidal, V.P.I.; Schley, G.; Wilhelm, D.; Schedl, A.; Englert, C.; Scholz, H. The Wilms' tumor gene Wt1 is required for normal development of the retina. *EMBO J.* **2002**, *21*, 1398–1405. [CrossRef] [PubMed]

24. Hanson, J.; Gorman, J.; Reese, J.; Fraizer, G. Regulation of vascular endothelial growth factor, VEGF, gene promoter by the tumor suppressor, WT1. *Front Biosci.* **2007**, *12*, 2279–2290. [CrossRef] [PubMed]
25. Sordello, S.; Bertrand, N.; Plouet, J. Vascular endothelial growth factor is up-regulated in vitro and in vivo by androgens. *Biochem. Biophys. Res. Commun.* **1998**, *251*, 287–290. [CrossRef] [PubMed]
26. Aslan, G.; Cimen, S.; Yorukoglu, K.; Tuna, B.; Sonmez, D.; Mungan, U.; Celebi, I. Vascular endothelial growth factor expression in untreated and androgen-deprived patients with prostate cancer. *Pathol. Res. Pract.* **2005**, *201*, 593–598. [CrossRef] [PubMed]
27. Smith, L.B.; Walker, W.H. The regulation of spermatogenesis by androgens. *Semin. Cell Dev. Biol.* **2014**, *30*, 2–13. [CrossRef] [PubMed]
28. Metzger, E.; Wissmann, M.; Yin, N.; Müller, J.M.; Schneider, R.; Peters, A.H.; Günther, T.; Buettner, R.; Schüle, R. LSD1 demethylates repressive histone marks to promote androgen-receptor-dependent transcription. *Nature* **2005**, *437*, 436–439. [CrossRef] [PubMed]
29. Kashyap, V.; Ahmad, S.; Nilsson, E.M.; Helczynski, L.; Kenna, S.; Persson, J.L.; Gudas, L.J.; Mongan, N.P. The lysine specific demethylase-1 (LSD1/KDM1A) regulates VEGF-A expression in prostate cancer. *Mol. Oncol.* **2013**, *7*, 555–566. [CrossRef] [PubMed]
30. Cai, C.; He, H.H.; Chen, S.; Coleman, I.; Wang, H.; Fang, Z.; Chen, S.; Nelson, P.S.; Liu, X.S.; Brown, M. Androgen receptor gene expression in prostate cancer is directly suppressed by the androgen receptor through recruitment of lysine-specific demethylase 1. *Cancer Cell* **2011**, *20*, 457–471. [CrossRef] [PubMed]
31. Deng, X.; Shao, G.; Zhang, H.; Li, C.; Zhang, D.; Cheng, L.; Elzey, B.; Pili, R.; Ratliff, T.; Huang, J. Protein arginine methyltransferase 5 functions as an epigenetic activator of the androgen receptor to promote prostate cancer cell growth. *Oncogene* **2016**, *36*, 1223–1231. [CrossRef] [PubMed]
32. Levy, A.P.; Levy, N.S.; Goldberg, M.A. Post-transcriptional regulation of vascular endothelial growth factor by hypoxia. *J. Biol. Chem.* **1996**, *271*, 2746–2753. [CrossRef] [PubMed]
33. Levy, N.S.; Chung, S.; Furneaux, H.; Levy, A.P. Hypoxic stabilization of vascular endothelial growth factor mRNA by the RNA-binding protein HuR. *J. Biol. Chem.* **1998**, *273*, 6417–6423. [CrossRef] [PubMed]
34. Shih, S.C.; Claffey, K.P. Regulation of human vascular endothelial growth factor mRNA stability in hypoxia by heterogeneous nuclear ribonucleoprotein L. *J. Biol. Chem.* **1999**, *274*, 1359–1365. [CrossRef] [PubMed]
35. Chang, S.H.; Lu, Y.C.; Li, X.; Hsieh, W.Y.; Xiong, Y.; Ghosh, M.; Evans, T.; Elemento, O.; Hla, T. Antagonistic function of the RNA-binding protein HuR and miR-200b in post-transcriptional regulation of vascular endothelial growth factor-A expression and angiogenesis. *J. Biol. Chem.* **2013**, *288*, 4908–4921. [CrossRef] [PubMed]
36. Ray, P.S.; Jia, J.; Yao, P.; Majumder, M.; Hatzoglou, M.; Fox, P.L. A stress-responsive RNA switch regulates VEGFA expression. *Nature* **2009**, *457*, 915–919. [CrossRef] [PubMed]
37. Jafarifar, F.; Yao, P.; Eswarappa, S.M.; Fox, P.L. Repression of VEGFA by CA-rich element-binding microRNAs is modulated by hnRNP L. *EMBO J.* **2011**, *30*, 1324–1334. [CrossRef] [PubMed]
38. Arcondeguy, T.; Lacazette, E.; Millevoi, S.; Prats, H.; Touriol, C. VEGF-A mRNA processing, stability and translation: A paradigm for intricate regulation of gene expression at the post-transcriptional level. *Nucleic Acids Res.* **2013**, *41*, 7997–8010. [CrossRef] [PubMed]
39. Sun, D.; Layer, R.; Mueller, A.C.; Cichewicz, M.A.; Negishi, M.; Paschal, B.M.; Dutta, A. Regulation of several androgen-induced genes through the repression of the miR-99a/let-7c/miR-125b-2 miRNA cluster in prostate cancer cells. *Oncogene* **2014**, *33*, 1448–1457. [CrossRef] [PubMed]
40. Morris, M.J.; Negishi, Y.; Pazsint, C.; Schonhoft, J.D.; Basu, S. An RNA G-quadruplex is essential for cap-independent translation initiation in human VEGF IRES. *J. Am. Chem. Soc.* **2010**, *132*, 17831–17839. [CrossRef] [PubMed]
41. Bornes, S.; Prado-Lourenco, L.; Bastide, A.; Zanibellato, C.; Iacovoni, J.S.; Lacazette, E.; Prats, A.C.; Touriol, C.; Prats, H. Translational induction of VEGF internal ribosome entry site elements during the early response to ischemic stress. *Circ. Res.* **2007**, *100*, 305–308. [CrossRef] [PubMed]
42. Sfar, S.; Hassen, E.; Saad, H.; Mosbah, F.; Chouchane, L. Association of VEGF genetic polymorphisms with prostate carcinoma risk and clinical outcome. *Cytokine* **2006**, *35*, 21–28. [CrossRef] [PubMed]
43. Bornes, S.; Boulard, M.; Hieblot, C.; Zanibellato, C.; Iacovoni, J.S.; Prats, H.; Touriol, C. Control of the Vascular Endothelial Growth Factor Internal Ribosome Entry Site (IRES) Activity and Translation Initiation by Alternatively Spliced Coding Sequences. *J. Biol. Chem.* **2004**, *279*, 18717–18726. [CrossRef] [PubMed]

44. Levine, A.C.; Liu, X.H.; Greenberg, P.D.; Eliashvili, M.; Schiff, J.D.; Aaronson, S.A.; Holland, J.F.; Kirschenbaum, A. Androgens induce the expression of vascular endothelial growth factor in human fetal prostatic fibroblasts. *Endocrinology* **1998**, *139*, 4672–4678. [CrossRef] [PubMed]
45. Li, J.; Wang, E.; Rinaldo, F.; Datta, K. Upregulation of VEGF-C by androgen depletion: the involvement of IGF-IR-FOXO pathway. *Oncogene* **2005**, *24*, 5510–5520. [CrossRef] [PubMed]
46. Mabjeesh, N.J.; Willard, M.T.; Frederickson, C.E.; Zhong, H.; Simons, J.W. Androgens stimulate hypoxia-inducible factor 1 activation via autocrine loop of tyrosine kinase receptor/phosphatidylinositol 3′-kinase/protein kinase B in prostate cancer cells. *Clin. Cancer Res.* **2003**, *9*, 2416. [PubMed]
47. Wang, Q.; Li, W.; Liu, X.S.; Carroll, J.S.; Jänne, O.A.; Keeton, E.K.; Chinnaiyan, A.M.; Pienta, K.J.; Brown, M. A hierarchical network of transcription factors governs androgen receptor-dependent prostate cancer growth. *Mol. Cell* **2007**, *27*, 380–392. [CrossRef] [PubMed]
48. Bolton, E.C.; So, A.Y.; Chaivorapol, C.; Haqq, C.M.; Li, H.; Yamamoto, K.R. Cell- and gene-specific regulation of primary target genes by the androgen receptor. *Genes Dev.* **2007**, *21*, 2005–2017. [CrossRef] [PubMed]
49. Massie, C.E.; Adryan, B.; Barbosa-Morais, N.L.; Lynch, A.G.; Tran, M.G.; Neal, D.E.; Mills, I.G. New androgen receptor genomic targets show an interaction with the ETS1 transcription factor. *EMBO Rep.* **2007**, *8*, 871. [CrossRef] [PubMed]
50. Eisermann, K.; Bazarov, A.; Brett, A.; Knapp, E.; Piontkivska, H.; Fraizer, G. Uncovering androgen responsive regulatory networks in prostate cancer. In Proceedings of the Ohio Collaborative Conference on Bioinformatics, Cleveland, OH, USA, 15–17 June 2009.
51. Mueller, M.D.; Vigne, J.L.; Minchenko, A.; Lebovic, D.I.; Leitman, D.C.; Taylor, R.N. Regulation of vascular endothelial growth factor (VEGF) gene transcription by estrogen receptors alpha and beta. *Proc. Natl. Acad. Sci. USA* **2000**, *97*, 10972–10977. [CrossRef] [PubMed]
52. Stoner, M.; Wormke, M.; Saville, B.; Samudio, I.; Qin, C.; Abdelrahim, M.; Safe, S. Estrogen regulation of vascular endothelial growth factor gene expression in ZR-75 breast cancer cells through interaction of estrogen receptor a and SP proteins. *Oncogene* **2004**, *23*, 1052–1063. [CrossRef] [PubMed]
53. Kimbro, K.S.; Simons, J.W. Hypoxia-inducible factor-1 in human breast and prostate cancer. *Endocr. Relat. Cancer* **2006**, *13*, 739–749. [CrossRef] [PubMed]
54. Zhong, H.; Semenza, G.L.; Simons, J.W.; De Marzo, A.M. Up-regulation of hypoxia-inducible factor 1α is an early event in prostate carcinogenesis. *Cancer Detect. Prev.* **2004**, *28*, 88–93. [CrossRef] [PubMed]
55. Ragnum, H.B.; Røe, K.; Holm, R.; Vlatkovic, L.; Nesland, J.M.; Aarnes, E.; Ree, A.H.; Flatmark, K.; Seierstad, T.; Lilleby, W. Hypoxia-independent downregulation of hypoxia-inducible factor 1 targets by androgen deprivation therapy in prostate cancer. *Int. J. Radiat. Oncol. Biol. Phys.* **2013**, *87*, 753–760. [CrossRef] [PubMed]
56. Horii, K.; Suzuki, Y.; Kondo, Y.; Akimoto, M.; Nishimura, T.; Yamabe, Y.; Sakaue, M.; Sano, T.; Kitagawa, T.; Himeno, S.; et al. Androgen-dependent gene expression of prostate-specific antigen is enhanced synergistically by hypoxia in human prostate cancer cells. *Mol. Cancer Res.* **2007**, *5*, 383–391. [CrossRef] [PubMed]
57. Mitani, T.; Harada, N.; Nakano, Y.; Inui, H.; Yamaji, R. Coordinated action of hypoxia-inducible factor-1alpha and beta-catenin in androgen receptor signaling. *J. Biol. Chem.* **2012**, *287*, 33594–33606. [CrossRef] [PubMed]
58. Antonarakis, E.; Armstrong, A.; Dehm, S.; Luo, J. Androgen receptor variant-driven prostate cancer: Clinical implications and therapeutic targeting. *Prostate Cancer Prostatic Dis.* **2016**, *19*, 231–241. [CrossRef] [PubMed]
59. Hörnberg, E.; Ylitalo, E.B.; Crnalic, S.; Antti, H.; Stattin, P.; Widmark, A.; Bergh, A.; Wikström, P. Expression of androgen receptor splice variants in prostate cancer bone metastases is associated with castration-resistance and short survival. *PLoS ONE* **2011**, *6*, e19059. [CrossRef] [PubMed]
60. Sun, S.; Sprenger, C.C.; Vessella, R.L.; Haugk, K.; Soriano, K.; Mostaghel, E.A.; Page, S.T.; Coleman, I.M.; Nguyen, H.M.; Sun, H.; et al. Castration resistance in human prostate cancer is conferred by a frequently occurring androgen receptor splice variant. *J. Clin. Investig.* **2010**, *120*, 2715–2730. [CrossRef] [PubMed]
61. Hu, R.; Dunn, T.A.; Wei, S.; Isharwal, S.; Veltri, R.W.; Humphreys, E.; Han, M.; Partin, A.W.; Vessella, R.L.; Isaacs, W.B.; et al. Ligand-independent androgen receptor variants derived from splicing of cryptic exons signify hormone-refractory prostate cancer. *Cancer Res.* **2009**, *69*, 16–22. [CrossRef] [PubMed]
62. Efstathiou, E.; Titus, M.; Wen, S.; Hoang, A.; Karlou, M.; Ashe, R.; Tu, S.M.; Aparicio, A.; Troncoso, P.; Mohler, J. Molecular characterization of enzalutamide-treated bone metastatic castration-resistant prostate cancer. *Eur. Urol.* **2015**, *67*, 53–60. [CrossRef] [PubMed]

63. Antonarakis, E.S.; Lu, C.; Wang, H.; Luber, B.; Nakazawa, M.; Roeser, J.C.; Chen, Y.; Mohammad, T.A.; Chen, Y.; Fedor, H.L. AR-V7 and resistance to enzalutamide and abiraterone in prostate cancer. *N. Engl. J. Med.* **2014**, *371*, 1028–1038. [CrossRef] [PubMed]
64. Dehm, S.M.; Schmidt, L.J.; Heemers, H.V.; Vessella, R.L.; Tindall, D.J. Splicing of a novel androgen receptor exon generates a constitutively active androgen receptor that mediates prostate cancer therapy resistance. *Cancer Res.* **2008**, *68*, 5469–5477. [CrossRef] [PubMed]
65. Wadosky, K.M.; Koochekpour, S. Molecular mechanisms underlying resistance to androgen deprivation therapy in prostate cancer. *Oncotarget* **2016**, *7*, 64447–64470. [CrossRef] [PubMed]
66. Ferrer, F.A.; Miller, L.J.; Andrawis, R.I.; Kurtzman, S.H.; Albertsen, P.C.; Laudone, V.P.; Kreutzer, D.L. Vascular endothelial growth factor (VEGF) expression in human prostate cancer: In situ and in vitro expression of VEGF by human prostate cancer cells. *J. Urol.* **1997**, *157*, 2329–2333. [CrossRef]
67. Duque, J.L.F.; Loughlin, K.R.; Adam, R.M.; Kantoff, P.W.; Zurakowski, D.; Freeman, M.R. Plasma levels of vascular endothelial growth factor are increased in patients with metastatic prostate cancer. *Urology* **1999**, *54*, 523–527. [CrossRef]
68. Duque, J.L.F.; Loughlin, K.R.; Adam, R.M.; Kantoff, P.; Mazzucchi, E.; Freeman, M.R. Measurement of plasma levels of vascular endothelial growth factor in prostate cancer patients: Relationship with clinical stage, Gleason score, prostate volume, and serum prostate-specific antigen. *Clinics* **2006**, *61*, 401–408. [CrossRef] [PubMed]
69. Kelly, W.K.; Halabi, S.; Carducci, M.; George, D.; Mahoney, J.F.; Stadler, W.M.; Morris, M.; Kantoff, P.; Monk, J.P.; Kaplan, E. Randomized, double-blind, placebo-controlled phase III trial comparing docetaxel and prednisone with or without bevacizumab in men with metastatic castration-resistant prostate cancer: CALGB 90401. *J. Clin. Oncol.* **2012**, *30*, 1534–1540. [CrossRef] [PubMed]

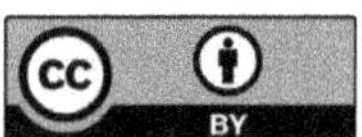

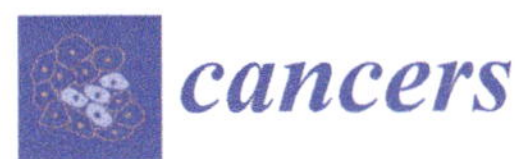

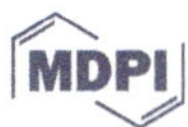

Review

Stromal Androgen Receptor in Prostate Cancer Development and Progression

Damien A. Leach [1,2,*] and Grant Buchanan [1,3]

1 The Basil Hetzel Institute for Translational Health Research, The University of Adelaide, Adelaide 5011, Australia; Grant.Buchanan@act.gov.au
2 Department of Surgery and Cancer, Imperial College London, Hammersmith Hospital Campus, Du Cane Road, London W12 0NN, UK
3 Department of Radiation Oncology, Canberra Teaching Hospital, Canberra 2605, Australia
* Correspondence: damien.leach@imperial.ac.uk; Tel.: +44-208-594-2821

Academic Editor: Emmanuel S. Antonarakis
Received: 30 November 2016; Accepted: 16 January 2017; Published: 22 January 2017

Abstract: Prostate cancer development and progression is the result of complex interactions between epithelia cells and fibroblasts/myofibroblasts, in a series of dynamic process amenable to regulation by hormones. Whilst androgen action through the androgen receptor (AR) is a well-established component of prostate cancer biology, it has been becoming increasingly apparent that changes in AR signalling in the surrounding stroma can dramatically influence tumour cell behavior. This is reflected in the consistent finding of a strong association between stromal AR expression and patient outcomes. In this review, we explore the relationship between AR signalling in fibroblasts/myofibroblasts and prostate cancer cells in the primary site, and detail the known functions, actions, and mechanisms of fibroblast AR signaling. We conclude with an evidence-based summary of how androgen action in stroma dramatically influences disease progression.

Keywords: prostate cancer; stroma; fibroblasts; androgen; androgen receptor

---

1. Introduction

Histological assessment of solid tumours has been used in combination with clinical parameters for many decades to inform both diagnosis and management decisions. In the emerging era of immunotherapeutics and personalized medicine, histology and molecular assessment is playing an increasingly important role in defining prognosis and individualised treatment options. Assessment now often includes protein activity and mutation status in addition to extent and level within a tumour sample, as well as markers of tumour activity, mitosis and turnover. For breast cancer, levels and extent of oestrogen receptor (ER), progesterone receptor (PR, as a marker of ER function) and HER2 are used to broadly categorize a tumour and inform on the benefit of anti-estrogen agents (e.g., tamoxifen) or tyrosine kinase inhibitors. Similarly, assessment of colon cancer includes EGRF, KNAS and UHA1; of melanoma, BRAF; of lung cancer, EGRF, ALK, KRAS and ROS-1; and of leukaemia a panel of markers for typing. Prostate cancer remains an anomaly in this regard. Despite being the most common, non-skin, cancer, and the leading cause of cancer related death, prognosis and treatment is generally defined using clinical and pathological parameters established decades ago. The predominant histological patterns of glandular disorganization are captured in the Gleason score, which together with clinical assessment and/or medical imaging regarding the extent of disease within the prostate and any extracapsular disease, are combined to provide prognostic information. Serum prostate specific antigen (PSA) testing was introduced over 20 years ago, and although useful in stratification of patients for investigation, risk of recurrence following definitive treatment and disease monitoring, is not a particularly useful in a prognostic sense. Intriguingly, the lack of prognostic markers available to patients and clinicians is predicted to have led to both over and under treatment of patients, with financial and social implications for both patients and the health care system. Currently, no histological markers are routinely used to determine prostate cancer prognosis, or inform on the usefulness of androgen ablation strategies. A key limitation in this regard is the multi-focal nature of most prostate cancers, and the inherent heterogeneity within cancerous epithelia of individual patients. One alternative being explored is the assessment of reactive changes occurring within the surrounding stroma.

Despite being generally regarded as a simple supportive structure for the specialised cells within an organ, the stroma is actually vital to organ development and homeostasis, and plays a significant role in both carcinogenesis and metastasis. The stroma is composed of a mixture of smooth muscle cells, fibroblasts, immune cells, lymphatics, vasculature and extracellular matrix (ECM) as well as via a rich array of secreted factors, hormones, enzymes and other soluble second messengers. Along with direct cell-cell interaction, these factors mediate communication between stromal constituents and bidirectional signalling between stromal and epithelial compartments, which is observed in all organs and is vital for normal development. With carcinogenesis and with tumour growth, substantial changes are found in stromal constituents and behaviour. Cancer stroma is characterised by a loss of smooth muscle cells and a predominance of activated myofibroblasts, termed cancer associated fibroblasts (CAFs), that enable carcinogenesis, stimulate tumour growth and contribute to invasion [1]. The CAFs which surround the cancerous gland development from multiple sources, circulating marrow derived progenitors, adipose tissue, and fibroblasts from distant organs, but a vast majority are reported to develop from the resident fibroblast population [2,3]. Indeed, the extent of transformation of the fibroblasts can associate with disease progression, potentially through providing paracrine cues to disrupt and disaffect homeostasis. The prostate provides a compelling example of intra-compartmental signalling that influences normal development and malignant cell behaviour. The growing appreciation of the role played by prostate stroma in carcinogenesis, tumour behaviour and response to conventional therapy is driving new innovation in research and treatment.

Prostate cancer remains the most commonly diagnosed non-skin malignancy and second leading cause of cancer related death in US men, with invasion and metastasis from the primary site reducing patient survival by 50%. Current clinical nomograms utilize imaging, clinico-pathological parameters and serum leak of epithelial produced PSA to broadly stratify cancers according to risk of progression following treatment, but cannot accurately predict tumour progression at the time of diagnosis, or the timeframe in which progression might be clinically significant. As a consequence, it is believed that many patients either incur treatments and their associated side effects unnecessarily, or are not receiving the appropriate therapy or monitoring for aggressive disease.

Androgens are a key factor in prostatic development, homeostasis and malignancy. With respect to the former, early in vivo studies showed that the absence of hormone responsive stroma prevented epithelial cell differentiation and organ and glandular development [4,5]. Nonetheless, the vast majority of androgen and androgen receptor (AR) research has been focussed on epithelial cancer cells because of the response of these cells, and prostate tumours, to androgen deprivation. The purpose of this review is to provide an emerging review of hormone signalling in the fibroblasts and myofibroblasts of the prostate (the most prominent stromal cells in prostate cancer) and how it controls stromal-epithelial interactions in the primary tumour setting, and to describe how changes in this pathway are emerging as a key determinants of prostate cancer progression and outcome.

2. Stromal AR in Prostate Cancer Outcome

Continued growth of metastatic prostate cancer cells during complete androgen blockade, in both clinical and experimental settings, is the result of mechanisms permissive for continued function of AR and/or those of its activated pathways despite combined AR/androgen targeting. Although increased AR expression in the epithelial cancer cells is one such mechanism, there is inconsistent evidence that it contributes to development or progression of the primary tumour. As reviewed in Tamburrino et al. [6], epithelial AR levels in primary prostate cancers has been inconsistently related to patient outcome, with 20% of studies suggesting high cancer AR as a prognostic marker of good outcome, 26% showing high AR as a prognostic marker of poor outcome, and the majority showing no relationship (Table 1). In comparison, for the smaller number of studies looking at stroma, a loss of stromal AR has universally been related to the cancerous state, high risk clinical parameters, disease progression and/or poor outcome (Table 2). In these studies, the term stroma refers to the cells directly adjacent to the epithelial or cancerous cells, which are usually noted for their fibroblast appearance. In a study of twenty patients, Mohler et al., showed lower intensity immunostaining of AR in cancer stroma compared to regions of benign prostatic hyperplasia [7], but there was no correlation with cancer progression, possibly due to the small cohort size. However, in larger studies, statistically significant associates were made. In four studies, in cohorts of 53 patients (radical prostatectomy (RP) samples), 152 patients (two separate cohorts, 78 transurethral resection of the prostate (TURP), and 74 biopsy), 96 patients (RP), and 53 patients (RP), low stromal AP was significantly associated with biochemical relapse and response to castration [8–11]. Other clinical parameters were also associated, including Gleason score and disease stage. We have shown in a cohort of 64 patients that low stromal AR expression inversely associates with patient outcome, to which we later added that the using FKBP5 as a marker of AR activity could be combined with AR levels to for an even stronger inverse relationship with patient outcome [12,13]. Importantly, this cohort had benign and cancers samples taken from each patient, which showed that the loss of AR was specific to the cancer associated stroma. Overall, all currently published patient-based studies indicate that lower AR in prostate cancer stroma is associated with disease progression and/or worse outcome, implying that stromal AR is protective. It will be important to know if this has prognostic significance, both in terms of patients most at risk of developing advanced disease and the potential response of an individual tumour to androgen deprivation. These findings are distinct from the potential beneficial effects of stromal AR in preventing caner initiation and development, which is discussed further below.

Table 1. Expression of AR in cancerous epithelial tissue and association with outcomes. RP = Radical prostatectomy; TURP = Transurethral resection of the prostate; IHC = Immunohistochemistry; RT-PCR = Real time polymerase chain reaction.

Authors	Specimens	Cohort Size	Methods	Effect on Prostate Cancer Outcome
[14]	Biopsies	62	IHC	Higher AR, better prognosis
[15]	Biopsy, RP and TURP	42	IHC	Higher AR, better prognosis
[16]	Biopsies	90	IHC	Higher AR, better prognosis
[17]	RP	197	IHC	Higher AR, better prognosis
[18]	RP	105	IHC	Higher AR, better prognosis
[19]	mixed RP, TURP, Biopsy	42	IHC	Higher AR, better prognosis
[9]	RP	96	IHC	Higher AR, biochemical relapse
[20]	RP	115	RT-PCR	Higher AR, biochemical relapse
[21]	RP	340	IHC	Higher AR, biochemical relapse
[22]	RP	52	IHC	Higher AR, biochemical relapse
[8]	RP	53	IHC	Higher AR, biochemical relapse
[22]	RP	52	IHC	Higher AR, worse prognosis
[23]	RP	640	IHC	Higher AR, worse prognosis
[24]	mixed RP/biopsy	66	IF	Higher AR, worse prognosis
[11]	RP	56	IHC	Not prognostic
[25]	RP	232	IHC	Not prognostic
[26]	TURP	68	IHC	Not prognostic
[27]	RP	64	IHC	Not prognostic
[28]	Biopsies	17	IHC	Not prognostic
[29]	RP	121	RT-PCR	Not prognostic
[30]	TURP and RP	81	IHC	Not prognostic
[31]	RP and metastases	119	IHC	Not prognostic
[32]	RP	2805	IHC and RT-PCR	Not prognostic
[33]	RP	172	IHC	Not prognostic
[34]	TURP	24	IHC	Not prognostic

Table 1. *Cont.*

Authors	Specimens	Cohort Size	Methods	Effect on Prostate Cancer Outcome
[10]	TURP + biopsy	154	IHC	Not prognostic
[35]	RP	43	IHC	Not prognostic
[7]	RP	20	IHC	Not prognostic
[12]	TURP	64	IHC	Not prognostic
[36]	RP	53	branched chain DNA	Not prognostic
[37]	RP	10	IHC	Unavailable
[38]	Biopsies	39	IHC	Unavailable
[39]	RP	26	IHC	Unavailable
[40]	RP	50	IHC	Unavailable

Table 2. Expression of AR in cancerous stroma and association with patient outcomes. RP = Radical prostatectomy; TURP = Transurethral resection of the prostate; IHC = Immunohistochemistry.

Authors	Specimens	Cohort Size	Methods	Effect on Prostate Cancer Outcome
[41]	RP	44	IHC	Low AR, biochemical relapse
[8]	RP	53	IHC	Low AR, biochemical relapse
[9]	RP	96	IHC	Low AR, biochemical relapse
[12]	TURP	64	IHC	Low AR, PCSM
[10]	TURP + biopsy	152	IHC	Low AR, worse prognosis
[11]	RP	56	IHC	Low AR, worse prognosis
[7]	RP	20	IHC	(low AR, no association with Gleason)

3. Androgen Signalling

Androgens act primarily through their cognate receptor, the androgen receptor (AR), which is a potent transcription factor with broad tissue distribution and a major mediator of cellular function and homeostasis. Androgens are vital for growth and maturation of the prostate. However, the mechanism, regulation, and outcomes of AR signalling are based primarily on whole body physiological responses, and molecular studies in predominantly cancerous epithelial cells. AR signalling (Figure 1), in most basic terms this starts with cellular internalization of circulating androgens such as testosterone (T). Androgens then bind directly to the AR with variable affinity, or in the case of T may be first metabolized to the more potent dihydrotestosterone (DHT) via the enzyme 5-alpha reductase. Steroid binding to the AR occurs in the cytoplasm, where the receptor resides in an inactive state in complex with molecular chaperones, such as HSP90, and other proteins. Binding and activation in the initiation of genomic signalling pathways including PI3K-AKT, and ERK. Activation of AR also results in alteration sin the interaction with chaperones, allowing for translocation to the nucleus via movement along microtubules. Nuclearisation culminates in the interaction of the AR with chromatin, and ultimately regulation of the cellular transcriptional profile. The transcriptional response to androgens is modulated by the availability of steroid and the cellular complement of pioneer, coregulatory and chaperone proteins.

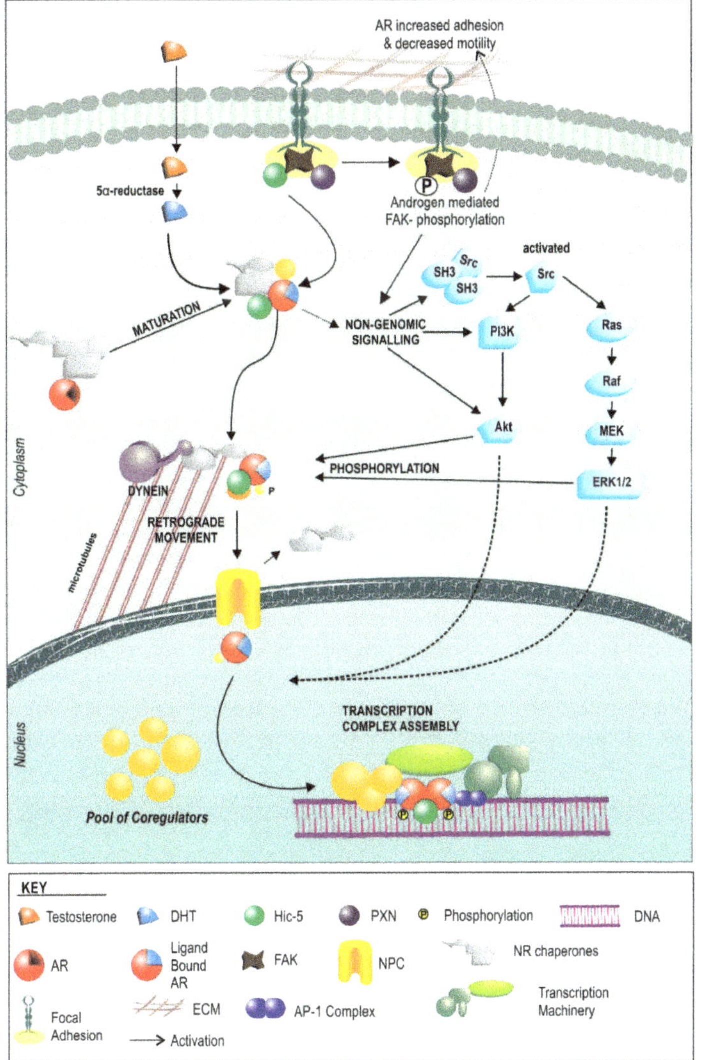

Figure 1. Schematic of androgen receptor (AR) signalling in fibroblasts/myofibroblasts. Serum testosterone enters the cell, converts, via the 5α-reductase enzyme, into dihydrotestosterone (DHT). This then binds to the AR which resides in the cytoplasm, bound to chaperones, causing a conformational change and activation of the AR. The AR can then cause a series of non-genomic effects via kinase pathways, but also shuttles via microtubules to the nucleus which it enters via nuclear pore complexes (NPC). Concomitantly, activated AR also causes nuclear translocation of focal adhesion proteins such as Hic-5 (thus altering adhesiveness and movement of cells) which it uses as a co-regulator, along with a pool of cofactors and other co-regulators (some of which are fibroblast/stroma specific) to combine with transcriptional machinery and regulate gene expression.

4. How AR Signaling in the Stroma Works

Despite observations of AR in the stroma being important in all stages of prostate development and carcinogenesis, until recently little was known about the mechanics of AR function in that cellular compartment. In the benign prostate the predominant stromal cells are smooth muscle cells, a majority of which strongly express AR. Myofibroblasts are the predominant cell type present in the tumour stroma, and although they can be seen to express AR and show physiological and molecular responses to androgens in vivo [12], primary human fibroblasts shed AR expression within 1–2 passages in culture. To overcome this limitation, two engineered human prostate myofibroblast cell lines have been developed, WPMY-1 and PShTert-ARs [41,42]. Of these two, only PShTert-AR cells stably express AR, which has a similar AR binding patterns and gene regulation to primary and in vivo mesenchyme [12,43], as well as being able to inhibit fibroblast proliferation replicative of in vivo studies of human prostate, as well as being able to excite epithelial cells proliferation just as mesenchyme in mouse recombination studies [12]. Furthermore, androgen action in these myofibroblast cells lines validates in patient NPF and CAFs [12].

In general terms, the molecular action of AR function in fibroblast lineage cells appears to follow the same general basic principles as AR in epithelial cells, but with some key differences that radically alter the cellular response (Figure 1). At the front end, HSP90 appears to be equally essential for AR function in both cell types [44], and the receptor traffics to the nucleus only following steroid binding [45]. Importantly however, when we recently compared the global transcriptional response to androgens, only around 10% of genes regulated by androgens in prostate myofibroblasts were common with those regulated in epithelial cells [12]. This appears to be the result of lineage-specific differences in the expression of co-regulators and pioneer factors. Cofactors are a diverse set of proteins that exert their effects on AR by influencing stability, ligand binding, interaction with other proteins, DNA interactions via modification to histone acetylation, methylation and sumoylation, recruitment of the transcriptional machinery or baseline activity. The expression and ratio of co-regulators are different between epithelial cells and non-epithelial cells of the prostate [46]. As an example, we have shown that the mesenchymal specific co-regulator, Hic-5 affects regulation of over 50% of genes targeted by androgen receptor in fibroblasts [45]. Pioneer factors are proteins that regulate targeting and/or activity of transcription factors to specific regions of DNA. Unlike epithelial cancer cells that utilize the forkhead protein, FOXA1 as the primary AR pioneer factor [47–50], we have shown that prostate fibroblasts appear to use the AP1 complex, and JUN in particular, leads to regulation of distinct molecular pathways in fibroblasts [43]. As one example, JUN driven fibroblast specific regulation of licensing factor FBXO32 by AR results in a switch to inhibiting of fibroblast proliferation by androgens.

5. Stromal AR in Prostate Development

In the embryonic/developing prostate the urogenital mesenchyme (UGM) is comprised of AR positive precursors to fibroblast and smooth muscle cells, similar to myofibroblasts [51–53]. Supporting a role for stromal androgen signalling throughout prostate development, expression of the AR occurs higher and earlier in this compartment than in epithelia, and is maintained throughout maturation. This has been demonstrated in tissue recombination models, where AR positive UGM leads to normal growth and glandular differentiation of urogenital epithelia (UGE). In contrast, AR negative mesenchyme from skin results in differentiation of UGE to stratified squamous epithelia [4,54] (Figure 2A). Studies utilizing cells extracted from testicular feminized (Tfm) mice, which have a non-functional AR, further clarify the importance of stromal androgen signalling. When wild type (WT) UGM is combined with UGE from Tfm mice, prostatic structures develop normally. In contrast, tissues generated from Tfm UGM and either WT UGE or Tfm UGE fail to generate glandular architecture [55] (Figure 2A). Additional studies demonstrate poor differentiation of prostatic ducts and glandular acini in mice that lack stromal AR [56] (Figure 2A). Although androgen signalling in the mature prostate epithelia is primarily responsible for secretion of seminal fluid constituents, including prostate specific antigen (PSA) [57], this process can also be modulated by the prostatic stroma [58,59]. In the mature prostate, AR positive smooth muscle cells are the predominant cell type. In vitro, AR action in fibroblasts increases epithelial AR activity, as measured by in vitro assays of AR activity [60], and results in increased in epithelial PSA production [61]. Collectively, these findings implicate stromal

AR activity in development, maintenance and biological function of adjacent epithelia. More broadly, there appears to be a universal role for mesenchymal hormone signalling in the development of both male and female reproductive organs, with expression of the appropriate hormone receptors in adjacent stroma critical for subsequent organ-specific responses to oestrogen, progesterone, and testosterone [62–65].

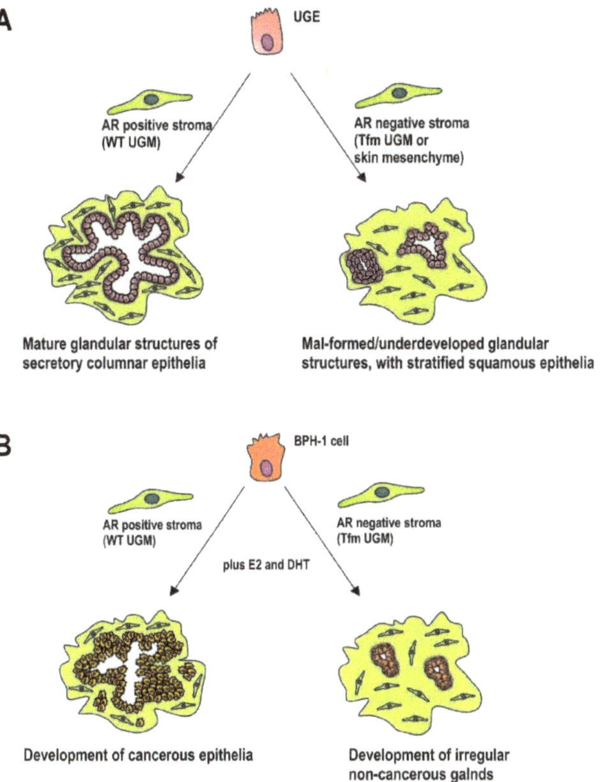

Figure 2. Impact of AR expression on prostate development and carcinogenesis. (**A**) Stromal AR is required for prostate development. In mouse models combining embryonic urogenital epithelia (UGE) with AR positive urogenital mesenchyme (UGM) results in normal epithelial structures, which doesn't occur when UGE is combined with AR negative or non-functionally AR containing mesenchyme; (**B**) AR is needed in stroma for cancer initiation. When transformed BPH-1 cells are grown in mice in the presence of AR positive mesenchyme cancer initiation and development can occur, but when combined with AR negative stroma, only small, irregular, non-cancerous glands form.

6. Stromal AR in Carcinogenesis

The role of stromal androgen signalling in prostate carcinogenesis is becoming more and more prominent [66–68]. Stromal AR activity is also required for tumour formation in prostatic epithelia in recombinant mouse models [69]. AR negative initiated epithelial cells were implanted into castrate mice flanks along with AR negative or positive UGM. Mice were then treated with or without androgen and estrogen. In mice implanted with epithelia alone, there was no tumour formation under any treatment condition. Where mice were implanted with initiated epithelium and AR positive UGM, tumour formation occurred in 36% (n = 30/84) of hormone treated mice but <0.5% (n = 1/218) of untreated mice [69]. Whilst that study did not specifically compare AR positive versus AR negative

UGM, it did demonstrated the importance of stroma in early stage cancer, and the potential role of stromal AR signalling in tumour formation. A role in early transformation was addressed more recently by implantation of initiated prostate epithelia (via knockdown of tumour suppressors PTEN and p53) with wild-type or Tfm mesenchyme [70]. When initiated, epithelia were combined with WT mesenchyme, tumour formation occurred following hormonal stimulation (Figure 2B). In contrast, when combined with the AR negative Tfm mesenchyme, the result was merely the development of small non-invasive growths (Figure 2B). Significantly, the presence of AR in the epithelial cells did not affect those processes [70]. Similarly, the spontaneous development of prostatic intraepithelial neoplasia seen in PTEN+/− mice, was decreased in offspring bred with stromal AR knockout mice (ARKO) [71]. Furthermore, inhibiting the AR chaperone, HSP90, in CAFs, thereby reducing the AR activity, retards growth of patient derived cancer cell and CAF recombinant xenografts in mice [44].

AR positive stroma is also capable of inducing prostate tumour formation from grafted AR negative benign prostatic hyperplasia (BPH)-1 cells [69], but is hindered in mice which lack stromal AR in comparison to stromal AR positive mice [72]. Perhaps significantly, in men of African descent where there is a higher incidence of prostate cancer compared to Caucasian men, there is reportedly higher stromal AR expression [73]. Regardless, the evidence collectively supports stromal AR signalling acting to induce prostate cancer cell proliferation and potentially play an important role in early prostate carcinogenesis. Thus, it would appear that stromal AR plays an important and often overlooked role in early prostate carcinogenesis. It is important, however, to distinguish this from the potential role of decreased stromal AR in cancer progression and metastasis (see Section 2).

7. Why Is Stromal AR Lost?

Despite the relationship between clinical outcome and stromal AR loss highlighted in Table 2, the mechanisms underpinning altered AR expression in this compartment in some, or perhaps all, prostate tumours are unknown. One hypothesis is AR negative/low CAFs represent a subgroup of an initial CAF population that undergoes clonal selection in some manner. We have previously reported that AR action in myofibroblasts inhibits their intrinsic proliferation [12], which might provide a selective pressure for the AR negative/low CAF population over those that highly express the receptor. A second tier question is how variable AR expression occurs in stroma in the first place. Cellular variability in ligand availability is one possibility. We know that AR signalling in stroma is less sensitive than in epithelial cells, and thus more vulnerable to systemic changes in androgen levels, or on altered supply based on local tumour microarchitecture and/or vascular supply. Decreased ligand availability will manifest as decreased AR stabilization and increased receptor turnover. An alternative and relatively unexplored possibility is that of stromal mutagenesis occurring distinct from genetic alterations within the cancer cells themselves. Some studies using mixed prostate tumour samples have, for example, paradoxically identified inactivating AR mutations that have been difficult to rationale in the context of almost invariable AR driven epithelial disease [74]. It is tempting to speculate that some of those mutations may have been captured from stromal components. Epigenetic regulation could also be involved, as changes in methylation state are known to regulate AR expression [75]. Alternatively, p53 has been show to negatively affect AR interactions leading to receptor stabilization and activity [76], and forms part of a stromal signature in prostate cancer associated with biochemical relapse [77]. However, down regulated genes weren't assessed as part of that study, so it is currently unclear if there is a direct relationship.

There is a clear need for a more contemporary analysis of cancer cells associated with high and low stromal AR content, and to track mutational and transcription events within each compartment. It is likely that events in one or both compartments of a tumour will can change the way cancer cells interact with their microenvironment. Paracrine factors such as interleukins, interferons, and miRNAs have all been reported to reduce AR levels [78–82]. Nitric oxide is a product of certain events within cancer cells, inhibits AR expression and activity, and plays a role in cancer progression and metastasis [83–85].

Given the potential prognostic importance of stromal AR expression, studies need to extend beyond speculative hypotheses to address in real time how AR levels fluctuate within a tumour sample.

8. Possible Mechanisms for the Involvement of Stromal AR Signalling in Cancer Progression and Outcome

The mechanisms by which stromal AR action influences response of adjacent epithelia are slowly emerging. Secretion of factors by fibroblasts in response to androgens activate intracellular signalling pathways in epithelia as well as post translational modification of AR, increased AR activity [12,86], and stimulation of epithelial proliferation [87,88]. In contrast however, in transgenic adenocarcinoma of the mouse prostate (TRAMP) mice co-inoculated with AR negative highly metastatic human prostate cancer PC3 cells and human WMPY fibroblasts, knockdown of fibroblast AR with a specific siRNA did not alter cancer cell proliferation based on Ki67 index [89]. Reconciling the paradox between the apparent need for stromal AR signalling in the initial stages of cancer development versus the apparent importance of lost stromal AR signalling with cancer progression and outcome may have previously been problematic as there has been limited research into the function of AR in stromal cells. This dichotomy can now be recognized as not mutually exclusive as detailed below and surmised in Figure 3.

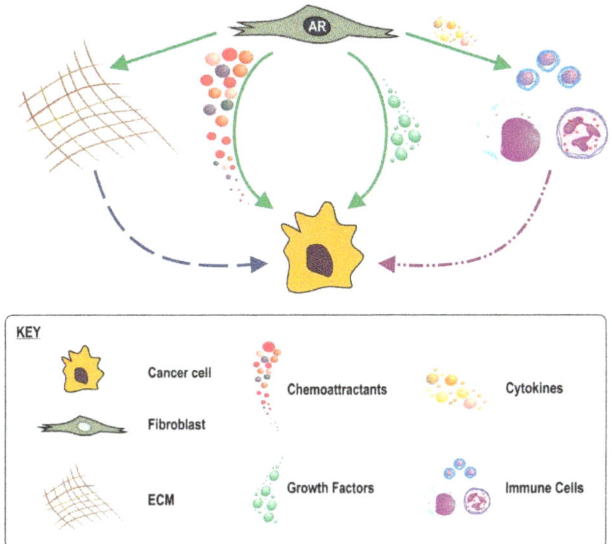

Figure 3. Potential mechanism for fibroblast AR influence on prostate cancer outcomes. AR signalling in fibroblasts regulates growth factors, chemoattractants, cytokines and ECM production. By regulating growth factors AR creates a hospitable environment for cancer, thus when AR is lost the local environment may drive cancer cells to metastasise elsewhere. AR regulates chemoattractant production, disruption of this may excite the migratory capacity of cancer cells. By regulating cytokine production, AR signalling in fibroblasts my influence immune response which may have significant effects on tumour cells. AR signalling in fibroblasts controls fibroblast production of ECM, when AR is lost, this could dysregulate the ECM and enhance the migratory potential of cancer by providing a transversable ECM microenvironment.

8.1. Loss of Stromal AR Creating Less Favourable Conditions

Fibroblasts produce a number of paracrine factors favourable for cancer cell growth (Table 3). A number of these paracrine factors are reported to be influential in cancer initiation and growth and their inhibition in fibroblasts is reported to alter cancer progression in vivo [90,91]. We and others have recently shown how fibroblast androgen action leads to regulation of a number of these paracrine factors in vitro, at least at an RNA level (Table) [12,87]. During prostate development moreover, androgen drives mesenchyme secretion of paracrine factors including FGFs, BMPs, WNTs, TGFBs and EPHs [92]. Furthermore stromal specific AR knockdown reduces mesenchymal production of key paracrine factors, IGF1, FGF7, FGF10, and HGF [56,71,93]. Indeed mouse models of androgen deprivation therapy (ADT) have reported marked reduction in stromal expression of FGF2 Il6, IGF1 and TGFB [91,94–96], all of which are capable of significantly increasing cancer cell proliferation and tumour growth [97], and acting to maintain terminal differentiation of the glandular epithelia [98]. An increased abundance of stimulatory growth factors by mesenchymal androgen action might thus contribute to the tumourigenic process. For initiated cancer cells however, decreased in local availability of paracrine mediators as the result of declining mesenchymal AR signalling could result in (i) de-differentiation and/or epithelial-mesenchymal transition (EMT); (ii) reduced epithelial AR function and PSA production that has implications for clinical monitoring via PSA and response to androgen deprivation therapy; and (iii) a less hospitable environment for epithelial cells thus driving pathways for epithelial movement and metastasis to more favourable sites.

Table 3. Stromal produced paracrine factors. Proliferative effect (P), Differential effect (D) supported by [97,99,100]. Androgen regulation (Y = yes, regulated by androgen, N = no, not regulated by androgen) determined from microarray data from [12,45,87].

Paracrine Factor	Effect	Androgen Regulation
CTGF	P	Y
FGF (2, 5, 7, 8, 9, 10)	P, D	Y (2, 5, 7), N (8), *N/A* (9, 10)
HGF	P, D	Y
IGF (1, 2)	P, D	Y (1, 2)
IL-6	P	Y
PDGF	P, D	Y
TGFb (1, 2, 3)	P, D	Y (1, 2, 3)
VEGF (A, B, C)	P	Y (A,C), N (B)
WNT	P	Y
CXCL12	P	N
EGF	P, D	*N/A*
TGFa	P, D	*N/A*

8.2. A Role for Stromal in AR Inflammatory Processes

A high abundance of inflammatory cells is associated with development of prostate cancer and with poor outcome [101], and there is an association between age induced decline in testosterone and increased prostatic inflammation [102–104]. Although an anti-inflammatory effect of androgens has been demonstrated for the whole prostate [105], the role of fibroblasts, and indeed fibroblast AR signalling, in this process is unclear. Significantly however, fibroblasts are known to interact with inflammatory immune cells [106], and testosterone action in synovial fibroblasts has been suggested to have an anti-inflammatory role by inhibition of pro-inflammatory cytokine production [107,108]. Moreover, CAFs themselves have been reported to activate immune responses via NFKB secretion, while AR in prostatic fibroblasts is believed to modulate the release of pro-inflammatory cytokines that affect initiation and development of BPH and PIN [71]. The above data are collectively compelling for immune regulation in the prostate and a role in the tumour process, but the specific mechanisms and role of fibroblast AR need direct elucidation.

8.3. AR in CAF Movement and a Subsequent Role in Cancer Invasion

Compared to normal fibroblasts, CAFs have been shown to modulate movement of cancer cells through a variety of distinct mechanisms and effectors [90,109–113], and in themselves are more migratory than NPFs [114]. On one level, changes in fibroblast maintenance of ECM can serve to enhance movement of cancerous epithelia directly via independent matrix interactions [115,116]. On another, the ability of fibroblasts to move, create guidance structures, and dictate cancer cell movement may a key determinant in cancer progression and metastasis [115,117,118]. We have previously reported in fibroblasts a non-genomic role for AR and its co-regulator, Hic-5, in controlling fibroblast movement. With decreased androgen action, Hic-5 associates preferentially with the focal adhesion complex to inhibit its activity, facilitating fibroblasts detachment from the extracellular matrix and increased movement. It can be predicted therefore, that the loss of fibroblast AR might increase fibroblast movement and stimulate direct guidance of cancer cells. Furthermore, chemotactic cues are reported to outweigh any other conflicting stimuli, and drive migration [119]. Androgen also regulates the fibroblast expression of the potent chemo attractant, CXC12 [12,87]. The role of CXCL12 in controlling cancer cell movement is well known [120]. Additionally there are a host of other chemokines produced by CAFs which may similarly be regulated any androgen [56,88,121,122], and could provide an avenue by which disruption of AR signaling in fibroblasts may change the migrationary potential of cancer cells thus affecting patient outcomes.

8.4. Stromal AR Regulation of ECM

We recently hypothesised that the inverse relationship between stromal AR level and prostate cancer outcome is the result, in part, of changes in the production and regulation of fibroblast ECM [12]. The ECM is an intricate matrix of proteins and glycans that provide structural support for tissue and organs, and acts as a repository of hormones, enzymes and second messengers. It has been shown that the ECM can stimulate tumour growth and encourage cell cycle progression of cancer cells through proliferative checkpoints [123]. The ECM can also drive cancer cell gene expression, signal transduction, cell morphology, cell survival, and motility [124]. Changes in ECM can also cause CAFs to secret pro-inflammatory markers, thereby enhancing cancer progression [125,126]. In physical terms, it appears that the ECM can regulate cancer cell invasion via multiple parameters, including density, orientation, stiffness, and organisation of the matrix fibres. Whilst the effects of these different ECM characteristics can be interdependent or combine to create effects, it should be noted that they are independently able to affect cancer cell behaviour [127].

The role of ECM density is potentially complicated as well as controversial. Accompanying the switch from benign to malignant tissue for a number of different cancers is an increase in certain ECM proteins such as collagen 1. However, these reactive changes also coincide with a change from a mainly smooth muscle stroma that doesn't produce much ECM, to one composed predominantly of high-ECM producing/maintaining fibroblasts and myofibroblast. These changes occur with all solid tumours, but nevertheless not every cancer will metastasise. In breast cancer, high collagen production is associated with cancer development and is reported to excite tumourigenesis and proliferation, and to alter intracellular processes to excite cancer cell movement [128–130]. While increased density may contribute to cancer initiation, it might conversely oppose tumour progression. As an example, hypoxia is a known driver of cancer progression and is associated with the ECM acquiring a loose and porous phenotype [131]. Although early 2-D ECM models suggested a relationship between density and cancer cell motility, more recent 3-D models show that cancer cells move more rapidly and easily through low density ECM [132–134]. The idea of androgen regulation is confirmed in vivo with a number of observations in ADT studies, noting changes in ECM volume [135–138] as well as changes in MMP levels [138,139]. Furthermore androgen regulates ECM component genes expression, and produces an ECM capable of altering cancer cell adhesion and migration [12].

The firmness or rigidity of the ECM fibres is also reported to affect cell movement. Traditionally, increased stiffness was believed to enhance migration by encouraging mesenchymal-type cell invasion [140], and by regulating cellular arrangement of integrins to control cell movement processes [129]. Conversely, increased stiffness and rigidity inhibits the ability of ECM fibres to be degraded by proteolytic enzymes such as MMP [141]. The recent move towards 3-D modelling has shed greater light on this process, specifically that maximal cell movement of cancer cells, such as human prostate DU145 cells, occurs in matrices exhibiting lesser stiffness [142].

Another aspect of the ECM that is accruing evidence for a major role in cancer progression is the orientation of the ECM fibres. In both in vitro and in vivo systems, cancer cells exhibit increased invasion and metastasis if ECM is arranged linearly to provide tunnels and tracts for cell movement. Similarly, the pore size, or space between ECM fibres can modulate cancer cell movement [132,134,143]. In in vitro 3D modelling, testing different poor sizes, widths, and arrangements, suggests that increased density and constricted poor sizes have an inhibitory effect on cell migration [140,144].

In summary, movement of cancer cells appears to be the culmination of intrinsic changes within the cell combined with the external influence and guidance of the ECM [145]. Fibroblasts AR has the ability to regulate the ECM, which when lost will create an environment favourable for cancer cell invasion and metastasis. This ability of AR signalling within fibroblasts to regulate the ECM may be key factor in stromal AR correlation with outcome and worthy of further investigation.

9. Potential Importance of Stromal AR in Neoadujant Hormone Therapy

As prostate cancers progress to hormone refractory metastatic disease, usually under conditions of androgen deprivation or complete androgen blockade, the epithelial AR is widely believed to have acquired the capacity to drive tumour growth. In early stage disease however, it appears as if the stromal AR is required in both tumour initiation and conversely as an inhibitor of progression and metastasis, and unlike its epithelial counterpart holds prognostic information. Additionally, in mouse recombinant models where patient cancer tissue is grown in the presence of either AR positive or negative fibroblasts, the apoptotic response of cancer cells to castration is significantly modulated by AR in the surrounding fibroblasts [12]. Given this dichotomy, we reviewed the use of ADT in a neoadjuvant setting for primary prostate cancer (Table 4). Despite ADT not usually deemed a standard treatment for organ confined prostate disease, the CaPSURE registry showed increasing trends since 1990 for the use of ADT in a neoadjuvant setting either alone or in conjunction with of other forms of treatment [146]. Neoadjuvant use of ADT does reduce primary tumour size by 25%–30% [147,148]. However, recent studies using pre-existing patient cohort information showed that neoadjuvant ADT as a front-line therapy led to greater relative mortality when compared to surgery or radiation in a cohort of 7538 prostate cancer patients [149]. In a second population-based study of over 1900 men with T1–T2 prostate cancer, the use of ADT as primary therapy was associated with a lower rate of prostate cancer-specific survival [150]. In a study of 16,000 men with well-to-moderately differentiated tumours, the use of primary ADT within the first six months of diagnosis was associated with worse rates of overall survival and prostate cancer specific mortality, regardless of any additional treatment after this first 6 months [151]. A similar finding was reported by the European Organization for Research and Treatment of Cancer (EORTC) clinical trial, which investigated immediate and delayed use of ADT for treatment of locally defined tumours [152]. The use of ADT for localized prostate cancer increased the subsequent need for chemotherapy [153]. Nonetheless, there have been other reports suggesting either no or a slight beneficial effect of primary ADT [154,155], but these have had significantly smaller cohorts of 176 and 57 patients, respectively. Likewise, in a larger study of 1006 patients with low to intermediate prostate cancer treated with low dose brachytherapy (LDB), the use of ADT either three months prior to or concomitantly with LDB did not affect disease free or overall patient survival [156]. Furthermore, studies that have reported unconventional forms of primary ADT (i.e., diethylstilbestrol) have had inconsistent results with benefit for T2 tumours but deleterious effects for T1 disease [157]. Overall, the evidence suggests that neoadjuvant use of ADT may produce harmful effects through unknown mechanisms. However as discussed above, ADT is of well proven benefit in metastatic disease so the adverse response of this treatment when used in a primary setting must be due to adverse targeting/response of the early stage tumours. It is entirely possible that this paradox is due to effects of androgen signalling in cancer fibroblasts associating with the primary/early stage lesions.

Table 4. Outcomes from studies investigating effects of neoadjuvant ADT and outcomes of patients with localized prostate cancer.

References	N	Pca Staging	ADT Use	Comparison	Outcome
[149]	7538	T1–T3	Neo	ADT vs. surgery or radiation	ADT increases hazard ratio
[150]	19,271	T1–T2	Neo (<180 days)	ADT vs. conservative management	Decreased PCSS
[151]	16,000	T1–T2	Neo (<first 6 months)	ADT in first 6months vs. no ADT in first 6 months	Increased PCSM
[153]	29,775	Localized	Neo	ADT vs. noADT	ADT increases need for subsequent treatments
[158]	844		Neo (<first 6 months)	Neo compared to WW, RP, radiotherapy	Neo had worse 10 year PCSS of all treatments
[159]	10,179	Localised	Neo	Neo compared to no treatment, RP, BT, ERBT	ADT worse PCSS
[160]	402	Localised	Neo (<first 3 months)	Neo compared to RP alone	Neo = pathological downstaging and lowers % of patients with positive margins
[161]	547	Localised	Neo	3-month vs. 8-month neo	Positive margin rates were significantly lower in the 8 than 3-month group
[162]	167	T1a–T2b	Neo (<first 3 months)	3-month neo vs. RP alone	Neo had less lymph node involvement, less positive margins
[163]	393	T2–T3	Neo (3–6 months)	Neo vs. RP alone	Neo had better positive margin rates
[164]	119	T2–T3a	Neo (<first 4 months)	4-month neo vs. RP alone	Neo had better positive margin rates
[154]	176	B2/T2–T3	Neo	1-year ADT vs. long term ADT	No measurable significant benefit
[155]	57		Neo		No benefit
[156]	1006	Low-intermediate	Neo ADT + LDB	ADT prior to or after LDB	No effect of PCSS
[165]	282	T2b	Neo (<first 3 months)	3-month neo vs. RP alone	No difference in 5 year BCR
[166]	126	T1b–T3aNXM0	Neo (<first 3 months)	3-month neo vs. RP alone	No difference in PSA progression-free survival (7 year follow up)
[167]	148	T1b–T3	Neo (<first 3 months)	3-month neo vs. RP alone	No significant difference in BCR-free (8 year followup)
[152]	985	Localized	ADT Immediately or upon symptoms of progression	Immediate ADT vs. delayed ADT	Delayed ADT increased risk of mortality
[157]	1903	T1–T2	Neo (diethylstilbesterol)	ADT in T1 vs. ADT in T2	benefit T2, deletrious in T1
[168]	213	T1b/c–T2c	Neo	Neo prior to surgery vs. surgery alone	Neo = less organ confinement, lower 7-year survival

10. Future of Stromal AR

10.1. Prognostic Tool

There is growing appreciation for the influence of stroma in cancer, so much so that a number of studies have looked to the stroma for prognostic utilisation. Morphological characterisation of prostate cancer has used the degree of desmoplatic stroma to predict biochemical recurrence and cancer related death [169–171]. Stromal signatures and protein profiles have been investigated, and have been used to predict relapse post prostatectomy and clinical outcome [77,172–174]. Clinically, no protein expression or gene profiles are used to aid prognosis, despite the various immunohistochemical markers used in other cancers, such as breast cancer where oestrogen and progesterone receptors are used to inform on disease coarse and management. Along these lines we, and others have studied the benefit of using stromal AR in clinical settings. Despite inconsistent findings for the prognostic values for epithelial AR, a loss of stromal AR is consistently associated with disease relapse and outcome [7–12,41] (Table 2). We have also found using FKBP51 in addition to AR, as a marker of functional AR activity is even more robust prognostic tool [13]. These studies have focus on tissue samples, development of serum markers for stromal AR changes may also be useful tool. From whole genome studies we know a number of genes targeted by AR fibroblasts code for secreted proteins so with further work there may be potential for development of serum markers.

10.2. Therapeutic Targets

Just like in the prognostic setting, the cancer stroma is being investigated for its therapeutic influence and even as a target. The important role of CAFs have led to monoclonal antibodies and drugs which target the CAF marker, fibroblast activated protein (FAP) [175–177]. The stroma surrounding the tumour is exposed to any serum administered therapeutic agent before said therapeutic agent reacts with the cancer. Indeed it has been postulated that the stroma will mediate the influence of the therapeutic agent [178].

Therapeutic antibodies and small molecule inhibitors delivered in nanoparticles as well as extracts from natural compounds are being investigated for disrupting paracrine communication between the stroma and cancer cells to treat solid cancers [179,180]. A number of stromal produced paracrine factors, regulated by AR have been targeted therapeutically to varying degrees of success. Androgen regulated paracrine factors such as TGFs, FGFs, EGF, HGFs produced by the stroma having agents capable of targeting them [178]. FGF targeting has been reported to be effective in both in vitro and in vivo studies for treating prostate cancer [181,182]. Similarly, agents targeting HGF in prostate cancer are in different phases of clinical trial [183,184].

However, no therapeutic agents have been developed to specifically target stromal AR. Indeed in cases of neoaduvent ADT or use of AR antagonists the effect on stromal AR and the subsequent effects of stromal AR inhibition is rarely considered. In review of studies investigating the use of ADT on primary prostate tumors, the neoadjuvant use of ADT predominantly produces worse outcomes for the patients, with relapse free survival and overall survival reduced. Given the relationship between reduced stromal AR and cancer related progression and death, it may be more important to investigate either anti-androgen which affect only epithelial cells, or developing drugs which will decrease epithelial AR but enrich stromal AR signalling. As we have previously shown a single co-regulator can have vast effects on global gene expression with the cell. One way to ensure specificity would be to target AR co-regulators and pioneer factors, a number of which are specific for one cell type or the other [46]. In comparison of prostatic and skin fibroblasts to cancer cell lines, a panel of 33 co-regulators were differentially expressed between the two cell types [46]. Cancer cell type specific co-regulators included SP1, NCOA1, NCOA2, and PIAS1. Importantly these are potentially targetable [185,186]. Pioneer factors are also targetable, and as we have shown FOXA1 is expressed and active only in epithelial cells and not fibroblasts [43,186]. However targeting Hic-5, AP-1, or other proteins which is also or highly expressed in the stroma should be avoided as inhibiting stromal AR may have detrimental side-effects. Taking into account stromal AR should become an important step in future development of treatments targeting AR signalling, especially in a neoadjuvent setting.

Acknowledgments: We are grateful for support from Prostate Cancer Foundation of Australia, Cancer Australia, and The Urology Foundation (UK).

Author Contributions: This review was conceived by Damien A. Leach, co-written and edited by Damien A. Leach and Grant Buchanan.

Conflicts of Interest: The authors declare no conflict of interest.

References

1. Tuxhorn, J.A.; Ayala, G.E.; Smith, M.J.; Smith, V.C.; Dang, T.D.; Rowley, D.R. Reactive stroma in human prostate cancer: Induction of myofibroblast phenotype and extracellular matrix remodeling. *Clin. Cancer Res.* **2002**, *8*, 2912–2923. [PubMed]
2. Rowley, D.R. What might a stromal response mean to prostate cancer progression? *Cancer Metastasis Rev.* **1998**, *17*, 411–419. [CrossRef] [PubMed]
3. Tuxhorn, J.A.; Ayala, G.E.; Rowley, D.R. Reactive stroma in prostate cancer progression. *J. Urol.* **2001**, *166*, 2472–2483. [CrossRef]
4. Cunha, G.R.; Chung, L.W. Stromal-epithelial interactions—I. Induction of prostatic phenotype in urothelium of testicular feminized (Tfm/y) mice. *J. Steroid Biochem.* **1981**, *14*, 1317–1324. [CrossRef]
5. Donjacour, A.A.; Cunha, G.R. The effect of androgen deprivation on branching morphogenesis in the mouse prostate. *Dev. Biol.* **1988**, *128*, 1–14. [CrossRef]
6. Tamburrino, L.; Salvianti, F.; Marchiani, S.; Pinzani, P.; Nesi, G.; Serni, S.; Forti, G.; Baldi, E. Androgen receptor (AR) expression in prostate cancer and progression of the tumor: Lessons from cell lines, animal models and human specimens. *Steroids* **2012**, *77*, 996–1001. [CrossRef] [PubMed]
7. Mohler, J.L.; Chen, Y.; Hamil, K.; Hall, S.H.; Cidlowski, J.A.; Wilson, E.M.; French, F.S.; Sar, M. Androgen and glucocorticoid receptors in the stroma and epithelium of prostatic hyperplasia and carcinoma. *Clin. Cancer Res.* **1996**, *2*, 889–895. [PubMed]
8. Ricciardelli, C.; Choong, C.S.; Buchanan, G.; Vivekanandan, S.; Neufing, P.; Stahl, J.; Marshall, V.R.; Horsfall, D.J.; Tilley, W.D. Androgen receptor levels in prostate cancer epithelial and peritumoral stromal cells identify non-organ confined disease. *Prostate* **2005**, *63*, 19–28. [CrossRef] [PubMed]
9. Henshall, S.M.; Quinn, D.I.; Lee, C.S.; Head, D.R.; Golovsky, D.; Brenner, P.C.; Delprado, W.; Stricker, P.D.; Grygiel, J.J.; Sutherland, R.L. Altered expression of androgen receptor in the malignant epithelium and adjacent stroma is associated with early relapse in prostate cancer. *Cancer Res.* **2001**, *61*, 423–427. [PubMed]
10. Wikstrom, P.; Marusic, J.; Stattin, P.; Bergh, A. Low stroma androgen receptor level in normal and tumor prostate tissue is related to poor outcome in prostate cancer patients. *Prostate* **2009**, *69*, 799–809. [CrossRef] [PubMed]
11. Olapade-Olaopa, E.O.; MacKay, E.H.; Taub, N.A.; Sandhu, D.P.; Terry, T.R.; Habib, F.K. Malignant transformation of human prostatic epithelium is associated with the loss of androgen receptor immunoreactivity in the surrounding stroma. *Clin. Cancer Res.* **1999**, *5*, 569–576. [PubMed]
12. Leach, D.A.; Need, E.F.; Toivanen, R.; Trotta, A.P.; Palenthorpe, H.M.; Tamblyn, D.J.; Kopsaftis, T.; England, G.M.; Smith, E.; Drew, P.A.; et al. Stromal androgen receptor regulates the composition of the microenvironment to influence prostate cancer outcome. *Oncotarget* **2015**, *6*, 16135–16150. [CrossRef] [PubMed]
13. Leach, D.A.; Trotta, A.P.; Need, E.F.; Risbridger, G.P.; Taylor, R.A.; Buchanan, G. The prognostic value of stromal FK506-binding protein 1 and androgen receptor in prostate cancer outcome. *Prostate* **2017**, *77*, 185–195. [CrossRef] [PubMed]
14. Takeda, H.; Akakura, K.; Masai, M.; Akimoto, S.; Yatani, R.; Shimazaki, J. Androgen receptor content of prostate carcinoma cells estimated by immunohistochemistry is related to prognosis of patients with stage D2 prostate carcinoma. *Cancer* **1996**, *77*, 934–940. [CrossRef]
15. Segawa, N.; Mori, I.; Utsunomiya, H.; Nakamura, M.; Nakamura, Y.; Shan, L.; Kakudo, K.; Katsuoka, Y. Prognostic significance of neuroendocrine differentiation, proliferation activity and androgen receptor expression in prostate cancer. *Pathol. Int.* **2001**, *51*, 452–459. [CrossRef] [PubMed]

16. Pertschuk, L.P.; Schaeffer, H.; Feldman, J.G.; Macchia, R.J.; Kim, Y.D.; Eisenberg, K.; Braithwaite, L.V.; Axiotis, C.A.; Prins, G.; Green, G.L. Immunostaining for prostate cancer androgen receptor in paraffin identifies a subset of men with a poor prognosis. *Lab. Investig.* **1995**, *73*, 302–305. [PubMed]
17. Sweat, S.D.; Pacelli, A.; Bergstralh, E.J.; Slezak, J.M.; Cheng, L.; Bostwick, D.G. Androgen receptor expression in prostate cancer lymph node metastases is predictive of outcome after surgery. *J. Urol.* **1999**, *161*, 1233–1237. [CrossRef]
18. Barboro, P.; Salvi, S.; Rubagotti, A.; Boccardo, S.; Spina, B.; Truini, M.; Carmignani, G.; Introini, C.; Ferrari, N.; Boccardo, F.; et al. Prostate cancer: Prognostic significance of the association of heterogeneous nuclear ribonucleoprotein K and androgen receptor expression. *Int. J. Oncol.* **2014**, *44*, 1589–1598. [CrossRef] [PubMed]
19. Segawa, N.; Nakamura, M.; Shan, L.; Utsunomiya, H.; Nakamura, Y.; Mori, I.; Katsuoka, Y.; Kakudo, K. Expression and somatic mutation on androgen receptor gene in prostate cancer. *Int. J. Urol.* **2002**, *9*, 545–553. [CrossRef] [PubMed]
20. Rosner, I.L.; Ravindranath, L.; Furusato, B.; Chen, Y.; Gao, C.; Cullen, J.; Sesterhenn, I.A.; McLeod, D.G.; Srivastava, S.; Petrovics, G. Higher tumor to benign ratio of the androgen receptor mRNA expression associates with prostate cancer progression after radical prostatectomy. *Urology* **2007**, *70*, 1225–1229. [CrossRef] [PubMed]
21. Cordon-Cardo, C.; Kotsianti, A.; Verbel, D.A.; Teverovskiy, M.; Capodieci, P.; Hamann, S.; Jeffers, Y.; Clayton, M.; Elkhettabi, F.; Khan, F.M.; et al. Improved prediction of prostate cancer recurrence through systems pathology. *J. Clin. Investig.* **2007**, *117*, 1876–1883. [CrossRef] [PubMed]
22. Inoue, T.; Segawa, T.; Shiraishi, T.; Yoshida, T.; Toda, Y.; Yamada, T.; Kinukawa, N.; Kinoshita, H.; Kamoto, T.; Ogawa, O. Androgen receptor, Ki67, and p53 expression in radical prostatectomy specimens predict treatment failure in Japanese population. *Urology* **2005**, *66*, 332–337. [CrossRef] [PubMed]
23. Li, R.; Wheeler, T.; Dai, H.; Frolov, A.; Thompson, T.; Ayala, G. High level of androgen receptor is associated with aggressive clinicopathologic features and decreased biochemical recurrence-free survival in prostate: Cancer patients treated with radical prostatectomy. *Am. J. Surg. Pathol.* **2004**, *28*, 928–934. [CrossRef] [PubMed]
24. Donovan, M.J.; Osman, I.; Khan, F.M.; Vengrenyuk, Y.; Capodieci, P.; Koscuiszka, M.; Anand, A.; Cordon-Cardo, C.; Costa, J.; Scher, H.I. Androgen receptor expression is associated with prostate cancer-specific survival in castrate patients with metastatic disease. *BJU Int.* **2010**, *105*, 462–467. [CrossRef] [PubMed]
25. Qiu, Y.Q.; Leuschner, I.; Braun, P.M. Androgen receptor expression in clinically localized prostate cancer: Immunohistochemistry study and literature review. *Asian J. Androl.* **2008**, *10*, 855–863. [CrossRef] [PubMed]
26. Noordzij, M.A.; Bogdanowicz, J.F.; van Krimpen, C.; van der Kwast, T.H.; van Steenbrugge, G.J. The prognostic value of pretreatment expression of androgen receptor and bcl-2 in hormonally treated prostate cancer patients. *J. Urol.* **1997**, *158*, 1880–1884. [CrossRef]
27. Rades, D.; Setter, C.; Dahl, O.; Schild, S.E.; Noack, F. The prognostic impact of tumor cell expression of estrogen receptor-alpha, progesterone receptor, and androgen receptor in patients irradiated for nonsmall cell lung cancer. *Cancer* **2012**, *118*, 157–163. [CrossRef] [PubMed]
28. Sadi, M.V.; Barrack, E.R. Image analysis of androgen receptor immunostaining in metastatic prostate cancer. Heterogeneity as a predictor of response to hormonal therapy. *Cancer* **1993**, *71*, 2574–2580. [CrossRef]
29. Sterbis, J.R.; Gao, C.; Furusato, B.; Chen, Y.; Shaheduzzaman, S.; Ravindranath, L.; Osborn, D.J.; Rosner, I.L.; Dobi, A.; McLeod, D.G.; et al. Higher expression of the androgen-regulated gene PSA/HK3 mRNA in prostate cancer tissues predicts biochemical recurrence-free survival. *Clin. Cancer Res.* **2008**, *14*, 758–763. [CrossRef] [PubMed]
30. Theodoropoulos, V.E.; Tsigka, A.; Mihalopoulou, A.; Tsoukala, V.; Lazaris, A.C.; Patsouris, E.; Ghikonti, I. Evaluation of neuroendocrine staining and androgen receptor expression in incidental prostatic adenocarcinoma: Prognostic implications. *Urology* **2005**, *66*, 897–902. [CrossRef] [PubMed]
31. Fleischmann, A.; Rocha, C.; Schobinger, S.; Seiler, R.; Wiese, B.; Thalmann, G.N. Androgen receptors are differentially expressed in Gleason patterns of prostate cancer and down-regulated in matched lymph node metastases. *Prostate* **2011**, *71*, 453–460. [CrossRef] [PubMed]
32. Minner, S.; Enodien, M.; Sirma, H.; Luebke, A.M.; Krohn, A.; Mayer, P.S.; Simon, R.; Tennstedt, P.; Muller, J.; Scholz, L.; et al. ERG status is unrelated to PSA recurrence in radically operated prostate cancer in the absence of antihormonal therapy. *Clin. Cancer Res.* **2011**, *17*, 5878–5888. [CrossRef] [PubMed]
33. Sweat, S.D.; Pacelli, A.; Bergstralh, E.J.; Slezak, J.M.; Bostwick, D.G. Androgen receptor expression in prostatic intraepithelial neoplasia and cancer. *J. Urol.* **1999**, *161*, 1229–1232. [CrossRef]

34. Ford, O.H., 3rd; Gregory, C.W.; Kim, D.; Smitherman, A.B.; Mohler, J.L. Androgen receptor gene amplification and protein expression in recurrent prostate cancer. *J. Urol.* **2003**, *170*, 1817–1821. [CrossRef] [PubMed]
35. Choucair, K.; Ejdelman, J.; Brimo, F.; Aprikian, A.; Chevalier, S.; Lapointe, J. PTEN genomic deletion predicts prostate cancer recurrence and is associated with low AR expression and transcriptional activity. *BMC Cancer* **2012**. [CrossRef] [PubMed]
36. Zhao, H.; Coram, M.A.; Nolley, R.; Reese, S.W.; Young, S.R.; Peehl, D.M. Transcript levels of androgen receptor variant AR-V1 or AR-V7 do not predict recurrence in patients with prostate cancer at indeterminate risk for progression. *J. Urol.* **2012**, *188*, 2158–2164. [CrossRef] [PubMed]
37. Miyamoto, K.K.; McSherry, S.A.; Dent, G.A.; Sar, M.; Wilson, E.M.; French, F.S.; Sharief, Y.; Mohler, J.L. Immunohistochemistry of the androgen receptor in human benign and malignant prostate tissue. *J. Urol.* **1993**, *149*, 1015–1019. [PubMed]
38. Schatzl, G.; Madersbacher, S.; Haitel, A.; Gsur, A.; Preyer, M.; Haidinger, G.; Gassner, C.; Ochsner, M.; Marberger, M. Associations of serum testosterone with microvessel density, androgen receptor density and androgen receptor gene polymorphism in prostate cancer. *J. Urol.* **2003**, *169*, 1312–1315. [CrossRef] [PubMed]
39. De Winter, J.A.; Trapman, J.; Brinkmann, A.O.; Boersma, W.J.; Mulder, E.; Schroeder, F.H.; Claassen, E.; van der Kwast, T.H. Androgen receptor heterogeneity in human prostatic carcinomas visualized by immunohistochemistry. *J. Pathol.* **1990**, *160*, 329–332. [CrossRef] [PubMed]
40. Gaston, K.E.; Kim, D.; Singh, S.; Ford, O.H., 3rd; Mohler, J.L. Racial differences in androgen receptor protein expression in men with clinically localized prostate cancer. *J. Urol.* **2003**, *170*, 990–993. [CrossRef] [PubMed]
41. Li, Y.; Li, C.X.; Ye, H.; Chen, F.; Melamed, J.; Peng, Y.; Liu, J.; Wang, Z.; Tsou, H.C.; Wei, J.; et al. Decrease in stromal androgen receptor associates with androgen-independent disease and promotes prostate cancer cell proliferation and invasion. *J. Cell. Mol. Med.* **2008**, *12*, 2790–2798. [CrossRef] [PubMed]
42. Webber, M.M.; Trakul, N.; Thraves, P.S.; Bello-DeOcampo, D.; Chu, W.W.; Storto, P.D.; Huard, T.K.; Rhim, J.S.; Williams, D.E. A human prostatic stromal myofibroblast cell line WPMY-1: A model for stromal-epithelial interactions in prostatic neoplasia. *Carcinogenesis* **1999**, *20*, 1185–1192. [CrossRef] [PubMed]
43. Leach, D.A.; Panagopoulos, V.; Nash, C.; Bevan, C.; Thomson, A.A.; Selth, L.A.; Buchanan, G. Cell-lineage specificity and role of AP-1 in the prostate fibroblast androgen receptor cistrome. *Mol. Cell. Endocrinol.* **2017**, *439*, 261–272. [CrossRef] [PubMed]
44. Henke, A.; Franco, O.E.; Stewart, G.D.; Riddick, A.C.; Katz, E.; Hayward, S.W.; Thomson, A.A. Reduced contractility and motility of prostatic cancer-associated fibroblasts after inhibition of heat shock protein 90. *Cancers* **2016**, *8*, 77. [CrossRef] [PubMed]
45. Leach, D.A.; Need, E.F.; Trotta, A.P.; Grubisha, M.J.; DeFranco, D.B.; Buchanan, G. Hic-5 influences genomic and non-genomic actions of the androgen receptor in prostate myofibroblasts. *Mol. Cell. Endocrinol.* **2014**, *384*, 185–199. [CrossRef] [PubMed]
46. Bebermeier, J.H.; Brooks, J.D.; DePrimo, S.E.; Werner, R.; Deppe, U.; Demeter, J.; Hiort, O.; Holterhus, P.M. Cell-line and tissue-specific signatures of androgen receptor-coregulator transcription. *J. Mol. Med. (Berl.)* **2006**, *84*, 919–931. [CrossRef] [PubMed]
47. Gerhardt, J.; Montani, M.; Wild, P.; Beer, M.; Huber, F.; Hermanns, T.; Muntener, M.; Kristiansen, G. FOXA1 promotes tumor progression in prostate cancer and represents a novel hallmark of castration-resistant prostate cancer. *Am. J. Pathol.* **2012**, *180*, 848–861. [CrossRef] [PubMed]
48. Jin, H.J.; Zhao, J.C.; Wu, L.; Kim, J.; Yu, J. Cooperativity and equilibrium with FOXA1 define the androgen receptor transcriptional program. *Nat. Commun.* **2014**. [CrossRef] [PubMed]
49. Robinson, J.L.; Carroll, J.S. FoxA1 is a key mediator of hormonal response in breast and prostate cancer. *Front. Endocrinol.* **2012**. [CrossRef] [PubMed]
50. Sahu, B.; Laakso, M.; Pihlajamaa, P.; Ovaska, K.; Sinielnikov, I.; Hautaniemi, S.; Janne, O.A. FoxA1 specifies unique androgen and glucocorticoid receptor binding events in prostate cancer cells. *Cancer Res.* **2013**, *73*, 1570–1580. [CrossRef] [PubMed]
51. Hayward, S.W.; Baskin, L.S.; Haughney, P.C.; Cunha, A.R.; Foster, B.A.; Dahiya, R.; Prins, G.S.; Cunha, G.R. Epithelial development in the rat ventral prostate, anterior prostate and seminal vesicle. *Acta Anat. (Basel)* **1996**, *155*, 81–93. [CrossRef] [PubMed]
52. Hayward, S.W.; Cunha, G.R.; Dahiya, R. Normal development and carcinogenesis of the prostate. A unifying hypothesis. *Ann. N. Y. Acad. Sci.* **1996**, *784*, 50–62. [CrossRef] [PubMed]

53. Bierhoff, E.; Walljasper, U.; Hofmann, D.; Vogel, J.; Wernert, N.; Pfeifer, U. Morphological analogies of fetal prostate stroma and stromal nodules in BPH. *Prostate* **1997**, *31*, 234–240. [CrossRef]
54. Cunha, G.R. Tissue interactions between epithelium and mesenchyme of urogenital and integumental origin. *Anat. Rec.* **1972**, *172*, 529–541. [CrossRef] [PubMed]
55. Chung, L.W.; Cunha, G.R. Stromal-epithelial interactions: II. Regulation of prostatic growth by embryonic urogenital sinus mesenchyme. *Prostate* **1983**, *4*, 503–511. [CrossRef] [PubMed]
56. Yu, S.; Zhang, C.; Lin, C.C.; Niu, Y.; Lai, K.P.; Chang, H.C.; Yeh, S. Altered prostate epithelial development and IGF-1 signal in mice lacking the androgen receptor in stromal smooth muscle cells. *Prostate* **2011**, *71*, 517–524. [CrossRef] [PubMed]
57. Donjacour, A.A.; Cunha, G.R. Assessment of prostatic protein secretion in tissue recombinants made of urogenital sinus mesenchyme and urothelium from normal or androgen-insensitive mice. *Endocrinology* **1993**, *132*, 2342–2350. [PubMed]
58. Cunha, G.R. Role of mesenchymal-epithelial interactions in normal and abnormal development of the mammary gland and prostate. *Cancer* **1994**, *74*, 1030–1044. [CrossRef]
59. Hayward, S.W.; Rosen, M.A.; Cunha, G.R. Stromal-epithelial interactions in the normal and neoplastic prostate. *Br. J. Urol.* **1997**, *79*, 18–26. [CrossRef] [PubMed]
60. Cano, P.; Godoy, A.; Escamilla, R.; Dhir, R.; Onate, S.A. Stromal-epithelial cell interactions and androgen receptor-coregulator recruitment is altered in the tissue microenvironment of prostate cancer. *Cancer Res.* **2007**, *67*, 511–519. [CrossRef] [PubMed]
61. Arnold, J.T.; Gray, N.E.; Jacobowitz, K.; Viswanathan, L.; Cheung, P.W.; McFann, K.K.; Le, H.; Blackman, M.R. Human prostate stromal cells stimulate increased PSA production in DHEA-treated prostate cancer epithelial cells. *J. Steroid Biochem. Mol. Biol.* **2008**, *111*, 240–246. [CrossRef] [PubMed]
62. Cooke, P.S.; Young, P.; Hess, R.A.; Cunha, G.R. Estrogen receptor expression in developing epididymis, efferent ductules, and other male reproductive organs. *Endocrinology* **1991**, *128*, 2874–2879. [CrossRef] [PubMed]
63. Cooke, P.S.; Young, P.; Cunha, G.R. Androgen receptor expression in developing male reproductive organs. *Endocrinology* **1991**, *128*, 2867–2873. [CrossRef] [PubMed]
64. Kurita, T.; Young, P.; Brody, J.R.; Lydon, J.P.; O'Malley, B.W.; Cunha, G.R. Stromal progesterone receptors mediate the inhibitory effects of progesterone on estrogen-induced uterine epithelial cell deoxyribonucleic acid synthesis. *Endocrinology* **1998**, *139*, 4708–4713. [CrossRef] [PubMed]
65. Sugimura, Y.; Cunha, G.R.; Bigsby, R.M. Androgenic induction of DNA synthesis in prostatic glands induced in the urothelium of testicular feminized (Tfm/Y) mice. *Prostate* **1986**, *9*, 217–225. [CrossRef] [PubMed]
66. Nieto, C.M.; Rider, L.C.; Cramer, S.D. Influence of stromal-epithelial interactions on androgen action. *Endocr. Relat. Cancer* **2014**, *21*, T147–T160. [CrossRef] [PubMed]
67. Wen, S.; Chang, H.C.; Tian, J.; Shang, Z.; Niu, Y.; Chang, C. Stromal androgen receptor roles in the development of normal prostate, benign prostate hyperplasia, and prostate cancer. *Am. J. Pathol.* **2015**, *185*, 293–301. [CrossRef] [PubMed]
68. Singh, M.; Jha, R.; Melamed, J.; Shapiro, E.; Hayward, S.W.; Lee, P. Stromal androgen receptor in prostate development and cancer. *Am. J. Pathol.* **2014**, *184*, 2598–2607. [CrossRef] [PubMed]
69. Wang, Y.; Sudilovsky, D.; Zhang, B.; Haughney, P.C.; Rosen, M.A.; Wu, D.S.; Cunha, T.J.; Dahiya, R.; Cunha, G.R.; Hayward, S.W. A human prostatic epithelial model of hormonal carcinogenesis. *Cancer Res.* **2001**, *61*, 6064–6072. [PubMed]
70. Ricke, E.A.; Williams, K.; Lee, Y.F.; Couto, S.; Wang, Y.; Hayward, S.W.; Cunha, G.R.; Ricke, W.A. Androgen hormone action in prostatic carcinogenesis: Stromal androgen receptors mediate prostate cancer progression, malignant transformation and metastasis. *Carcinogenesis* **2012**, *33*, 1391–1398. [CrossRef] [PubMed]
71. Lai, K.P.; Yamashita, S.; Huang, C.K.; Yeh, S.; Chang, C. Loss of stromal androgen receptor leads to suppressed prostate tumourigenesis via modulation of pro-inflammatory cytokines/chemokines. *EMBO Mol. Med.* **2012**, *4*, 791–807. [CrossRef] [PubMed]
72. Niu, Y.; Altuwaijri, S.; Yeh, S.; Lai, K.P.; Yu, S.; Chuang, K.H.; Huang, S.P.; Lardy, H.; Chang, C. Targeting the stromal androgen receptor in primary prostate tumors at earlier stages. *Proc. Natl. Acad. Sci. USA* **2008**, *105*, 12188–12193. [CrossRef] [PubMed]
73. Olapade-Olaopa, E.O.; Muronda, C.A.; MacKay, E.H.; Danso, A.P.; Sandhu, D.P.; Terry, T.R.; Habib, F.K. Androgen receptor protein expression in prostatic tissues in Black and Caucasian men. *Prostate* **2004**, *59*, 460–468. [CrossRef] [PubMed]

74. Hay, C.W.; McEwan, I.J. The impact of point mutations in the human androgen receptor: Classification of mutations on the basis of transcriptional activity. *PLoS ONE* **2012**, *7*, e32514. [CrossRef] [PubMed]
75. Keil, K.P.; Abler, L.L.; Laporta, J.; Altmann, H.M.; Yang, B.; Jarrard, D.F.; Hernandez, L.L.; Vezina, C.M. Androgen receptor DNA methylation regulates the timing and androgen sensitivity of mouse prostate ductal development. *Dev. Biol.* **2014**, *396*, 237–245. [CrossRef] [PubMed]
76. Shenk, J.L.; Fisher, C.J.; Chen, S.Y.; Zhou, X.F.; Tillman, K.; Shemshedini, L. p53 represses androgen-induced transactivation of prostate-specific antigen by disrupting hAR amino- to carboxyl-terminal interaction. *J. Biol. Chem.* **2001**, *276*, 38472–38479. [CrossRef] [PubMed]
77. Jia, Z.; Rahmatpanah, F.B.; Chen, X.; Lernhardt, W.; Wang, Y.; Xia, X.Q.; Sawyers, A.; Sutton, M.; McClelland, M.; Mercola, D. Expression changes in the stroma of prostate cancer predict subsequent relapse. *PLoS ONE* **2012**, *7*, e41371. [CrossRef]
78. Lee, S.O.; Chun, J.Y.; Nadiminty, N.; Lou, W.; Gao, A.C. Interleukin-6 undergoes transition from growth inhibitor associated with neuroendocrine differentiation to stimulator accompanied by androgen receptor activation during LNCaP prostate cancer cell progression. *Prostate* **2007**, *67*, 764–773. [CrossRef] [PubMed]
79. Jia, L.; Choong, C.S.; Ricciardelli, C.; Kim, J.; Tilley, W.D.; Coetzee, G.A. Androgen receptor signaling: Mechanism of interleukin-6 inhibition. *Cancer Res.* **2004**, *64*, 2619–2626. [CrossRef] [PubMed]
80. Kumar, B.; Khaleghzadegan, S.; Mears, B.; Hatano, K.; Kudrolli, T.A.; Chowdhury, W.H.; Yeater, D.B.; Ewing, C.M.; Luo, J.; Isaacs, W.B.; et al. Identification of miR-30b-3p and miR-30d-5p as direct regulators of Androgen Receptor Signaling in Prostate Cancer by complementary functional microRNA library screening. *Oncotarget* **2016**, *7*, 72593–72607. [CrossRef] [PubMed]
81. Ostling, P.; Leivonen, S.K.; Aakula, A.; Kohonen, P.; Makela, R.; Hagman, Z.; Edsjo, A.; Kangaspeska, S.; Edgren, H.; Nicorici, D.; et al. Systematic analysis of microRNAs targeting the androgen receptor in prostate cancer cells. *Cancer Res.* **2011**, *71*, 1956–1967. [CrossRef] [PubMed]
82. Fletcher, C.E.; Dart, D.A.; Bevan, C.L. Interplay between steroid signalling and microRNAs: Implications for hormone-dependent cancers. *Endocr. Relat. Cancer* **2014**, *21*, R409–R429. [CrossRef] [PubMed]
83. Bhowmick, R.; Girotti, A.W. Pro-survival and pro-growth effects of stress-induced nitric oxide in a prostate cancer photodynamic therapy model. *Cancer Lett.* **2014**, *343*, 115–122. [CrossRef] [PubMed]
84. Fahey, J.M.; Girotti, A.W. Accelerated migration and invasion of prostate cancer cells after a photodynamic therapy-like challenge: Role of nitric oxide. *Nitric Oxide* **2015**, *49*, 47–55. [CrossRef] [PubMed]
85. Cronauer, M.V.; Ince, Y.; Engers, R.; Rinnab, L.; Weidemann, W.; Suschek, C.V.; Burchardt, M.; Kleinert, H.; Wiedenmann, J.; Sies, H.; et al. Nitric oxide-mediated inhibition of androgen receptor activity: Possible implications for prostate cancer progression. *Oncogene* **2007**, *26*, 1875–1884. [CrossRef] [PubMed]
86. Shigemura, K.; Isotani, S.; Wang, R.; Fujisawa, M.; Gotoh, A.; Marshall, F.F.; Zhau, H.E.; Chung, L.W. Soluble factors derived from stroma activated androgen receptor phosphorylation in human prostate LNCaP cells: Roles of ERK/MAP kinase. *Prostate* **2009**, *69*, 949–955. [CrossRef] [PubMed]
87. Tanner, M.J.; Welliver, R.C., Jr.; Chen, M.; Shtutman, M.; Godoy, A.; Smith, G.; Mian, B.M.; Buttyan, R. Effects of androgen receptor and androgen on gene expression in prostate stromal fibroblasts and paracrine signaling to prostate cancer cells. *PLoS ONE* **2011**, *6*, e16027. [CrossRef] [PubMed]
88. Yu, S.; Xia, S.; Yang, D.; Wang, K.; Yeh, S.; Gao, Z.; Chang, C. Androgen receptor in human prostate cancer-associated fibroblasts promotes prostate cancer epithelial cell growth and invasion. *Med. Oncol.* **2013**. [CrossRef] [PubMed]
89. Niu, Y.; Altuwaijri, S.; Lai, K.P.; Wu, C.T.; Ricke, W.A.; Messing, E.M.; Yao, J.; Yeh, S.; Chang, C. Androgen receptor is a tumor suppressor and proliferator in prostate cancer. *Proc. Natl. Acad. Sci. USA* **2008**, *105*, 12182–12187. [CrossRef] [PubMed]
90. Aprelikova, O.; Palla, J.; Hibler, B.; Yu, X.; Greer, Y.E.; Yi, M.; Stephens, R.; Maxwell, G.L.; Jazaeri, A.; Risinger, J.I.; et al. Silencing of miR-148a in cancer-associated fibroblasts results in WNT10B-mediated stimulation of tumor cell motility. *Oncogene* **2013**, *32*, 3246–3253. [CrossRef] [PubMed]
91. Placencio, V.R.; Sharif-Afshar, A.R.; Li, X.; Huang, H.; Uwamariya, C.; Neilson, E.G.; Shen, M.M.; Matusik, R.J.; Hayward, S.W.; Bhowmick, N.A. Stromal transforming growth factor-beta signaling mediates prostatic response to androgen ablation by paracrine Wnt activity. *Cancer Res.* **2008**, *68*, 4709–4718. [CrossRef] [PubMed]
92. Murashima, A.; Kishigami, S.; Thomson, A.; Yamada, G. Androgens and mammalian male reproductive tract development. *Biochim. Biophys. Acta* **2015**, *1849*, 163–170. [CrossRef] [PubMed]

93. Yu, S.; Yeh, C.R.; Niu, Y.; Chang, H.C.; Tsai, Y.C.; Moses, H.L.; Shyr, C.R.; Chang, C.; Yeh, S. Altered prostate epithelial development in mice lacking the androgen receptor in stromal fibroblasts. *Prostate* **2012**, *72*, 437–449. [CrossRef] [PubMed]
94. Saylor, P.J.; Kozak, K.R.; Smith, M.R.; Ancukiewicz, M.A.; Efstathiou, J.A.; Zietman, A.L.; Jain, R.K.; Duda, D.G. Changes in biomarkers of inflammation and angiogenesis during androgen deprivation therapy for prostate cancer. *Oncologist* **2012**, *17*, 212–219. [CrossRef] [PubMed]
95. Saylor, P.J.; Karoly, E.D.; Smith, M.R. Prospective study of changes in the metabolomic profiles of men during their first three months of androgen deprivation therapy for prostate cancer. *Clin. Cancer Res.* **2012**, *18*, 3677–3685. [CrossRef] [PubMed]
96. Ohlson, N.; Bergh, A.; Stattin, P.; Wikstrom, P. Castration-induced epithelial cell death in human prostate tissue is related to locally reduced IGF-1 levels. *Prostate* **2007**, *67*, 32–40. [CrossRef] [PubMed]
97. Bhowmick, N.A.; Neilson, E.G.; Moses, H.L. Stromal fibroblasts in cancer initiation and progression. *Nature* **2004**, *432*, 332–337. [CrossRef] [PubMed]
98. Diener, K.R.; Need, E.F.; Buchanan, G.; Hayball, J.D. TGF-beta signalling and immunity in prostate tumourigenesis. *Expert Opin. Ther. Targets* **2010**, *14*, 179–192. [CrossRef] [PubMed]
99. Berry, P.A.; Maitland, N.J.; Collins, A.T. Androgen receptor signalling in prostate: Effects of stromal factors on normal and cancer stem cells. *Mol. Cell. Endocrinol.* **2008**, *288*, 30–37. [CrossRef] [PubMed]
100. Kwabi-Addo, B.; Ozen, M.; Ittmann, M. The role of fibroblast growth factors and their receptors in prostate cancer. *Endocr. Relat. Cancer* **2004**, *11*, 709–724. [CrossRef] [PubMed]
101. Tidehag, V.; Hammarsten, P.; Egevad, L.; Granfors, T.; Stattin, P.; Leanderson, T.; Wikstrom, P.; Josefsson, A.; Hagglof, C.; Bergh, A. High density of S100A9 positive inflammatory cells in prostate cancer stroma is associated with poor outcome. *Eur. J. Cancer* **2014**, *50*, 1829–1835. [CrossRef] [PubMed]
102. Bernoulli, J.; Yatkin, E.; Konkol, Y.; Talvitie, E.M.; Santti, R.; Streng, T. Prostatic inflammation and obstructive voiding in the adult Noble rat: Impact of the testosterone to estradiol ratio in serum. *Prostate* **2008**, *68*, 1296–1306. [CrossRef] [PubMed]
103. Bernoulli, J.; Yatkin, E.; Laakso, A.; Anttinen, M.; Bosland, M.; Vega, K.; Kallajoki, M.; Santti, R.; Pylkkanen, L. Histopathological evidence for an association of inflammation with ductal pin-like lesions but not with ductal adenocarcinoma in the prostate of the noble rat. *Prostate* **2008**, *68*, 728–739. [CrossRef] [PubMed]
104. Kaufman, J.M.; Vermeulen, A. The decline of androgen levels in elderly men and its clinical and therapeutic implications. *Endocr. Rev.* **2005**, *26*, 833–876. [CrossRef] [PubMed]
105. Jia, Y.L.; Liu, X.; Yan, J.Y.; Chong, L.M.; Li, L.; Ma, A.C.; Zhou, L.; Sun, Z.Y. The alteration of inflammatory markers and apoptosis on chronic prostatitis induced by estrogen and androgen. *Int. Urol. Nephrol.* **2015**, *47*, 39–46. [CrossRef] [PubMed]
106. Comito, G.; Giannoni, E.; Segura, C.P.; Barcellos-de-Souza, P.; Raspollini, M.R.; Baroni, G.; Lanciotti, M.; Serni, S.; Chiarugi, P. Cancer-associated fibroblasts and M2-polarized macrophages synergize during prostate carcinoma progression. *Oncogene* **2014**, *33*, 2423–2431. [CrossRef] [PubMed]
107. Ganesan, K.; Balachandran, C.; Manohar, B.M.; Puvanakrishnan, R. Effects of testosterone, estrogen and progesterone on TNF-alpha mediated cellular damage in rat arthritic synovial fibroblasts. *Rheumatol. Int.* **2012**, *32*, 3181–3188. [CrossRef] [PubMed]
108. Xu, J.; Itoh, Y.; Hayashi, H.; Takii, T.; Miyazawa, K.; Onozaki, K. Dihydrotestosterone inhibits interleukin-1alpha or tumor necrosis factor alpha-induced proinflammatory cytokine production via androgen receptor-dependent inhibition of nuclear factor-kappaB activation in rheumatoid fibroblast-like synovial cell line. *Biol. Pharm. Bull.* **2011**, *34*, 1724–1730. [CrossRef] [PubMed]
109. De Wever, O.; Nguyen, Q.D.; van Hoorde, L.; Bracke, M.; Bruyneel, E.; Gespach, C.; Mareel, M. Tenascin-C and SF/HGF produced by myofibroblasts in vitro provide convergent pro-invasive signals to human colon cancer cells through RhoA and Rac. *FASEB J.* **2004**, *18*, 1016–1018. [PubMed]
110. Denys, H.; Derycke, L.; Hendrix, A.; Westbroek, W.; Gheldof, A.; Narine, K.; Pauwels, P.; Gespach, C.; Bracke, M.; De Wever, O. Differential impact of TGF-beta and EGF on fibroblast differentiation and invasion reciprocally promotes colon cancer cell invasion. *Cancer Lett.* **2008**, *266*, 263–274. [CrossRef] [PubMed]
111. Zhang, Y.; Xie, R.L.; Croce, C.M.; Stein, J.L.; Lian, J.B.; van Wijnen, A.J.; Stein, G.S. A program of microRNAs controls osteogenic lineage progression by targeting transcription factor Runx2. *Proc. Natl. Acad. Sci. USA* **2011**, *108*, 9863–9868. [CrossRef] [PubMed]

112. Cai, J.; Tang, H.; Xu, L.; Wang, X.; Yang, C.; Ruan, S.; Guo, J.; Hu, S.; Wang, Z. Fibroblasts in omentum activated by tumor cells promote ovarian cancer growth, adhesion and invasiveness. *Carcinogenesis* **2012**, *33*, 20–29. [CrossRef] [PubMed]
113. Fuyuhiro, Y.; Yashiro, M.; Noda, S.; Matsuoka, J.; Hasegawa, T.; Kato, Y.; Sawada, T.; Hirakawa, K. Cancer-associated orthotopic myofibroblasts stimulates the motility of gastric carcinoma cells. *Cancer Sci.* **2012**, *103*, 797–805. [CrossRef] [PubMed]
114. Alcoser, T.A.; Bordeleau, F.; Carey, S.P.; Lampi, M.C.; Kowal, D.R.; Somasegar, S.; Varma, S.; Shin, S.J.; Reinhart-King, C.A. Probing the biophysical properties of primary breast tumor-derived fibroblasts. *Cell. Mol. Bioeng.* **2015**, *8*, 76–85. [CrossRef] [PubMed]
115. Gaggioli, C.; Hooper, S.; Hidalgo-Carcedo, C.; Grosse, R.; Marshall, J.F.; Harrington, K.; Sahai, E. Fibroblast-led collective invasion of carcinoma cells with differing roles for RhoGTPases in leading and following cells. *Nat. Cell Biol.* **2007**, *9*, 1392–1400. [CrossRef] [PubMed]
116. Coulson-Thomas, V.J.; Gesteira, T.F.; Coulson-Thomas, Y.M.; Vicente, C.M.; Tersariol, I.L.; Nader, H.B.; Toma, L. Fibroblast and prostate tumor cell cross-talk: Fibroblast differentiation, TGF-beta, and extracellular matrix down-regulation. *Exp. Cell Res.* **2010**, *316*, 3207–3226. [CrossRef] [PubMed]
117. Dang, T.T.; Prechtl, A.M.; Pearson, G.W. Breast cancer subtype-specific interactions with the microenvironment dictate mechanisms of invasion. *Cancer Res.* **2011**, *71*, 6857–6866. [CrossRef] [PubMed]
118. Shieh, A.C.; Rozansky, H.A.; Hinz, B.; Swartz, M.A. Tumor cell invasion is promoted by interstitial flow-induced matrix priming by stromal fibroblasts. *Cancer Res.* **2011**, *71*, 790–800. [CrossRef] [PubMed]
119. Lin, B.; Yin, T.; Wu, Y.I.; Inoue, T.; Levchenko, A. Interplay between chemotaxis and contact inhibition of locomotion determines exploratory cell migration. *Nat. Commun.* **2015**. [CrossRef] [PubMed]
120. Sun, X.; Cheng, G.; Hao, M.; Zheng, J.; Zhou, X.; Zhang, J.; Taichman, R.S.; Pienta, K.J.; Wang, J. CXCL12/CXCR4/CXCR7 chemokine axis and cancer progression. *Cancer Metastasis Rev.* **2010**, *29*, 709–722. [CrossRef] [PubMed]
121. Grimm, S.; Jennek, S.; Singh, R.; Enkelmann, A.; Junker, K.; Rippaus, N.; Berndt, A.; Friedrich, K. Malignancy of bladder cancer cells is enhanced by tumor-associated fibroblasts through a multifaceted cytokine-chemokine loop. *Exp. Cell Res.* **2015**, *335*, 1–11. [CrossRef] [PubMed]
122. Li, X.; Sterling, J.A.; Fan, K.H.; Vessella, R.L.; Shyr, Y.; Hayward, S.W.; Matrisian, L.M.; Bhowmick, N.A. Loss of TGF-beta responsiveness in prostate stromal cells alters chemokine levels and facilitates the development of mixed osteoblastic/osteolytic bone lesions. *Mol. Cancer Res.* **2012**, *10*, 494–503. [CrossRef] [PubMed]
123. Aragona, M.; Panciera, T.; Manfrin, A.; Giulitti, S.; Michielin, F.; Elvassore, N.; Dupont, S.; Piccolo, S. A mechanical checkpoint controls multicellular growth through YAP/TAZ regulation by actin-processing factors. *Cell* **2013**, *154*, 1047–1059. [CrossRef] [PubMed]
124. Hynes, R.O. The extracellular matrix: Not just pretty fibrils. *Science* **2009**, *326*, 1216–1219. [CrossRef] [PubMed]
125. Chao, Y.H.; Tsuang, Y.H.; Sun, J.S.; Sun, M.G.; Chen, M.H. Centrifugal force induces human ligamentum flavum fibroblasts inflammation through activation of JNK and p38 pathways. *Connect. Tissue Res.* **2012**, *53*, 422–429. [CrossRef] [PubMed]
126. Chao, Y.H.; Yang, H.S.; Sun, M.G.; Sun, J.S.; Chen, M.H. Elastin-derived peptides induce inflammatory responses through the activation of NF-kappaB in human ligamentum flavum cells. *Connect. Tissue Res.* **2012**, *53*, 407–414. [CrossRef] [PubMed]
127. Maller, O.; DuFort, C.C.; Weaver, V.M. YAP forces fibroblasts to feel the tension. *Nat. Cell Biol.* **2013**, *15*, 570–572. [CrossRef] [PubMed]
128. Provenzano, P.P.; Inman, D.R.; Eliceiri, K.W.; Knittel, J.G.; Yan, L.; Rueden, C.T.; White, J.G.; Keely, P.J. Collagen density promotes mammary tumor initiation and progression. *BMC Med.* **2008**. [CrossRef] [PubMed]
129. Levental, K.R.; Yu, H.; Kass, L.; Lakins, J.N.; Egeblad, M.; Erler, J.T.; Fong, S.F.; Csiszar, K.; Giaccia, A.; Weninger, W.; et al. Matrix crosslinking forces tumor progression by enhancing integrin signaling. *Cell* **2009**, *139*, 891–906. [CrossRef] [PubMed]
130. Nguyen-Ngoc, K.V.; Cheung, K.J.; Brenot, A.; Shamir, E.R.; Gray, R.S.; Hines, W.C.; Yaswen, P.; Werb, Z.; Ewald, A.J. ECM microenvironment regulates collective migration and local dissemination in normal and malignant mammary epithelium. *Proc. Natl. Acad. Sci. USA* **2012**, *109*, E2595–E2604. [CrossRef] [PubMed]
131. Kakkad, S.M.; Solaiyappan, M.; O'Rourke, B.; Stasinopoulos, I.; Ackerstaff, E.; Raman, V.; Bhujwalla, Z.M.; Glunde, K. Hypoxic tumor microenvironments reduce collagen I fiber density. *Neoplasia* **2010**, *12*, 608–617. [CrossRef] [PubMed]

132. Carey, S.P.; Kraning-Rush, C.M.; Williams, R.M.; Reinhart-King, C.A. Biophysical control of invasive tumor cell behavior by extracellular matrix microarchitecture. *Biomaterials* **2012**, *33*, 4157–4165. [CrossRef] [PubMed]
133. Carey, S.P.; D'Alfonso, T.M.; Shin, S.J.; Reinhart-King, C.A. Mechanobiology of tumor invasion: Engineering meets oncology. *Crit. Rev. Oncol. Hematol.* **2012**, *83*, 170–183. [CrossRef] [PubMed]
134. Wolf, K.; Te Lindert, M.; Krause, M.; Alexander, S.; Te Riet, J.; Willis, A.L.; Hoffman, R.M.; Figdor, C.G.; Weiss, S.J.; Friedl, P. Physical limits of cell migration: Control by ECM space and nuclear deformation and tuning by proteolysis and traction force. *J. Cell Biol.* **2013**, *201*, 1069–1084. [CrossRef] [PubMed]
135. Bruni-Cardoso, A.; Augusto, T.M.; Pravatta, H.; Damas-Souza, D.M.; Carvalho, H.F. Stromal remodelling is required for progressive involution of the rat ventral prostate after castration: Identification of a matrix metalloproteinase-dependent apoptotic wave. *Int. J. Androl.* **2010**, *33*, 686–695. [CrossRef] [PubMed]
136. Justulin, L.A., Jr.; Delella, F.K.; Felisbino, S.L. Doxazosin reduces cell proliferation and increases collagen fibers in rat prostatic lobes. *Cell Tissue Res.* **2008**, *332*, 171–183. [CrossRef] [PubMed]
137. Justulin, L.A., Jr.; Acquaro, C.; Carvalho, R.F.; Silva, M.D.; Felisbino, S.L. Combined effect of the finasteride and doxazosin on rat ventral prostate morphology and physiology. *Int. J. Androl.* **2010**, *33*, 489–499. [CrossRef] [PubMed]
138. Delella, F.K.; Justulin, L.A., Jr.; Felisbino, S.L. Finasteride treatment alters MMP-2 and -9 gene expression and activity in the rat ventral prostate. *Int. J. Androl.* **2010**, *33*, e114–e122. [CrossRef] [PubMed]
139. Li, S.C.; Chen, G.F.; Chan, P.S.; Choi, H.L.; Ho, S.M.; Chan, F.L. Altered expression of extracellular matrix and proteinases in Noble rat prostate gland after long-term treatment with sex steroids. *Prostate* **2001**, *49*, 58–71. [CrossRef] [PubMed]
140. Charras, G.; Sahai, E. Physical influences of the extracellular environment on cell migration. *Nat. Rev. Mol. Cell Biol.* **2014**, *15*, 813–824. [CrossRef] [PubMed]
141. Sieh, S.; Taubenberger, A.V.; Rizzi, S.C.; Sadowski, M.; Lehman, M.L.; Rockstroh, A.; An, J.; Clements, J.A.; Nelson, C.C.; Hutmacher, D.W. Phenotypic characterization of prostate cancer LNCaP cells cultured within a bioengineered microenvironment. *PLoS ONE* **2012**, *7*, e40217. [CrossRef] [PubMed]
142. Zaman, M.H.; Trapani, L.M.; Sieminski, A.L.; Mackellar, D.; Gong, H.; Kamm, R.D.; Wells, A.; Lauffenburger, D.A.; Matsudaira, P. Migration of tumor cells in 3D matrices is governed by matrix stiffness along with cell-matrix adhesion and proteolysis. *Proc. Natl. Acad. Sci. USA* **2006**, *103*, 10889–10894. [CrossRef] [PubMed]
143. Sabeh, F.; Shimizu-Hirota, R.; Weiss, S.J. Protease-dependent versus -independent cancer cell invasion programs: Three-dimensional amoeboid movement revisited. *J. Cell Biol.* **2009**, *185*, 11–19. [CrossRef] [PubMed]
144. Tozluoglu, M.; Tournier, A.L.; Jenkins, R.P.; Hooper, S.; Bates, P.A.; Sahai, E. Matrix geometry determines optimal cancer cell migration strategy and modulates response to interventions. *Nat. Cell Biol.* **2013**, *15*, 751–762. [CrossRef] [PubMed]
145. Sahai, E. Mechanisms of cancer cell invasion. *Curr. Opin. Genet. Dev.* **2005**, *15*, 87–96. [CrossRef] [PubMed]
146. Cooperberg, M.R.; Broering, J.M.; Kantoff, P.W.; Carroll, P.R. Contemporary trends in low risk prostate cancer: Risk assessment and treatment. *J. Urol.* **2007**, *178*, S14–S19. [CrossRef] [PubMed]
147. Zelefsky, M.J.; Leibel, S.A.; Burman, C.M.; Kutcher, G.J.; Harrison, A.; Happersett, L.; Fuks, Z. Neoadjuvant hormonal therapy improves the therapeutic ratio in patients with bulky prostatic cancer treated with three-dimensional conformal radiation therapy. *Int. J. Radiat. Oncol. Biol. Phys.* **1994**, *29*, 755–761. [CrossRef]
148. Henderson, A.; Laing, R.W.; Langley, S.E. Identification of pubic arch interference in prostate brachytherapy: Simplifying the transrectal ultrasound technique. *Brachytherapy* **2003**, *2*, 240–245. [CrossRef] [PubMed]
149. Cooperberg, M.R.; Vickers, A.J.; Broering, J.M.; Carroll, P.R. Comparative risk-adjusted mortality outcomes after primary surgery, radiotherapy, or androgen-deprivation therapy for localized prostate cancer. *Cancer* **2010**, *116*, 5226–5234. [CrossRef] [PubMed]
150. Lu-Yao, G.L.; Albertsen, P.C.; Moore, D.F.; Shih, W.; Lin, Y.; DiPaola, R.S.; Yao, S.L. Survival following primary androgen deprivation therapy among men with localized prostate cancer. *JAMA* **2008**, *300*, 173–181. [CrossRef] [PubMed]
151. Wong, Y.N.; Freedland, S.J.; Egleston, B.; Vapiwala, N.; Uzzo, R.; Armstrong, K. The role of primary androgen deprivation therapy in localized prostate cancer. *Eur. Urol.* **2009**, *56*, 609–616. [CrossRef] [PubMed]
152. Studer, U.E.; Whelan, P.; Albrecht, W.; Casselman, J.; de Reijke, T.; Hauri, D.; Loidl, W.; Isorna, S.; Sundaram, S.K.; Debois, M.; et al. Immediate or deferred androgen deprivation for patients with prostate cancer not suitable for local treatment with curative intent: European Organisation for Research and Treatment of Cancer (EORTC) Trial 30891. *J. Clin. Oncol.* **2006**, *24*, 1868–1876. [CrossRef] [PubMed]

153. Lu-Yao, G.L.; Albertsen, P.C.; Li, H.; Moore, D.F.; Shih, W.; Lin, Y.; Dipaola, R.S.; Yao, S.L. Does primary androgen-deprivation therapy delay the receipt of secondary cancer therapy for localized prostate cancer? *Eur. Urol.* **2012**, *62*, 966–972. [CrossRef] [PubMed]
154. Labrie, F.; Candas, B.; Gomez, J.L.; Cusan, L. Can combined androgen blockade provide long-term control or possible cure of localized prostate cancer? *Urology* **2002**, *60*, 115–119. [CrossRef]
155. Akaza, H.; Homma, Y.; Usami, M.; Hirao, Y.; Tsushima, T.; Okada, K.; Yokoyama, M.; Ohashi, Y.; Aso, Y. Efficacy of primary hormone therapy for localized or locally advanced prostate cancer: Results of a 10-year follow-up. *BJU Int.* **2006**, *98*, 573–579. [CrossRef] [PubMed]
156. Morris, M.J.; Eisenberger, M.A.; Pili, R.; Denmeade, S.R.; Rathkopf, D.; Slovin, S.F.; Farrelly, J.; Chudow, J.J.; Vincent, M.; Scher, H.I.; et al. A phase I/IIA study of AGS-PSCA for castration-resistant prostate cancer. *Ann. Oncol.* **2012**, *23*, 2714–2719. [CrossRef] [PubMed]
157. Byar, D.P.; Corle, D.K. Hormone therapy for prostate cancer: Results of the Veterans Administration Cooperative Urological Research Group studies. *NCI Monogr.* **1988**, *7*, 165–170.
158. Merglen, A.; Schmidlin, F.; Fioretta, G.; Verkooijen, H.M.; Rapiti, E.; Zanetti, R.; Miralbell, R.; Bouchardy, C. Short- and long-term mortality with localized prostate cancer. *Arch. Intern. Med.* **2007**, *167*, 1944–1950. [CrossRef] [PubMed]
159. Zhou, E.H.; Ellis, R.J.; Cherullo, E.; Colussi, V.; Xu, F.; Chen, W.D.; Gupta, S.; Whalen, C.C.; Bodner, D.; Resnick, M.I.; et al. Radiotherapy and survival in prostate cancer patients: A population-based study. *Int. J. Radiat. Oncol. Biol. Phys.* **2009**, *73*, 15–23. [CrossRef] [PubMed]
160. Schulman, C.C.; Debruyne, F.M.; Forster, G.; Selvaggi, F.P.; Zlotta, A.R.; Witjes, W.P. 4-Year follow-up results of a European prospective randomized study on neoadjuvant hormonal therapy prior to radical prostatectomy in T2-3N0M0 prostate cancer. European Study Group on Neoadjuvant Treatment of Prostate Cancer. *Eur. Urol.* **2000**, *38*, 706–713. [CrossRef] [PubMed]
161. Gleave, M.E.; Goldenberg, S.L.; Chin, J.L.; Warner, J.; Saad, F.; Klotz, L.H.; Jewett, M.; Kassabian, V.; Chetner, M.; Dupont, C.; et al. Randomized comparative study of 3 versus 8-month neoadjuvant hormonal therapy before radical prostatectomy: Biochemical and pathological effects. *J. Urol.* **2001**, *166*, 500–506. [CrossRef]
162. Prezioso, D.; Lotti, T.; Polito, M.; Montironi, R. Neoadjuvant hormone treatment with leuprolide acetate depot 3.75 mg and cyproterone acetate, before radical prostatectomy: A randomized study. *Urol. Int.* **2004**, *72*, 189–195. [CrossRef] [PubMed]
163. Selli, C.; Montironi, R.; Bono, A.; Pagano, F.; Zattoni, F.; Manganelli, A.; Selvaggi, F.P.; Comeri, G.; Fiaccavento, G.; Guazzieri, S.; et al. Effects of complete androgen blockade for 12 and 24 weeks on the pathological stage and resection margin status of prostate cancer. *J. Clin. Pathol.* **2002**, *55*, 508–513. [CrossRef] [PubMed]
164. Gravina, G.L.; Festuccia, C.; Galatioto, G.P.; Muzi, P.; Angelucci, A.; Ronchi, P.; Costa, A.M.; Bologna, M.; Vicentini, C. Surgical and biologic outcomes after neoadjuvant bicalutamide treatment in prostate cancer. *Urology* **2007**, *70*, 728–733. [CrossRef] [PubMed]
165. Soloway, M.S.; Pareek, K.; Sharifi, R.; Wajsman, Z.; McLeod, D.; Wood, D.P., Jr.; Puras-Baez, A. Lupron Depot Neoadjuvant Prostate Cancer Study Group. Neoadjuvant androgen ablation before radical prostatectomy in cT2bNxMo prostate cancer: 5-year results. *J. Urol.* **2002**, *167*, 112–116. [CrossRef]
166. Aus, G.; Abrahamsson, P.A.; Ahlgren, G.; Hugosson, J.; Lundberg, S.; Schain, M.; Schelin, S.; Pedersen, K. Three-month neoadjuvant hormonal therapy before radical prostatectomy: A 7-year follow-up of a randomized controlled trial. *BJU Int.* **2002**, *90*, 561–566. [CrossRef] [PubMed]
167. Yee, D.S.; Lowrance, W.T.; Eastham, J.A.; Maschino, A.C.; Cronin, A.M.; Rabbani, F. Long-term follow-up of 3-month neoadjuvant hormone therapy before radical prostatectomy in a randomized trial. *BJU Int.* **2010**, *105*, 185–190. [CrossRef] [PubMed]
168. Klotz, L.H.; Goldenberg, S.L.; Jewett, M.A.; Fradet, Y.; Nam, R.; Barkin, J.; Chin, J.; Chatterjee, S. Canadian Uro-Oncology Group. Long-term followup of a randomized trial of 0 versus 3 months of neoadjuvant androgen ablation before radical prostatectomy. *J. Urol.* **2003**, *170*, 791–794. [CrossRef] [PubMed]
169. Ayala, G.E.; Muezzinoglu, B.; Hammerich, K.H.; Frolov, A.; Liu, H.; Scardino, P.T.; Li, R.; Sayeeduddin, M.; Ittmann, M.M.; Kadmon, D.; et al. Determining prostate cancer-specific death through quantification of stromogenic carcinoma area in prostatectomy specimens. *Am. J. Pathol.* **2011**, *178*, 79–87. [CrossRef] [PubMed]

170. Tomas, D.; Spajic, B.; Milosevic, M.; Demirovic, A.; Marusic, Z.; Kruslin, B. Intensity of stromal changes predicts biochemical recurrence-free survival in prostatic carcinoma. *Scand. J. Urol. Nephrol.* **2010**, *44*, 284–290. [CrossRef] [PubMed]
171. Yanagisawa, N.; Li, R.; Rowley, D.; Liu, H.; Kadmon, D.; Miles, B.J.; Wheeler, T.M.; Ayala, G.E. Stromogenic prostatic carcinoma pattern (carcinomas with reactive stromal grade 3) in needle biopsies predicts biochemical recurrence-free survival in patients after radical prostatectomy. *Hum. Pathol.* **2007**, *38*, 1611–1620. [CrossRef] [PubMed]
172. Kinseth, M.A.; Jia, Z.; Rahmatpanah, F.; Sawyers, A.; Sutton, M.; Wang-Rodriguez, J.; Mercola, D.; McGuire, K.L. Expression differences between African American and Caucasian prostate cancer tissue reveals that stroma is the site of aggressive changes. *Int. J. Cancer* **2014**, *134*, 81–91. [CrossRef] [PubMed]
173. Planche, A.; Bacac, M.; Provero, P.; Fusco, C.; Delorenzi, M.; Stehle, J.C.; Stamenkovic, I. Identification of prognostic molecular features in the reactive stroma of human breast and prostate cancer. *PLoS ONE* **2011**, *6*, e18640. [CrossRef] [PubMed]
174. Rodriguez-Berriguete, G.; Sanchez-Espiridion, B.; Cansino, J.R.; Olmedilla, G.; Martinez-Onsurbe, P.; Sanchez-Chapado, M.; Paniagua, R.; Fraile, B.; Royuela, M. Clinical significance of both tumor and stromal expression of components of the IL-1 and TNF-alpha signaling pathways in prostate cancer. *Cytokine* **2013**, *64*, 555–563. [CrossRef] [PubMed]
175. Scott, A.M.; Wiseman, G.; Welt, S.; Adjei, A.; Lee, F.T.; Hopkins, W.; Divgi, C.R.; Hanson, L.H.; Mitchell, P.; Gansen, D.N.; et al. A Phase I dose-escalation study of sibrotuzumab in patients with advanced or metastatic fibroblast activation protein-positive cancer. *Clin. Cancer Res.* **2003**, *9*, 1639–1647. [PubMed]
176. LeBeau, A.M.; Brennen, W.N.; Aggarwal, S.; Denmeade, S.R. Targeting the cancer stroma with a fibroblast activation protein-activated promelittin protoxin. *Mol. Cancer Ther.* **2009**, *8*, 1378–1386. [CrossRef] [PubMed]
177. Brennen, W.N.; Rosen, D.M.; Wang, H.; Isaacs, J.T.; Denmeade, S.R. Targeting carcinoma-associated fibroblasts within the tumor stroma with a fibroblast activation protein-activated prodrug. *J. Natl. Cancer Inst.* **2012**, *104*, 1320–1334. [CrossRef] [PubMed]
178. Sluka, P.; Davis, I.D. Cell mates: Paracrine and stromal targets for prostate cancer therapy. *Nat. Rev. Urol.* **2013**, *10*, 441–451. [CrossRef] [PubMed]
179. Killian, P.H.; Kronski, E.; Michalik, K.M.; Barbieri, O.; Astigiano, S.; Sommerhoff, C.P.; Pfeffer, U.; Nerlich, A.G.; Bachmeier, B.E. Curcumin inhibits prostate cancer metastasis in vivo by targeting the inflammatory cytokines CXCL1 and -2. *Carcinogenesis* **2012**, *33*, 2507–2519. [CrossRef] [PubMed]
180. Yeung, T.L.; Leung, C.S.; Li, F.; Wong, S.S.; Mok, S.C. Targeting stromal-cancer cell crosstalk networks in ovarian cancer treatment. *Biomolecules* **2016**. [CrossRef] [PubMed]
181. Aigner, A.; Renneberg, H.; Bojunga, J.; Apel, J.; Nelson, P.S.; Czubayko, F. Ribozyme-targeting of a secreted FGF-binding protein (FGF-BP) inhibits proliferation of prostate cancer cells in vitro and in vivo. *Oncogene* **2002**, *21*, 5733–5742. [CrossRef] [PubMed]
182. Herbert, C.; Schieborr, U.; Saxena, K.; Juraszek, J.; De Smet, F.; Alcouffe, C.; Bianciotto, M.; Saladino, G.; Sibrac, D.; Kudlinzki, D.; et al. Molecular mechanism of SSR128129E, an extracellularly acting, small-molecule, allosteric inhibitor of fgf receptor signaling. *Cancer Cell.* **2016**, *30*, 176–178. [CrossRef] [PubMed]
183. Cecchi, F.; Bottaro, D.P. Novel antagonists of heparin binding growth factors. *Oncotarget* **2012**, *3*, 911–912. [CrossRef] [PubMed]
184. Cecchi, F.; Rabe, D.C.; Bottaro, D.P. Targeting the HGF/Met signaling pathway in cancer therapy. *Expert Opin. Ther. Targets* **2012**, *16*, 553–572. [CrossRef] [PubMed]
185. Chen, J.; Wu, F.X.; Luo, H.L.; Liu, J.J.; Luo, T.; Bai, T.; Li, L.Q.; Fan, X.H. Berberine upregulates miR-22-3p to suppress hepatocellular carcinoma cell proliferation by targeting Sp1. *Am. J. Transl. Res.* **2016**, *8*, 4932–4941. [PubMed]
186. Foley, C.; Mitsiades, N. Moving beyond the androgen receptor (AR): Targeting AR-interacting proteins to treat prostate cancer. *Horm. Cancer* **2016**, *7*, 84–103. [CrossRef] [PubMed]

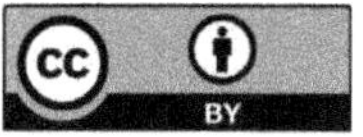

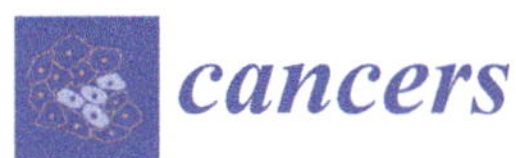

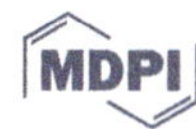

Review

Epigenomic Regulation of Androgen Receptor Signaling: Potential Role in Prostate Cancer Therapy

Vito Cucchiara [1,2], Joy C. Yang [1], Vincenzo Mirone [2], Allen C. Gao [1,4], Michael G. Rosenfeld [3] and Christopher P. Evans [1,4,*]

1 Department of Urology, School of Medicine, University of California, Davis, 4860 Y Street, Suite 3500, Sacramento, CA 95817, USA; vito.cucchiara89@gmail.com (V.C.); jcyang@ucdavis.edu (J.C.Y.); acgao@ucdavis.edu (A.C.G.)

2 Department of Neurosciences, Reproductive Sciences and Odontostomatology, University Federico II, Naples 80131, Italy; mirone@unina.it

3 Department of Medicine, Howard Hughes Medical Institute, University of California San Diego, La Jolla, CA 92093, USA; mrosenfeld@ucsd.edu

4 Comprehensive Cancer Center, UC Davis School of Medicine, University of California, Davis, Sacramento, CA 95817, USA

* Correspondence: cpevans@ucdavis.edu; Tel.: +1-916-734-7520; Fax: +1-916-734-8094

Academic Editor: Emmanuel S. Antonarakis
Received: 30 November 2016; Accepted: 11 January 2017; Published: 16 January 2017

Abstract: Androgen receptor (AR) signaling remains the major oncogenic pathway in prostate cancer (PCa). Androgen-deprivation therapy (ADT) is the principle treatment for locally advanced and metastatic disease. However, a significant number of patients acquire treatment resistance leading to castration resistant prostate cancer (CRPC). Epigenetics, the study of heritable and reversible changes in gene expression without alterations in DNA sequences, is a crucial regulatory step in AR signaling. We and others, recently described the technological advance Chem-seq, a method to identify the interaction between a drug and the genome. This has permitted better understanding of the underlying regulatory mechanisms of AR during carcinogenesis and revealed the importance of epigenetic modifiers. In screening for new epigenomic modifiying drugs, we identified SD-70, and found that this demethylase inhibitor is effective in CRPC cells in combination with current therapies. The aim of this review is to explore the role of epigenetic modifications as biomarkers for detection, prognosis, and risk evaluation of PCa. Furthermore, we also provide an update of the recent findings on the epigenetic key processes (DNA methylation, chromatin modifications and alterations in noncoding RNA profiles) involved in AR expression and their possible role as therapeutic targets.

Keywords: epigenetics; prostate cancer; androgen receptor; methylation; acetylation; non-coding RNA; biomarkers; novel treatments

---

1. Introduction

Prostate cancer (PCa) is the most prevalent cancer in men and the third cause of cancer-specific mortality in Western countries [1]. To understand the cornerstone of prostate carcinogenesis, many authors have pointed towards the central role of the androgen receptor (AR). AR, a member of the nuclear receptor superfamily and located at chromosome Xq11-12, contains three major functional domains. The first, highly unstructured, and largest domain is the N-terminal domain (NTD), which comprises the activation function 1 (AF1) motif. The DNA binding domain (DBD) is the second AR-region and contains two zinc fingers that cooperate with the androgen-response element (ARE), and allow dimerization. The hinge region is a bridge between the DBD and the ligand binding domain

(LBD), which accommodates the second activation function (AF2) motif [2]. It is well established that sustained AR activity is inexorable from PCa cell survival and disease progression, even following androgen deprivation therapy (ADT) [3,4]. Since the discovery in the 1940s that PCa is dependent on androgens [5], the central therapy for patients with locally advanced or metastatic disease targets the AR. After an initial period of therapeutic response, PCa become insensitive to these therapies and progresses to the castration resistant prostate cancer (CRPC) [6]. To date, in addition to the well- known genetic mutations, epigenetics is considered fundamental in the molecular pathogenesis of PCa. Epigenetics has been described as "the stable transmission of cellular information due to a modification of the DNA without a change in DNA sequence" [7,8]. It has been demonstrated that alteration of epigenetic marks may determine cancer initiation, development, and subsequent progression [9,10]. This review focuses on the role of epigenetic processes such as histone methylation, histone acetylation and non-coding RNA that play a central role in the regulation of AR in PCa pathogenesis and progression and discusses further modalities of treatment.

2. Histone Methylation

Histone methylation is an important and complex method of transcriptional control mediated by histone methyltransferase (HMT) and histone demethylase (HDM) enzymes. Methylation changes to the local chromatin encourage or repress transcription according to the site of modification [11]. For example, methylation of lysine residues 4 and 36 in histone H3 (H3K4, H3K36) generally preserves euchromatic domains [12,13] whereas the modification of H3K9 and H3K27 [14,15] forms heterochromatic regions. Arginine methylation is an alternative method of histone modification. Protein arginine methyltransferase (PRMT) family members such as PRMT6 [16] and coactivator associated arginine methyltransferase 1 (CARM1) [17], are enzymes responsible for histone methylation at arginine residues. Several articles [2,18] suggest that the histone methylation of AR can regulate the transcriptional activity of AR.

One of the most extensively studied HMT enzymes in PCa is SET9, which seems to improve gene expression by inducing histone H3K4me1 and obstructing histone H3K9 methylation and the nucleosome remodeling deacetylase (NURD) complex [19–21]. Different groups have observed elevated levels of this enzyme in malignant epithelial cells from PCa patients [22,23]. To explore its role in the regulation of the AR, many works describe that SET9 is responsible for N–C inter-domain cooperation that is important for AR transcriptional activity [24–26]. It was subsequently found that the hinge region of AR contains a motif (KLKK) that is comparable to the sites modified by the methyltransferase SET9 in other proteins [22,23]. Even if SET9 was shown to methylate AR, a consensus could still remain elusive about the sensitivity of this interaction. It is also unclear which Lys is methylated; one study shows Lys 630 [23] and another Lys 632 [22].

The nuclear receptor-binding SET domain-protein 2 (NSD2) is a histone methyltransferase that cooperates with the DBD of the AR [27]. High levels of NSD2 are related to the expression of PSA (prostate specific antigen) [27]. A paper by Asangani et al. reported that high levels of NSD2 correlate with aggressive characteristics in PCa [28]. The mechanism of action is linked to the enhancer of zeste homolog 2 (EZH2), a component of Polycomb repressive complex 2 (PRC2) [4]. The enhancement of EZH2 leads to the transcriptional inhibition of miR-203, miR-31 and miR-26, which are repressors of NSD2. This complex mechanism facilitates an over expression of NSD2 with the generation of the active histone mark, H3K36me2. Moreover, the study by Yang et al. [29] shows that NSD2 acts as a transcriptional coactivator of NF-κB for activation of target genes, such as *IL-6*, *IL-8*, *VEGFA* and *survivin* in CRPC cells.

Historically, EZH2 has been considered an AR transcriptional repressor. This peculiarity has been related to the ability of EZH2 to catalyze two repressive histone markers, H3K27me3 and H3K4me3, via AR recruitment [30]. Other works with conflicting findings have established a strong correlation between increased EZH2 and more aggressive [31], neuroendocrine [32] or metastatic [33] PCa. The role of EZH2 as an AR coactivator has been described to be AKT dependent. In fact, the phosphorylation of EZH2 serine 21 mediated by PI3K/AKT obstructs the methylation of H3K27 [34]. Xu et al. [35] confirmed these previous reports and showed that the phosphorylation of EZH2 at serine 21 defines the oncogenic function of EZH2 as a coactivator of AR in advanced PCa. This mechanism is independent of PCRC2 and H3K27me3 and suggests that EZH2 can methylate other proteins or other histone residues.

Another methyltransferase involved in PCa growth is PRMT6 [36]. PRMT6 has a high affinity for H3 and provides H3R2me2, a well-known repressive mark [36] but at the same time it was widely detected in a cohort of patients affected by PCa [37]. Almeida-Rios et al. [38] recently showed that PRMT6 silencing in PC-3 cells downregulates the PI3K/AKT/mTOR pathway and increases AR signaling.

A relevant enzyme for the AR regulation is the lysine specific demethylase 1 (LSD1). It has been targeted for its dual ability to suppress or stimulate AR expression [18]. The explanation of its role as a transcriptional coactivator can be the de-methylation of H3K9me1,2 [39]. The activity of this methyltransferase could be regulated by other post-transcriptional modifications. For example, it was discovered that H3 phosphorylation mediated by the protein kinase C-related kinase 1 (PRK1) [40] and the protein kinase C 1 (PKC1) [41] changes the substrate of LSD1 from H3K4me1,2 to H3K9me1,2 with an enhancement of AR related gene expression. Recently, Yang et al. [42] described an alternative mechanism of LSD1 that involves the generation of ROS leading to DNA damage. The authors report that this ROS generation occurs after androgen stimulation, which determines the demethylation of H3K4me1,2 on ARE regions, resulting in DNA damage. This DNA damage releases DNA and facilitates DNA loop formation, which is critical for miRNA expression and transcription. Subsequently, OGG1 and APEX1, DNA damage repair factors, are recruited to these ARE regions in an androgen and LSD1 dependent manner, suggesting that LSD1-mediated AR targets transcription relies on H3K4 demethylation and DNA oxidation [42].

Historically, despite its aforementioned role as coactivator, LSD1 has been considered a corepressor. LSD1 acts as a demethylase for H3K4me1,2 [43] enhancing the recruitment of corepressor complexes. Moreover, has been reported that LSD1 can reduce the expression of several genes such as the AR gene or *AKR1C3* and *HSD17B6*, two genes responsible for the androgen synthesis [18,44]. The overexpression of AKR1C3 have been correlated with PCa progression and aggressiveness [45,46] and recent findings describe the activation of AKR1C3 as a mechanism of resistance to Enzalutamide and Abiraterone [47,48].

Furthermore, it has been shown that other HMT enzymes such as the lysine demethylase 4B (KDM4B) [49], KDM4C [50], and KDM3A [51] can enhance the AR transcription activity. KDM4B, an enzyme that can de-methylate H3K9me3, has a duplex function. It can stimulate the AR activity directly through the demethylation of H3K9me3, or indirectly reducing the ubiquitylation and degradation of AR [49].

It is well known that one of the tumorigenic mechanisms in PCa cells is the fusion gene *TMPRSS2-ERG* [52] and several works highlight the causal relationship between the AR signaling and these genomic rearrangements [53]. Androgen stimulation facilitates the co-recruitment of the AR and the topoisomerase II beta (TOP2B) at *TMPRSS2* and *ERG* loci near genomic breakpoints, leading to TOP2B-mediated DNA double strand break formation [54].

Yu et al. [55], through the use of a chromatin precipitation (ChIP) technique, discovered that ERG expression increases the recruitment of EZH2 which may then mediate the repression of AR transcription activity through H3K27 methylation [55]. Using a global proteomics approach to unravel the mechanism that might control androgen-dependent *TMPRSS2-ERG* fusion, Metzeger et al. [56] showed that the di-methylation of K114 mediated by LSD1 is executed by the histone mehylatransferase EHMT2. LSD1-K114me2 allows for interactions with the chromodomain helicase DNA-binding protein 1 (CHD1). The complex (EHMT2-LSD1 K114me2-CHD1) controls chromatin binding of AR, and it was found to play an important role in regulating the *TMPRSS2-ERG* oncogenic fusion [56]. The mechanisms of action of the principal methyltransferases and demethylases involved in the regulation of AR gene expression are presented in Figure 1.

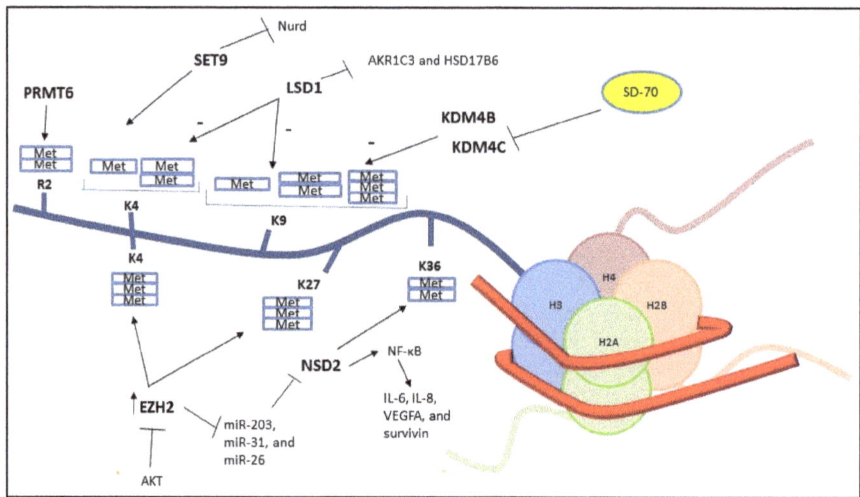

Figure 1. Schematic overview of AR histone 3 methylation status. SD70 inhibits the demethylase activity of KDM4C and is effective in CRPC cells both in vitro and in vivo. NURD: nucleosome remodeling deacetylase complex; EZH2: enhancer of zeste homolog 2; LSD1: lysine specific demethylase 1; NSD2: nuclear receptor-binding SET domain-protein 2; PRMT6: protein arginine methyltransferase 6; KDM4B and KDM4C: Lysine Demethylase 4B and 4C.

3. Histone Acetylation

The histone acetyltransferases (HAT) and histone deacetylases (HDAC) are two groups of enzymes that regulate acetylation and deacetylation [57]. In general, active euchromatin is relatively hyperacetylated whereas inactive heterochromatin is hypoacetylated [58]. In 2000, Fu et al. discovered within the flexible hinge region of AR a short sequence (KLKK), with the property of an acetylation motif [59].

As described in other reviews [18,60–62], the histone acetylation status is a reversible process of placing and removing covalent acetyl groups that can improve or reduce the AR transcriptional activity, respectively. To study the fundamental role of AR acetylation, several groups used two different models in which the acetyl acceptor sites were mutated to be non-functional or acetylation mimetic. In these two scenarios, when the AR is non-functional, the AR takes on a repressed form, which increases binding to co-repressor proteins including NCoR [59,63,64]. In the other case, when the acetylation acceptor mutated sites mimic acetylation, we can observe a completely different result; an improvement of the transcriptional activity and a reduction of the interaction with co-repressor proteins [60,63].

3.1. *AR Activation Mediated by Histone Acetylation*

Many works have described several co-regulators of the AR transcription machinery with a HAT activity such as p300/CAF [59], p160/SRC [65], Tat-interactive protein, 60 kDa (TIP60) [66], and *N*-acetyltransferase arrest-defect 1 protein (ARD1) [67].

CBP and p300 are proteins with HAT activity, and they are able to regulate transcription [68,69]. It was discovered that AR is acetylated by p300 and p300/cAMP-response element-binding protein associated factor (PCAF) both in vitro and in vivo [59]. Recently, Zhong et al. [70] explained an interesting pathway involving PTEN and AKT. The authors show that the inactivation or deletion of PTEN and the subsequent phosphorylation of AR at the serine 81 stimulates the acetylation of the AR by p300. Furthermore, it has been described that p300 can affect the AR activity indirectly. In fact, the acetylation of b-catenin provided by p300, determines a different interaction with the AR leading to an enhanced AR transcription [71].

The Steroid Receptor Coactivator-1 (SRC1) is responsible for the activation of AR due to its HAT domain [72]. Moreover, it has not only been shown that SRC1 can interact directly with AR, but it can recruit other coactivators (p300/CBP) in order to stimulate the transcriptional activity of the AR [73]. A recent study describes the possible role of the SCR1/p160 binding site as a novel therapeutic target. In fact, using two overlapping SRC1 peptides the authors show an inhibition of AR-dependent genes, such as *PSA* and *TMPRSS2* [74].

As previously suggested in another review [60], in addition to androgens, various other factors can stimulate the levels of AR acetylation mediated by CBP/p300 or SRC1. Despite the fact that the mechanism of action is not well-understood, it has been proposed that bombesin, via Src and PKC signaling pathways, can activate p300 activity. This interaction leads to enhanced acetylation of AR resulting in increased expression of AR-regulated genes (*PSA*) [75]. At the same time, IL-4 increases CBP/p300 protein expression and enhances interaction of AR with CBP/p300 proteins through a recruitment of p300 protein to the androgen responsive elements (AREs) in the promoters of androgen responsive genes [76]. IL-6 is another cytokine important for cell growth and survival in PCa both in vitro and in vivo [77], and it has been reported that SRC-1 can improve its ligand independent stimulation of AR by IL-6 via MAPK [78].

TIP60, an AR factor acetyl transferase (FAT), has a specificity for the LBD of the AR [79]. More recently, it has been shown that TIP60 may be directly responsible for the acetylation of AR and it can interplay with HDACs at the PSA promoter gene. The equilibrium between these can lead to activation or suppression of AR transcription [80]. Shiota et al. [81] explained that TIP60 overexpression facilitates the acetylated form of AR and, consequently, the AR localization in the nucleus in absence of an androgen enriched environment.

Arrest defective-1 protein (ARD1) is another acetyltransferase [82] which has important functions in several types of cancer through acetylating different target proteins [83–85]. Wang et al. [67] reported that the level of ARD1 is consistently higher in PCa, and recently, a work by DePaolo et al. [86] revealed that ARD1 not only acetylates AR at lysine 618 but also creates a ternary complex with AR and HSP90, playing a role in the AR-HS90 dissociation.

Interestingly, another study suggests that the levels of AR potentiate the recruitment of AR and the components of the transcription machinery to chromatin in order to enhance the acetylation on H3K9 and on H3K14 in CRPC cells even in an androgen deprivation environment [87]. These finding are in line with other works [88], which report how an enhanced acetylation in cells that overexpress AR is linked to the development of a castration resistant condition.

3.2. AR Inhibition Mediated by Histone Acetylation

As mentioned above, acetylation of particular residues determines the enhancement of the AR activity, and it is normal to expect that the opposite process can lead to inhibition. Within the HDAC family, we encounter several proteins with a similar enzymatic activity. For example, HDAC1 interacts with the PSA promoter and suppresses AR signaling [66] while HDAC7 has the similar ability to inhibit AR, but in this case the mechanism of action is independent of AR acetyl acceptor sites [89]. Moreover, several studies describe that HDAC6 regulates the correct folding of the AR mainly via modulating HSP90 acetylation. The acetylation of HSP90 results in a destabilization of the AR and subsequently in its degradation by the proteasome [90].

Sirtuin 1 (SIRT1), a NAD-dependent deacetylase, has been described as a repressor of AR activity [91]. Fu et al. extended precious observations and established a role for SIRT1 in regulating cellular growth by repressing and deacetylating the AR directly [91]. Moreover, the same group highlighted a "functional antagonism" between SIRT1 and p300 at the same site of the hinge region avoiding the N-C terminal interaction [61,91]. Figure 2 depicts the molecular communication between AR and acetylation status in order to enhance or reduce AR gene expression.

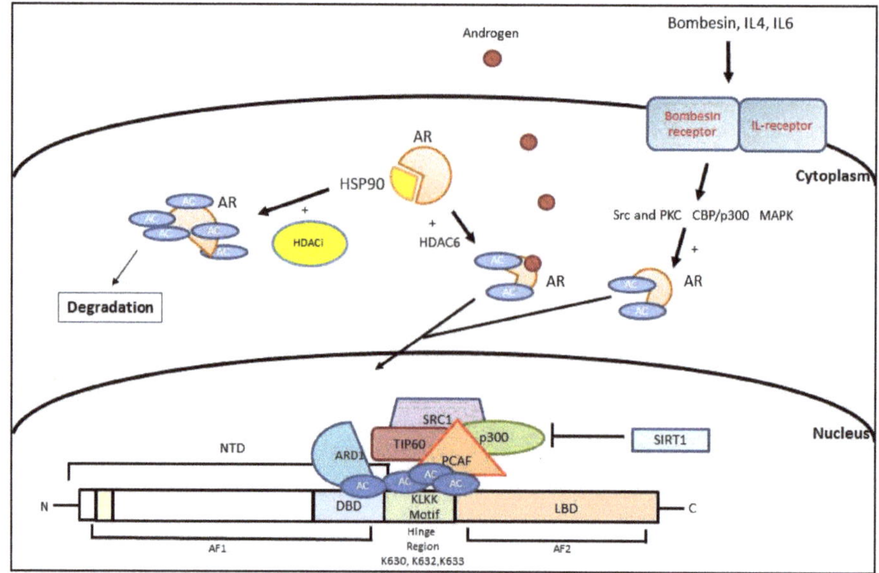

Figure 2. Graphic representation of the balance between acetylation and deacetylation in the regulation of androgen receptor (AR) gene expression. The mechanism of action of histone deacetylase inhibitors (HDACi) such as romidepsin and panobinostat is related to the heat shock protein-90 (HSP90). NTD: N-terminal domain; DBD: DNA binding domain; LBD: ligand binding domain; AF1 and AF2: activation function 1 and 2; PKC: protein kinase C; SRC1: steroid receptor coactivator-1; TIP60: Tat-interactive protein, 60 kDa; ARD1: *N*-acetyltransferase arrest-defect 1; SIRT1: Sirtuin 1; PCAF: p300/cAMP-response element-binding protein associated factor.

4. Non-Coding RNA

In the last decade, several articles corroborated by the use of new technologies to reveal that a major portion of the non-coding genome is transcribed with many regulatory functions. This brought about a change in thinking that non-coding RNA can have a role in cancer [92]. Non-coding RNAs (ncRNAs) are divided into two major groups based on their size: small ncRNA (<200 bp) and long ncRNA (>200 bp) [93].

4.1. MicroRNA and AR

MicroRNAs (miRNAs) are a class of small non-coding RNAs with an important role in cell development, differentiation and signal transduction. Generally, miRNAs cause mRNA translational repression or mRNA degradation by binding to the 3′ untranslated region (3′-UTR) [94]. Furthermore, recent studies have reported that the 5′-UTR of mRNAs might be involved in the gene regulation by miRNA, and it has been shown that miRNA can activate gene expression rather than repress it [95,96]. Based on the central role of AR signaling in the normal and neoplastic growth of the prostate cell, many reports describe the existence of feedback loops between miRNAs and AR [97].

4.1.1. Androgen Regulation of miRNA Expression

In 2011, Waltering et al. presented one of the first miR microarray studies to examine androgen regulation of miRNAs [98], and they showed that dihydrotestosterone (DHT) positively modulates 17 miRNAs in VCaP cells whereas castration causes high levels of 42 miRNAs. The work of several independent groups demonstrates that miRNAs such as miR-19a, miR-148, and miR-27a are androgen inducible miRNAs [99–101]. Indeed, androgen-mediated overexpression of miR-27a results in the reduction of prohibitin, a well-known tumor-suppressor gene and co-repressor of the AR, with a subsequently increased expression of AR genes and increased PCa cell growth [101].

Genome-wide screenings of androgen target genes have identified miR-125b as androgen-inducible miRNA [102] and in particular have been shown that androgens carry out this action by binding the promoter region of the miR-125b gene. Moreover, Sun et al. [103] reported that AR targets the miR-99a/let7c/125b-2 cluster genes region LNC00478 and subsequently represses the level of this cluster. The authors also explain the role of two chromatin modifiers EZH2 or JMJD3, that can suppress or enhance the levels of the miR-99a/let7c/125b-2 cluster depending on the presence or the absence of androgen [103]. The downregulation of the miR-99a/let7c/125b-2 cluster has been shown to protect many of their target mRNAs from degradation. On the contrary, when miR-125b is overexpressed, it cooperates with the insulin-like growth factor 1 (IGF1R) to enhance PCa cell development [103]. MiR-125b has been reported to stimulate the PCa cells growth without androgen stimulation through down-regulating the expression of Bak1 (Bcl-2 homologous antagonist/killer 1) [104] and by targeting the Bcl-2-binding component 3 (BBC3) and p53 [105–107]. MiR-125b, as described in another work [108], is connected to Her2-AR pathway and could have a function in inducing CRPC.

MiR-135a has been found to be upregulated in androgen sensitive PCa cells and AR, as previously reported for miR-125, directly activates transcription by using a functional ARE in the miR-135a promoter region [109]. To explore the biological effects of miR-135a in prostate cells, the researchers overexpressed miR-135a in LNCaP cells and demonstrated that miR-135a can down-regulate the expression of the Rho-associated protein kinase 1 (*ROCK1*) and *ROCK2* (implicated in cytoskeleton regulation) at mRNA and protein levels [109]. Coarfa et al. [110] also found AR recruitment to the ARE in the promoter region under androgen stimulation. They additionally identified stronger co-recruitment of AR and coactivators to a region immediately downstream of the miR-135a-5p gene without the addition of androgen. Combined with the inhibitory effect of miR-135a-5p on expression of AR and its coactivators, this suggests a negative feedback loop that can de-repress AR axis transcriptional output upon androgen deprivation. A recent study by Wan et al. [111] describes a downregulation of miR-135a in CRPC. The authors found that RB-associated KRAB zinc finger (*RBAK*) and matrix metalloproteinase 11 (*MMP11*), two genes involved in migration pathway, are controlled by miR-135a. They showed that PCa progression is associated with low levels of miR-135a and high levels of RBAK and MMP11.

MiR-32 is also reportedly an androgen-regulated miRNA. The transfection of pre-miR-32 into LNCaP cells confers significant cell growth and reduces apoptosis. In CRPC, miR-32 is regulated by androgen through targeting the B-cell translocation gene 2 (*BTG2*), a member of the antiproliferative (APRO) gene family [112]. BTG2 regulates several cellular mechanisms such as cell cycle progression, DNA damage repair, and apoptosis, and thus it has been shown that its levels are suppressed in many human cancers [113].

AR acts as a stimulus for miR-21 transcription by targeting miPPR-21, the miR-21 promoter [114]. AR is not the only enhancer of miR-21. In fact, mir-21 can be stimulated by two other transcriptional factors, the activator protein 1 (AP-1) and the signal transducer and activator of transcription 3 (STAT3) [115,116]. Furthermore, Mishra et al. [117] described a positive feedback loop between miR-21 and AR. The AR and miR-21 axis negatively alters the TGFBR2 pathway, and in this way inhibits the tumor-suppressive activity of TGFβ. Mir-21 is implicated even in the regulation of the cell cycle, and the same group further revealed that miR-21 is not only able to reduce the level of a cyclin-dependent kinase inhibitor p57Kip2, but it is also able to attenuate p57Kip2-mediated responses [118].

MiR-221 and miR-222 are encoded on the X chromosome [119], but curiously they are downregulated by AR in an androgen enriched environment [112]. A recent review by Shih et al. [97] highlighted the mutual interaction between miR-221 and AR. Even though miR-221 has been extensively studied, we still do not have a clear idea on what its expression pattern in PCa is. For example, work by Gordanpour et al. [120] shows low levels of miR-221 in aggressive PCa with an inverse association with the Gleason Score, clinical recurrence, and metastasis. On the other hand, another study revealed a linear correlation between miR-221 expression and the pathological stage, lymph node involvement, Gleason Score, and biochemical recurrence (BCR) [121]. Yang et al. [122] confirmed that miR-221 and miR-222 are highly expressed in an androgen insensitive cell line (PC-3), and the experimental down-regulation of miR-221 or miR-222 inhibits migration and increases apoptosis in PC-3 cells. At the same time, the authors describe that the expression of SIRT1, a histone deacetylase, is increased in PCa cells after the inhibition of miR-221 and miR-222, suggesting that SIRT1 may play a suppressive role against the tumorigenic action of these miRNAs. To explore another possible mechanism of action of miR-221, a systematic biochemical and bioinformatical study has been performed [123]. It reveals two miR-221 targets, HECT domain E3 ubiquitin protein ligase 2 (*HECTD2*) and member RAS oncogene family (*RAB1A*). In this study, downregulation of HECTD2 affected androgen related transcription, and downregulation of HECTD2 and RAB1A altered the expression of many cell cycle genes and pathways, promoting tumor metastasis and leading to the development or maintenance of the CRPC phenotype.

4.1.2. MiRNA Regulation of Androgen Signaling

Many investigations have been conducted for documenting the role of miRs in controlling the AR pathway. By using a miR library in 2011, Ostling et al. demonstrated the ability of 71 unique miRs (52 decreasing and 19 increasing) to influence the AR [124]. Since then several miRNAs have been described as having a role in the regulation of AR activity directly or through co-regulators [97,125].

MiR-205 is deregulated in PCa compared to benign prostate tissues, it is inversely associated to advanced disease and short life expectancy, and miR-205 levels exhibit a negative correlation to AR [126]. Moreover, miR-205 was also found to be lower in CRPC patients in comparison with men who had not initiated ADT. Hagman et al. [126] reported that mir-205 directly targets AR and reduces both AR transcript and proteins. The role of miR-205 is not only related to AR, but it has been found that this miRNA can regulate several genes. Some of these genes (*IL-8* and *EDN1*) are responsible for improving the expression of the AR, and others are involved in the MAPK/ERK, mTOR, and IL-6 signaling pathways [97].

MiR-34 family includes three miRNAs that have been previously reported to suppress tumorigenesis by different mechanisms, including modulation of cell cycle, epithelial to mesenchymal transition, or metastasis [127]. In PCa, all miR-34 family members are downregulated, and the expression of miR-34a or miR-34c correlates with the tumor grade, advanced disease, and life expectancy [128,129]. This down-regulation has been linked to several mechanisms such as methylation of the CpG islands in the promoter region of this miRNAs, regulation by p53 in response to DNA stress, and a mechanism involving the p38- MAPK/MK2 pathway [129–132]. As reported in the study by Ostling et al., in PCa cells a statistically significant inverse association exists between miR-34a and AR [124]. Recently, Fang et al. [133] demonstrated that the long non-coding RNA PlncRNA-1, known to be enhanced by AR, can preserve AR from miR-34c-mediated suppression in PCa cells. According to the theory of competing endogenous RNAs, some kind of RNAs may "titrate" other ribonucleic acids such as miRNAs [133].

LET7 levels are frequently decreased in human cancers [134,135]. The most important and well known targets of this miRNA are the oncogenes *RAS* and *MYC* [136,137]. A work by Nadiminty et al. explain that LET7c determines PCa tumor suppression through AR, and this mechanism is linked to the ability of this tumor-suppressing miRNA to target *c-MYC*, a molecule required for the correct transcription of AR [138]. In detail, the same group also found that LET7c reduces AR activity and decreases growth of C4-2B cells, and it can be attributable to the association of this miRNA with c-MYC 3′-UTR and the subsequent reduction of AR transcription [138]. These results are corroborated by other studies. Gao et al. [139] reported that the suppression of the AR and c-MYC diminishes PCa cell proliferation, but at the same time, an ectopic overexpression of c-MYC mitigates the tumor progression due to AR suppression, supporting an intense molecular relation between the AR and c-MYC.

Not only do miRNAs have direct effects, but they can also use other pathways to control androgen signaling. Two of these pathways are mediated by the ERBB-2 and PI3K/AKT. The tyrosine receptor ERBB-2 is often elevated in PCa, whereas the activation of PI3K/AKT signaling is linked to proliferation, metastasis, apoptosis resistance and angiogenesis in PCa [140]. A work by Epis et al. demonstrates that the *ERBB-2* mRNA 3′-UTR contains two specific miR-331-3p target sites and that miR-331-3p suppresses ERBB-2 expression at both the transcript and protein levels. MiR-331-3p expression was found to be lower in ERBB-2 overexpressing PCa tissue compared to normal adjacent tissue. The same group also explained that miR-331-3p is involved in the downstream PI3K/AKT signaling in multiple PCa cell lines. Interestingly, it has been shown that miR-331-3p acts specifically to decrease PSA promoter activity and PSA levels without reducing AR expression [140].

MiR-488* directly targets AR by targeting the AR in 3′-UTR. MiR-488* down-regulates AR protein expression in both androgen-sensitive and insensitive PCa cells, inhibiting cellular growth and increasing apoptosis as observed after the transfection of miR-488* [141].

MiR-17-5p has been shown to target PCAF, a coactivator of AR, and to support PCa development [142]. The authors found that the overexpression of PCAF in PCa cells is inversely associated with miR-17-5p levels, suggesting that low levels of miR-17-5p can enhance AR signaling in PCa cells indirectly by modulating PCAF expression. Moreover, circulating miRNAs of the miR-17 family have been recently associated with a reduction of PSA levels and overall survival in CRPC patients [143].

MiR-124 has been described as a tumor suppressor miRNA in several cancer types including PCa [144–146]. In accordance with its role in many biological processes, different authors examined the mechanism of action of miR-124. As reported in a recent review [97], the reduction of miR-124 levels in PCa cells is due to hypermethylation of the promoter. As a consequence of this event, both cell lines or clinical prostate samples showed an elevation in AR expression. Mechanistically, the presence of the miR-124-binding site in the AR 3′-UTR seems to explain the reason why miR-124 is involved in the negative regulation of the AR [147]. Moreover, Shi et al. reported that miR-124 can induce the upregulation of p53, causing cell death and apoptosis in AR-positive PCa cells [147].

The same authors propose an explanation of this phenomenon. The upregulation of p53 may in part be due to the capacity of miR-124 to inhibit the AR/miR-125b signaling pathway or by targeting the 3′-UTR of the high mobility group A (*HMGA*) gene which, as previously reported, can inactivate p53 [147]. A recent study shows that miR-124 can inhibit AR expression and suppress PCa cells proliferation and, on the other hand, that miR-124 is an androgen/AR responsive gene [148].

Finally, in the same class of small ncRNA we can include miR-145. MiR-145 has consistently been found to be downregulated in several types of cancer, including PCa [149,150], and it is inversely correlated with metastasis, survival and ADT response [151]. The reason for its downregulation is not completely clear. It could be due to the methylation of the miR-145 promoter, to the mutation of p53 that is a transcriptional activator of miR-145, or to the effect of IL-6 [151]. Larne et al. [151] theorized that miR-145 may determine a reduction of the AR and its target genes, *PSA* and *TMPRSS2*, at both transcription and protein levels by direct binding because the AR 3′-UTR contains a predicted miR-145 binding site. Moreover, using clinical prostate specimens the authors confirmed the same promising results, suggesting a future role of this miRNA as a novel therapeutic intervention. Our findings regarding the role of miRNAs in AR transcriptional activity are summarized in Figure 3.

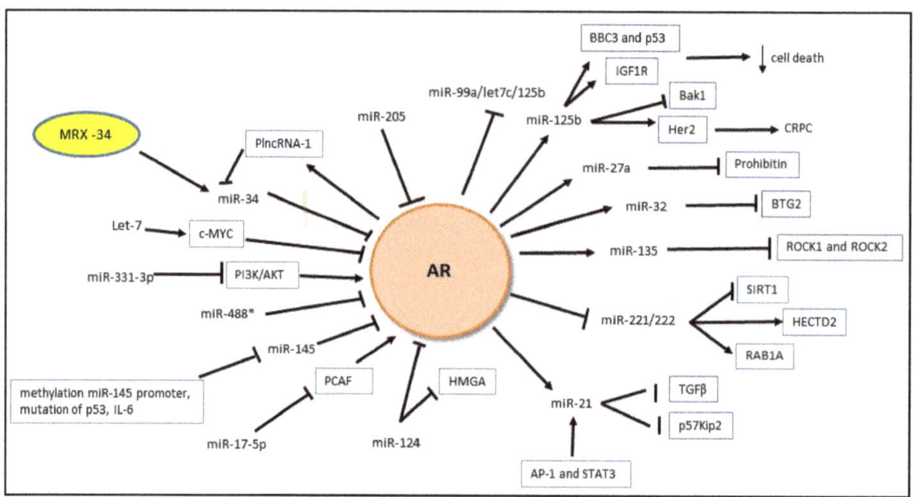

Figure 3. Mutual regulatory model of miRNAs and androgen receptor (AR). The graphic also shows MRX-34, the first miRNA based therapy for cancer. BBC3: Bcl-2-binding component 3; IGF1R: Insulin-like growth factor 1; Bak1: Bcl-2 homologous antagonist/killer 1; HER2: human epidermal growth factor receptor 2; p57Kip2: cyclin-dependent kinase inhibitor; AP-1: activator protein 1; STAT3: signal transducer and activator of transcription 3; HMGA: high mobility group A gene; PCAF: p300/cAMP-response element-binding protein associated factor; PI3K: phosphatidylinositol-3-kinases; PlncRNA-1: prostate cancer-up-regulated long noncoding RNA 1.

4.2. Long Non Coding RNA and AR

Given the growing body of evidence documenting the role of long non coding RNA (lncRNA) in controlling various biological processes or having a central role in various cancers [152–154], it is reasonable to assume that lncRNAs may have a significant role in PCa as well. Several investigations in PCa suggest that specific lncRNAs can modulate AR activity through various mechanisms [97].

In 2000, Srikantan et al. [155] characterized the prostate cancer gene expression marker 1 (PCGEM1). PCGEM1 is overexpressed in more than half of PCa tissues [156], and its upregulation has been associated with high-risk PCa [157]. Moreover, the ectopic expression of PCGEM1 may be a cause of resistance to doxorubicin-induced apoptosis [158], and this can explain why a gene expression analysis found its levels upregulated in CRPC [159]. The prostate cancer noncoding RNA1 (PRNCR1) is transcribed from the "gene desert" region of chromosome 8q24. It is a 13 kb intron less lncRNA, and although the role of PRNCR1 is not well known, its knockdown reportedly inhibits cell viability [160]. Several works confirm that PCGEM1 is an androgen-regulated prostate-specific gene [155,161] and that PCGEM1 [162] as well as PRNCR1 [160] are involved in prostate carcinogenesis through AR activation.

An elegant study performed by Yang et al. [156] discovered a particular chromatin mechanism for AR transactivation mediated by PRNCR1 and PCGEM1. The authors explain that binding of PRNCR1 to the AR enhancer region and its association with DOT1L is fundamental for the enrollment of PCGEM1. As reported in the article, PCGEM1 needs the recruitment of Pygo2 to form a selective looping of the enhancer region in order to induce transcription of the target genes. Moreover, the authors state that PRNCR1 and PCGEM1 are indispensable for the activation of both truncated and full-length AR. Confirming these results, the knockdown of these lncRNAs in the CRPC cell line strongly suppresses the growth of the cancer in a xenograft model [156].

Nevertheless, the efficacy of these findings has been questioned. In fact, Prensner et al. [163] disagreed with these reports because they found that only PCGEM1 is associated with PCa. Moreover, using a large cohort of high-risk PCa patients, they showed the lack of an association of these lncRNAs with poor disease outcomes.

Recently, Ho et al. [164] described a new mechanism through which PCGEM1 can regulate AR expression in CRPC. They demonstrate that androgen deprivation induces the elevation of PCGEM1 through p54/nrb (engaged in RNA splicing and gene regulation) leading to expression of the splice variant AR3 and castration resistance disease.

The lncRNA PCA3, one of the most important prostate-specific genes, has been extensively studied as a tumor biomarker [165] due to its specific expression in both PCa and high-grade prostatic intraepithelial neoplasia [166]. PCA3 has been demonstrated to have a role in the regulation of AR signaling. Several experiments silencing PCA3 showed a reduction of AR target genes and a higher number of cells in the sub G0/G1 phase of the cell cycle [167]. Lemos et al. recently explained that PCA3 can be considered a significant marker to detect the "epithelial to mesenchymal transition" process [168].

Another lncRNA named CTBP1 antisense (CTBP1-AS) has been identified as a promoter of the AR transcriptional activity [169]. To explore the function of CTBP1, the authors use an antisense non-coding RNA. Thanks to this, it has been shown that CTBP1-AS works by repressing CTBP1 in two different scenarios. Firstly, CTBP1-AS acts with the RNA-binding transcriptional repressor PSF to recruit the HDAC–Sin3A complexes to CTBP1 promoter in cis with the loss of activating histone marks. Secondly, in the trans-regulatory pathway, CTBP1-AS also enhances PSF complexes to the regulatory regions of target genes, leading to the transcriptional repression of suppressive genes [169]. Despite the fact that its mechanism of action has been elucidated, we have opposing results regarding the effective levels of CTBP-1 in PCa. Takayama et al. [169] revealed the suppressive role of CTBP1 in AR-positive PCa cells, but there is another work describing not only that CTBP1 is upregulated in metastatic PCa but also that CTBP1 has a sort of stimulatory effect in PCa cells [170]. As suggested by the authors, this debate can be solved by analyzing tumor samples or cell lines used in these works. In fact, the experiments of Wang et al. were performed predominantly in AR-negative cells while Takayama et al. showed that CTBP1 exerts tumor suppressive effects in AR-positive PCa cell lines.

Cui et al. [171] firstly demonstrated that the expression of PlncRNA-1 is significantly higher in PCa cells compared to normal cells but also, more interestingly, that PlncRNA-1 silencing decreases AR mRNA- and AR-related genes. The authors give the same results in both androgen-dependent (LNCaP) and androgen-independent cell lines (LNCaP-AI). As above mentioned, the same group recently discovered that PlncRNA-1 can deregulate the expression of miR-34c and miR-297. At the same time, these two miRNAs have the ability to reduce PlncRNA-1 expression, creating a reciprocal inhibitory feedback loop [133].

The lncRNA HOTAIR is a 2.2-kb-long transcript localized to the boundaries of the HOXC gene cluster [172]. Tsai et al. [173] elucidated the role of HOTAIR as a scaffold protein that interacts at the 5′ domain with PRC2 and at the 3′ domain with the LSD1/CoREST/REST complex. This allows the concomitant methylation of H3K27 and the demethylation of H3K4 [173]. Zhang et al. [172] recently investigated the role of HOTAIR interacting with the AR. They discovered high levels of HOTAIR after ADT and further confirmed that its knockdown decreased cell proliferation. In the same work, one of the possible mechanisms underlying the effect of this lncRNA has been explained. HOTAIR seems to limit the AR ubiquitination and degradation, reducing the interaction between AR and the E3 ubiquitin ligase MDM2, and this can explain why the overexpression of HOTAIR can led to a CRPC condition [172].

Prostate cancer transcript-associated 18 (PCAT18) is a lncRNA reported to be prostate specific and up-regulated in PCa compared to other tumors [174]. An RNA sequencing on paired metastatic/non-metastatic PCa xenografts derived from clinical specimens showed the upregulation of PCAT18 in metastatic PCa. Furthermore, the same group discovered not only that AR can improve PCAT18 overexpression but that this lncRNA can be involved in PCa cell proliferation, cell migration and cell invasion [174].

Another novel lncRNA, PCAT29, was recently discovered, and its relationship to the AR explained. Malik et al. [175] described a different behavior of this lncRNA in presence or in absence of androgens. Specifically, PCAT29 is suppressed by dihydrotestosterone (DHT) and increased after ADT. Low or repressed levels of PCAT29 show an improvement in proliferation and migration of PCa cells; whereas PCAT29 overexpression confers the opposite effect and attenuates growth and metastasis of prostate tumors [175]. Moreover, Sakurai et al. [176] proposed a mechanism of regulation for this lncRNA based on an equilibrium between different molecules. In androgen-dependent cells, androgen stimulates AR to bind to the PCAT29 locus suppressing its expression. On the contrary, FOXA1 and NKX3-1 can balance the effect mediated by AR and prevent the repression of PCAT29. Interestingly, in castration resistant cells low levels of FOXA1 and NKX3-1 together with an anomalous activation of AR determine the decrease of PCAT29 [176].

5. Novel PCa Biomarkers

Prostate specific antigen (PSA) is the most important screening technique used for PCa diagnosis and tumor monitoring. Despite being organ specific, PSA is not cancer specific, and its level changes in the presence of several conditions such as prostatitis, hyperplasia, prostate biopsies and surgeries [177]. All of these pitfalls may determine over-diagnosis and over-treatment especially for low or very low-risk PCa patients [178–180]. Despite the fact that in the last decade innumerable molecules have been discovered, the inconsistency of some findings, the difficulty of reproducibility, and the lack of clinical studies with a significant number of patients can explain the reason why only a very small number of these markers have been used in clinical practice.

The epigenetic alterations in PCa, as in part described above, can provide effective biomarkers for early detection and cancer relapse, for prognosis and, finally, to predict then response to specific therapies [181]. In this section, we present the epigenetic biomarkers with a consistent role and use in clinical practice.

5.1. Epigenetic Signature as Biomarkers

Several reviews report the role of the DNA methylation asset as a biomarker for PCa detection/diagnosis or prognosis and response to therapy [181,182].

One of the most frequent epigenetic alterations in PCa is the aberrant promoter methylation of the glutathione S-transferase pi 1 (*GSTP1*) gene. In fact, *GSTP1* has been considered one of the most promising candidates for a DNA methylation biomarker because it appears in more than 90% of cases [183].

In 2011, Wu et al. [184] published a meta-analysis on GSTP1 methylation in body fluids. The authors highlight an excellent specificity (86.8%–100%) but a lower sensitivity in urine (18.8%–83.2%) and serum or plasma (13.0%–71.9%) samples. These findings suggest the possible role of GSTP1 methylation as a biomarker for PCa diagnosis [185]. In 2014, a review by Strand et al. [186] studied the ability of GSTPI methylation as a biomarker for disease prognosis. In this case the authors did not find strong evidence for the use of this gene in cancer tissues for predicting early disease outcomes [185].

In order to enhance the predictive power of this biomarker, several gene panels have been studied. The combination of GSTP1 with other DNA methylation biomarkers showed an improvement in the detection rate (86% for urine and 42%–47% for serum) [181].

Moreover, the combination of the methylation pattern of three genes (*GSTP1*, *APC*, and *RARB2*) has been evaluated in a prospective study named ProCaM [187]. The test performed on urine samples collected after DRE presented a higher predictive accuracy than simply using PSA and clinical characteristics [188].

A methylation marker genetic test, ConfirmMDx (MDxHealth, Inc., Irvine, CA, USA), is a tissue-based assay that studies the epigenetic alteration surrounding the tumor lesions. This test identifies the methylation pattern of three genes (*GSTP1*, *APC*, and *RASSF1*) in men with a low risk for disease after a negative biopsy. ConfirmMDx, after a validation in a European and a US population, achieved a negative predictive value of 88%–90% [189,190]. Furthermore, the 2016 Clinical Guide of the National Comprehensive Cancer Network [191] recommended this test for the early detection of PCa in patients with an elevated PSA and prior negative biopsy.

To explore the biological role of DNA methylation alterations and to understand the utility of these epigenetic modifications as future biomarkers or as therapeutic targets, Aryee et al. [192] used a genome-scale analysis of DNA methylation among metastatic PCa patients. Although a consistent inter-individual heterogeneity in DNA methylation alterations was found, the authors showed that the methylation signatures are preserved in each patients' metastases. This interesting intra-individual homogeneity is a promising finding in the development of personalized treatments against all lethal metastatic PCa cell clones [192].

5.2. Long Non-Coding RNA as Biomarkers

Prostate cancer antigen 3 (PCA3) is a prostate cancer-specific antigen mapped to chromosome 9q21-22 [193]. It is a lncRNA of unknown function identified by Bussemakers et al. in 1999 [194]. More than 95% of PCa specimens show PCA3 over-expression [194], and in addition to cancer tissue, PCA3 transcripts have also been identified in urine samples of patients with benign enlargement and malignant disease of the prostate [165]. The Progensa PCA3 test (Hologic Gen-Probe, Marlborough, MA, USA), an in vitro amplification test, attained Conformiteé Européenne (CE) in 2006, and it was approved by the US FDA in 2012 for use in men older than 50 years old with one or more negative biopsies [195].

The PCA3-test involves collection of a urine sample after DRE to mobilize prostatic cells. The PCA3 score is a mathematical operation, and it can be acquired by dividing PCA3 RNA by PSA RNA levels in order to normalize PCA3 signals.

Despite these suggestive findings, the best cut-off to use is still controversial. A urine PCA3 score more of than 35 has been linked with a sensitivity comprised between 47%–57% and a specificity around 70% [196,197]. A recent meta-analysis by Lu et al. describes a sensitivity and specificity of 72% and 53%, respectively, with a PCA3 score cut-off of 20 [198]. Crawford et al. in a large multicenter study showed that a cut-off of 35 is correlated with a large number of false negatives, even though it can reduce the number of re-biopsies by 77% [199]. Controversial results have been reported regarding the relationship between PCA3 score and aggressive features. Some studies describe a correlation with the Gleason Score, the tumor volume, and extracapsular extension [200,201], but others didn't find any correlation with the aggressiveness of the tumor [202,203]. Despite these conflicting results, PCA3 score has been considered a more specific indicator with a better predictive value than the PSA [204].

In 2013, GenomeDx Biosciences (Vancouver, BC, Canada) and Mayo Clinic (Rochester, MN, USA) co-developed and validated a tissue-based genomic classifier that is able to evaluate the risk of developing clinical metastases at 5 years postoperatively named Decipher [205]. The authors used a high-density transcriptome-wide microarray to assess the expression of over 1.4 million markers including protein-coding genes and ncRNAs in 545 PCa patients samples including 213 who experienced early metastasis [205]. This test, whose result is expressed as a continuous risk score ranging from 0 to 1, is based on 22 RNA biomarkers related to cell proliferation, differentiation, motility, immune modulation and AR signaling. Decipher has been studied by several groups with varying cohorts of patients [206]. Karnes et al. [207] evaluated the prognostic role of Decipher in 219 high-risk PCa patients with a median follow up of 6.7 years after surgery. On multivariable analyses, higher decipher scores resulted in the highest prognostic predictor of metastasis with an area under the curve (AUC) of 0.79. 85 high-risk patients with PSA failure after radical prostatectomy (RP) were evaluated by Ross et al. in 2014 [208]. The genomic classifier showed an AUC of 0.82 compared to 0.64 of Gleason Score and 0.69 of PSA doubling time. The prognostic value of Decipher has also been studied in PCa patients undergoing adjuvant or salvage radiation therapy following RP. Den et al. [209] demonstrated that the AUC of this genomic test is 0.78 and 0.80 to predict BCR and metastasis, respectively, in a cohort of 139 patients treated by RP and adjuvant radiotherapy. Patients with a higher genomic score mainly benefit from this adjuvant treatment. With a median follow-up of 10 years, the same group followed 188 patients from two different institutions treated with RP and adjuvant or salvage radiotherapy [210]. Decipher predicts the occurrence of metastases on multivariable analyses and confirmed the previous results suggesting that adjuvant radiotherapy should be taken into consideration for PCa patients with high genomic score. Approved in the United States for patients with positive margins, pT3 disease, or PSA failure after surgery [211], Decipher could help physicians in the clinical decision making in order to improve accuracy in predicting patient outcomes.

5.3. MicroRNA as Biomarkers

Several studies suggest the use of miRNAs in the clinical setting and many reviews have been published about the argument [97,212,213]. The exploitation of different technological platforms, the examination of different samples (tissues, sera, urine), the retrospective design of many studies, the use of endogenous or exogenous controls, and the presence of contaminating non-neoplastic cells are all potential explanations for controversial results reported until now. Despite these obstacles, miRNAs have been reported to have a promising role as novel biomarkers in PCa. In the last few decades, many miRNAs profiles have been presented, but there is not a large consensus in the expression of a single signature in different groups. For this reason, many efforts have been undertaken to discover a panel of small RNAs in order to reduce the inter-individualities between several settings.

Larne et al. [149] focused their attention on a combination of four miRNAs. These four discriminatory miRNAs (miR-96-5p, miR-183-5p, miR-145-5p, and miR-221-5p), characterize the miR index quote (miQ). This test seems to predict PCa (AUC = 0.931) after a validation in four external cohorts. In addition, miQ was investigated to predict the manifestation of metastases (AUC = 0.827) and unfavorable disease behavior (AUC = 0.895).

As mentioned above, several miRNAs, regulated by or involved in AR transcriptional activity, are able to predict biochemical failure, clinical relapse, and castration resistant status. Interestingly, the overexpression of miR-21 has been reported in patients with castration-resistant disease [214], and it is reported to be an independent predictor of BCR in patients with a Gleason Score of 6 [215]. In the same way, miR-221 and miR-222 have been found to be upregulated in CRPC patients [216], and other studies demonstrate that miR-221 is also able to predict both recurrence and cancer related death [217,218].

6. Novel Treatments

Androgen deprivation therapy (ADT) is the principle treatment for advanced PCa and induces remission in 80%–90% of patients [219]. Despite an initial response, cancer cells are able to escape, and they subsequently continue to proliferate. This condition is termed castration resistant prostate cancer (CRPC), and it reportedly has a median overall survival rate of 23–37 months from the start of ADT [220]. The mechanisms governing the reactivation of AR despite castrated levels of testosterone have been widely studied. Although several alternative pathways have been observed and reported [221,222], the predominant mechanisms for cancer cell proliferation under deprivation conditions are due to reactivation, overexpression or mutation of the AR [223]. Therefore, therapies aimed to block the AR or to block the crosstalk of this steroid receptor with other molecular pathways are considered promising approaches to treat CRPCs. Here, we present three examples of how the regulation of AR epigenomic mechanisms could offer a novel therapeutic target to limit PCa proliferation.

6.1. Demethylase Inhibitor

Uncovering the locations of proteins throughout the genome helped physicians to understand the biology of both healthy and tumoral prostates. Chromatin immunoprecipitation (ChIP) followed by high-throughput DNA sequencing (ChIP-seq) is considered a novel technique to discover transcription factor binding sites, chromatin regulators, and the identification of genomic histone marks. Moreover, mapping the interactions of small molecules with chromatin, a technique named Chem-seq, has not only helped build the understanding of novel mechanisms underlying the biology of diseases but in discovering new specific treatments [224].

Chem-seq, ChIP-seq, and RNA-seq methods were used to evaluate the role of a small molecule, termed SD70, originally recognized as an inhibitor of DHT and chromosomal translocations events in PCa [225]. The 8-hydroxyquinoline domain of SD70 has been found to be similar to other molecules considered as competitive inhibitors of the histone demethylase KDM4 family and in particular KDM4C [226]. A biotinylated derivative of SD70 (B-SD70) has been observed as having the ability to bind the AR regulatory enhancers in an androgen-dependent manner. Further experiments show that SD70 was able to suppress DHT-regulated gene transcriptions in androgen dependent and independent cell lines, but at the same time, AR localization was not altered. As a consequence of its structure and analogy with other histone demethylase inhibitors, SD70 was found to inhibit the demethylase activity of KDM4C (Figure 1). KDM4C, as aforementioned above, plays a role in AR transcriptional program, mainly regulating the histone H3K9me3/me2 demethylase activity [50,227,228]. Using a Chem-seq assay on AR target gene enhancers, the authors reveal that KDM4C is located on the same gene enhancers that are co-occupied by B-SD70.

RNA-seq analysis in KDM4C knockdown cells confirmed the central role of KDM4C on AR target-gene regulation. Moreover, a Chip-seq in androgen dependent cells revealed that SD70 represses the methylation activity of KDM4C at the AR-regulated enhancers [225]. In consideration of the fact that "in vivo" experiments with a xenograft model unveiled a conspicuous inhibitor effect of SD70 on tumor cell growth without any particular toxicity, SD70 should be considered a potential candidate therapy in PCa patients.

6.2. Deacetylase Inhibitor

Histone deacetylase inhibitors (HDACi) are a group of molecules with anticancer activity against hematologic and solid tumors [229]. Different classes of HDAC, as previously described, modulate the acetylation profile of numerous genes including AR. Several studies have reported that HDAC inhibitors, such as trichostatin A (TSA), suberoylanilide hydroxamic acid (SAHA), and valproic acid, may reduce AR expression [230–232], but their mechanisms of action are not completely clear. One of them is undoubtedly correlated to the heat shock protein-90 (HSP90). HSP90 is a chaperone protein indispensable for molecular stability and the right folding and function of steroid hormone receptors such as the AR [233,234] (Figure 2).

A recent review [235] extensively reported the activity of several HDACi as novel therapeutic options in CRPC but here we might focus our attention on the efficacy of HDACi which mainly affect the HSP90-AR signaling.

Romidepsin is a cyclic depsipeptide, enhancing the acetylation of HSP90, that reportedly interferes with the correct folding of AR determining its degradation [236]. Despite these encouraging pre-clinical data and two phase I clinical trials that did not show a particular toxicity, a phase II study (NCT00106418) unveiled a very low clinical activity in 35 metastatic CRPC patients. In particular, only two enrolled patients displayed a PSA reduction more than 50% in a period of time longer than 6 months. Moreover, a substantial proportion of patients (31%) interrupted the trial due to several toxic effects [237]. As suggested by the same authors, these data do not support the use of single-agent romidepsin in unselected CRPC patients.

Panobinostat is a cinnamic hydroxamic acid class molecule with an HDACi activity. In vivo studies in AR-positive PCa cell lines showed a significant degradation of the AR mediated by the acetylation and subsequent inhibition of the HSP90 chaperone function [238]. In 2010, Rathkopf et al. reported the first results of a phase I clinical trial (NCT00663832) of oral panobinostat versus oral panobinostat plus docetaxel in patients with advanced disease. Despite the fact that all patients being solely treated with panobinostat displayed a clinical progression, 63% of patients treated with a combination therapy exhibited a biochemical response greater than 50% [238]. The same group examined the effect of intravenous panobinostat in a phase II trial (NCT00667862). Of the 35 enrolled patients, none of them exhibited a significant PSA reduction [239]. Again, despite promising preclinical data and a strong scientific rationale, panobinostat has not shown a sufficient level of clinical activity as a single agent in metastatic patients.

6.3. Non Coding RNA Therapy

In the last decade, several findings have documented the role of miRNAs as new oncogenes or tumor suppressor genes, thus supporting their use as therapeutic tools. Artificial miRNA mimics and inhibitors are considered a good way in which to "block or boost" the production of several proteins [240]. MiRNA mimics have been used to reintroduce tumor suppressor miRNAs, and miRNA inhibitors serve to reduce the levels of oncogenic miRNAs. Interesting results from preclinical studies using mouse models demonstrate the possible therapeutic application of miRNA mimics in PCa [241]. The bi-univocal correlation between p53, one of the most important tumor suppressor genes, and miR-34 highlighted the role of this miRNA as an encouraging therapy for cancer [242]. MiR-34a seems to be a promising target in PCa because "in vivo" studies proved that its reintroduction decreases the growth of prostate xenografts [243]. In April 2013, a liposome-formulated miRNA34a mimic (MRX34), sponsored by Mirna Therapeutics (Austin, TX, USA), was tested in a phase I clinical trial (NCT01829971) [244] (Figure 3). This was the first attempt to use a miRNA as an innovative therapy for cancer.

7. Conclusions

The androgen receptor is the central regulator of nominal and tumor prostate biology. Prostate carcinogenesis is a complex event due to genetic mutations and epigenetic alterations. In the past decade, the role of epigenetic regulation has become evident, and considerable progress has been made defining its role in the onset and progression of prostate cancer. In this review we focused our attention mainly on the AR epigenetic alterations. A better understanding of AR transcriptional pathway is indispensable to develop diagnostic and therapeutic procedures exploiting these epigenetic changes. Although PSA remains the prevalent test for prostate cancer screening and prognosis, the new generation of biomarkers can help physicians in their clinical decisions. The PCA3 test is widely used in clinical practice but chromatin remodeling marks and miRNA panels, as well as genomic tests, are becoming new promising predictive tools. New technologies for global epigenomic analyses and integration with genomic and transcriptomic data are extending our knowledge on prostate tumorigenesis. A new approach named "Chem-seq" permitted us to uncover the site and the mechanism of action of a small molecule named SD70. The demethylase SD70, targeting a key regulator of AR function, is effective in CRPC cells in combination with current therapies. Furthermore, the optimization of the stability of miRNAs and the improvement of the efficacy of HDAC inhibitors are also challenges for the future treatment of prostate cancer. Knowing the specific molecular mechanisms underlying tumors will be desiderable for the identification of more effective approaches allowing to personalize therapy.

Acknowledgments: The authors did not receive any founds in support of this research work.

Author Contributions: Vito Cucchiara performed the data analysis and wrote the paper; Joy C. Yang, Vincenzo Mirone, Allen C. Gao and Christopher P. Evans helped in drafting the manuscript; Michael G. Rosenfeld and Christopher P. Evans conceived and designed the project.

Conflicts of Interest: The authors declare no conflict of interest.

References

1. Torre, L.A.; Bray, F.; Siegel, R.L.; Ferlay, J.; Lortet-Tieulent, J.; Jemal, A. Global cancer statistics, 2012. *CA Cancer J. Clin.* **2015**, *65*, 87–108. [CrossRef] [PubMed]
2. Van der Steen, T.; Tindall, D.J.; Huang, H. Posttranslational modification of the androgen receptor in prostate cancer. *Int. J. Mol. Sci.* **2013**, *14*, 14833–14859. [CrossRef] [PubMed]
3. Sharifi, N.; Gulley, J.L.; Dahut, W.L. Androgen deprivation therapy for prostate cancer. *J. Am. Med. Assoc.* **2005**, *294*, 238–244. [CrossRef] [PubMed]
4. Mills, I.G. Maintaining and reprogramming genomic androgen receptor activity in prostate cancer. *Nat. Rev. Cancer* **2014**, *14*, 187–198. [CrossRef] [PubMed]
5. Huggins, C.; Stevens, R.E., Jr.; Hodges, C.V. Studies on prostatic cancer: The effects of castration on advanced carcinoma of the prostate gland. *Arch. Surg.* **1941**, *43*, 209–223. [CrossRef]
6. Masson, S.; Bahl, A. Metastatic castrate-resistant prostate cancer: Dawn of a new age of management. *BJU Int.* **2012**, *110*, 1110–1114. [CrossRef] [PubMed]
7. Bernstein, B.E.; Meissner, A.; Lander, E.S. The mammalian epigenome. *Cell* **2007**, *128*, 669–681. [CrossRef] [PubMed]
8. Probst, A.V.; Dunleavy, E.; Almouzni, G. Epigenetic inheritance during the cell cycle. *Nat. Rev. Mol. Cell Biol.* **2009**, *10*, 192–206. [CrossRef] [PubMed]
9. Kanwal, R.; Gupta, S. Epigenetics and cancer. *J. Appl. Physiol. (1985)* **2010**, *109*, 598–605. [CrossRef] [PubMed]
10. Sharma, S.; Kelly, T.K.; Jones, P.A. Epigenetics in cancer. *Carcinogenesis* **2010**, *31*, 27–36. [CrossRef] [PubMed]
11. Peterson, C.L.; Laniel, M.A. Histones and histone modifications. *Curr. Biol.* **2004**, *14*, R546–R551. [CrossRef] [PubMed]
12. Strahl, B.D.; Ohba, R.; Cook, R.G.; Allis, C.D. Methylation of histone H3 at lysine 4 is highly conserved and correlates with transcriptionally active nuclei in tetrahymena. *Proc. Natl. Acad. Sci. USA* **1999**, *96*, 14967–14972. [CrossRef] [PubMed]
13. Bannister, A.J.; Schneider, R.; Myers, F.A.; Thorne, A.W.; Crane-Robinson, C.; Kouzarides, T. Spatial distribution of Di- and Tri-methyl Lysine 36 of histone H3 at active genes. *J. Biol. Chem.* **2005**, *280*, 17732–17736. [CrossRef] [PubMed]
14. Heard, E.; Rougeulle, C.; Arnaud, D.; Avner, P.; Allis, C.D.; Spector, D.L. Methylation of histone H3 at Lys-9 is an early mark on the X chromosome during X inactivation. *Cell* **2001**, *107*, 727–738. [CrossRef]
15. Rougeulle, C.; Chaumeil, J.; Sarma, K.; Allis, C.D.; Reinberg, D.; Avner, P.; Heard, E. Differential histone H3 Lys-9 and Lys-27 methylation profiles on the X chromosome. *Mol. Cell. Biol.* **2004**, *24*, 5475–5484. [CrossRef] [PubMed]
16. Obianyo, O.; Thompson, P.R. Kinetic mechanism of protein arginine methyltransferase 6 (PRMT6). *J. Biol. Chem.* **2012**, *287*, 6062–6071. [CrossRef] [PubMed]
17. Schurter, B.T.; Koh, S.S.; Chen, D.; Bunick, G.J.; Harp, J.M.; Hanson, B.L.; Henschen-Edman, A.; Mackay, D.R.; Stallcup, M.R.; Aswad, D.W. Methylation of histone H3 by coactivator-associated arginine methyltransferase 1. *Biochemistry* **2001**, *40*, 5747–5756. [CrossRef] [PubMed]
18. Cai, C.; Yuan, X.; Balk, S.P. Androgen receptor epigenetics. *Transl. Androl. Urology* **2013**, *2*, 148–157.
19. Nishioka, K.; Chuikov, S.; Sarma, K.; Erdjument-Bromage, H.; Allis, C.D.; Tempst, P.; Reinberg, D. Set9, a novel histone H3 methyltransferase that facilitates transcription by precluding histone tail modifications required for heterochromatin formation. *Genes Dev.* **2002**, *16*, 479–489. [CrossRef] [PubMed]
20. Sonderstrup, I.M.; Nygard, S.B.; Poulsen, T.S.; Linnemann, D.; Stenvang, J.; Nielsen, H.J.; Bartek, J.; Brunner, N.; Norgaard, P.; Riis, L. Topoisomerase-1 and -2a gene copy numbers are elevated in mismatch repair-proficient colorectal cancers. *Mol. Oncol.* **2015**, *9*, 1207–1217. [CrossRef] [PubMed]
21. Wilson, J.R.; Jing, C.; Walker, P.A.; Martin, S.R.; Howell, S.A.; Blackburn, G.M.; Gamblin, S.J.; Xiao, B. Crystal structure and functional analysis of the histone methyltransferase set7/9. *Cell* **2002**, *111*, 105–115. [CrossRef]
22. Gaughan, L.; Stockley, J.; Wang, N.; McCracken, S.R.; Treumann, A.; Armstrong, K.; Shaheen, F.; Watt, K.; McEwan, I.J.; Wang, C.; et al. Regulation of the androgen receptor by SET9-mediated methylation. *Nucleic Acids Res.* **2011**, *39*, 1266–1279. [CrossRef] [PubMed]
23. Ko, S.; Ahn, J.; Song, C.S.; Kim, S.; Knapczyk-Stwora, K.; Chatterjee, B. Lysine methylation and functional modulation of androgen receptor by SET9 methyltransferase. *Mol. Endocrinol.* **2011**, *25*, 433–444. [CrossRef] [PubMed]

24. Langley, E.; Kemppainen, J.A.; Wilson, E.M. Intermolecular NH2-/carboxyl-terminal interactions in androgen receptor dimerization revealed by mutations that cause androgen insensitivity. *J. Biol. Chem.* **1998**, *273*, 92–101. [CrossRef] [PubMed]
25. Langley, E.; Zhou, Z.X.; Wilson, E.M. Evidence for an anti-parallel orientation of the ligand-activated human androgen receptor dimer. *J. Biol. Chem.* **1995**, *270*, 29983–29990. [PubMed]
26. He, B.; Gampe, R.T., Jr.; Kole, A.J.; Hnat, A.T.; Stanley, T.B.; An, G.; Stewart, E.L.; Kalman, R.I.; Minges, J.T.; Wilson, E.M. Structural basis for androgen receptor interdomain and coactivator interactions suggests a transition in nuclear receptor activation function dominance. *Mol. Cell* **2004**, *16*, 425–438. [CrossRef] [PubMed]
27. Kang, H.B.; Choi, Y.; Lee, J.M.; Choi, K.C.; Kim, H.C.; Yoo, J.Y.; Lee, Y.H.; Yoon, H.G. The histone methyltransferase, NSD2, enhances androgen receptor-mediated transcription. *FEBS Lett.* **2009**, *583*, 1880–1886. [CrossRef] [PubMed]
28. Asangani, I.A.; Ateeq, B.; Cao, Q.; Dodson, L.; Pandhi, M.; Kunju, L.P.; Mehra, R.; Lonigro, R.J.; Siddiqui, J.; Palanisamy, N.; et al. Characterization of the EZH2-MMSET histone methyltransferase regulatory axis in cancer. *Mol. Cell* **2013**, *49*, 80–93. [CrossRef] [PubMed]
29. Yang, P.; Guo, L.; Duan, Z.J.; Tepper, C.G.; Xue, L.; Chen, X.; Kung, H.J.; Gao, A.C.; Zou, J.X.; Chen, H.W. Histone methyltransferase NSD2/Mmset mediates constitutive NF-κB signaling for cancer cell proliferation, survival, and tumor growth via a feed-forward loop. *Mol. Cell. Biol.* **2012**, *32*, 3121–3131. [CrossRef] [PubMed]
30. Zhao, J.C.; Yu, J.; Runkle, C.; Wu, L.; Hu, M.; Wu, D.; Liu, J.S.; Wang, Q.; Qin, Z.S.; Yu, J. Cooperation between polycomb and androgen receptor during oncogenic transformation. *Genome Res.* **2012**, *22*, 322–331. [CrossRef] [PubMed]
31. Varambally, S.; Dhanasekaran, S.M.; Zhou, M.; Barrette, T.R.; Kumar-Sinha, C.; Sanda, M.G.; Ghosh, D.; Pienta, K.J.; Sewalt, R.G.; Otte, A.P.; et al. The polycomb group protein EZH2 is involved in progression of prostate cancer. *Nature* **2002**, *419*, 624–629. [CrossRef] [PubMed]
32. Dardenne, E.; Beltran, H.; Benelli, M.; Gayvert, K.; Berger, A.; Puca, L.; Cyrta, J.; Sboner, A.; Noorzad, Z.; MacDonald, T.; et al. *N*-Myc induces an EZH2-mediated transcriptional program driving neuroendocrine prostate cancer. *Cancer Cell* **2016**, *30*, 563–577. [CrossRef] [PubMed]
33. Tolkach, Y.; Merseburger, A.; Herrmann, T.; Kuczyk, M.; Serth, J.; Imkamp, F. Signatures of adverse pathological features, androgen insensitivity and metastatic potential in prostate cancer. *Anticancer Res.* **2015**, *35*, 5443–5451. [PubMed]
34. Cha, T.L.; Zhou, B.P.; Xia, W.; Wu, Y.; Yang, C.C.; Chen, C.T.; Ping, B.; Otte, A.P.; Hung, M.C. Akt-mediated phosphorylation of EZH2 suppresses methylation of Lysine 27 in histone H3. *Science* **2005**, *310*, 306–310. [CrossRef] [PubMed]
35. Xu, K.; Wu, Z.J.; Groner, A.C.; He, H.H.; Cai, C.; Lis, R.T.; Wu, X.; Stack, E.C.; Loda, M.; Liu, T.; et al. EZH2 oncogenic activity in castration-resistant prostate cancer cells is polycomb-independent. *Science* **2012**, *338*, 1465–1469. [CrossRef] [PubMed]
36. Hyllus, D.; Stein, C.; Schnabel, K.; Schiltz, E.; Imhof, A.; Dou, Y.; Hsieh, J.; Bauer, U.M. PRMT6-mediated methylation of R2 in histone H3 antagonizes H3 K4 trimethylation. *Genes Dev.* **2007**, *21*, 3369–3380. [CrossRef] [PubMed]
37. Vieira, F.Q.; Costa-Pinheiro, P.; Ramalho-Carvalho, J.; Pereira, A.; Menezes, F.D.; Antunes, L.; Carneiro, I.; Oliveira, J.; Henrique, R.; Jeronimo, C. Deregulated expression of selected histone methylases and demethylases in prostate carcinoma. *Endocr. Relat. Cancer* **2014**, *21*, 51–61. [CrossRef] [PubMed]
38. Almeida-Rios, D.; Graca, I.; Vieira, F.Q.; Ramalho-Carvalho, J.; Pereira-Silva, E.; Martins, A.T.; Oliveira, J.; Goncalves, C.S.; Costa, B.M.; Henrique, R.; et al. Histone methyltransferase PRMT6 plays an oncogenic role of in prostate cancer. *Oncotarget* **2016**, *7*, 53018–53028. [CrossRef] [PubMed]
39. Metzger, E.; Wissmann, M.; Yin, N.; Muller, J.M.; Schneider, R.; Peters, A.H.; Gunther, T.; Buettner, R.; Schule, R. Lsd1 demethylates repressive histone marks to promote androgen-receptor-dependent transcription. *Nature* **2005**, *437*, 436–439. [CrossRef] [PubMed]
40. Metzger, E.; Yin, N.; Wissmann, M.; Kunowska, N.; Fischer, K.; Friedrichs, N.; Patnaik, D.; Higgins, J.M.; Potier, N.; Scheidtmann, K.H.; et al. Phosphorylation of histone H3 at threonine 11 establishes a novel chromatin mark for transcriptional regulation. *Nat. Cell Biol.* **2008**, *10*, 53–60. [CrossRef] [PubMed]

41. Metzger, E.; Imhof, A.; Patel, D.; Kahl, P.; Hoffmeyer, K.; Friedrichs, N.; Muller, J.M.; Greschik, H.; Kirfel, J.; Ji, S.; et al. Phosphorylation of histone H3T6 by PKCbeta(i) controls demethylation at histone H3K4. *Nature* **2010**, *464*, 792–796. [CrossRef] [PubMed]
42. Yang, S.; Zhang, J.; Zhang, Y.; Wan, X.; Zhang, C.; Huang, X.; Huang, W.; Pu, H.; Pei, C.; Wu, H.; et al. Kdm1a triggers androgen-induced miRNA transcription via H3K4me2 demethylation and DNA oxidation. *Prostate* **2015**, *75*, 936–946. [CrossRef] [PubMed]
43. Shi, Y.; Lan, F.; Matson, C.; Mulligan, P.; Whetstine, J.R.; Cole, P.A.; Casero, R.A.; Shi, Y. Histone demethylation mediated by the nuclear amine oxidase homolog LSD1. *Cell* **2004**, *119*, 941–953. [CrossRef] [PubMed]
44. Cai, C.; He, H.H.; Chen, S.; Coleman, I.; Wang, H.; Fang, Z.; Chen, S.; Nelson, P.S.; Liu, X.S.; Brown, M.; et al. Androgen receptor gene expression in prostate cancer is directly suppressed by the androgen receptor through recruitment of lysine-specific demethylase 1. *Cancer Cell* **2011**, *20*, 457–471. [CrossRef] [PubMed]
45. Stanbrough, M.; Bubley, G.J.; Ross, K.; Golub, T.R.; Rubin, M.A.; Penning, T.M.; Febbo, P.G.; Balk, S.P. Increased expression of genes converting adrenal androgens to testosterone in androgen-independent prostate cancer. *Cancer Res.* **2006**, *66*, 2815–2825. [CrossRef] [PubMed]
46. Wako, K.; Kawasaki, T.; Yamana, K.; Suzuki, K.; Jiang, S.; Umezu, H.; Nishiyama, T.; Takahashi, K.; Hamakubo, T.; Kodama, T.; et al. Expression of androgen receptor through androgen-converting enzymes is associated with biological aggressiveness in prostate cancer. *J. Clin. Pathol.* **2008**, *61*, 448–454. [CrossRef] [PubMed]
47. Liu, C.; Lou, W.; Zhu, Y.; Yang, J.C.; Nadiminty, N.; Gaikwad, N.W.; Evans, C.P.; Gao, A.C. Intracrine androgens and AKR1C3 activation confer resistance to enzalutamide in prostate cancer. *Cancer Res.* **2015**, *75*, 1413–1422. [CrossRef] [PubMed]
48. Liu, C.; Armstrong, C.M.; Lou, W.; Lombard, A.; Evans, C.P.; Gao, A.C. Inhibition of AKR1C3 activation overcomes resistance to abiraterone in advanced prostate cancer. *Mol. Cancer Ther.* **2016**, *16*, 35–44. [CrossRef] [PubMed]
49. Coffey, K.; Rogerson, L.; Ryan-Munden, C.; Alkharaif, D.; Stockley, J.; Heer, R.; Sahadevan, K.; O'Neill, D.; Jones, D.; Darby, S.; et al. The lysine demethylase, KDM4B, is a key molecule in androgen receptor signalling and turnover. *Nucleic Acids Res.* **2013**, *41*, 4433–4446. [CrossRef] [PubMed]
50. Wissmann, M.; Yin, N.; Muller, J.M.; Greschik, H.; Fodor, B.D.; Jenuwein, T.; Vogler, C.; Schneider, R.; Gunther, T.; Buettner, R.; et al. Cooperative demethylation by JMJD2C and LSD1 promotes androgen receptor-dependent gene expression. *Nat. Cell Biol.* **2007**, *9*, 347–353. [CrossRef] [PubMed]
51. Yamane, K.; Toumazou, C.; Tsukada, Y.; Erdjument-Bromage, H.; Tempst, P.; Wong, J.; Zhang, Y. JHDM2A, a JmjC-containing H3K9 demethylase, facilitates transcription activation by androgen receptor. *Cell* **2006**, *125*, 483–495. [CrossRef] [PubMed]
52. Tomlins, S.A.; Rhodes, D.R.; Perner, S.; Dhanasekaran, S.M.; Mehra, R.; Sun, X.W.; Varambally, S.; Cao, X.; Tchinda, J.; Kuefer, R.; et al. Recurrent fusion of TMPRSS2 and ETS transcription factor genes in prostate cancer. *Science* **2005**, *310*, 644–648. [CrossRef] [PubMed]
53. Haffner, M.C.; de Marzo, A.M.; Meeker, A.K.; Nelson, W.G.; Yegnasubramanian, S. Transcription-induced DNA double strand breaks: Both oncogenic force and potential therapeutic target? *Clin. Cancer Res.* **2011**, *17*, 3858–3864. [CrossRef] [PubMed]
54. Haffner, M.C.; Aryee, M.J.; Toubaji, A.; Esopi, D.M.; Albadine, R.; Gurel, B.; Isaacs, W.B.; Bova, G.S.; Liu, W.; Xu, J.; et al. Androgen-induced TOP2B-mediated double-strand breaks and prostate cancer gene rearrangements. *Nat. Genet.* **2010**, *42*, 668–675. [CrossRef] [PubMed]
55. Yu, J.; Yu, J.; Mani, R.S.; Cao, Q.; Brenner, C.J.; Cao, X.; Wang, X.; Wu, L.; Li, J.; Hu, M.; et al. An integrated network of androgen receptor, polycomb, and TMPRSS2-ERG gene fusions in prostate cancer progression. *Cancer Cell* **2010**, *17*, 443–454. [CrossRef] [PubMed]
56. Metzger, E.; Willmann, D.; McMillan, J.; Forne, I.; Metzger, P.; Gerhardt, S.; Petroll, K.; von Maessenhausen, A.; Urban, S.; Schott, A.K.; et al. Assembly of methylated KDM1A and CHD1 drives androgen receptor-dependent transcription and translocation. *Nat. Struct. Mol. Biol.* **2016**, *23*, 132–139. [CrossRef] [PubMed]
57. Fu, M.; Rao, M.; Wu, K.; Wang, C.; Zhang, X.; Hessien, M.; Yeung, Y.G.; Gioeli, D.; Weber, M.J.; Pestell, R.G. The androgen receptor acetylation site regulates cAMP and Akt but not ERK-induced activity. *J. Biol. Chem.* **2004**, *279*, 29436–29449. [CrossRef] [PubMed]
58. Grant, P.A.; Berger, S.L. Histone acetyltransferase complexes. *Semin. Cell Dev. Biol.* **1999**, *10*, 169–177. [CrossRef] [PubMed]

59. Fu, M.; Wang, C.; Reutens, A.T.; Wang, J.; Angeletti, R.H.; Siconolfi-Baez, L.; Ogryzko, V.; Avantaggiati, M.L.; Pestell, R.G. P300 and p300/cAMP-response element-binding protein-associated factor acetylate the androgen receptor at sites governing hormone-dependent transactivation. *J. Biol. Chem.* **2000**, *275*, 20853–20860. [CrossRef] [PubMed]
60. Coffey, K.; Robson, C.N. Regulation of the androgen receptor by post-translational modifications. *J. Endocrinol.* **2012**, *215*, 221–237. [CrossRef] [PubMed]
61. Lavery, D.N.; Bevan, C.L. Androgen receptor signalling in prostate cancer: The functional consequences of acetylation. *J. Biomed. Biotechnol.* **2011**. [CrossRef] [PubMed]
62. Culig, Z. Androgen receptor coactivators in regulation of growth and differentiation in prostate cancer. *J. Cell. Physiol.* **2016**, *231*, 270–274. [CrossRef] [PubMed]
63. Fu, M.; Rao, M.; Wang, C.; Sakamaki, T.; Wang, J.; di Vizio, D.; Zhang, X.; Albanese, C.; Balk, S.; Chang, C.; et al. Acetylation of androgen receptor enhances coactivator binding and promotes prostate cancer cell growth. *Mol. Cell. Biol.* **2003**, *23*, 8563–8575. [CrossRef] [PubMed]
64. Xu, K.; Shimelis, H.; Linn, D.E.; Jiang, R.; Yang, X.; Sun, F.; Guo, Z.; Chen, H.; Li, W.; Chen, H.; et al. Regulation of androgen receptor transcriptional activity and specificity by rnf6-induced ubiquitination. *Cancer Cell* **2009**, *15*, 270–282. [CrossRef] [PubMed]
65. Xu, J.; Wu, R.C.; O'Malley, B.W. Normal and cancer-related functions of the p160 steroid receptor co-activator (SRC) family. *Nat. Rev. Cancer* **2009**, *9*, 615–630. [CrossRef] [PubMed]
66. Gaughan, L.; Logan, I.R.; Cook, S.; Neal, D.E.; Robson, C.N. Tip60 and histone deacetylase 1 regulate androgen receptor activity through changes to the acetylation status of the receptor. *J. Biol. Chem.* **2002**, *277*, 25904–25913. [CrossRef] [PubMed]
67. Wang, Z.; Wang, Z.; Guo, J.; Li, Y.; Bavarva, J.H.; Qian, C.; Brahimi-Horn, M.C.; Tan, D.; Liu, W. Inactivation of androgen-induced regulator ard1 inhibits androgen receptor acetylation and prostate tumorigenesis. *Proc. Natl. Acad. Sci. USA* **2012**, *109*, 3053–3058. [CrossRef] [PubMed]
68. Bannister, A.J.; Kouzarides, T. The CBP co-activator is a histone acetyltransferase. *Nature* **1996**, *384*, 641–643. [CrossRef] [PubMed]
69. Ogryzko, V.V.; Schiltz, R.L.; Russanova, V.; Howard, B.H.; Nakatani, Y. The transcriptional coactivators p300 and CBP are histone acetyltransferases. *Cell* **1996**, *87*, 953–959. [CrossRef]
70. Zhong, J.; Ding, L.; Bohrer, L.R.; Pan, Y.; Liu, P.; Zhang, J.; Sebo, T.J.; Karnes, R.J.; Tindall, D.J.; van Deursen, J.; et al. P300 acetyltransferase regulates androgen receptor degradation and pten-deficient prostate tumorigenesis. *Cancer Res.* **2014**, *74*, 1870–1880. [CrossRef] [PubMed]
71. Levy, L.; Wei, Y.; Labalette, C.; Wu, Y.; Renard, C.A.; Buendia, M.A.; Neuveut, C. Acetylation of beta-catenin by p300 regulates beta-catenin-Tcf4 interaction. *Mol. Cell. Biol.* **2004**, *24*, 3404–3414. [CrossRef] [PubMed]
72. Spencer, T.E.; Jenster, G.; Burcin, M.M.; Allis, C.D.; Zhou, J.; Mizzen, C.A.; McKenna, N.J.; Onate, S.A.; Tsai, S.Y.; Tsai, M.J.; et al. Steroid receptor coactivator-1 is a histone acetyltransferase. *Nature* **1997**, *389*, 194–198. [PubMed]
73. McKenna, N.J.; Lanz, R.B.; O'Malley, B.W. Nuclear receptor coregulators: Cellular and molecular biology. *Endocr. Rev.* **1999**, *20*, 321–344. [CrossRef] [PubMed]
74. Nakka, M.; Agoulnik, I.U.; Weigel, N.L. Targeted disruption of the p160 coactivator interface of androgen receptor (AR) selectively inhibits AR activity in both androgen-dependent and castration-resistant ar-expressing prostate cancer cells. *Int. J. Biochem. Cell Biol.* **2013**, *45*, 763–772. [CrossRef] [PubMed]
75. Gong, J.; Zhu, J.; Goodman, O.B., Jr.; Pestell, R.G.; Schlegel, P.N.; Nanus, D.M.; Shen, R. Activation of p300 histone acetyltransferase activity and acetylation of the androgen receptor by bombesin in prostate cancer cells. *Oncogene* **2006**, *25*, 2011–2021. [CrossRef] [PubMed]
76. Lee, S.O.; Chun, J.Y.; Nadiminty, N.; Lou, W.; Feng, S.; Gao, A.C. Interleukin-4 activates androgen receptor through CBP/p300. *Prostate* **2009**, *69*, 126–132. [CrossRef] [PubMed]
77. Malinowska, K.; Neuwirt, H.; Cavarretta, I.T.; Bektic, J.; Steiner, H.; Dietrich, H.; Moser, P.L.; Fuchs, D.; Hobisch, A.; Culig, Z. Interleukin-6 stimulation of growth of prostate cancer in vitro and in vivo through activation of the androgen receptor. *Endocr.-Relat. Cancer* **2009**, *16*, 155–169. [CrossRef] [PubMed]
78. Ueda, T.; Mawji, N.R.; Bruchovsky, N.; Sadar, M.D. Ligand-independent activation of the androgen receptor by interleukin-6 and the role of steroid receptor coactivator-1 in prostate cancer cells. *J. Biol. Chem.* **2002**, *277*, 38087–38094. [CrossRef] [PubMed]

79. Brady, M.E.; Ozanne, D.M.; Gaughan, L.; Waite, I.; Cook, S.; Neal, D.E.; Robson, C.N. Tip60 is a nuclear hormone receptor coactivator. *J. Biol. Chem.* **1999**, *274*, 17599–17604. [CrossRef] [PubMed]
80. Gaughan, L.; Logan, I.R.; Neal, D.E.; Robson, C.N. Regulation of androgen receptor and histone deacetylase 1 by mdm2-mediated ubiquitylation. *Nucleic Acids Res.* **2005**, *33*, 13–26. [CrossRef] [PubMed]
81. Shiota, M.; Yokomizo, A.; Masubuchi, D.; Tada, Y.; Inokuchi, J.; Eto, M.; Uchiumi, T.; Fujimoto, N.; Naito, S. Tip60 promotes prostate cancer cell proliferation by translocation of androgen receptor into the nucleus. *Prostate* **2010**, *70*, 540–554. [CrossRef] [PubMed]
82. Park, E.C.; Szostak, J.W. Ard1 and nat1 proteins form a complex that has N-terminal acetyltransferase activity. *EMBO J.* **1992**, *11*, 2087–2093. [PubMed]
83. Hua, K.T.; Tan, C.T.; Johansson, G.; Lee, J.M.; Yang, P.W.; Lu, H.Y.; Chen, C.K.; Su, J.L.; Chen, P.B.; Wu, Y.L.; et al. *N*-alpha-acetyltransferase 10 protein suppresses cancer cell metastasis by binding PIX proteins and inhibiting Cdc42/Rac1 activity. *Cancer Cell* **2011**, *19*, 218–231. [CrossRef] [PubMed]
84. Jeong, J.W.; Bae, M.K.; Ahn, M.Y.; Kim, S.H.; Sohn, T.K.; Bae, M.H.; Yoo, M.A.; Song, E.J.; Lee, K.J.; Kim, K.W. Regulation and destabilization of HIF-1alpha by ARD1-mediated acetylation. *Cell* **2002**, *111*, 709–720. [CrossRef]
85. Lee, C.F.; Ou, D.S.; Lee, S.B.; Chang, L.H.; Lin, R.K.; Li, Y.S.; Upadhyay, A.K.; Cheng, X.; Wang, Y.C.; Hsu, H.S.; et al. HNaa10p contributes to tumorigenesis by facilitating DNMT1-mediated tumor suppressor gene silencing. *J. Clin. Investig.* **2010**, *120*, 2920–2930. [CrossRef] [PubMed]
86. DePaolo, J.S.; Wang, Z.; Guo, J.; Zhang, G.; Qian, C.; Zhang, H.; Zabaleta, J.; Liu, W. Acetylation of androgen receptor by ARD1 promotes dissociation from HSP90 complex and prostate tumorigenesis. *Oncotarget* **2016**, *7*, 71417–71428. [CrossRef] [PubMed]
87. Urbanucci, A.; Marttila, S.; Janne, O.A.; Visakorpi, T. Androgen receptor overexpression alters binding dynamics of the receptor to chromatin and chromatin structure. *Prostate* **2012**, *72*, 1223–1232. [CrossRef] [PubMed]
88. Jia, L.; Shen, H.C.; Wantroba, M.; Khalid, O.; Liang, G.; Wang, Q.; Gentzschein, E.; Pinski, J.K.; Stanczyk, F.Z.; Jones, P.A.; et al. Locus-wide chromatin remodeling and enhanced androgen receptor-mediated transcription in recurrent prostate tumor cells. *Mol. Cell. Biol.* **2006**, *26*, 7331–7341. [CrossRef] [PubMed]
89. Karvonen, U.; Janne, O.A.; Palvimo, J.J. Androgen receptor regulates nuclear trafficking and nuclear domain residency of corepressor HDAC7 in a ligand-dependent fashion. *Exp. Cell Res.* **2006**, *312*, 3165–3183. [CrossRef] [PubMed]
90. Ai, J.; Wang, Y.; Dar, J.A.; Liu, J.; Liu, L.; Nelson, J.B.; Wang, Z. Hdac6 regulates androgen receptor hypersensitivity and nuclear localization via modulating HSP90 acetylation in castration-resistant prostate cancer. *Mol. Endocrinol.* **2009**, *23*, 1963–1972. [CrossRef] [PubMed]
91. Fu, M.; Liu, M.; Sauve, A.A.; Jiao, X.; Zhang, X.; Wu, X.; Powell, M.J.; Yang, T.; Gu, W.; Avantaggiati, M.L.; et al. Hormonal control of androgen receptor function through SIRT1. *Mol. Cell. Biol.* **2006**, *26*, 8122–8135. [CrossRef] [PubMed]
92. Zhang, A.; Zhang, J.; Kaipainen, A.; Lucas, J.M.; Yang, H. Long non-coding RNA: A newly deciphered "code" in prostate cancer. *Cancer Lett.* **2016**, *375*, 323–330. [CrossRef] [PubMed]
93. Brosnan, C.A.; Voinnet, O. The long and the short of noncoding RNAs. *Curr. Opin. Cell Biol.* **2009**, *21*, 416–425. [CrossRef] [PubMed]
94. Bartel, D.P. MicroRNAs: Genomics, biogenesis, mechanism, and function. *Cell* **2004**, *116*, 281–297. [CrossRef]
95. Bartel, D.P. MicroRNAs: Target recognition and regulatory functions. *Cell* **2009**, *136*, 215–233. [CrossRef] [PubMed]
96. Tay, Y.; Zhang, J.; Thomson, A.M.; Lim, B.; Rigoutsos, I. MicroRNAs to nanog, Oct4 and Sox2 coding regions modulate embryonic stem cell differentiation. *Nature* **2008**, *455*, 1124–1128. [CrossRef] [PubMed]
97. Shih, J.W.; Wang, L.Y.; Hung, C.L.; Kung, H.J.; Hsieh, C.L. Non-coding RNAs in castration-resistant prostate cancer: Regulation of androgen receptor signaling and cancer metabolism. *Int. J. Mol. Sci.* **2015**, *16*, 28943–28978. [CrossRef] [PubMed]
98. Waltering, K.K.; Porkka, K.P.; Jalava, S.E.; Urbanucci, A.; Kohonen, P.J.; Latonen, L.M.; Kallioniemi, O.P.; Jenster, G.; Visakorpi, T. Androgen regulation of micro-RNAs in prostate cancer. *Prostate* **2011**, *71*, 604–614. [CrossRef] [PubMed]

99. Mo, W.; Zhang, J.; Li, X.; Meng, D.; Gao, Y.; Yang, S.; Wan, X.; Zhou, C.; Guo, F.; Huang, Y.; et al. Identification of novel AR-targeted microRNAs mediating androgen signalling through critical pathways to regulate cell viability in prostate cancer. *PLoS ONE* **2013**, *8*, e56592. [CrossRef] [PubMed]
100. Murata, T.; Takayama, K.; Katayama, S.; Urano, T.; Horie-Inoue, K.; Ikeda, K.; Takahashi, S.; Kawazu, C.; Hasegawa, A.; Ouchi, Y.; et al. MiR-148a is an androgen-responsive microRNA that promotes LNCaP prostate cell growth by repressing its target cand1 expression. *Prostate Cancer Prostatic Dis.* **2010**, *13*, 356–361. [CrossRef] [PubMed]
101. Fletcher, C.E.; Dart, D.A.; Sita-Lumsden, A.; Cheng, H.; Rennie, P.S.; Bevan, C.L. Androgen-regulated processing of the oncomir miR-27a, which targets prohibitin in prostate cancer. *Hum. Mol. Genet.* **2012**, *21*, 3112–3127. [CrossRef] [PubMed]
102. Takayama, K.; Tsutsumi, S.; Katayama, S.; Okayama, T.; Horie-Inoue, K.; Ikeda, K.; Urano, T.; Kawazu, C.; Hasegawa, A.; Ikeo, K.; et al. Integration of cap analysis of gene expression and chromatin immunoprecipitation analysis on array reveals genome-wide androgen receptor signaling in prostate cancer cells. *Oncogene* **2011**, *30*, 619–630. [CrossRef] [PubMed]
103. Sun, D.; Layer, R.; Mueller, A.C.; Cichewicz, M.A.; Negishi, M.; Paschal, B.M.; Dutta, A. Regulation of several androgen-induced genes through the repression of the miR-99a/let-7c/miR-125b-2 miRNA cluster in prostate cancer cells. *Oncogene* **2014**, *33*, 1448–1457. [CrossRef] [PubMed]
104. Pang, Y.; Young, C.Y.; Yuan, H. MicroRNAs and prostate cancer. *Acta Biochim. Biophys. Sin.* **2010**, *42*, 363–369. [CrossRef] [PubMed]
105. Catto, J.W.; Alcaraz, A.; Bjartell, A.S.; de Vere White, R.; Evans, C.P.; Fussel, S.; Hamdy, F.C.; Kallioniemi, O.; Mengual, L.; Schlomm, T.; et al. MicroRNA in prostate, bladder, and kidney cancer: A systematic review. *Eur. Urol.* **2011**, *59*, 671–681. [CrossRef] [PubMed]
106. Yang, X.; Bemis, L.; Su, L.J.; Gao, D.; Flaig, T.W. Mir-125b regulation of androgen receptor signaling via modulation of the receptor complex co-repressor NCOR2. *Biores. Open Access* **2012**, *1*, 55–62. [CrossRef] [PubMed]
107. ChunJiao, S.; Huan, C.; ChaoYang, X.; GuoMei, R. Uncovering the roles of miRNAs and their relationship with androgen receptor in prostate cancer. *IUBMB Life* **2014**, *66*, 379–386. [CrossRef] [PubMed]
108. Xu, X.; Lv, Y.G.; Yan, C.Y.; Yi, J.; Ling, R. Enforced expression of hsa-miR-125a-3p in breast cancer cells potentiates docetaxel sensitivity via modulation of BRCA1 signaling. *Biochem. Biophys. Res. Commun.* **2016**, *479*, 893–900. [CrossRef] [PubMed]
109. Kroiss, A.; Vincent, S.; Decaussin-Petrucci, M.; Meugnier, E.; Viallet, J.; Ruffion, A.; Chalmel, F.; Samarut, J.; Allioli, N. Androgen-regulated microRNA-135a decreases prostate cancer cell migration and invasion through downregulating rock1 and rock2. *Oncogene* **2015**, *34*, 2846–2855. [CrossRef] [PubMed]
110. Coarfa, C.; Fiskus, W.; Eedunuri, V.K.; Rajapakshe, K.; Foley, C.; Chew, S.A.; Shah, S.S.; Geng, C.; Shou, J.; Mohamed, J.S.; et al. Comprehensive proteomic profiling identifies the androgen receptor axis and other signaling pathways as targets of microRNAs suppressed in metastatic prostate cancer. *Oncogene* **2016**, *35*, 2345–2356. [CrossRef] [PubMed]
111. Wan, X.; Pu, H.; Huang, W.; Yang, S.; Zhang, Y.; Kong, Z.; Yang, Z.; Zhao, P.; Li, A.; Li, T.; et al. Androgen-induced miR-135a acts as a tumor suppressor through downregulating RBAK and MMP11, and mediates resistance to androgen deprivation therapy. *Oncotarget* **2016**, *7*, 51284–51300. [CrossRef] [PubMed]
112. Jalava, S.E.; Urbanucci, A.; Latonen, L.; Waltering, K.K.; Sahu, B.; Janne, O.A.; Seppala, J.; Lahdesmaki, H.; Tammela, T.L.; Visakorpi, T. Androgen-regulated miR-32 targets BTG2 and is overexpressed in castration-resistant prostate cancer. *Oncogene* **2012**, *31*, 4460–4471. [CrossRef] [PubMed]
113. Mao, B.; Zhang, Z.; Wang, G. BTG2: A rising star of tumor suppressors (review). *Int. J. Oncol.* **2015**, *46*, 459–464. [CrossRef] [PubMed]
114. Ribas, J.; Ni, X.; Haffner, M.; Wentzel, E.A.; Salmasi, A.H.; Chowdhury, W.H.; Kudrolli, T.A.; Yegnasubramanian, S.; Luo, J.; Rodriguez, R.; et al. MiR-21: An androgen receptor-regulated microRNA that promotes hormone-dependent and hormone-independent prostate cancer growth. *Cancer Res.* **2009**, *69*, 7165–7169. [CrossRef] [PubMed]
115. Fujita, S.; Ito, T.; Mizutani, T.; Minoguchi, S.; Yamamichi, N.; Sakurai, K.; Iba, H. MiR-21 gene expression triggered by AP-1 is sustained through a double-negative feedback mechanism. *J. Mol. Biol.* **2008**, *378*, 492–504. [CrossRef] [PubMed]

116. Iliopoulos, D.; Jaeger, S.A.; Hirsch, H.A.; Bulyk, M.L.; Struhl, K. STAT3 activation of miR-21 and miR-181b-1 via PTEN and CYLD are part of the epigenetic switch linking inflammation to cancer. *Mol. Cell* **2010**, *39*, 493–506. [CrossRef] [PubMed]
117. Mishra, S.; Deng, J.J.; Gowda, P.S.; Rao, M.K.; Lin, C.L.; Chen, C.L.; Huang, T.; Sun, L.Z. Androgen receptor and microRNA-21 axis downregulates transforming growth factor beta receptor II (TGFBR2) expression in prostate cancer. *Oncogene* **2014**, *33*, 4097–4106. [CrossRef] [PubMed]
118. Mishra, S.; Lin, C.L.; Huang, T.H.; Bouamar, H.; Sun, L.Z. MicroRNA-21 inhibits p57kip2 expression in prostate cancer. *Mol. Cancer* **2014**. [CrossRef] [PubMed]
119. Garofalo, M.; Quintavalle, C.; Romano, G.; Croce, C.M.; Condorelli, G. MiR221/222 in cancer: Their role in tumor progression and response to therapy. *Curr. Mol. Med.* **2012**, *12*, 27–33. [CrossRef] [PubMed]
120. Gordanpour, A.; Stanimirovic, A.; Nam, R.K.; Moreno, C.S.; Sherman, C.; Sugar, L.; Seth, A. MiR-221 is down-regulated in tmprss2:Erg fusion-positive prostate cancer. *Anticancer Res.* **2011**, *31*, 403–410. [PubMed]
121. Li, T.; Li, R.S.; Li, Y.H.; Zhong, S.; Chen, Y.Y.; Zhang, C.M.; Hu, M.M.; Shen, Z.J. MiR-21 as an independent biochemical recurrence predictor and potential therapeutic target for prostate cancer. *J. Urol.* **2012**, *187*, 1466–1472. [CrossRef] [PubMed]
122. Yang, X.; Yang, Y.; Gan, R.; Zhao, L.; Li, W.; Zhou, H.; Wang, X.; Lu, J.; Meng, Q.H. Down-regulation of miR-221 and miR-222 restrain prostate cancer cell proliferation and migration that is partly mediated by activation of sirt1. *PLoS ONE* **2014**, *9*, e98833. [CrossRef] [PubMed]
123. Sun, T.; Wang, X.; He, H.H.; Sweeney, C.J.; Liu, S.X.; Brown, M.; Balk, S.; Lee, G.S.; Kantoff, P.W. MiR-221 promotes the development of androgen independence in prostate cancer cells via downregulation of HECTD2 and RAB1A. *Oncogene* **2014**, *33*, 2790–2800. [CrossRef] [PubMed]
124. Ostling, P.; Leivonen, S.K.; Aakula, A.; Kohonen, P.; Makela, R.; Hagman, Z.; Edsjo, A.; Kangaspeska, S.; Edgren, H.; Nicorici, D.; et al. Systematic analysis of microRNAs targeting the androgen receptor in prostate cancer cells. *Cancer Res.* **2011**, *71*, 1956–1967. [CrossRef] [PubMed]
125. Gao, L.; Alumkal, J. Epigenetic regulation of androgen receptor signaling in prostate cancer. *Epigenetics* **2010**, *5*, 100–104. [CrossRef] [PubMed]
126. Hagman, Z.; Haflidadottir, B.S.; Ceder, J.A.; Larne, O.; Bjartell, A.; Lilja, H.; Edsjo, A.; Ceder, Y. MiR-205 negatively regulates the androgen receptor and is associated with adverse outcome of prostate cancer patients. *Br. J. Cancer* **2013**, *108*, 1668–1676. [CrossRef] [PubMed]
127. Choi, Y.J.; Lin, C.P.; Ho, J.J.; He, X.; Okada, N.; Bu, P.; Zhong, Y.; Kim, S.Y.; Bennett, M.J.; Chen, C.; et al. MiR-34 miRNAs provide a barrier for somatic cell reprogramming. *Nat. Cell Biol.* **2011**, *13*, 1353–1360. [CrossRef] [PubMed]
128. Hagman, Z.; Larne, O.; Edsjo, A.; Bjartell, A.; Ehrnstrom, R.A.; Ulmert, D.; Lilja, H.; Ceder, Y. MiR-34c is downregulated in prostate cancer and exerts tumor suppressive functions. *Int. J. Cancer* **2010**, *127*, 2768–2776. [CrossRef] [PubMed]
129. Kong, D.; Heath, E.; Chen, W.; Cher, M.; Powell, I.; Heilbrun, L.; Li, Y.; Ali, S.; Sethi, S.; Hassan, O.; et al. Epigenetic silencing of miR-34a in human prostate cancer cells and tumor tissue specimens can be reversed by br-dim treatment. *Am. J. Transl. Res.* **2012**, *4*, 14–23. [PubMed]
130. Cannell, I.G.; Kong, Y.W.; Johnston, S.J.; Chen, M.L.; Collins, H.M.; Dobbyn, H.C.; Elia, A.; Kress, T.R.; Dickens, M.; Clemens, M.J.; et al. P38 mapk/mk2-mediated induction of miR-34c following DNA damage prevents myc-dependent DNA replication. *Proc. Natl. Acad. Sci. USA* **2010**, *107*, 5375–5380. [CrossRef] [PubMed]
131. Corney, D.C.; Flesken-Nikitin, A.; Godwin, A.K.; Wang, W.; Nikitin, A.Y. MicroRNA-34b and microRNA-34c are targets of p53 and cooperate in control of cell proliferation and adhesion-independent growth. *Cancer Res.* **2007**, *67*, 8433–8438. [CrossRef] [PubMed]
132. Toyota, M.; Suzuki, H.; Sasaki, Y.; Maruyama, R.; Imai, K.; Shinomura, Y.; Tokino, T. Epigenetic silencing of microRNA-34b/c and B-cell translocation gene 4 is associated with cpg island methylation in colorectal cancer. *Cancer Res.* **2008**, *68*, 4123–4132. [CrossRef] [PubMed]
133. Fang, Z.; Xu, C.; Li, Y.; Cai, X.; Ren, S.; Liu, H.; Wang, Y.; Wang, F.; Chen, R.; Qu, M.; et al. A feed-forward regulatory loop between androgen receptor and PlncRNA-1 promotes prostate cancer progression. *Cancer Lett.* **2016**, *374*, 62–74. [CrossRef] [PubMed]

134. Calin, G.A.; Liu, C.G.; Sevignani, C.; Ferracin, M.; Felli, N.; Dumitru, C.D.; Shimizu, M.; Cimmino, A.; Zupo, S.; Dono, M.; et al. MicroRNA profiling reveals distinct signatures in B cell chronic lymphocytic leukemias. *Proc. Natl. Acad. Sci. USA* **2004**, *101*, 11755–11760. [CrossRef] [PubMed]
135. Ozen, M.; Creighton, C.J.; Ozdemir, M.; Ittmann, M. Widespread deregulation of microRNA expression in human prostate cancer. *Oncogene* **2008**, *27*, 1788–1793. [CrossRef]
136. Johnson, S.M.; Grosshans, H.; Shingara, J.; Byrom, M.; Jarvis, R.; Cheng, A.; Labourier, E.; Reinert, K.L.; Brown, D.; Slack, F.J. RAS is regulated by the let-7 microRNA family. *Cell* **2005**, *120*, 635–647. [CrossRef] [PubMed]
137. Kumar, M.S.; Lu, J.; Mercer, K.L.; Golub, T.R.; Jacks, T. Impaired microRNA processing enhances cellular transformation and tumorigenesis. *Nat. Genet.* **2007**, *39*, 673–677. [CrossRef] [PubMed]
138. Nadiminty, N.; Tummala, R.; Lou, W.; Zhu, Y.; Zhang, J.; Chen, X.; eVere White, R.W.; Kung, H.J.; Evans, C.P.; Gao, A.C. MicroRNA let-7c suppresses androgen receptor expression and activity via regulation of myc expression in prostate cancer cells. *J. Biol. Chem.* **2012**, *287*, 1527–1537. [CrossRef]
139. Gao, L.; Schwartzman, J.; Gibbs, A.; Lisac, R.; Kleinschmidt, R.; Wilmot, B.; Bottomly, D.; Coleman, I.; Nelson, P.; McWeeney, S.; et al. Androgen receptor promotes ligand-independent prostate cancer progression through c-Myc upregulation. *PLoS ONE* **2013**, *8*, e63563. [CrossRef] [PubMed]
140. Epis, M.R.; Giles, K.M.; Barker, A.; Kendrick, T.S.; Leedman, P.J. Mir-331–3p regulates erbb-2 expression and androgen receptor signaling in prostate cancer. *J. Biol. Chem.* **2009**, *284*, 24696–24704. [CrossRef] [PubMed]
141. Sikand, K.; Slaibi, J.E.; Singh, R.; Slane, S.D.; Shukla, G.C. Mir 488* inhibits androgen receptor expression in prostate carcinoma cells. *Int. J. Cancer* **2011**, *129*, 810–819. [CrossRef] [PubMed]
142. Gong, A.Y.; Eischeid, A.N.; Xiao, J.; Zhao, J.; Chen, D.; Wang, Z.Y.; Young, C.Y.; Chen, X.M. Mir-17–5p targets the p300/cbp-associated factor and modulates androgen receptor transcriptional activity in cultured prostate cancer cells. *BMC Cancer* **2012**. [CrossRef] [PubMed]
143. Lin, H.M.; Castillo, L.; Mahon, K.L.; Chiam, K.; Lee, B.Y.; Nguyen, Q.; Boyer, M.J.; Stockler, M.R.; Pavlakis, N.; Marx, G.; et al. Circulating microRNAs are associated with docetaxel chemotherapy outcome in castration-resistant prostate cancer. *Br. J. Cancer* **2014**, *110*, 2462–2471. [CrossRef] [PubMed]
144. Lujambio, A.; Ropero, S.; Ballestar, E.; Fraga, M.F.; Cerrato, C.; Setien, F.; Casado, S.; Suarez-Gauthier, A.; Sanchez-Cespedes, M.; Git, A.; et al. Genetic unmasking of an epigenetically silenced microRNA in human cancer cells. *Cancer Res.* **2007**, *67*, 1424–1429. [CrossRef] [PubMed]
145. Agirre, X.; Vilas-Zornoza, A.; Jimenez-Velasco, A.; Martin-Subero, J.I.; Cordeu, L.; Garate, L.; San Jose-Eneriz, E.; Abizanda, G.; Rodriguez-Otero, P.; Fortes, P.; et al. Epigenetic silencing of the tumor suppressor microRNA Hsa-miR-124a regulates CDK6 expression and confers a poor prognosis in acute lymphoblastic leukemia. *Cancer Res.* **2009**, *69*, 4443–4453. [CrossRef] [PubMed]
146. Mitchell, P.S.; Parkin, R.K.; Kroh, E.M.; Fritz, B.R.; Wyman, S.K.; Pogosova-Agadjanyan, E.L.; Peterson, A.; Noteboom, J.; O'Briant, K.C.; Allen, A.; et al. Circulating microRNAs as stable blood-based markers for cancer detection. *Proc. Natl. Acad. Sci. USA* **2008**, *105*, 10513–10518. [CrossRef] [PubMed]
147. Shi, X.B.; Xue, L.; Ma, A.H.; Tepper, C.G.; Gandour-Edwards, R.; Kung, H.J.; deVere White, R.W. Tumor suppressive miR-124 targets androgen receptor and inhibits proliferation of prostate cancer cells. *Oncogene* **2013**, *32*, 4130–4138. [CrossRef] [PubMed]
148. Chu, M.; Chang, Y.; Guo, Y.; Wang, N.; Cui, J.; Gao, W.Q. Regulation and methylation of tumor suppressor miR-124 by androgen receptor in prostate cancer cells. *PLoS ONE* **2015**, *10*, e0116197. [CrossRef] [PubMed]
149. Larne, O.; Martens-Uzunova, E.; Hagman, Z.; Edsjo, A.; Lippolis, G.; den Berg, M.S.; Bjartell, A.; Jenster, G.; Ceder, Y. Miq—A novel microRNA based diagnostic and prognostic tool for prostate cancer. *Int. J. Cancer* **2013**, *132*, 2867–2875. [CrossRef] [PubMed]
150. Wach, S.; Nolte, E.; Szczyrba, J.; Stohr, R.; Hartmann, A.; Orntoft, T.; Dyrskjot, L.; Eltze, E.; Wieland, W.; Keck, B.; et al. MicroRNA profiles of prostate carcinoma detected by multiplatform microRNA screening. *Int. J. Cancer* **2012**, *130*, 611–621. [CrossRef] [PubMed]
151. Larne, O.; Hagman, Z.; Lilja, H.; Bjartell, A.; Edsjo, A.; Ceder, Y. Mir-145 suppress the androgen receptor in prostate cancer cells and correlates to prostate cancer prognosis. *Carcinogenesis* **2015**, *36*, 858–866. [CrossRef] [PubMed]
152. Gutschner, T.; Diederichs, S. The hallmarks of cancer: A long non-coding RNA point of view. *RNA Biol.* **2012**, *9*, 703–719. [CrossRef] [PubMed]

153. Prensner, J.R.; Chinnaiyan, A.M. The emergence of lncRNAs in cancer biology. *Cancer Discov.* **2011**, *1*, 391–407. [CrossRef] [PubMed]
154. Guttman, M.; Rinn, J.L. Modular regulatory principles of large non-coding RNAs. *Nature* **2012**, *482*, 339–346. [CrossRef] [PubMed]
155. Srikantan, V.; Zou, Z.; Petrovics, G.; Xu, L.; Augustus, M.; Davis, L.; Livezey, J.R.; Connell, T.; Sesterhenn, I.A.; Yoshino, K.; et al. *PCGEM1*, a prostate-specific gene, is overexpressed in prostate cancer. *Proc. Natl. Acad. Sci. USA* **2000**, *97*, 12216–12221. [CrossRef] [PubMed]
156. Yang, L.; Lin, C.; Jin, C.; Yang, J.C.; Tanasa, B.; Li, W.; Merkurjev, D.; Ohgi, K.A.; Meng, D.; Zhang, J.; et al. LncRNA-dependent mechanisms of androgen-receptor-regulated gene activation programs. *Nature* **2013**, *500*, 598–602. [CrossRef] [PubMed]
157. Petrovics, G.; Zhang, W.; Makarem, M.; Street, J.P.; Connelly, R.; Sun, L.; Sesterhenn, I.A.; Srikantan, V.; Moul, J.W.; Srivastava, S. Elevated expression of *PCGEM1*, a prostate-specific gene with cell growth-promoting function, is associated with high-risk prostate cancer patients. *Oncogene* **2004**, *23*, 605–611. [CrossRef] [PubMed]
158. Fu, X.; Ravindranath, L.; Tran, N.; Petrovics, G.; Srivastava, S. Regulation of apoptosis by a prostate-specific and prostate cancer-associated noncoding gene, PCGEM1. *DNA Cell Biol.* **2006**, *25*, 135–141. [CrossRef] [PubMed]
159. Romanuik, T.L.; Wang, G.; Morozova, O.; Delaney, A.; Marra, M.A.; Sadar, M.D. LNCaP Atlas: Gene expression associated with in vivo progression to castration-recurrent prostate cancer. *BMC Med. Genom.* **2010**. [CrossRef] [PubMed]
160. Chung, S.; Nakagawa, H.; Uemura, M.; Piao, L.; Ashikawa, K.; Hosono, N.; Takata, R.; Akamatsu, S.; Kawaguchi, T.; Morizono, T.; et al. Association of a novel long non-coding RNA in 8q24 with prostate cancer susceptibility. *Cancer Sci.* **2011**, *102*, 245–252. [CrossRef] [PubMed]
161. Parolia, A.; Crea, F.; Xue, H.; Wang, Y.; Mo, F.; Ramnarine, V.R.; Liu, H.H.; Lin, D.; Saidy, N.R.; Clermont, P.L.; et al. The long non-coding RNA *PCGEM1* is regulated by androgen receptor activity in vivo. *Mol. Cancer* **2015**. [CrossRef] [PubMed]
162. Hung, C.L.; Wang, L.Y.; Yu, Y.L.; Chen, H.W.; Srivastava, S.; Petrovics, G.; Kung, H.J. A long noncoding RNA connects c-Myc to tumor metabolism. *Proc. Natl. Acad. Sci. USA* **2014**, *111*, 18697–18702. [CrossRef] [PubMed]
163. Prensner, J.R.; Sahu, A.; Iyer, M.K.; Malik, R.; Chandler, B.; Asangani, I.A.; Poliakov, A.; Vergara, I.A.; Alshalalfa, M.; Jenkins, R.B.; et al. The IncRNAs *PCGEM1* and *PRNCR1* are not implicated in castration resistant prostate cancer. *Oncotarget* **2014**, *5*, 1434–1438. [CrossRef] [PubMed]
164. Ho, T.T.; Huang, J.; Zhou, N.; Zhang, Z.; Koirala, P.; Zhou, X.; Wu, F.; Ding, X.; Mo, Y.Y. Regulation of PCGEM1 by p54/nrb in prostate cancer. *Sci. Rep.* **2016**. [CrossRef] [PubMed]
165. Hessels, D.; Klein Gunnewiek, J.M.; van Oort, I.; Karthaus, H.F.; van Leenders, G.J.; van Balken, B.; Kiemeney, L.A.; Witjes, J.A.; Schalken, J.A. DD3(PCA3)-based molecular urine analysis for the diagnosis of prostate cancer. *Eur. Urol.* **2003**, *44*, 8–15, discussion 15–16. [CrossRef]
166. Popa, I.; Fradet, Y.; Beaudry, G.; Hovington, H.; Beaudry, G.; Tetu, B. Identification of PCA3 (DD3) in prostatic carcinoma by in situ hybridization. *Mod. Pathol.* **2007**, *20*, 1121–1127. [CrossRef] [PubMed]
167. Ferreira, L.B.; Palumbo, A.; de Mello, K.D.; Sternberg, C.; Caetano, M.S.; de Oliveira, F.L.; Neves, A.F.; Nasciutti, L.E.; Goulart, L.R.; Gimba, E.R. PCA3 noncoding RNA is involved in the control of prostate-cancer cell survival and modulates androgen receptor signaling. *BMC Cancer* **2012**. [CrossRef] [PubMed]
168. Lemos, A.E.; Ferreira, L.B.; Batoreu, N.M.; de Freitas, P.P.; Bonamino, M.H.; Gimba, E.R. PCA3 long noncoding RNA modulates the expression of key cancer-related genes in lncap prostate cancer cells. *Tumour Biol.* **2016**, *37*, 11339–11348. [CrossRef] [PubMed]
169. Takayama, K.; Horie-Inoue, K.; Katayama, S.; Suzuki, T.; Tsutsumi, S.; Ikeda, K.; Urano, T.; Fujimura, T.; Takagi, K.; Takahashi, S.; et al. Androgen-responsive long noncoding RNA CTBP1-AS promotes prostate cancer. *EMBO J.* **2013**, *32*, 1665–1680. [CrossRef] [PubMed]
170. Wang, R.; Asangani, I.A.; Chakravarthi, B.V.; Ateeq, B.; Lonigro, R.J.; Cao, Q.; Mani, R.S.; Camacho, D.F.; McGregor, N.; Schumann, T.E.; et al. Role of transcriptional corepressor CtBP1 in prostate cancer progression. *Neoplasia* **2012**, *14*, 905–914. [CrossRef] [PubMed]

171. Cui, Z.; Ren, S.; Lu, J.; Wang, F.; Xu, W.; Sun, Y.; Wei, M.; Chen, J.; Gao, X.; Xu, C.; et al. The prostate cancer-up-regulated long noncoding RNA PlncRNA-1 modulates apoptosis and proliferation through reciprocal regulation of androgen receptor. *Urol. Oncol.* **2013**, *31*, 1117–1123. [CrossRef] [PubMed]
172. Zhang, A.; Zhao, J.C.; Kim, J.; Fong, K.W.; Yang, Y.A.; Chakravarti, D.; Mo, Y.Y.; Yu, J. LncRNA hotair enhances the androgen-receptor-mediated transcriptional program and drives castration-resistant prostate cancer. *Cell Rep.* **2015**, *13*, 209–221. [CrossRef] [PubMed]
173. Tsai, M.C.; Manor, O.; Wan, Y.; Mosammaparast, N.; Wang, J.K.; Lan, F.; Shi, Y.; Segal, E.; Chang, H.Y. Long noncoding RNA as modular scaffold of histone modification complexes. *Science* **2010**, *329*, 689–693. [CrossRef] [PubMed]
174. Crea, F.; Watahiki, A.; Quagliata, L.; Xue, H.; Pikor, L.; Parolia, A.; Wang, Y.; Lin, D.; Lam, W.L.; Farrar, W.L.; et al. Identification of a long non-coding RNA as a novel biomarker and potential therapeutic target for metastatic prostate cancer. *Oncotarget* **2014**, *5*, 764–774. [CrossRef] [PubMed]
175. Malik, R.; Patel, L.; Prensner, J.R.; Shi, Y.; Iyer, M.K.; Subramaniyan, S.; Carley, A.; Niknafs, Y.S.; Sahu, A.; Han, S.; et al. The lncRNA PCAT29 inhibits oncogenic phenotypes in prostate cancer. *Mol. Cancer Res.* **2014**, *12*, 1081–1087. [CrossRef] [PubMed]
176. Sakurai, K.; Reon, B.J.; Anaya, J.; Dutta, A. The IncRNA DRAIC/PCAT29 locus constitutes a tumor-suppressive nexus. *Mol. Cancer Res.* **2015**, *13*, 828–838. [CrossRef] [PubMed]
177. Saini, S. Psa and beyond: Alternative prostate cancer biomarkers. *Cell. Oncol. (Dordr.)* **2016**, *39*, 97–106. [CrossRef] [PubMed]
178. Cary, K.C.; Cooperberg, M.R. Biomarkers in prostate cancer surveillance and screening: Past, present, and future. *Ther. Adv. Urol.* **2013**, *5*, 318–329. [CrossRef] [PubMed]
179. Walter, L.C.; Bertenthal, D.; Lindquist, K.; Konety, B.R. PSA screening among elderly men with limited life expectancies. *J. Am. Med. Assoc.* **2006**, *296*, 2336–2342. [CrossRef] [PubMed]
180. Strope, S.A.; Andriole, G.L. Prostate cancer screening: Current status and future perspectives. *Nat. Rev. Urol.* **2010**, *7*, 487–493. [CrossRef] [PubMed]
181. Jeronimo, C.; Henrique, R. Epigenetic biomarkers in urological tumors: A systematic review. *Cancer Lett.* **2014**, *342*, 264–274. [CrossRef] [PubMed]
182. Massie, C.E.; Mills, I.G.; Lynch, A.G. The importance of DNA methylation in prostate cancer development. *J. Steroid Biochem. Mol. Biol.* **2016**, *37*, 11339–11348. [CrossRef] [PubMed]
183. Henrique, R.; Jeronimo, C. Molecular detection of prostate cancer: A role for GSTP1 hypermethylation. *Eur. Urol.* **2004**, *46*, 660–669, discussion 669. [CrossRef] [PubMed]
184. Wu, T.; Giovannucci, E.; Welge, J.; Mallick, P.; Tang, W.Y.; Ho, S.M. Measurement of GSTP1 promoter methylation in body fluids may complement PSA screening: A meta-analysis. *Br. J. Cancer* **2011**, *105*, 65–73. [CrossRef] [PubMed]
185. Blute, M.L., Jr.; Damaschke, N.A.; Jarrard, D.F. The epigenetics of prostate cancer diagnosis and prognosis: Update on clinical applications. *Curr. Opin. Urol.* **2015**, *25*, 83–88. [CrossRef] [PubMed]
186. Strand, S.H.; Orntoft, T.F.; Sorensen, K.D. Prognostic DNA methylation markers for prostate cancer. *Int. J. Mol. Sci.* **2014**, *15*, 16544–16576. [CrossRef] [PubMed]
187. Baden, J.; Green, G.; Painter, J.; Curtin, K.; Markiewicz, J.; Jones, J.; Astacio, T.; Canning, S.; Quijano, J.; Guinto, W.; et al. Multicenter evaluation of an investigational prostate cancer methylation assay. *J. Urol.* **2009**, *182*, 1186–1193. [CrossRef] [PubMed]
188. Baden, J.; Adams, S.; Astacio, T.; Jones, J.; Markiewicz, J.; Painter, J.; Trust, C.; Wang, Y.; Green, G. Predicting prostate biopsy result in men with prostate specific antigen 2.0 to 10.0 ng/mL using an investigational prostate cancer methylation assay. *J. Urol.* **2011**, *186*, 2101–2106. [CrossRef] [PubMed]
189. Stewart, G.D.; Van Neste, L.; Delvenne, P.; Delree, P.; Delga, A.; McNeill, S.A.; O'Donnell, M.; Clark, J.; Van Criekinge, W.; Bigley, J.; et al. Clinical utility of an epigenetic assay to detect occult prostate cancer in histopathologically negative biopsies: Results of the matloc study. *J. Urol.* **2013**, *189*, 1110–1116. [CrossRef] [PubMed]
190. Partin, A.W.; Van Neste, L.; Klein, E.A.; Marks, L.S.; Gee, J.R.; Troyer, D.A.; Rieger-Christ, K.; Jones, J.S.; Magi-Galluzzi, C.; Mangold, L.A.; et al. Clinical validation of an epigenetic assay to predict negative histopathological results in repeat prostate biopsies. *J. Urol.* **2014**, *192*, 1081–1087. [CrossRef] [PubMed]

191. Carroll, P.R.; Parsons, J.K.; Andriole, G.; Bahnson, R.R.; Castle, E.P.; Catalona, W.J.; Dahl, D.M.; Davis, J.W.; Epstein, J.I.; Etzioni, R.B.; et al. NCCN guidelines insights: Prostate cancer early detection, version 2.2016. *J. Natl. Compr. Cancer Netw.* **2016**, *14*, 509–519.
192. Aryee, M.J.; Liu, W.; Engelmann, J.C.; Nuhn, P.; Gurel, M.; Haffner, M.C.; Esopi, D.; Irizarry, R.A.; Getzenberg, R.H.; Nelson, W.G.; et al. DNA methylation alterations exhibit intraindividual stability and interindividual heterogeneity in prostate cancer metastases. *Sci. Transl. Med.* **2013**. [CrossRef] [PubMed]
193. Romero Otero, J.; Garcia Gomez, B.; Campos Juanatey, F.; Touijer, K.A. Prostate cancer biomarkers: An update. *Urol. Oncol.* **2014**, *32*, 252–260. [CrossRef] [PubMed]
194. Bussemakers, M.J.; van Bokhoven, A.; Verhaegh, G.W.; Smit, F.P.; Karthaus, H.F.; Schalken, J.A.; Debruyne, F.M.; Ru, N.; Isaacs, W.B. DD3: A new prostate-specific gene, highly overexpressed in prostate cancer. *Cancer Res.* **1999**, *59*, 5975–5979. [PubMed]
195. Sartori, D.A.; Chan, D.W. Biomarkers in prostate cancer: What's new? *Curr. Opin. Oncol.* **2014**, *26*, 259–264. [CrossRef] [PubMed]
196. Haese, A.; de la Taille, A.; van Poppel, H.; Marberger, M.; Stenzl, A.; Mulders, P.F.; Huland, H.; Abbou, C.C.; Remzi, M.; Tinzl, M.; et al. Clinical utility of the PCA3 urine assay in european men scheduled for repeat biopsy. *Eur. Urol.* **2008**, *54*, 1081–1088. [CrossRef] [PubMed]
197. Hu, B.; Yang, H.; Yang, H. Diagnostic value of urine prostate cancer antigen 3 test using a cutoff value of 35 ug/L in patients with prostate cancer. *Tumour Biol.* **2014**, *35*, 8573–8580. [CrossRef] [PubMed]
198. Luo, Y.; Gou, X.; Huang, P.; Mou, C. The PCA3 test for guiding repeat biopsy of prostate cancer and its cut-off score: A systematic review and meta-analysis. *Asian J. Androl.* **2014**, *16*, 487–492. [PubMed]
199. Crawford, E.D.; Rove, K.O.; Trabulsi, E.J.; Qian, J.; Drewnowska, K.P.; Kaminetsky, J.C.; Huisman, T.K.; Bilowus, M.L.; Freedman, S.J.; Glover, W.L., Jr.; et al. Diagnostic performance of PCA3 to detect prostate cancer in men with increased prostate specific antigen: A prospective study of 1962 cases. *J. Urol.* **2012**, *188*, 1726–1731. [CrossRef] [PubMed]
200. Merola, R.; Tomao, L.; Antenucci, A.; Sperduti, I.; Sentinelli, S.; Masi, S.; Mandoj, C.; Orlandi, G.; Papalia, R.; Guaglianone, S.; et al. PCA3 in prostate cancer and tumor aggressiveness detection on 407 high-risk patients: A national cancer institute experience. *J. Exp. Clin. Cancer Res.* **2015**. [CrossRef] [PubMed]
201. Chevli, K.K.; Duff, M.; Walter, P.; Yu, C.; Capuder, B.; Elshafei, A.; Malczewski, S.; Kattan, M.W.; Jones, J.S. Urinary PCA3 as a predictor of prostate cancer in a cohort of 3073 men undergoing initial prostate biopsy. *J. Urol.* **2014**, *191*, 1743–1748. [CrossRef] [PubMed]
202. Hessels, D.; van Gils, M.P.; van Hooij, O.; Jannink, S.A.; Witjes, J.A.; Verhaegh, G.W.; Schalken, J.A. Predictive value of PCA3 in urinary sediments in determining clinico-pathological characteristics of prostate cancer. *Prostate* **2010**, *70*, 10–16. [CrossRef] [PubMed]
203. Van Gils, M.P.; Hessels, D.; Hulsbergen-van de Kaa, C.A.; Witjes, J.A.; Jansen, C.F.; Mulders, P.F.; Rittenhouse, H.G.; Schalken, J.A. Detailed analysis of histopathological parameters in radical prostatectomy specimens and PCA3 urine test results. *Prostate* **2008**, *68*, 1215–1222. [CrossRef] [PubMed]
204. Vlaeminck-Guillem, V.; Ruffion, A.; Andre, J.; Devonec, M.; Paparel, P. Urinary prostate cancer 3 test: Toward the age of reason? *Urology* **2010**, *75*, 447–453. [CrossRef] [PubMed]
205. Erho, N.; Crisan, A.; Vergara, I.A.; Mitra, A.P.; Ghadessi, M.; Buerki, C.; Bergstralh, E.J.; Kollmeyer, T.; Fink, S.; Haddad, Z.; et al. Discovery and validation of a prostate cancer genomic classifier that predicts early metastasis following radical prostatectomy. *PLoS ONE* **2013**, *8*, e66855. [CrossRef] [PubMed]
206. Moschini, M.; Spahn, M.; Mattei, A.; Cheville, J.; Karnes, R.J. Incorporation of tissue-based genomic biomarkers into localized prostate cancer clinics. *BMC Med.* **2016**. [CrossRef] [PubMed]
207. Karnes, R.J.; Bergstralh, E.J.; Davicioni, E.; Ghadessi, M.; Buerki, C.; Mitra, A.P.; Crisan, A.; Erho, N.; Vergara, I.A.; Lam, L.L.; et al. Validation of a genomic classifier that predicts metastasis following radical prostatectomy in an at risk patient population. *J. Urol.* **2013**, *190*, 2047–2053. [CrossRef] [PubMed]
208. Ross, A.E.; Feng, F.Y.; Ghadessi, M.; Erho, N.; Crisan, A.; Buerki, C.; Sundi, D.; Mitra, A.P.; Vergara, I.A.; Thompson, D.J.; et al. A genomic classifier predicting metastatic disease progression in men with biochemical recurrence after prostatectomy. *Prostate Cancer Prostatic Dis.* **2014**, *17*, 64–69. [CrossRef] [PubMed]
209. Den, R.B.; Feng, F.Y.; Showalter, T.N.; Mishra, M.V.; Trabulsi, E.J.; Lallas, C.D.; Gomella, L.G.; Kelly, W.K.; Birbe, R.C.; McCue, P.A.; et al. Genomic prostate cancer classifier predicts biochemical failure and metastases in patients after postoperative radiation therapy. *Int. J. Radiat. Oncol. Biol. Phys.* **2014**, *89*, 1038–1046. [CrossRef] [PubMed]

210. Den, R.B.; Yousefi, K.; Trabulsi, E.J.; Abdollah, F.; Choeurng, V.; Feng, F.Y.; Dicker, A.P.; Lallas, C.D.; Gomella, L.G.; Davicioni, E.; et al. Genomic classifier identifies men with adverse pathology after radical prostatectomy who benefit from adjuvant radiation therapy. *J. Clin. Oncol.* **2015**, *33*, 944–951. [CrossRef] [PubMed]
211. Mohler, J.L.; Armstrong, A.J.; Bahnson, R.R.; D'Amico, A.V.; Davis, B.J.; Eastham, J.A.; Enke, C.A.; Farrington, T.A.; Higano, C.S.; Horwitz, E.M.; et al. Prostate cancer, version 1.2016. *J. Natl. Compr. Cancer Network* **2016**, *14*, 19–30.
212. Fabris, L.; Ceder, Y.; Chinnaiyan, A.M.; Jenster, G.W.; Sorensen, K.D.; Tomlins, S.; Visakorpi, T.; Calin, G.A. The potential of microRNAs as prostate cancer biomarkers. *Eur. Urol.* **2016**, *70*, 312–322. [CrossRef] [PubMed]
213. Schubert, M.; Junker, K.; Heinzelmann, J. Prognostic and predictive miRNA biomarkers in bladder, kidney and prostate cancer: Where do we stand in biomarker development? *J. Cancer Res. Clin. Oncol.* **2016**, *142*, 1673–1695. [CrossRef] [PubMed]
214. Shen, J.; Hruby, G.W.; McKiernan, J.M.; Gurvich, I.; Lipsky, M.J.; Benson, M.C.; Santella, R.M. Dysregulation of circulating microRNAs and prediction of aggressive prostate cancer. *Prostate* **2012**, *72*, 1469–1477. [CrossRef] [PubMed]
215. Melbo-Jorgensen, C.; Ness, N.; Andersen, S.; Valkov, A.; Donnem, T.; Al-Saad, S.; Kiselev, Y.; Berg, T.; Nordby, Y.; Bremnes, R.M.; et al. Stromal expression of MiR-21 predicts biochemical failure in prostate cancer patients with gleason score 6. *PLoS ONE* **2014**, *9*, e113039. [CrossRef] [PubMed]
216. Sun, T.; Yang, M.; Chen, S.; Balk, S.; Pomerantz, M.; Hsieh, C.L.; Brown, M.; Lee, G.S.; Kantoff, P.W. The altered expression of MiR-221/-222 and MiR-23b/-27b is associated with the development of human castration resistant prostate cancer. *Prostate* **2012**, *72*, 1093–1103. [CrossRef] [PubMed]
217. Kneitz, B.; Krebs, M.; Kalogirou, C.; Schubert, M.; Joniau, S.; van Poppel, H.; Lerut, E.; Kneitz, S.; Scholz, C.J.; Strobel, P.; et al. Survival in patients with high-risk prostate cancer is predicted by MiR-221, which regulates proliferation, apoptosis, and invasion of prostate cancer cells by inhibiting IRF2 and SOCS3. *Cancer Res.* **2014**, *74*, 2591–2603. [CrossRef] [PubMed]
218. Spahn, M.; Joniau, S.; Gontero, P.; Fieuws, S.; Marchioro, G.; Tombal, B.; Kneitz, B.; Hsu, C.Y.; van Der Eeckt, K.; Bader, P.; et al. Outcome predictors of radical prostatectomy in patients with prostate-specific antigen greater than 20 ng/mL: A european multi-institutional study of 712 patients. *Eur. Urol.* **2010**, *58*, 1–7, discussion 10–11. [CrossRef] [PubMed]
219. Denis, L.; Murphy, G.P. Overview of phase III trials on combined androgen treatment in patients with metastatic prostate cancer. *Cancer* **1993**, *72*, 3888–3895. [CrossRef]
220. Hellerstedt, B.A.; Pienta, K.J. The truth is out there: An overall perspective on androgen deprivation. *Urol. Oncol.* **2003**, *21*, 272–281. [CrossRef]
221. Rojas, A.; Liu, G.; Coleman, I.; Nelson, P.S.; Zhang, M.; Dash, R.; Fisher, P.B.; Plymate, S.R.; Wu, J.D. Il-6 promotes prostate tumorigenesis and progression through autocrine cross-activation of IGF-IR. *Oncogene* **2011**, *30*, 2345–2355. [CrossRef] [PubMed]
222. Dai, Y.; Desano, J.; Tang, W.; Meng, X.; Meng, Y.; Burstein, E.; Lawrence, T.S.; Xu, L. Natural proteasome inhibitor celastrol suppresses androgen-independent prostate cancer progression by modulating apoptotic proteins and nf-kappab. *PLoS ONE* **2010**, *5*, e14153. [CrossRef] [PubMed]
223. Chandrasekar, T.; Yang, J.C.; Gao, A.C.; Evans, C.P. Mechanisms of resistance in castration-resistant prostate cancer (crpc). *Transl. Androl. Urol.* **2015**, *4*, 365–380. [PubMed]
224. Anders, L.; Guenther, M.G.; Qi, J.; Fan, Z.P.; Marineau, J.J.; Rahl, P.B.; Loven, J.; Sigova, A.A.; Smith, W.B.; Lee, T.I.; et al. Genome-wide localization of small molecules. *Nat. Biotechnol.* **2014**, *32*, 92–96. [CrossRef] [PubMed]
225. Jin, C.; Yang, L.; Xie, M.; Lin, C.; Merkurjev, D.; Yang, J.C.; Tanasa, B.; Oh, S.; Zhang, J.; Ohgi, K.A.; et al. Chem-seq permits identification of genomic targets of drugs against androgen receptor regulation selected by functional phenotypic screens. *Proc. Natl. Acad. Sci. USA* **2014**, *111*, 9235–9240. [CrossRef] [PubMed]
226. King, O.N.; Li, X.S.; Sakurai, M.; Kawamura, A.; Rose, N.R.; Ng, S.S.; Quinn, A.M.; Rai, G.; Mott, B.T.; Beswick, P.; et al. Quantitative high-throughput screening identifies 8-hydroxyquinolines as cell-active histone demethylase inhibitors. *PLoS ONE* **2010**, *5*, e15535. [CrossRef] [PubMed]
227. Cloos, P.A.; Christensen, J.; Agger, K.; Maiolica, A.; Rappsilber, J.; Antal, T.; Hansen, K.H.; Helin, K. The putative oncogene GASC1 demethylates tri- and dimethylated lysine 9 on histone H3. *Nature* **2006**, *442*, 307–311. [CrossRef] [PubMed]

228. Whetstine, J.R.; Nottke, A.; Lan, F.; Huarte, M.; Smolikov, S.; Chen, Z.; Spooner, E.; Li, E.; Zhang, G.; Colaiacovo, M.; et al. Reversal of histone lysine trimethylation by the JMJD2 family of histone demethylases. *Cell* **2006**, *125*, 467–481. [CrossRef] [PubMed]
229. Piekarz, R.L.; Frye, R.; Turner, M.; Wright, J.J.; Allen, S.L.; Kirschbaum, M.H.; Zain, J.; Prince, H.M.; Leonard, J.P.; Geskin, L.J.; et al. Phase ii multi-institutional trial of the histone deacetylase inhibitor romidepsin as monotherapy for patients with cutaneous t-cell lymphoma. *J. Clin. Oncol.* **2009**, *27*, 5410–5417. [CrossRef] [PubMed]
230. Wheler, J.J.; Janku, F.; Falchook, G.S.; Jackson, T.L.; Fu, S.; Naing, A.; Tsimberidou, A.M.; Moulder, S.L.; Hong, D.S.; Yang, H.; et al. Phase I study of anti-VEGF monoclonal antibody bevacizumab and histone deacetylase inhibitor valproic acid in patients with advanced cancers. *Cancer Chemother. Pharmacol.* **2014**, *73*, 495–501. [CrossRef] [PubMed]
231. Welsbie, D.S.; Xu, J.; Chen, Y.; Borsu, L.; Scher, H.I.; Rosen, N.; Sawyers, C.L. Histone deacetylases are required for androgen receptor function in hormone-sensitive and castrate-resistant prostate cancer. *Cancer Res.* **2009**, *69*, 958–966. [CrossRef] [PubMed]
232. Rokhlin, O.W.; Glover, R.B.; Guseva, N.V.; Taghiyev, A.F.; Kohlgraf, K.G.; Cohen, M.B. Mechanisms of cell death induced by histone deacetylase inhibitors in androgen receptor-positive prostate cancer cells. *Mol. Cancer Res.* **2006**, *4*, 113–123. [CrossRef] [PubMed]
233. Fang, Y.; Fliss, A.E.; Robins, D.M.; Caplan, A.J. Hsp90 regulates androgen receptor hormone binding affinity in vivo. *J. Biol. Chem.* **1996**, *271*, 28697–28702. [CrossRef] [PubMed]
234. Solit, D.B.; Scher, H.I.; Rosen, N. Hsp90 as a therapeutic target in prostate cancer. *Semin. Oncol.* **2003**, *30*, 709–716. [CrossRef]
235. Kaushik, D.; Vashistha, V.; Isharwal, S.; Sediqe, S.A.; Lin, M.F. Histone deacetylase inhibitors in castration-resistant prostate cancer: Molecular mechanism of action and recent clinical trials. *Ther. Adv. Urol.* **2015**, *7*, 388–395. [CrossRef] [PubMed]
236. Yu, X.; Guo, Z.S.; Marcu, M.G.; Neckers, L.; Nguyen, D.M.; Chen, G.A.; Schrump, D.S. Modulation of p53, ErbB1, ErbB2, and Raf-1 expression in lung cancer cells by depsipeptide FR901228. *J. Natl. Cancer Inst.* **2002**, *94*, 504–513. [CrossRef] [PubMed]
237. Molife, L.R.; Attard, G.; Fong, P.C.; Karavasilis, V.; Reid, A.H.; Patterson, S.; Riggs, C.E., Jr.; Higano, C.; Stadler, W.M.; McCulloch, W.; et al. Phase II, two-stage, single-arm trial of the histone deacetylase inhibitor (HDACi) romidepsin in metastatic castration-resistant prostate cancer (CRPC). *Ann. Oncol.* **2010**, *21*, 109–113. [CrossRef] [PubMed]
238. Rathkopf, D.; Wong, B.Y.; Ross, R.W.; Anand, A.; Tanaka, E.; Woo, M.M.; Hu, J.; Dzik-Jurasz, A.; Yang, W.; Scher, H.I. A phase I study of oral panobinostat alone and in combination with docetaxel in patients with castration-resistant prostate cancer. *Cancer Chemother. Pharmacol.* **2010**, *66*, 181–189. [CrossRef] [PubMed]
239. Rathkopf, D.E.; Picus, J.; Hussain, A.; Ellard, S.; Chi, K.N.; Nydam, T.; Allen-Freda, E.; Mishra, K.K.; Porro, M.G.; Scher, H.I.; et al. A phase 2 study of intravenous panobinostat in patients with castration-resistant prostate cancer. *Cancer Chemother. Pharmacol.* **2013**, *72*, 537–544. [CrossRef] [PubMed]
240. Garzon, R.; Marcucci, G.; Croce, C.M. Targeting microRNAs in cancer: Rationale, strategies and challenges. Nature reviews. *Drug Discov.* **2010**, *9*, 775–789. [CrossRef] [PubMed]
241. Li, X.J.; Ren, Z.J.; Tang, J.H. MicroRNA-34a: A potential therapeutic target in human cancer. *Cell Death Dis.* **2014**, *5*, e1327. [CrossRef] [PubMed]
242. Zhang, D.G.; Zheng, J.N.; Pei, D.S. P53/microRNA-34-induced metabolic regulation: New opportunities in anticancer therapy. *Mol. Cancer* **2014**. [CrossRef] [PubMed]
243. Yamamura, S.; Saini, S.; Majid, S.; Hirata, H.; Ueno, K.; Deng, G.; Dahiya, R. MicroRNA-34a modulates c-myc transcriptional complexes to suppress malignancy in human prostate cancer cells. *PLoS ONE* **2012**, *7*, e29722. [CrossRef] [PubMed]
244. Bouchie, A. First microRNA mimic enters clinic. *Nat. Biotechnol.* **2013**. [CrossRef] [PubMed]

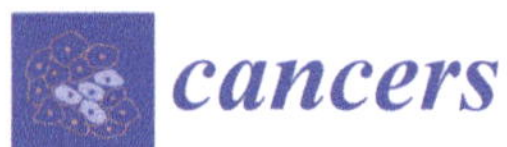

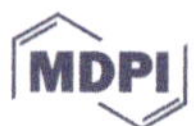

Review

A Tale of Two Signals: AR and WNT in Development and Tumorigenesis of Prostate and Mammary Gland

Hubert Pakula [1,2], Dongxi Xiang [1,2] and Zhe Li [1,2,*]

1 Division of Genetics, Brigham and Women's Hospital, 77 Avenue Louis Pasteur, Room 466, Boston, MA 02115, USA; hpakula@partners.org (H.P.); dxiang@bwh.harvard.edu (D.X.)
2 Department of Medicine, Harvard Medical School, Boston, MA 02115, USA
* Correspondence: zli4@rics.bwh.harvard.edu; Tel.: +1-617-525-4740; Fax: +1-617-525-4705

Academic Editor: Emmanuel S. Antonarakis
Received: 6 December 2016; Accepted: 24 January 2017; Published: 27 January 2017

Abstract: Prostate cancer (PCa) is one of the most common cancers and among the leading causes of cancer deaths for men in industrialized countries. It has long been recognized that the prostate is an androgen-dependent organ and PCa is an androgen-dependent disease. Androgen action is mediated by the androgen receptor (AR). Androgen deprivation therapy (ADT) is the standard treatment for metastatic PCa. However, almost all advanced PCa cases progress to castration-resistant prostate cancer (CRPC) after a period of ADT. A variety of mechanisms of progression from androgen-dependent PCa to CRPC under ADT have been postulated, but it remains largely unclear as to when and how castration resistance arises within prostate tumors. In addition, AR signaling may be modulated by extracellular factors among which are the cysteine-rich glycoproteins WNTs. The WNTs are capable of signaling through several pathways, the best-characterized being the canonical WNT/β-catenin/TCF-mediated canonical pathway. Recent studies from sequencing PCa genomes revealed that CRPC cells frequently harbor mutations in major components of the WNT/β-catenin pathway. Moreover, the finding of an interaction between β-catenin and AR suggests a possible mechanism of cross talk between WNT and androgen/AR signaling pathways. In this review, we discuss the current knowledge of both AR and WNT pathways in prostate development and tumorigenesis, and their interaction during development of CRPC. We also review the possible therapeutic application of drugs that target both AR and WNT/β-catenin pathways. Finally, we extend our review of AR and WNT signaling to the mammary gland system and breast cancer. We highlight that the role of AR signaling and its interaction with WNT signaling in these two hormone-related cancer types are highly context-dependent.

Keywords: androgen receptor; AR; WNT; prostate; prostate cancer; castration-resistant prostate cancer; CRPC; mammary gland; breast cancer

---

1. Introduction

For the men in the United States, prostate cancer (PCa) is not only one of the most commonly diagnosed cancers, but also one of the most predominant causes of death from cancer [1,2]. The American Cancer Society estimates that in 2016, there will be 180,890 newly diagnosed cases and 26,120 deaths due to PCa in the United States, making it the second leading cause of cancer death in men [3]. Since the prostate gland development depends on androgens and androgen receptor (AR) signaling [4,5], human PCa initially responds to androgen-deprivation therapy (ADT) [6,7]. However, the cancer often reappears, and is accompanied by rising levels of serum prostate-specific antigen (PSA) [8,9]. PSA (KLK3) is encoded by an androgen-dependent gene, and increased expression of PSA in an environment of castrate levels of circulating androgens indicates that adaptive androgen signaling has emerged in the tumor [10,11]. Accordingly, in the majority of cases, an initially hormone-sensitive

PCa will evolve to a lethal castration-resistant prostate cancer (CRPC) [12–15]. The underlying molecular basis for how PCa cells escape from the growth control by exogenous androgens remains poorly understood. Recent studies, however, pointed to the AR and its actions as a key factor in many CRPCs, despite the reduction in circulating testosterone. The mechanisms involved in this change include increased expression and stability of the AR protein, activating mutations in this receptor that alter its ligand specificity, and changes in the expression of transcriptional co-regulators of the AR [16,17]. In addition, AR and its cognate ligands interact with potent oncogenic systems, such as WNT signaling, to elicit changes in cellular adhesion and oncogenesis [18–21].

WNT signaling is an evolutionary highly conserved signaling system throughout the eukaryotic kingdom. During embryonic and postnatal development, WNT signaling controls many cellular processes, including proliferation, survival and differentiation [22–26]. Deregulation in WNT signaling leads to an imbalance of such processes, often resulting in aberrant development or disease [27,28]; in particular, deregulated WNT signaling is common in human cancers, including malignancies of the intestine [29–31], liver [32–35], skin [36,37], breast [38–41] and prostate [42,43].

The term Wnt is an amalgam of Wg and Int [44], as the genes *Wingless* (*Wg*) and *integration 1 (Int1)* are homologues in *Drosophila* and mouse, respectively [45,46]. *Wg* was genetically characterized as a segment polarity gene in *Drosophila* in 1980 by Nüsslein-Volhard and Wieschaus [47]. The proto-oncogene *Int1* was first identified in 1982 by Nusse and Varmus as a preferential site for proviral integration of the mouse mammary tumor virus (MMTV) in a mouse mammary cancer model [48]. Since the identification of *Wnt1*, genome sequencing has revealed the existence of 19 *Wnt* genes in mammals. All WNT proteins share common features that are essential for their function, including a signal peptide for secretion, many potential glycosylation sites, and WNT ligands interact with seven-pass transmembrane receptors of the Frizzled (FZD) family and/or single-pass transmembrane co-receptors, such as lipoprotein receptor-related protein 5/6 (LRP5/6), ROR2, and RYK [49–54]. Co-factors such as R-spondin and Wise also take part in WNT-receptor complex activity [55–57]. R-spondin/LGR (leucine-rich repeat-containing G-protein coupled-like receptor) complexes and WNT ligands directly interact with FZD-LRP-receptor complexes on target cells to activate downstream signaling. This leads to the activation of various intracellular signaling cascades that can be cross-connected or act independently. The intracellular signaling activated by WNT proteins is organized into two categories: canonical and non-canonical. Canonical WNT signaling is often referred to as the WNT/β-catenin pathway, as it relies on β-catenin-dependent transcriptional activation triggered by WNT-stimulated signals. In contrast, non-canonical WNT pathways, including the WNT/$Ca2^+$ (calcium) and WNT/JNK (c-Jun N-terminal kinase), WNT/Rho pathways, are β-catenin-independent and activate a variety of downstream intracellular signaling cascades [26,58–60]. These mechanisms have been the subject of numerous reviews [22–26], and therefore will only be briefly described here.

In this review, we will discuss the multifaceted manner with which both the canonical and non-canonical WNT pathways influence and modulate AR signaling in CRPC development. We will consider the possible therapeutic application of drugs that target both pathways. We will also discuss these under the context of recurrent mutations in both pathways identified from PCa genomes. Finally, we will extend our review of these two pathways to the mammary gland system and breast cancer.

2. An Overview of the Canonical and Non-Canonical WNT Signaling Pathways

The known molecular components and the cascade of the canonical WNT signaling pathway are summarized in Figure 1. Canonical WNT signaling strictly controls the level of the cytoplasmic protein β-catenin. β-Catenin, encoded by the *CTNNB1* gene [61], is a member of the armadillo family of proteins. β-Catenin consists of an N-terminal region of 149 amino acids, followed by a central domain of 515 residues composed of 12 armadillo repeats, and a C-terminal region of 108 residues [62]. The N-terminal region contains phosphorylation sites recognized by GSK3β and CK1α and an α-catenin binding site, whereas the C-terminal region works as a transcriptional co-activator-binding domain (CBD) that interacts with histone modifiers such as histone acetyltransferases CBP/P300 [63]. β-Catenin has dual functions. It acts as a transcription cofactor with the T cell factor/lymphoid enhancer factor (TCF/LEF) in the WNT pathway [64–67]. It is also a structural adaptor protein that binds E-cadherin and α-catenin through its Armadillo repeats and N-terminal domain, respectively (E-cadherin is a core transmembrane adhesion protein, and α-catenin is a protein that binds actin and other actin-regulators) [68–72]. The multifaceted functions of β-catenin are regulated by three cellular pools of this molecule that are under strict regulation: a membrane pool of cadherin-associated β-catenin, a cytoplasmic pool, and a nuclear pool [73]. Canonical WNT signaling works in the following fashion: in the absence of WNT signals, β-catenin is efficiently captured by scaffold proteins, the AXINs, which are present within a destruction complex containing glycogen synthase kinase (GSK3β), adenomatous polyposis coli (APC) and the casein kinase-1 (CK1). The resident CK1 and GSK3β protein kinases sequentially phosphorylate conserved serine and threonine residues in the N-terminus of the captured β-catenin, generating a binding site for an E3 ubiquitin ligase. Ubiquitination targets β-catenin into proteasomes for rapid degradation [74–77]. Therefore, in the absence of WNT, cytoplasmic β-catenin levels remain low, and the transcription factors LEF1 and TCF interact with Grouchos in the nucleus to repress WNT pathway-specific target genes [78,79]. In contrast, upon the interaction of canonical WNT ligands to its receptors, FZD, and co-receptor, LRP5/6, the destruction complex is disassembled through phosphorylation of LRP5/6 by CK1γ and binding of AXIN to LRP, which prevents β-catenin degradation [80,81]. The inactivation of the destruction complex allows cytoplasmic stabilization and translocation of β-catenin to the nucleus, where it interacts with members of the TCF/LEF family [64–66] and converts the TCF/LEF proteins into potent transcriptional activators. It achieves this by displacing Grouchos [82] and by recruiting other co-activators such as B-cell lymphoma 9 (BCL9) [83,84], Pygopus [85,86], CREB-binding protein (CBP) [87,88] or Hyrax [89], ensuring efficient activation of WNT target genes encoding c-Myc [90], Cyclin D1 [91,92], urokinase-type plasminogen activator (uPA) [93], CD44 [94], Cox-2 and Cox-9 [95], and the *AR* gene [96,97], as well as genes that encode key components of the WNT pathway (e.g., FZDs, DKKs (Dickkopf), LRPs, AXIN2, β-TrCP and TCF/LEF) (Figure 1). These WNT target genes then influence cell cycle regulation, stem cell function and development, as well as invasion and metastasis of cancer cells. For an updated overview of the WNT pathway and its target genes, see the WNT homepage at http://www.stanford.edu/group/nusselab/cgi-bin/wnt/.

In addition to promoting the WNT activity, a series of biochemical experiments indicated that R-spondins (RSPOs) are able to synergize with the WNT pathway in the presence of canonical WNT ligands [98]. Similar to the WNT proteins, RSPOs are also cysteine-rich. However, unlike WNTs, the cysteine residues found in RSPOs are organized into two adjacent furin-like domains, which have been suggested to be sufficient for inducing β-catenin stabilization [98]. Recently, LGR4, LGR5 and LGR6, three closely related LGR proteins, have been identified as receptors for RSPOs. *LGR5* is a WNT target gene and although originally discovered as an intestinal stem cell marker [99], it has also become an ideal candidate marker for understanding stem cell and cancer biology of other epithelial cell types in mice and human [56,99–101]. The LGR5 protein had previously been identified as an orphan receptor, among LGRs. The LGR family is defined by a large extracellular N-terminal domain composed of a string of leucine-rich repeat units, a 7-transmembrane domains (7TM) and a cytoplasmic region. Specifically, LGR5, together with LGR4 and LGR6, belong to the B-class LGRs [100,102]. Close relatives are the LGRs for the follicle stimulating hormone (FSH), the luteinizing hormone (LH) and the thyroid-stimulating hormone (TSH), which are true G-protein coupled receptors. Recently, it was found that instead of binding hormones, the LGR4/5/6 receptors interact with RSPOs and do not activate G-proteins; instead, they promote WNT/β-catenin signaling. Specifically, the interaction of RSPOs and LGR5 has been assessed in cell surface binding assays, cell-free co-immunoprecipitation and tandem affinity purification mass spectrometry [55,102,103]. As their potentiating ability depends on the presence of a WNT ligand, the WNT secretion machinery can thus indirectly affect their role on WNT signaling.

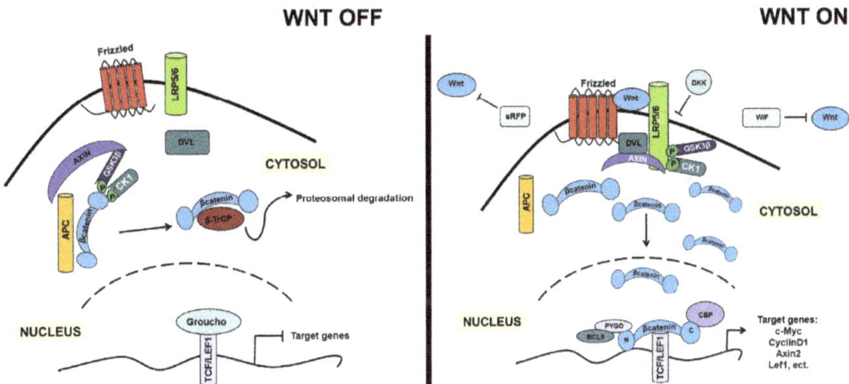

Figure 1. Schematic diagram of the canonical WNT signaling pathway. (left panel) the "WNT-Off" state: In the absence of a WNT signal, β-catenin levels in the cytoplasm are kept low through proteosomal degradation induced by the β-catenin destruction complex. Grouchos (transcriptional co-repressors) interact with TCF/LEF proteins and prevent the expression of WNT target genes. (right panel) the "WNT-On" state: When WNT ligands bind to their receptors Frizzled (FZD) and LRP5/6, the receptor complex can recruit components of the β-catenin destruction complex, resulting in accumulation of β-catenin in the cytoplasm. β-catenin will then translocate into the nucleus, replace Grouchos and recruit transcriptional co-activators to form the transcription complex with TCF/LEF proteins, which eventually promote expression of the WNT target genes.

The activation of canonical WNT signaling can also be blocked by extracellular proteins. These include the sFRP family (secreted frizzled related protein; sFRP1, 2, 4, and 5) [104], WIF (Wnt inhibitory factor) [105], the DKK family of proteins (DKK1–4 and DKKL1) [106], and the cysteine knot family proteins SOST [107] and WISE [108]. These soluble inhibitors bind to WNT, the FZD receptor in the case of sFRP, or to the co-receptor LRP5/6 in the case of DKK1 and SOST/WISE, thereby interfering with ligand–receptor complex formation and blocking WNT signaling [109].

While the canonical WNT signaling pathway has been extensively dissected biochemically and at the molecular level, non-canonical WNT signaling has been less focused on. The best characterized non-canonical WNT pathways include the WNT/$Ca2^+$ pathway, which was first described in vertebrates [58], and the planar polarity pathway (PCP), which was first identified in *Drosophila* [110]. Other non-canonical pathways include WNT/JNK and WNT/Rho signaling [111].

In the WNT/$Ca2^+$ pathway, the interaction of non-canonical WNT ligands and receptors recruits Dishevelled (DVL) and G protein, which activates phospholipase C (PLC), leading to production of 1,2-diacylglycerol (DAG); 1,2-DAG then activates protein kinase C (PKC), and inositol 1,4,5-triphosphate (IP3), thereby triggering intracellular calcium release from the endoplasmic reticulum [112,113]. Calcium release activates calcineurin (CNA) and Ca^{2+}/calmodulin-dependent protein kinase II (CAMKII), which increase expression of nuclear factor of activated T cells (NFAT)-dependent genes and inhibit canonical WNT signaling through nemo-like kinase (NLK), respectively [114,115]. Activated NFAT may boost the expression of several genes in neurons, cardiac and skeletal muscle cells, prostate, and pro-inflammatory genes in lymphocytes [116–118]. In the WNT-PCP pathway, FZD receptors activate a signaling cascade that involves the small GTPases Rho and Rac and c-Jun N-terminal kinase (JNK) [119]. In contrast to calcium-regulated non-canonical signaling, WNT/JNK signaling uses ROR2-dependent circuitry to activate downstream effectors of the activating protein-1 (AP-1) family of transcription factors [59,60]. In addition, a new β-catenin-independent aspect of WNT signaling was recently reported in proliferating cells: WNT signaling was found to peak at the G2/M phase of the cell cycle to produce the so-called WNT-dependent stabilization of proteins (WNT/STOP) [120,121]. This appears to be a dominant mode of WNT signaling in several cancer cell lines, where it is required for cell growth. Of note, boundaries of both canonical and non-canonical WNT pathways are not stringent and there are considerable degrees of overlapping between them [122].

3. WNT Signaling in Prostate Development and Stem Cells

In both human and rodents, the prostate gland surrounds the urethra at the base of the bladder and functions by contributing secretory proteins to the seminal fluid. In men, the prostate gland is a walnut-sized tissue with a zonal architecture, corresponding to central, periurethral transition, and peripheral zones, together with an anterior fibromuscular stroma [123]. Importantly, the outermost peripheral zone occupies the most volume, and harbors the majority of prostate carcinomas. In contrast, benign prostatic hyperplasia (BPH), a common nonmalignant condition found in older men, arises from the transition zone [124]. Unlike the human prostate that is a compact gland, the mouse prostate includes four paired lobes situated circumferentially around the urethra: anterior (AP), dorsal (DP), lateral (LP), and ventral (VP) prostate. The DP and LP are sometimes collectively referred to as the dorsolateral lobes of the prostate (DLP). At birth, each lobe of the VP consists of 1–3 main ducts with secondary and tertiary branches, whereas the more complex DLP initially has 9–12 unbranched proximal main ducts on each side [125,126].

In all species, formation of the prostate gland initiates during embryogenesis. During mid-gestation, the primitive urogenital sinus (UGS) is separated from the terminal region of the hindgut through division of the cloaca by the urorectal septum. The most rostral region (vesiculo-urethral part) of the primitive UGS forms the urinary bladder, whereas the most caudal region (phallic part) forms the penile urethra. The prostate gland originates from a sub-compartment of the lower urogenital tract (LUT), known as the definitive UGS [127,128]. The endodermal UGS is surrounded by embryonic connective tissue called urogenital sinus mesenchyme (UGM). Prostate development, growth and function is androgen dependent; however, other steroid receptors, such as estrogen receptors (ER) and retinoid receptors (RARs and RXRs), also contribute to prostate morphogenesis and differentiation. Prior to sexual differentiation of the UGS, UGM expresses AR in both sexes and thus acquires the capacity to undergo masculine development [129–131]. Over 30-year of research by Cunha and colleagues has shown that an AR-dependent signal from the urogenital mesenchyme is required for prostate formation, while AR is not initially required in the urogenital epithelium (UGE) for prostate organogenesis, but is subsequently necessary for epithelial differentiation and secretory protein expression [124,132–134]. In mouse, the prostatic ducts start to form after embryonic day 17 (E17) as solid epithelial buds formed from the UGE that invades the surrounding UGM [126]. During perinatal and neonatal development, prostatic buds undergo primary, secondary, and tertiary branching morphogenesis in a pattern unique to each pair of the DP, VP, LP, and AP lobes in rodents [125]. The rate of new VP ductal tip formation in Balb/c mice, a hallmark of branching morphogenesis, peaks at about postnatal day 5 (P5). Concurrent with branching morphogenesis, epithelial buds canalize in a proximal to distal direction along the developing ducts, giving rise to two distinct cell layers: a superficial layer of secretory columnar luminal epithelium lining prostatic ducts and a deep layer of basal epithelium including the rare neuroendocrine cells [135,136]. Basic prostatic architecture is established during puberty, upon an androgen-driven increase in prostate gland size. After that the prostatic epithelium reorganizes into a layer of outer cuboidal basal cells and inner tall columnar luminal cells. Human prostate development proceeds by a similar series of morphogenetic events, but gives rise to a mature prostate that contains a single capsulated structure divided into peripheral, central, and transitional zones. The basal cells express cytokeratins 5 and 14, and p63 and are localized along the basement membrane, but express AR at low or undetectable levels [137]. The luminal cells express cytokeratins 8 and 18 as well as high levels of AR [138]. In humans, mature luminal cells constitute the exocrine part of the prostate and secrete PSA and PAP (prostate acid phosphatase) [139,140]. The third epithelial cell type in the prostate is the androgen-independent neuroendocrine cell, which makes up only a small proportion of the prostate epithelial cells and is characterized by expression of functional markers such as chromogranin A and synaptophysin [141,142]. In addition, intermediate or transit-amplifying cells that express both the basal and luminal lineage markers are detectable during the developmental stage, under pathological conditions in adults, or when prostate epithelial cells are cultured in vitro [137,143–146].

The use of transgenic mice combined with molecular analyses have demonstrated the importance of several developmental signaling pathways during prostate organogenesis, including bone morphogenetic protein (BMP), transforming growth factor beta (TGFβ), Notch, sonic hedgehog (SHH), and WNT pathways [147]. Evidence that WNT signaling is involved in prostate morphogenesis comes from studies by Zhang et al. [148]. By creating six LongSAGE libraries at three key stages of prostate organogenesis: E16.5 UGS (i.e., a stage just before the first prostate buds are formed), P0 prostates (i.e., a stage when branching morphogenesis has begun), and 12-week adult prostates (i.e., a time of relative growth quiescence), Zhang and colleagues evaluated sex and cell-type specific genes associated with prostate induction and found expression changes of multiple WNT-related genes, such as *Sfrp2, Wnt4, Wnt5a, Wnt11, Fzd1, Fzd7, Fzd10, Lrp5, Axin1, Lef1, Nkd1*, and *RhoA* [148,149]. Accordingly, in vivo studies using *Sfrp1*-overexpressing transgenic mice and *Sfrp1*-null mice confirmed that this WNT modulator stimulates prostate branching morphogenesis, epithelial cell proliferation and secretory gene expression [150]. Additionally, in vitro studies by Prins and colleagues showed that the WNT signaling inhibitor DKK1 also stimulated growth and branching of cultured newborn rat VP lobes over a four-day period, suggesting that canonical WNT signaling suppresses prostate growth [147]. This was supported by another recent study where WNT3A, a canonical WNT ligand, reduced ductal branching of cultured neonatal rodent (rat) prostates and active canonical WNT signaling in epithelial progenitor cells maintaining their undifferentiated state [151]. In addition, *Wnt5a* was found to be indispensable during the UGS development. High levels of *Wnt5a* expression has been observed at the distal tips and along the centro-distal periductal mesenchyme during the period of postnatal branching morphogenesis, with a rapid decline thereafter in the VP but not the DP and LP [152]. Another study further demonstrated that loss of *Wnt5a* impeded buds branching during morphogenesis [153].

β-Catenin has been identified in both epithelial and mesenchymal structures that undergo a budding program; its activation is necessary and/or sufficient for specification of hair follicle, mammary gland and tooth buds [154–156]. Of note, an absolute requirement for this protein has been shown in prostatic induction. While conditional expression of a constitutively active form of β-catenin in developing prostate epithelium prevents epithelial differentiation [136,157], conditional deletion of the β-catenin gene (*Ctnnb1*) in the mouse prostate during embryonic stages results in significantly decreased prostatic budding and abrogates prostatic development [158]. Furthermore, a recent study by Mehta et al. demonstrated the importance of WNT-activators RSPOs in murine prostatic bud formation [136]. By in situ hybridization (ISH), Mehta et al. unveiled the expression pattern of *R-spondin1-4* (*Rspo1-4*) in developing and neonatal mouse LUT. They found that *Rspo3*, together with *Wnt4, Wnt10b, Wnt11* and *Wnt16*, appear to be more abundant in male versus female UGS and they stimulate prostatic development [136].

Although development of the adult prostate is largely completed at puberty, it must possess a mechanism to assure the homeostasis of its epithelium. To achieve this, prostate, similar to other epithelial organs, sets aside a life-long reservoir of somatic stem cells that retain self-renewal. The regenerative capacity of prostate epithelial stem cells (PSCs) has been shown in the experiment with repeated rounds of androgen ablation and restoration; thus PSCs are androgen-sensitive but not dependent, are capable of self-regeneration, and give rise to transit-amplifying cells that differentiate into various specialized epithelial cells of the prostate [159]. To date, the best approach to identify and characterize murine and human PSCs is to combine flow cytometry with functional assays, such as genetic lineage tracing experiments, tissue culture and renal capsule implantation. Specifically, first prostate epithelial cells are fractionated based on their surface antigenic profiles and then functional assays are used to determine whether different subpopulations possess stem cell activity or not. Based on this approach, the basal cell subpopulation appeared to be bipotent, i.e., capable of generating both luminal and basal lineages, thus indicating that basal cells have stem cell-like potential [160–162]. Independent studies by the two laboratories of Witte and Wilson showed that makers such as CD49f, Trop2 and CD166 could enrich prostate cells for the PSC activity among the Sca-1^{+} cells [145,163–167]. Similarly, Richardson et al. isolated human prostate cells expressing a stem cell marker CD133 and showed that $\alpha2\beta1$integrin^{+}CD133^{+} basal cells also correspond to an enriched stem cell fraction in the human prostate epithelium [168]. Finally, Leong et al. reported successful regeneration of prostatic tissues from single Lin^{-}Sca-1^{+}CD133^{+}CD44^{+}CD117^{+} cells, which are predominantly basal in mice and are exclusively basal in humans [169]. In addition to the cellular hierarchy of the prostatic epithelium in mice, Wang et al. showed in the lineage tracing experiments that rare luminal cells (i.e., castration-resistant *Nkx3-1* expressing cells (CARNs)) are bipotential and can self-renew in vivo [170]. Nevertheless, a full understanding the properties of prostate luminal epithelial cells has been hampered by the lack of suitable in vitro model systems. In comparison to the basal epithelial cells, luminal epithelial cells are indeed more sensitive for tissue dissociation, after which they fail to survive in explant culture or grafts [170,171]. To circumvent this technical difficulty, three-dimensional (3D) organoid culture was developed recently [172]. By using testosterone-responsive culture conditions, Karthaus et al. confirmed that human prostate luminal cells have potential to generate both basal and luminal lineages. Moreover, they showed that basal and luminal cells can each generate a complete multilayer prostate organoids, suggesting that both lineages have stem cell-like potentials [173]. Of note, the 3D organoid system, although mimicking a testosterone-naïve environment for the single stem cells, relies also on the addition of LGR4/5 ligand R-spondin1, a potent WNT/β-catenin agonist. This might shed a new light on the role of WNT activity in the maintenance and expansion of PSCs and their progeny. In fact, evidence of the importance of WNT activity in the maintenance of PSCs and their progeny was provided in two consecutive studies by the laboratory of Wilson; in one study, Blum et al. determined the transcriptional profiles of four populations of prostate cells: (i) urogenital epithelium from 16-day embryos, that represent fetal PSCs; (ii) Sca-1^{High} cells, enriched in adult PSCs; (iii) Sca-1^{Low} cells, that represent transit-amplifying cells; and (iv) Sca-1^{Negative} cells representing terminally differentiated population with no regenerative potential [174]. Upregulation of WNT signaling was observed in both fetal and adult PSCs. However, WNT signaling acts differently in these two populations, as the fetal PSC population is highly proliferating, whereas the adult PSC population is quiescent [174]. In another work, the same group reported that WNT receptors such as FZD6 and ligands such as WNT2 and WNT4 also control the stem cell niche activity [175]. Similarly, other WNT ligand has been shown to be critical in controlling self-renewal of PSCs in a prostasphere culture system [94]. Interestingly, activation of canonical WNT pathway through WNT3A results in a significant increase of the expression of nuclear β-catenin [94]. This is consistent with other reports showing that WNT3A signaling can preserve an undifferentiated phenotype in CD133^{+} human cord blood-derived cells [176] and it supports embryonic stem cell self-renewal [177]. Furthermore, the importance of β-catenin in the self-renewal of Lin^{-}Sca^{-}CD49f^{high} mouse prostate stem and progenitor cells has been provided in the study by Lukacs et al. [178]. This group reported that cells expressing the BMI-1 (polycomb group) protein require constitutively active β-catenin for increased self-renewal. This suggests that BMI-1 may be a mediator of WNT/FZD signaling in normal PSCs [178].

4. An Overview of AR and AR Signaling

The most critical molecular component of the androgen signaling pathway is the AR protein. Upon activation by androgens, AR mediates transcription of target genes that modulate growth and differentiation of prostate epithelial cells. AR plays a vital role in the development of male reproductive organs. Of note, its dysregulation contributes to the male pattern of baldness, development of prostatic hyperplasia, and later in life to PCa.

The *AR* gene is located on chromosome Xq11-12. It consists eight exons that encode an 110 kDa nuclear receptor that is a unique member of the nuclear steroid receptor gene family (Figure 2) [179,180]. The AR protein has four functional domains (Figure 2). The N-terminal domain (NTD) is the most variable and least conserved domain; it is needed to form a transcriptionally active molecule. Precisely, the NTD contains the activation function 1 (AF-1) domain that includes two overlapping transcription activation units (TAUs): TAU-1 (amino acids 1–370), which supports AR transcriptional activity upon stimulation by full agonist, and TAU-5 (amino acids 360–528), which confers a constitutive activity to the AR in the absence of its ligand-binding domain (LBD) (Figure 2) [181–183]. Next to the NTD lies the DNA-binding domain (DBD), which is the most conserved region in this protein. This DBD consists of two zinc finger modules that are responsible for binding to the hormone response elements [184,185]. The carboxy-terminal end of AR contains the LBD and the activation function 2 (AF-2) domain [183]. Lastly, the region between the DBD and LBD of AR is termed the hinge region (HR) (Figure 2). It provides the main portion of the nuclear translocation signal and regulates the transactivation potential as a result of posttranslational modifications. Interestingly, it serves as an integrator for signals coming from different pathways [185].

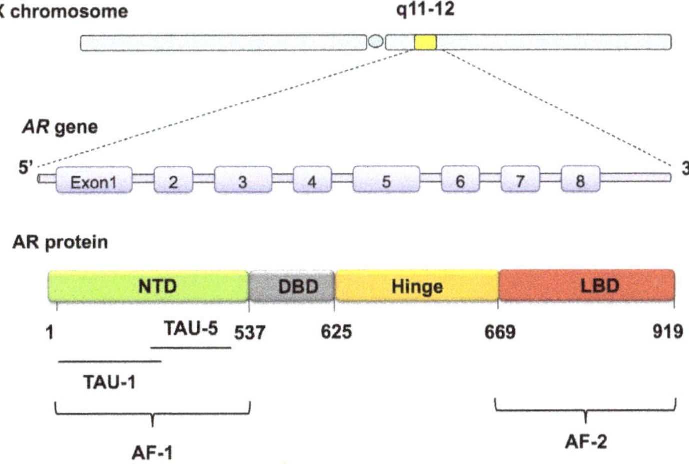

Figure 2. Schematic representation of the androgen receptor (AR) gene and protein, with indications of its specific motifs and domains. The *AR* gene is located on human X chromosome and is composed of 8 exons. The domains and motifs in the AR protein include: the N-terminal domain (NTD), the DNA-binding domain (DBD), the hinge region, and the ligand-binding domain (LBD), as well as the activation function 1 (AF-1) domain and the activation function 2 (AF-2) domain, and two transcription activation units (TAUs): TAU-1 and TAU-5.

In mammalian cells, AR is sequestered in the cytoplasm and is bound to heat shock protein complex consisting of Hsp70 (hsc70), Hsp40 (Ydj1), Hop (p60), Hsp90 and p23. The main role of this complex is to maintain AR in a conformation capable of ligand binding and to protect it from proteolysis [182,186–188]. Upon binding to testosterone or dihydrotestosterone (DHT), the chaperone heterocomplex mediates AR translocation to the nucleus (Figure 3). In the canonical genomic pathway, once in the nucleus, AR, as a homodimer, interacts with androgen response elements (ARE); by recruiting co-regulators to form a pre-initiation complex and together with the basal transcriptional machinery, it initiates transcription of its target genes (Figure 3A) [189–191]. Of note, nuclear targeting of AR is influenced by its HR, where a deletion markedly reduces ligand-induced nuclear translocation, but does not totally block signaling [192–194]. Subsequently, loss of bound ligand allows the nuclear export signal (NES) to coordinate AR shuttling to the cytoplasm where AR can be tethered again to cytoskeletal proteins in preparation for ligand binding [195,196].

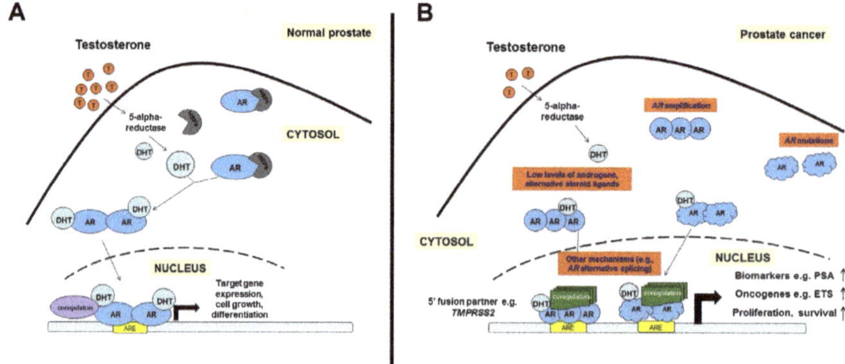

Figure 3. Schematic representation of AR signaling in normal prostate tissue and prostate cancer. (**A**) The AR is complexed to heat shock proteins (HSPs), principally HSP90, in the absence of steroid hormones. Upon binding to dihydrotestosterone (DHT), AR dimerizes and translocates to the nucleus. In the nucleus, AR binds to DNA via the androgen-responsive element (ARE). This occurs both by direct binding to DNA and by association with other transcription factors and co-regulators, leading to expression of its target genes that control growth and differentiation of prostate cells; (**B**) In PCa cells, AR signaling is maintained through other mechanisms such as *AR* amplification, *AR* mutations, or *AR* alternative splicing. AR can also be transactivated in the absence or under very low levels of androgens. In the nucleus, AR can drive expression of oncogenes such as those encoding the ETS transcription factors (e.g., ERG, ETV1), as a consequence of gene rearrangements (e.g., *TMPRSS2-ERG* gene fusion); it also controls expression of its target genes that support proliferation and survival of PCa cells.

Regulation of the AR activity occurs, in part, by posttranslational modifications, such as phosphorylation at several serine residues with or without a bound ligand [197]. Precisely, AR is phosphorylated at serine residues (Ser80, Ser93 and Ser641) that are believed to function by protecting AR from proteolytic degradation [196,198]. Degradation of AR plays a pivotal role in the regulation of AR function. AR is a direct target for MDM2-mediated ubiquitylation and proteolysis [199]. The NEDD4 ubiquitin ligase recruiting protein PMEPA1 may also play important roles in this pathway [200,201].

5. The Emergence of Castration Resistance

Although the preferred ligand for AR is DHT (Figure 3A), it has been reported that mutations frequently detected in both human PCa and in PCa cell lines may alter the ligand specificity of AR, leading to its promiscuous activity in the presence of alternative steroid ligands that do not bind to the wild-type AR [202,203]. In addition to mutations of *AR* found in PCa, important recent studies have shown that AR can drive expression of oncogenes such as those encoding the ETS transcription factors (e.g., ERG, ETV1) as a consequence of gene rearrangements [204]. The most common form of these rearrangements creates a *TMPRSS2-ERG* gene fusion, resulting in expression of an N-terminally truncated ERG protein under the control of the androgen-responsive promoter of *TMPRSS2* (Figure 3B) [204,205]. Furthermore, a recent whole-genome chromatin immunoprecipitation (ChIP) analysis showed that ERG could bind to AR downstream target genes and disturb AR signaling in PCa cells through epigenetic silencing [206]. By characterizing human PCa cell lines and knockin mouse models ectopically expressing ERG or ETV1, we demonstrated that ERG negatively regulates the AR transcriptional program, whereas ETV1 cooperates with AR signaling by favoring activation of the AR transcriptional program [207].

Prostate gland development and PCa are critically dependent on AR signaling. The ADT remains the most widely used treatment for patients with advanced PCa. In fact, androgen deprivation causes reduced AR expression, apoptosis and decreased tumor cell volume; however most PCas eventually develop the capacity for recurrent growth in the absence of testicular androgen (i.e., CRPC) [208–210]. The postulated mechanisms to explain the emergence of CRPC can be separated into three general categories, most of which center on AR signaling, including *AR* amplification, *AR* mutation, and overexpression of *AR* splice isoforms (Figure 3B). Another mechanism for increased AR signaling activity is the endogenous expression of androgen synthetic enzymes by tumor tissues, which leads to de novo androgen synthesis or conversion of weaker adrenal androgens into testosterone and DHT [124,211–214]. Up to 80% of CRPCs display a marked increase in AR mRNA and protein [215–218]. Studies by Kim et al. have shown that AR protein expression is increased in recurrent tumor samples compared to paired androgen-sensitive samples in tumor xenograft models [210]. Specifically, in CWR22 xenograft tumors, castration initially induced growth arrest in tumor cells. However, foci of Ki-67 immunopositive cells were detected by 120 days after castration [210]. In nearly one-third of patients progressing after castration or antiandrogen treatments, the mechanism for increased AR expression is through amplification of the *AR* gene at Xq11-12 [183,215,216,219–221]. Additionally, the most recent analysis of whole-exome sequencing of 150 metastatic CRPC (mCRPC) biopsies revealed 63% of *AR* gene amplification and mutation in comparison to that of 440 primary PCa tissues [222]. This amplification leads to an increase in *AR* gene expression and enhances AR activation by low levels of androgens. It remains unclear, however, whether amplification of the *AR* gene in hormone-refractory tumors results in an increase in AR protein levels. In fact, contradicting results have been obtained. Studies by Koivisto et al. have shown that hormone-refractory prostate tumors carrying an amplified *AR* express a higher level of *AR* mRNA compared to untreated primary tumors with a single copy of *AR* per cell [220]. In contrast, studies by Linja et al. have revealed that hormone-refractory tumors carrying *AR* amplification were not found to express a higher level of *AR* mRNA than those with a normal *AR* copy number [217]. Therefore, the significance of *AR* amplification in PCa remains unclear. In addition, alternative splicing of *AR* mRNA is another mechanism implicated in progression to CRPC. Multiple aberrantly spliced AR variants (ARV) that miss the C-terminal LBD were detected in CRPCs [222–224]. Importantly, all ARVs retain the amino-terminal transactivation and DNA-binding domains. AR-V7 (AR1/2/3/CE3 variant) is constitutively active and the most abundant variant detected to date in CRPC [225]. Interestingly, elevated AR-V7 induces expression of a unique set of target genes [225]. Furthermore, recent findings suggested that AR-V7 could have value as a predictive biomarker in CRPC. Antonarakis et al. showed that AR-V7 mRNA in circulating tumor cells (CTCs) might be enhanced by AR-directed therapies including abiraterone acetate and enzalutamide, and its expression was associated with poor prognosis [226]. Of note, the full-length AR and AR-Vs appear to almost always coexist in PCa cells; thus, it remains highly challenging to dissect their corresponding roles in driving AR signaling in translational studies of clinical specimens [183].

6. Interaction between AR and WNT Signaling in Prostate Cancer

The paradigm that PCa development and emergence of therapy resistance are a consequence of the restoration of embryonic developmental programs (e.g., WNT signaling) has shed a new light on understanding the molecular mechanisms underlying epithelial invasion in prostate development and development of CRPC. While the (aberrant) AR signaling pathway is considered as the most critical player in CRPCs, as intracellular signaling pathways are often interconnected, other pathways, in particular, the WNT pathway, can also play key roles. As noted in the previous section, considerable evidence indicates that the WNT pathway plays a central role in the development of prostate tissues, by providing developmental growth inductive signals during embryonic/neonatal organogenesis. In PCa, studies by Schaeffer et al. have reported that androgen exposure regulates genes previously implicated in prostate carcinogenesis; these genes included those related to developmental pathways, such as WNT signaling, along with cellular programs regulating such "hallmarks" of cancer as angiogenesis, apoptosis, migration and proliferation [227]. This observation was in line with the previously published data showing that aberrant activation of the WNT/β-catenin pathway contributes to progression of several other major human cancer types [27,30,35,56,90,100,228]. The prime example is colorectal cancer, in which approximately 85% of cases display *loss-of-function* mutations in the tumor suppressor *APC* gene [229–232]. APC protein recruits β-catenin to the degradation complex and its loss leads to upregulation of β-catenin signaling (Figure 1). In addition, mutations of serine/threonine residues within the N-terminal domain of β-catenin suppress β-catenin degradation, leading to constitutive activation of WNT signaling even in the absence of WNT ligands. In PCa, mutations in the *APC* or *CTNNB1* (β-catenin) genes, which lead to constitutive activation of WNT signaling, similar to those found in colon cancer, have also been identified [202,233–236].

Accumulating evidence has supported that the WNT/β-catenin pathway plays an important role in CRPC, by interacting with AR signaling [234,237–239]. Several groups have focused on studying the role of β-catenin in CRPC compared to hormone-naïve PCa. Findings of a protein-protein interaction between AR and β-catenin have supported the biological significance of β-catenin in PCa cells. In 2000, Truica et al. showed that β-catenin could directly bind to AR to enhance its transcriptional activity stimulated by androgen, androstenedione, or estradiol, in LNCaP cells [240]. In 2002, Yang et al. demonstrated that β-catenin preferentially and directly bound to the LBD of AR in the presence of DHT over several other steroid hormone receptors [241]. Further studies revealed that β-catenin bound to the AF-2 region of the AR LBD, and modulated the transcriptional effects of the AR NTD as well as the p160 coactivator transcriptional intermediary factor 2 (TIF2); importantly, a single AR lysine residue (K720) has been shown to be necessary for the AR/β-catenin and TIF2/β-catenin interactions [242,243]. In β-catenin, early mapping experiments suggested that the NH2 terminus and the first six armadillo repeats of β-catenin were involved in its interaction with AR. In particular, deletion of repeat 6 fully abolished the physical interaction between AR and β-catenin, suggesting a key role of this repeat in the interaction [241]. Phenotypically, transient over-expression of β-catenin in AR^+ PCa cell lines CWR22-Rv1 and LAPC-4 enhanced AR-mediated transcription of its target genes, in an androgen-dependent manner [244]. Hence, β-catenin (wild-type or mutated) is considered as a ligand-dependent co-activator of the AR-driven transcription (Figure 4). Binding of β-catenin to ligand-engaged AR also facilitates the movement of β-catenin into the nucleus [245]. Furthermore, it was shown that WNT/β-catenin signaling could increase *AR* gene expression via the TCF/LEF-1 binding sites in the *AR* promoter [246]. Thus, in hormone-naïve PCa, WNT/β-catenin signaling serves as a positive regulator of AR signaling in an androgen-dependent manner (Figure 4A).

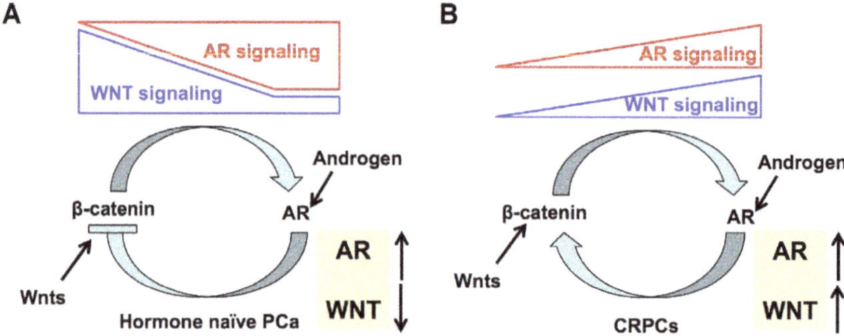

Figure 4. A simplified model of interaction between WNT and AR signaling during PCa development and progression. (**A**) In hormone naïve PCa cells, AR signaling inhibits the transcription of WNT/β-catenin target genes, while WNT/β-catenin signaling promotes transcription of AR target genes. Relative levels (i.e., anti-correlation but may reach to an equilibrium) of WNT (blue) and AR (red) signaling are indicated; (**B**) In CRPCs, AR and WNT/β-catenin signaling pathways stimulate each other to activate specific target genes for promoting androgen-independent growth and progression of PCa cells. Relative levels (i.e., positive correlation) of WNT (blue) and AR (red) signaling are indicated.

In the other hand, the effect of AR signaling on WNT/β-catenin signaling is more complicated. Early studies in gonadotropin-releasing hormone neuronal cells showed that in the presence of DHT, liganded AR repressed β-catenin/TCF-responsive reporter gene activity [247]. In androgen-dependent LNCaP PCa cells, androgen treatment repressed target genes of WNT/β-catenin, whereas inhibition of AR activity enhanced WNT/β-catenin-responsive transcription; this data suggested that under the hormone-naïve condition, AR signaling could repress β-catenin/TCF-mediated transcription induced by androgen [96] (Figure 4A). Mechanistically, as β-catenin interacts with TCF4 to control transcription of WNT/β-catenin target genes, this could be due to preferential interaction of β-catenin with AR rather than TCF4 in hormone-naïve PCa cells. While WNT/β-catenin pathway is repressed by AR in the androgen-dependent LNCaP cell line, upon repression of AR activity or in the androgen-independent subline of LNCaP cells (LNCaP-abl), the WNT/β-catenin responsive transcription appeared to be largely activated, suggesting a likely role of WNT signaling in PCa progression to CRPC [96] (Figure 4B). This could be due to an increased interaction of β-catenin with TCF4 (rather than AR), which could promote WNT/β-catenin-target gene expression [96]. Therapeutically, pharmacological and genetic inhibition of the WNT/β-catenin pathway (using siRNA against β-catenin or a small molecule β-catenin inhibitor) in LNCaP-abl cells re-established their sensitivity to enzalutamide, a synthetic non-steroidal antiandrogen [96]. Thus, this study implies that inhibition of the WNT/β-catenin pathway may be translated into an effective therapeutic approach to treat enzalutamide-resistant CRPC.

To add another layer of the complexity of interaction between AR and WNT/β-catenin signaling, it was shown that when PCa cells had been adapted to the low androgen environment (e.g., upon ADT), β-catenin could act as a co-activator of AR as well to enhance AR transcriptional activity in the presence of androstenedione, a weaker adrenal androgen remaining present in CRPC patients [239,241–243]. This direct interaction between AR and β-catenin seemed to elicit a specific expression of a set of target genes in low androgen conditions in CRPC, which is consistent with the previous finding that target genes regulated by AR signaling are different in CRPC cells compared to those in hormone-naïve PCa cells [248]. Thus, it seems the effect of AR signaling on WNT/β-catenin signaling is PCa stage-dependent: it suppresses WNT/β-catenin signaling in hormone-naïve PCa, but in CRPC, both AR signaling and WNT/β-catenin signaling work together to positively support each other and to control a unique set of genes for sustaining CRPC cells (Figure 4). Lastly and most importantly, the significance of WNT/β-catenin and AR pathways in CRPCs was further demonstrated in studies by Robinson et al [222]. Their clinical sequencing analysis of PCa genomes has revealed that the majority of individuals with CRPCs harbor molecular alternations in the *AR* gene, as well as in genes encoding the main components of the WNT/β-catenin pathway, such as APC, β-catenin and R-spondins, leading to overactivation of WNT/β-catenin signaling [222].

As described in the previous section, WNT ligands are highly conserved secreted molecules that play critical but pleiotropic roles in cell-cell signaling during embryogenesis. Interestingly, expression levels of several WNT ligands were found to be up- or down-regulated in advanced PCa. For instance, Chen et al. demonstrated that high levels of WNT1 and β-catenin expression were associated with advanced, metastatic, hormone-refractory prostate carcinoma, in which they could serve as markers for disease progression [236]. In two independent studies, another WNT ligand, WNT3A, has been shown to modulate growth of PCa cells [20,249]. Importantly, the activity of AR signaling in the presence of low concentrations of androgens was increased by application of purified WNT3A, suggesting an important role of the canonical WNT3A signaling on the AR program [20]. As to the non-canonical WNT pathways, elevated levels of WNT5A have been found to increase free intracellular calcium and CaMKII in PCa cell lines, indicating that the WNT/Ca2+ pathway operates via CaMKII in PCa [250]. Yamamoto et al. showed that WNT5A overexpression enhanced invasion of the PC3 PCa cell line, and the invasion activity required the expression of WNT receptors FZD2 and ROR2 [251]. Interestingly, the very recent clinical studies by Miyamoto et al. have shown the importance of non-canonical WNT in the maintenance of metastatic CRPC [252]. In details, they used RNA-in-situ hybridization (RNA-ISH) to identify the source of WNT production in tumor specimens and CTCs. Metastatic tumor biopsies from patients with CRPC had readily detectable *WNT5A* and *WNT7B*. Similarly, *WNT5A* or *WNT7B* mRNA was detected by RNA-ISH in a subset of CTCs from patients with CRPC [252]. This demonstrates that a subset of PCa cells express non-canonical WNT ligands, which may provide survival signals in the context of AR inhibition. Furthermore, elevated expression of another WNT ligand, WNT11, has also been detected in PCa tissues versus normal samples [21]. Interestingly, WNT11 induced expression of neuroendocrine differentiation (NED) markers NSE and ASCL1, while silencing of WNT11 in androgen-depleted LNCaP and androgen-independent PC3 cells prevented NED and resulted in apoptosis [19].

Secreted WNT antagonists, including the sFRP family, DKK family, and Wnt inhibitory factor-1 (WIF1), are negative modulators of WNT signaling [239,253–255]. Thus, their expression is expected to be downregulated in advanced PCa. Indeed, a recent study reported downregulation of sFRP2 in PCa [256]. *WIF1* mRNA appears to be downregulated in a considerable percentage of PCa samples [257]. Interestingly, laboratories of Zi and Hoang have demonstrated that ectopic expression of sFRP3 (FRZB) or WIF1 in a CRPC cell line PC3 caused a reversal of epithelial-to-mesenchymal transition and inhibition of tumor growth by inhibition of the canonical WNT pathway [258,259]. The role of the DKK family of WNT antagonist (e.g., DKK1) in PCa is arguably even more complex than that of the sFRP family or WIF1. DKK1 inhibits WNT signaling by disrupting the binding of LRP6 to the WNT/FZD ligand-receptor complex [239,255]. Although DKK1 is upregulated in early PCa, it is downregulated during progression from primary tumor to metastasis; however, its expression can also inhibit WNT-induced osteoblastic activity and thus reduces bone metastases [260,261]. Altogether, these results suggest that WNT ligands and antagonists may play different roles during PCa progression in a context-dependent manner.

7. Therapeutic Applications for Targeting WNT/β-catenin-AR Interactions in CRPC

Cancer stem cells (CSCs) have been proposed to contribute to therapy resistance and cancer recurrence [262]. In addition to its higher activity in CRPC, the WNT/β-catenin signaling pathway has also been linked to prostate CSCs. For instance, Jiang et al. showed that activation of the WNT pathway via inhibition of GSK3β promoted LNCaP C4-2B and DU145 cell-derived xenograft tumor growth, as well as C4-2B cell-derived bone metastasis [263]. Interestingly, they reported an increase of the $ALDH^+/CD133^+$ CSC-like subpopulation in these PCa cell lines. Previous studies have shown that PCa cells with these markers exhibited tumor-initiating and metastasis-initiation cell properties, although it was not absolutely clear whether the $ALDH^+/CD133^+$ subpopulation represented CSCs definitively [263–265]. In a recent study [266], it was shown that knockdown of a prostate tumor suppressor, DAB2IP, transformed normal prostate epithelial cells into CSCs, which exhibited enriched $CD44^+/CD24^-$ populations. Interestingly, they reported that it was the WNT/β-catenin signaling pathway that mediated upregulation of CD44 by *DAB2IP* knockdown. In this setting, CD44 not only served as a marker for CSCs, but also played a key role in facilitating the onset of prostate CSCs and increasing their chemoresistance [266]. Importantly, combination therapy based on WNT inhibitors (e.g., LGK974) and conventional drugs (e.g., docetaxel) synergistically enhanced their efficacy and robustly inhibited growth of xenograft tumors [266]. In another study, Rajan et al. reported a gene expression profiling study of seven patients with advanced PCa, with paired samples before and after ADT [267]. By using RNA sequencing combined with bioinformatic approaches, the authors identified alterations in the WNT/β-catenin signaling pathway following ADT. Additionally, they showed that the tankyrase inhibitor XAV939 (which promotes β-catenin degradation) reduced growth of the androgen-independent LNCaP-abl cell line, compared with the androgen-responsive LNCaP cells [267]. Similarly, Lee et al. demonstrated that iCRT-3, a novel compound that disrupts both β-catenin/TCF and β-catenin/AR protein-protein interactions, inhibited PCa growth in vivo and blocked bicalutamide-resistant prostate sphere-forming cells [268]. Overall, it seems that targeting CSCs via inhibition of WNT signaling may have the potential to reduce the self-renewal and aggressive behavior of PCa [162].

As to the non-canonical WNT pathway, the most recent clinical studies by Miyamoto et al. have shown that activation of this pathway in CTCs from patients with metastatic CRPC correlates with reduced effectiveness of antiandrogen treatment [252]. In particular, significant enrichment of non-canonical WNT signaling was observed in CTCs from patients whose PCa progressed in the presence of enzalutamide, particularly among CTCs with reduced glucocorticoid receptor expression. To test whether activation of non-canonical WNT signaling modulates enzalutamide sensitivity, they ectopically expressed the ligands for non-canonical WNT signaling, including WNT4, WNT5A, WNT7B, or WNT11, in LNCaP PCa cells, which express these ligands at low endogenous levels. They found that ectopic expression of a range of these WNT proteins in androgen-sensitive LNCaP cells enhanced their survival in the presence of enzalutamide, with WNT5A to be particularly effective in this regard [252]. Conversely, its knockdown resulted in reduced cell proliferation. This data suggests that the non-canonical WNT signaling pathway may serve as a potential new therapeutic target in PCa that is resistant to antiandrogen therapy.

Taken together, WNT signaling interacts with AR signaling using distinct mechanisms at different stages of PCa progression. In hormone-naïve PCa cells, WNT/β-catenin signaling promotes transcription of AR target genes, whereas AR signaling inhibits the transcription of WNT/β-catenin target genes (Figure 4A). However, in CRPCs, the AR and WNT/β-catenin signaling pathways stimulate each other to activate a unique set of target genes for promoting androgen-independent growth and progression of PCa cells (Figure 4B). The interaction between AR and WNT signaling provides a growth advantage to PCa cells at the castration level of androgens. Inhibition of the WNT/β-catenin pathway would thus offer a novel therapeutic strategy to target CRPC cells and CSCs [239].

8. AR and WNT Signaling in Mammary Gland Development and Breast Cancer

8.1. AR and WNT Signaling in Mammary Gland Development

WNT signaling plays key roles in both mammary gland development and breast cancer (BCa), largely through regulating mammary stem cell maintenance and basal mammary epithelial cell fate determination. An excellent review for this topic was published in this journal recently [41]. As to the AR signaling pathway, AR-mediated androgen actions play a direct or indirect role in mammary physiology (Figure 5). AR can interact with estrogen receptor alpha (ERα) and their interactions have inhibitory effects on their transactivational properties [269]. AR can also compete with ERα for binding to specific estrogen-responsive element (ERE) [270]. Thus, the effect of AR signaling in mammary gland development may be largely related to its effect on estrogen signaling. In fact, androgen treatment could inhibit estrogen-induced proliferation of mammary epithelial cells, particularly during puberty, leading to retarded mammary ductal extension and reduced expression of ERα [271–273]. Conversely, inactivation of AR resulted in accelerated mammary ductal growth and increased expression of ERα during puberty [273]. However, in addition to its inhibitory role on the ERα pathway, the role of AR signaling in mammary epithelial cells may be also mediated by inhibition of WNT/β-catenin signaling, a mechanism similar to that in hormone-naïve prostate cells (Figure 4). This is supported by the finding that loss of AR led to activation of the WNT/β-catenin pathway in the pubertal mammary gland [273]. In adult females, inhibition of AR signaling could also increase mammary ductal branching and mammary epithelial cell proliferation; however, this phenotype was not due to changes in serum estradiol levels or ERα expression, but was attributed to increased AR expression and consequently an increase in the ratio of AR to ERα (as ERα level remained constant) [271]. Relating to BCa, disruption of the inhibitory influence of androgen/AR signaling on mammary epithelial cells at either puberty or adult stage, as well as the crosstalk between AR signaling and estrogen or WNT signaling, are likely to have important implications for breast tumorigenesis [270,273].

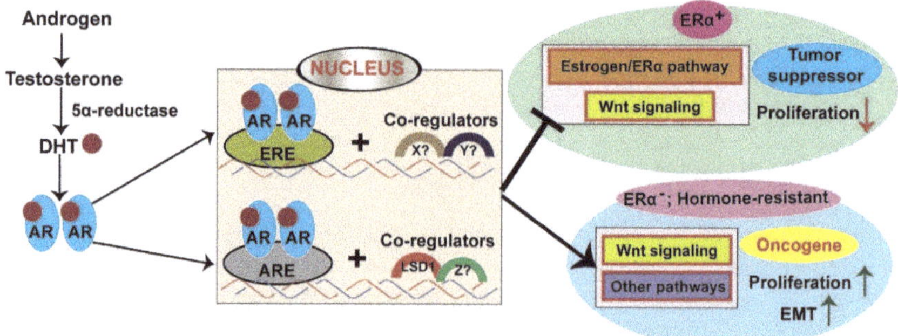

Figure 5. Proposed roles of AR and WNT signaling in mammary gland development and breast cancer. In breast cells, activated androgen/AR binds to ARE or ERE in its target genes. In ERα^+ cells, it largely works as a tumor suppressor by inhibiting estrogen/ERα signaling and/or WNT signaling; in ERα^- cells or even in ERα^+ cells that have become resistant to hormone therapy (targeting the estrogen/ER pathway), AR may function as an oncoprotein by activating WNT signaling and/or other oncogenic pathways. Under different cellular contexts, AR may utilize different co-regulators (e.g., LSD1, or other co-regulators remain to be defined (X?, Y?, or Z?)) to control distinct downstream programs.

8.2. AR Signaling in Breast Cancer

Unlike PCa, our understanding of AR signaling in BCa is still at its infancy. Some studies report that overexpression of AR is associated with better outcomes in BCa, while others illustrate a positive correlation of circulating androgens with high risk, recurrence and metastasis of BCa [274–279]. Historically, therapeutics targeting AR were considered beneficial for women diagnosed with advanced BCa [280]. In the "older generation" of androgen-related therapy for the treatment of BCa, including DHT, testosterone, and fluoxymesterone, certain clinical efficacies were observed [281–283]. However, androgen-related therapy gradually lost its attraction for the treatment of BCa, due to aromatization of androgens to estrogens, inconsistent clinical trials, undesirable virilizing side effects, and the broad utilization of estrogen-targeted therapy such as tamoxifen [284–287]. With improved preclinical interpretation of heterogeneity toward mammary epithelial cells and BCa subtypes, AR signaling-directed therapies, and resistance mechanisms of anti-estrogen therapies, there have been renewed enthusiasms in utilizing androgens and targeting AR for BCa [280,288].

In breast tissues, androgen can be converted to DHT, which subsequently activates AR. The liganded AR direct or indirectly (possibly together with distinct co-regulators under different ERα settings) interacts with either ARE or ERE in its target genes (Figure 5). In the presence of comparable levels of AR and ERα, AR competes with ERα, leading to inhibition of the estrogen/ER pathway [270,274]. In the absence of ERα (or under the conditional of resistance to hormone therapy), the ratio of AR to ERα increases and AR functions as an oncoprotein by recruiting different co-factors (e.g., lysine-specific demethylase 1 (LSD1)), leading to regulation of a different set of target genes, which may contribute to BCa cell proliferation and/or epithelial–mesenchymal transition (EMT) [270,289] (Figure 5).

BCa is often classified clinically into four subtypes based on expression of ER, progesterone receptor (PR), and human epidermal growth factor receptor 2 (HER2, also known as ERBB2): ER$^+$/PR$^+$/HER2$^-$, ER$^+$/PR$^+$/HER2$^+$, ER$^-$/PR$^-$/HER2$^+$, and ER$^-$/PR$^-$/HER2$^-$ (also known as triple negative breast cancer, TNBC). Relating to the ER status, AR likely plays distinct roles in BCa in a subtype-specific manner.

Positive expression of AR was clinically defined as immunohistochemical (IHC) nuclear staining $\geq$1% or $\geq$10% according to various studies [281,290–292]. AR is highly expressed in both primary (~80%) and metastatic (~60%) breast tumors [280]. AR expression varies in BCa across different subtypes; the prevalence of AR is approximately 70%–95%, 50%−81%, and 10%–53%, in ER^+, ER^-/$HER2^+$, and TNBC subtypes, respectively [275,281,282,293–298].

Modulation of AR signaling, either inhibitory or stimulatory, exhibits somewhat contradictory observations in different subtypes of BCa, particularly when interacting with ER signaling [283,299]. When prescribed to non-selected BCa patients, testosterone contributed to a response rate of about 20%–25%; due to broad side effects, this strategy has quickly been replaced by multiple ER-directed therapies [300–303]. However, a retrospective study reported a promising tumor control rate of 58.5% (tumor regression and stableness, $n = 53$) with testosterone therapy in patients with metastatic ER^+ BCa [304]. Androgen, together with tamoxifen, synergically increased response rates when treating advanced ER^+ BCa, but this study is still at the beginning stage [280,305]. Recently developed AR antagonists have demonstrated more potent and better clinical efficacies than those of the early-generations, which have generally been disappointing for combating BCa [280,288,306,307]. Here we will highlight the key AR-based therapeutics for treatment of BCa, in a subtype-specific manner.

8.2.1. AR in ER^+ Breast Cancer

AR is highly expressed in ER^+ BCa with a frequency of ~70%–95% [281,295,296,298,308]. In this BCa subtype, ER signaling functions as a dominant oncogenic driver; thus, clarifying its functional relationship with AR signaling would be beneficial for exploring the role of anti-estrogen therapies [309]. AR and ER can interact (and interfere) with each other functionally by sharing (and competing for) similar cofactors and nuclear binding sites [274,310]. AR expression may have contradicting functional consequences in ER^+ BCa in a treatment-dependent manner: some studies indicated that higher AR expression is associated with better therapy outcomes, whereas others have reported that AR plays an oncogenic role in tamoxifen-resistant subjects [294,311–314]. Nevertheless, AR signaling may mainly play an anti-proliferative effect in ER^+ BCa initially, due to its ability to antagonize the growth-promoting role of ER signaling [302]. Accordingly, androgens and androgen agonists have been evaluated for the efficacies of treating ER^+/AR^+ BCas [302]. But combination therapy based on enzalutamide (antiandrogen) and agents that target ER signaling (e.g., exemestane, anastrozole, or fulvestrant) has also been tested in clinical trials for potentially overcoming resistance to hormone therapy [294].

8.2.2. AR Signaling in ER^-/$HER2^+$ Breast Cancer

AR is highly expressed in ER^- BCa and the functional crosstalk between AR and HER2 is critical for the tumor cell survival and expansion [282,297,315]. In this subtype of BCa, the proliferative role of AR signaling has been well investigated [275,280]. Mechanisms underlying this functional interplay include direct transcriptional upregulation of HER2 signaling by AR via its heterodimer HER3, which in turn activates *AR* transcription in a positive feedback loop [297,316,317]. AR signaling also induces ligand-dependent stimulation of WNT signaling, via direct transcriptional upregulation of *WNT7B*, which activates β-catenin, resulting in *HER3* transcriptional activation [297]. HER2 signaling is the key oncogenic driver in this subtype of BCa and effective HER2-targeted therapies are crucial for treating patients with this BCa subtype. As AR antagonists can efficiently reduce cell proliferation [297,318], clinical trials are ongoing to explore whether combination of AR and HER2-directed therapies could result in any synergic outcomes [318].

8.2.3. AR Signaling in TNBC

The frequency of AR expression in TNBC is around 10% to 53% [281,296,298]. A molecular subtype of BCa referred to as the molecular apocrine subtype, which included those non-basal-like ER^- breast tumors that were also AR^+, was defined based on microarray expression profiling [319]. Later on, also based on gene expression profiling data, TNBCs were classified as six subtypes and those with AR expression were defined as the luminal androgen receptor (LAR) subtype [298]. Differentially expressed genes that characterize this subtype are heavily enriched in hormonally regulated pathways, including steroid synthesis, porphyrin metabolism, and androgen/estrogen metabolism [298,320]. AR signaling in TNBC was reported to maintain cell proliferation and AR also acted as a biomarker for sensitivity to both PI3K and ERK inhibition [318,321]. The functional role of AR in TNBC was further established based on the finding that LAR BCa cells were sensitive to AR antagonists and Hsp90 inhibitors [322]. An encouraging case for using AR-targeted therapy for treatment of AR^+ TNBC was reported recently, in which a patient with this BCa subtype had progressive disease following six cycles of cytotoxic chemotherapy, but attained a 100% response to bicalutamide (an antiandrogen) [323]. With the development of potent AR-directed therapies and promising combined therapeutic approaches, more clinical trials targeting AR^+ TNBC are being developed [318,321].

8.3. Interaction between AR and WNT Signaling in Breast Cancer

Overexpression of WNT induces aberrant activities of the WNT signaling pathway, which is a main driving force in BCa progression [297,324]. WNT ligands are associated with normal mammary gland development and overexpression of *WNT1* is oncogenic for BCa [325]. The interplay of AR and WNT signaling has been mainly studied in the ER^-/$HER2^+$ BCa subtype. Using gene set enrichment analysis (GSEA), Ni et al. observed that androgen (DHT)-stimulated genes in ER^-/$HER2^+$ BCa cells were mainly those involved in WNT signaling [297]. Furthermore, they found that AR upregulated *WNT7B* transcription in a ligand-dependent manner. WNT7B is a canonical WNT ligand and may play roles in the normal mammary gland development during the stages of ductal formation and involution [326,327]. Elevated expression of *WNT7B* has been found in ~10% of BCa cases [328]. In addition to activation of WNT signaling via the androgen/AR-WNT7B pathway, Ni et al. showed that similar to PCa, AR and WNT/β-catenin signaling also cooperated functionally; in this case, β-catenin cooperated with AR to promote the progression and maintenance of ER^-/$HER2^+$ BCa cells by upregulating *HER3*, which encodes a key co-receptor of HER2 in $HER2^+$ BCa [297]. Importantly, by targeting the AR pathway using bicalutamide, the growth of DHT-stimulated ER^-/$HER2^+$ breast tumor cells in vivo was inhibited [297].

Thus, in both PCa and BCa, AR signaling appears to regulate distinct sets of target genes in hormone-dependent cancers (i.e., hormone-naïve PCa, ER^+ BCa) and hormone-refractory cancers (i.e., CRPC, ER^- BCa, hormone therapy-resistant ER^+ BCa). Accordingly, both AR agonists and AR (and/or WNT) antagonists may be beneficial for BCa therapy, but in a BCa subtype and therapy stage-dependent manner. In particular, as both the AR and WNT signaling pathways drive progression and maintenance of AR^+ TNBCs, inhibitors for these two pathways may prove to be useful for targeting this TNBC subtype. In addition, AR antagonists and anti-HER2 agents may also be used in combination to treat ER^-/$HER2^+$ BCa with AR expression, and inhibitors for WNT signaling may offer another therapeutic opportunity, particularly when ER^-/$HER2^+$ BCa cells develop resistance to the anti-HER2/AR agents.

9. Concluding Remarks

As two key pathways regulating both normal development and tumorigenesis in hormone-responsive prostate and mammary glands, the context-dependent interplay of AR and WNT signaling pathways provides a unique opportunity to explore therapeutic options for treating prostate and breast cancers, particularly when under the setting of therapeutic resistance. As both CRPCs and ER^- BCas (i.e., TNBC and ER^-/$HER2^+$ BCa, or even ER^+ BCas that become resistant to hormone therapy) are refractory or unresponsive to hormone therapy, a better understanding of roles of AR and WNT pathways and their interactions in these hormone-refractory diseases should open a new avenue for improving their treatment and for combating the inevitable challenge of therapy resistance.

Acknowledgments: This work was supported by a Prostate Cancer Research Program Idea Development Award (W81XWH-15-1-0546) and a Breast cancer Research Program Breakthrough Award (W81XWH-15-1-0100) from Department of Defense (to Zhe Li).

Conflicts of Interest: The authors declare no conflict of interest.

References

1. Siegel, R.; Naishadham, D.; Jemal, A. Cancer statistics, 2013. *CA: Cancer J. Clin.* **2013**, *63*, 11–30. [CrossRef] [PubMed]
2. Ahmed, A.; Ali, S.; Sarkar, F.H. Advances in androgen receptor targeted therapy for prostate cancer. *J. Cell. Physiol.* **2014**, *229*, 271–276. [CrossRef] [PubMed]
3. Siegel, R.L.; Miller, K.D.; Jemal, A. Cancer statistics, 2016. *CA: Cancer J. Clin.* **2016**, *66*, 7–30. [CrossRef] [PubMed]
4. Brown, T.R.; Lubahn, D.B.; Wilson, E.M.; Joseph, D.R.; French, F.S.; Migeon, C.J. Deletion of the steroid-binding domain of the human androgen receptor gene in one family with complete androgen insensitivity syndrome: Evidence for further genetic heterogeneity in this sy ndrome. *Proc. Natl. Acad. Sci. USA* **1988**, *85*, 8151–8155. [CrossRef] [PubMed]
5. Lubahn, D.B.; Brown, T.R.; Simental, J.A.; Higgs, H.N.; Migeon, C.J.; Wilson, E.M.; French, F.S. Sequence of the intron/exon junctions of the coding region of the human androgen receptor gene and identification of a point mutation in a family with complete androgen insensitivity. *Proc. Natl. Acad. Sci. USA* **1989**, *86*, 9534–9538. [CrossRef] [PubMed]
6. Huggins, C.; Hodges, C.V. Studies on prostatic cancer. I. The effect of castration, of estrogen and androgen injection on serum phosphatases in metastatic carcinoma of the prostate. *CA: Cancer J. Clin.* **1972**, *22*, 232–240. [CrossRef]
7. Heidenreich, A.; Bastian, P.J.; Bellmunt, J.; Bolla, M.; Joniau, S.; van der Kwast, T.; Mason, M.; Matveev, V.; Wiegel, T.; Zattoni, F.; et al. Eau guidelines on prostate cancer. Part ii: Treatment of advanced, relapsing, and castration-resistant prostate cancer. *Eur. Urol.* **2014**, *65*, 467–479. [CrossRef] [PubMed]
8. Prensner, J.R.; Rubin, M.A.; Wei, J.T.; Chinnaiyan, A.M. Beyond psa: The next generation of prostate cancer biomarkers. *Sci. Transl. Med.* **2012**. [CrossRef] [PubMed]
9. Holzbeierlein, J.; Lal, P.; LaTulippe, E.; Smith, A.; Satagopan, J.; Zhang, L.; Ryan, C.; Smith, S.; Scher, H.; Scardino, P.; et al. Gene expression analysis of human prostate carcinoma during hormonal therapy identifies androgen-responsive genes and mechanisms of therapy resistance. *Am. J. Pathol.* **2004**, *164*, 217–227. [CrossRef]
10. Penney, K.L.; Schumacher, F.R.; Kraft, P.; Mucci, L.A.; Sesso, H.D.; Ma, J.; Niu, Y.; Cheong, J.K.; Hunter, D.J.; Stampfer, M.J.; et al. Association of KLK3 (PSA) genetic variants with prostate cancer risk and PSA levels. *Carcinogenesis* **2011**, *32*, 853–859. [CrossRef] [PubMed]
11. Parikh, H.; Wang, Z.; Pettigrew, K.A.; Jia, J.; Daugherty, S.; Yeager, M.; Jacobs, K.B.; Hutchinson, A.; Burdett, L.; Cullen, M.; et al. Fine mapping the KLK3 locus on chromosome 19q13.33 associated with prostate cancer susceptibility and psa levels. *Hum. Genet.* **2011**, *129*, 675–685. [CrossRef] [PubMed]
12. Feldman, B.J.; Feldman, D. The development of androgen-independent prostate cancer. *Nat. Rev. Cancer* **2001**, *1*, 34–45. [CrossRef] [PubMed]
13. Nieto, M.; Finn, S.; Loda, M.; Hahn, W.C. Prostate cancer: Re-focusing on androgen receptor signaling. *Int. J. Biochem. Cell Biol.* **2007**, *39*, 1562–1568. [CrossRef] [PubMed]
14. Snoek, R.; Cheng, H.; Margiotti, K.; Wafa, L.A.; Wong, C.A.; Wong, E.C.; Fazli, L.; Nelson, C.C.; Gleave, M.E.; Rennie, P.S. In vivo knockdown of the androgen receptor results in growth inhibition and regression of well-established, castration-resistant prostate tumors. *Clin. Cancer Res.* **2009**, *15*, 39–47. [CrossRef] [PubMed]
15. Sharma, N.L.; Massie, C.E.; Ramos-Montoya, A.; Zecchini, V.; Scott, H.E.; Lamb, A.D.; MacArthur, S.; Stark, R.; Warren, A.Y.; Mills, I.G.; et al. The androgen receptor induces a distinct transcriptional program in castration-resistant prostate cancer in man. *Cancer Cell* **2013**, *23*, 35–47. [CrossRef] [PubMed]
16. Pienta, K.J.; Bradley, D. Mechanisms underlying the development of androgen-independent prostate cancer. *Clin. Cancer Res.* **2006**, *12*, 1665–1671. [CrossRef] [PubMed]
17. Kypta, R.M.; Waxman, J. Wnt/beta-Catenin signalling in prostate cancer. *Nat. Rev. Urol.* **2012**, *9*, 418–428. [CrossRef] [PubMed]
18. Takahashi, S.; Watanabe, T.; Okada, M.; Inoue, K.; Ueda, T.; Takada, I.; Watabe, T.; Yamamoto, Y.; Fukuda, T.; Nakamura, T.; et al. Noncanonical wnt signaling mediates androgen-dependent tumor growth in a mouse model of prostate cancer. *Proc. Natl. Acad. Sci. USA* **2011**, *108*, 4938–4943. [CrossRef] [PubMed]

19. Uysal-Onganer, P.; Kawano, Y.; Caro, M.; Walker, M.M.; Diez, S.; Darrington, R.S.; Waxman, J.; Kypta, R.M. Wnt-11 promotes neuroendocrine-like differentiation, survival and migration of prostate cancer cells. *Mol. Cancer* **2010**. [CrossRef] [PubMed]
20. Verras, M.; Brown, J.; Li, X.; Nusse, R.; Sun, Z. Wnt3a growth factor induces androgen receptor-mediated transcription and enhances cell growth in human prostate cancer cells. *Cancer Res.* **2004**, *64*, 8860–8866. [CrossRef] [PubMed]
21. Zhu, H.; Mazor, M.; Kawano, Y.; Walker, M.M.; Leung, H.Y.; Armstrong, K.; Waxman, J.; Kypta, R.M. Analysis of wnt gene expression in prostate cancer: Mutual inhibition by wnt11 and the androgen receptor. *Cancer Res.* **2004**, *64*, 7918–7926. [CrossRef] [PubMed]
22. Nelson, W.J.; Nusse, R. Convergence of WNT, β-catenin, and cadherin pathways. *Science* **2004**, *303*, 1483–1487. [CrossRef] [PubMed]
23. Logan, C.Y.; Nusse, R. The WNT signaling pathway in development and disease. *Ann. Rev. Cell Dev. Biol.* **2004**, *20*, 781–810. [CrossRef] [PubMed]
24. Grigoryan, T.; Wend, P.; Klaus, A.; Birchmeier, W. Deciphering the function of canonical wnt signals in development and disease: Conditional loss- and gain-of-function mutations of beta-catenin in mice. *Genes Dev.* **2008**, *22*, 2308–2341. [CrossRef] [PubMed]
25. Klaus, A.; Birchmeier, W. Wnt signalling and its impact on development and cancer. *Nat. Rev. Cancer* **2008**, *8*, 387–398. [CrossRef] [PubMed]
26. Lien, W.H.; Fuchs, E. Wnt some lose some: Transcriptional governance of stem cells by WNT/β-catenin signaling. *Genes Dev.* **2014**, *28*, 1517–1532. [CrossRef] [PubMed]
27. Clevers, H. Wnt/ β-catenin signaling in development and disease. *Cell* **2006**, *127*, 469–480. [CrossRef] [PubMed]
28. Polakis, P. The many ways of WNT in cancer. *Curr. Opin. Genet. Dev.* **2007**, *17*, 45–51. [CrossRef] [PubMed]
29. Taketo, M.M. Shutting down wnt signal-activated cancer. *Nat. Genet.* **2004**, *36*, 320–322. [CrossRef] [PubMed]
30. White, B.D.; Chien, A.J.; Dawson, D.W. Dysregulation of Wnt/β-catenin signaling in gastrointestinal cancers. *Gastroenterology* **2012**, *142*, 219–232. [CrossRef] [PubMed]
31. Krausova, M.; Korinek, V. Wnt signaling in adult intestinal stem cells and cancer. *Cell. Signal.* **2014**, *26*, 570–579. [CrossRef] [PubMed]
32. Satoh, S.; Daigo, Y.; Furukawa, Y.; Kato, T.; Miwa, N.; Nishiwaki, T.; Kawasoe, T.; Ishiguro, H.; Fujita, M.; Tokino, T.; et al. AXIN1 mutations in hepatocellular carcinomas, and growth suppression in cancer cells by virus-mediated transfer of AXIN1. *Nat. Genet.* **2000**, *24*, 245–250. [CrossRef] [PubMed]
33. Guan, C.N.; Chen, X.M.; Lou, H.Q.; Liao, X.H.; Chen, B.Y.; Zhang, P.W. Clinical significance of axin and beta-catenin protein expression in primary hepatocellular carcinomas. *Asian Pac. J. Cancer Prev.: APJCP* **2012**, *13*, 677–681. [CrossRef] [PubMed]
34. Ishizaki, Y.; Ikeda, S.; Fujimori, M.; Shimizu, Y.; Kurihara, T.; Itamoto, T.; Kikuchi, A.; Okajima, M.; Asahara, T. Immunohistochemical analysis and mutational analyses of beta-catenin, axin family and APC genes in hepatocellular carcinomas. *Int. J. Oncol.* **2004**, *24*, 1077–1083. [PubMed]
35. Clevers, H. Axin and hepatocellular carcinomas. *Nat. Genet.* **2000**, *24*, 206–208. [CrossRef] [PubMed]
36. Sherwood, V.; Leigh, I.M. WNT signaling in cutaneous squamous cell carcinoma: A future treatment strategy? *J. Investig. Dermatol.* **2016**, *136*, 1760–1767. [CrossRef] [PubMed]
37. Chan, E.F.; Gat, U.; McNiff, J.M.; Fuchs, E. A common human skin tumour is caused by activating mutations in beta-catenin. *Nat. Genet.* **1999**, *21*, 410–413. [PubMed]
38. Shulewitz, M.; Soloviev, I.; Wu, T.; Koeppen, H.; Polakis, P.; Sakanaka, C. Repressor roles for TCF-4 and SFRP1 in WNT signaling in breast cancer. *Oncogene* **2006**, *25*, 4361–4369. [CrossRef] [PubMed]
39. Schlange, T.; Matsuda, Y.; Lienhard, S.; Huber, A.; Hynes, N.E. Autocrine wnt signaling contributes to breast cancer cell proliferation via the canonical wnt pathway and EGFR transactivation. *Breast Cancer Res.: BCR* **2007**, *9*, R63. [CrossRef] [PubMed]
40. Lindvall, C.; Bu, W.; Williams, B.O.; Li, Y. Wnt signaling, stem cells, and the cellular origin of breast cancer. *Stem Cell Rev.* **2007**, *3*, 157–168. [CrossRef] [PubMed]
41. Yu, Q.C.; Verheyen, E.M.; Zeng, Y.A. Mammary development and breast cancer: A WNT perspective. *Cancers* **2016**, *8*. [CrossRef] [PubMed]

42. Davies, G.; Jiang, W.G.; Mason, M.D. The interaction between beta-catenin, GSK3β and APC after motogen induced cell-cell dissociation, and their involvement in signal transduction pathways in prostate cancer. *Int. J. Oncol.* **2001**, *18*, 843–847. [PubMed]
43. Hu, B.R.; Fairey, A.S.; Madhav, A.; Yang, D.; Li, M.; Groshen, S.; Stephens, C.; Kim, P.H.; Virk, N.; Wang, L.; et al. AXIN2 expression predicts prostate cancer recurrence and regulates invasion and tumor growth. *Prostate* **2016**, *76*, 597–608. [CrossRef] [PubMed]
44. Nusse, R.; Brown, A.; Papkoff, J.; Scambler, P.; Shackleford, G.; McMahon, A.; Moon, R.; Varmus, H. A new nomenclature for INT-1 and related genes: The Wnt gene family. *Cell* **1991**. [CrossRef] [PubMed]
45. Cabrera, C.V.; Alonso, M.C.; Johnston, P.; Phillips, R.G.; Lawrence, P.A. Phenocopies induced with antisense RNA identify the wingless gene. *Cell* **1987**, *50*, 659–663. [CrossRef]
46. Rijsewijk, F.; Schuermann, M.; Wagenaar, E.; Parren, P.; Weigel, D.; Nusse, R. The Drosophila homolog of the mouse mammary oncogene int-1 is identical to the segment polarity gene wingless. *Cell* **1987**, *50*, 649–657. [CrossRef]
47. Nusslein-Volhard, C.; Wieschaus, E. Mutations affecting segment number and polarity in drosophila. *Nature* **1980**, *287*, 795–801. [CrossRef] [PubMed]
48. Nusse, R.; Varmus, H.E. Many tumors induced by the mouse mammary tumor virus contain a provirus integrated in the same region of the host genome. *Cell* **1982**, *31*, 99–109. [CrossRef]
49. Vinson, C.R.; Conover, S.; Adler, P.N. A Drosophila tissue polarity locus encodes a protein containing seven potential transmembrane domains. *Nature* **1989**, *338*, 263–264. [CrossRef] [PubMed]
50. Tamai, K.; Semenov, M.; Kato, Y.; Spokony, R.; Liu, C.; Katsuyama, Y.; Hess, F.; Saint-Jeannet, J.P.; He, X. LDL-receptor-related proteins in WNT signal transduction. *Nature* **2000**, *407*, 530–535. [PubMed]
51. Wehrli, M.; Dougan, S.T.; Caldwell, K.; O'Keefe, L.; Schwartz, S.; Vaizel-Ohayon, D.; Schejter, E.; Tomlinson, A.; DiNardo, S. Arrow encodes an LDL-receptor-related protein essential for wingless signalling. *Nature* **2000**, *407*, 527–530. [PubMed]
52. Mikels, A.J.; Nusse, R. WNTs as ligands: Processing, secretion and reception. *Oncogene* **2006**, *25*, 7461–7468. [CrossRef] [PubMed]
53. Huang, H.; He, X. Wnt/β-catenin signaling: New (and old) players and new insights. *Curr. Opin. Cell Biol.* **2008**, *20*, 119–125. [CrossRef] [PubMed]
54. Liu, Y.; Rubin, B.; Bodine, P.V.; Billiard, J. WNT5A induces homodimerization and activation of ROR2 receptor tyrosine kinase. *Journal of cellular biochemistry* **2008**, *105*, 497–502. [CrossRef] [PubMed]
55. Carmon, K.S.; Gong, X.; Lin, Q.; Thomas, A.; Liu, Q. R-spondins function as ligands of the orphan receptors LGR4 and LGR5 to regulate wnt/β-catenin signaling. *Proc. Natl. Acad. Sci. USA* **2011**, *108*, 11452–11457. [CrossRef] [PubMed]
56. de Lau, W.; Barker, N.; Low, T.Y.; Koo, B.K.; Li, V.S.; Teunissen, H.; Kujala, P.; Haegebarth, A.; Peters, P.J.; van de Wetering, M.; et al. LGR5 homologues associate with wnt receptors and mediate R-spondin signalling. *Nature* **2011**, *476*, 293–297. [CrossRef] [PubMed]
57. Holland, J.D.; Klaus, A.; Garratt, A.N.; Birchmeier, W. Wnt signaling in stem and cancer stem cells. *Curr. Opin. Cell Biol.* **2013**, *25*, 254–264. [CrossRef] [PubMed]
58. Kuhl, M.; Geis, K.; Sheldahl, L.C.; Pukrop, T.; Moon, R.T.; Wedlich, D. Antagonistic regulation of convergent extension movements in xenopus by WNT/β-catenin and WNT/Ca2+ signaling. *Mech. Dev.* **2001**, *106*, 61–76. [CrossRef]
59. Oishi, I.; Suzuki, H.; Onishi, N.; Takada, R.; Kani, S.; Ohkawara, B.; Koshida, I.; Suzuki, K.; Yamada, G.; Schwabe, G.C.; et al. The receptor tyrosine kinase ROR2 is involved in non-canonical WNT5A/JNK signalling pathway. *Genes Cells: Devot. Mol. Cell. Mech.* **2003**, *8*, 645–654. [CrossRef]
60. Schambony, A.; Wedlich, D. Wnt-5a/ROR2 regulate expression of xpapc through an alternative noncanonical signaling pathway. *Dev. Cell* **2007**, *12*, 779–792. [CrossRef] [PubMed]
61. Kraus, C.; Liehr, T.; Hulsken, J.; Behrens, J.; Birchmeier, W.; Grzeschik, K.H.; Ballhausen, W.G. Localization of the human β-catenin gene (*CTNNB1*) to 3p21: A region implicated in tumor development. *Genomics* **1994**, *23*, 272–274. [CrossRef] [PubMed]
62. Huber, A.H.; Weis, W.I. The structure of the beta-catenin/e-cadherin complex and the molecular basis of diverse ligand recognition by β-catenin. *Cell* **2001**, *105*, 391–402. [CrossRef]
63. Willert, K.; Nusse, R. β-catenin: A key mediator of wnt signaling. *Curr. Opin. Genet. Dev.* **1998**, *8*, 95–102. [CrossRef]

64. Behrens, J.; von Kries, J.P.; Kuhl, M.; Bruhn, L.; Wedlich, D.; Grosschedl, R.; Birchmeier, W. Functional interaction of β-catenin with the transcription factor LEF-1. *Nature* **1996**, *382*, 638–642. [CrossRef] [PubMed]
65. Molenaar, M.; van de Wetering, M.; Oosterwegel, M.; Peterson-Maduro, J.; Godsave, S.; Korinek, V.; Roose, J.; Destree, O.; Clevers, H. XTCF-3 transcription factor mediates beta-catenin-induced axis formation in xenopus embryos. *Cell* **1996**, *86*, 391–399. [CrossRef]
66. Huber, O.; Korn, R.; McLaughlin, J.; Ohsugi, M.; Herrmann, B.G.; Kemler, R. Nuclear localization of beta-catenin by interaction with transcription factor LEF-1. *Mech. Dev.* **1996**, *59*, 3–10. [CrossRef]
67. Riese, J.; Yu, X.; Munnerlyn, A.; Eresh, S.; Hsu, S.C.; Grosschedl, R.; Bienz, M. LEF-1, a nuclear factor coordinating signaling inputs from wingless and decapentaplegic. *Cell* **1997**, *88*, 777–787. [CrossRef]
68. Kemler, R. From cadherins to catenins: Cytoplasmic protein interactions and regulation of cell adhesion. *Trends Genet.: TIG* **1993**, *9*, 317–321. [CrossRef]
69. Rimm, D.L.; Koslov, E.R.; Kebriaei, P.; Cianci, C.D.; Morrow, J.S. Alpha 1(E)-catenin is an actin-binding and -bundling protein mediating the attachment of F-actin to the membrane adhesion complex. *Proc. Natl. Acad. Sci. USA* **1995**, *92*, 8813–8817. [CrossRef] [PubMed]
70. Drees, F.; Pokutta, S.; Yamada, S.; Nelson, W.J.; Weis, W.I. Alpha-Catenin is a molecular switch that binds E-cadherin-β-catenin and regulates actin-filament assembly. *Cell* **2005**, *123*, 903–915. [CrossRef] [PubMed]
71. Yamada, S.; Pokutta, S.; Drees, F.; Weis, W.I.; Nelson, W.J. Deconstructing the cadherin-catenin-actin complex. *Cell* **2005**, *123*, 889–901. [CrossRef] [PubMed]
72. Meng, W.; Takeichi, M. Adherens junction: Molecular architecture and regulation. *Cold Spring Harb. Perspect. Biol.* **2009**, *1*, a002899. [CrossRef] [PubMed]
73. Barth, A.I.; Nathke, I.S.; Nelson, W.J. Cadherins, catenins and apc protein: Interplay between cytoskeletal complexes and signaling pathways. *Curr. Opin. Cell Biol.* **1997**, *9*, 683–690. [CrossRef]
74. Behrens, J.; Jerchow, B.A.; Wurtele, M.; Grimm, J.; Asbrand, C.; Wirtz, R.; Kuhl, M.; Wedlich, D.; Birchmeier, W. Functional interaction of an axin homolog, conductin, with β-catenin, APC, and GSK3beta. *Science* **1998**, *280*, 596–599. [CrossRef] [PubMed]
75. Salomon, D.; Sacco, P.A.; Roy, S.G.; Simcha, I.; Johnson, K.R.; Wheelock, M.J.; Ben-Ze'ev, A. Regulation of β-catenin levels and localization by overexpression of plakoglobin and inhibition of the ubiquitin-proteasome system. *J. Cell Biol.* **1997**, *139*, 1325–1335. [CrossRef] [PubMed]
76. Liu, C.; Li, Y.; Semenov, M.; Han, C.; Baeg, G.H.; Tan, Y.; Zhang, Z.; Lin, X.; He, X. Control of β-catenin phosphorylation/degradation by a dual-kinase mechanism. *Cell* **2002**, *108*, 837–847. [CrossRef]
77. Zeng, X.; Tamai, K.; Doble, B.; Li, S.; Huang, H.; Habas, R.; Okamura, H.; Woodgett, J.; He, X. A dual-kinase mechanism for WNT co-receptor phosphorylation and activation. *Nature* **2005**, *438*, 873–877. [CrossRef] [PubMed]
78. Aberle, H.; Bauer, A.; Stappert, J.; Kispert, A.; Kemler, R. Beta-Catenin is a target for the ubiquitin-proteasome pathway. *EMBO J.* **1997**, *16*, 3797–3804. [CrossRef] [PubMed]
79. Roose, J.; Molenaar, M.; Peterson, J.; Hurenkamp, J.; Brantjes, H.; Moerer, P.; van de Wetering, M.; Destree, O.; Clevers, H. The Xenopus Wnt effector XTCF-3 interacts with groucho-related transcriptional repressors. *Nature* **1998**, *395*, 608–612. [PubMed]
80. Davidson, G.; Wu, W.; Shen, J.; Bilic, J.; Fenger, U.; Stannek, P.; Glinka, A.; Niehrs, C. Casein kinase 1 gamma couples wnt receptor activation to cytoplasmic signal transduction. *Nature* **2005**, *438*, 867–872. [CrossRef] [PubMed]
81. Bilic, J.; Huang, Y.L.; Davidson, G.; Zimmermann, T.; Cruciat, C.M.; Bienz, M.; Niehrs, C. Wnt induces LRP6 signalosomes and promotes dishevelled-dependent LRP6 phosphorylation. *Science* **2007**, *316*, 1619–1622. [CrossRef] [PubMed]
82. Daniels, D.L.; Weis, W.I. Beta-catenin directly displaces groucho/TLE repressors from TCF/LEF in wnt-mediated transcription activation. *Nat. Struct. Mol. Biol.* **2005**, *12*, 364–371. [CrossRef] [PubMed]
83. Kramps, T.; Peter, O.; Brunner, E.; Nellen, D.; Froesch, B.; Chatterjee, S.; Murone, M.; Zullig, S.; Basler, K. Wnt/Wingless signaling requires BCL9/legless-mediated recruitment of pygopus to the nuclear beta-catenin-TCF complex. *Cell* **2002**, *109*, 47–60. [CrossRef]
84. Brembeck, F.H.; Schwarz-Romond, T.; Bakkers, J.; Wilhelm, S.; Hammerschmidt, M.; Birchmeier, W. Essential role of BCL9-2 in the switch between beta-catenin's adhesive and transcriptional functions. *Genes Dev.* **2004**, *18*, 2225–2230. [CrossRef] [PubMed]

85. De la Roche, M.; Bienz, M. Wingless-Independent association of pygopus with DTCF target genes. *Curr. Biol.: CB* **2007**, *17*, 556–561. [CrossRef] [PubMed]
86. Belenkaya, T.Y.; Han, C.; Standley, H.J.; Lin, X.; Houston, D.W.; Heasman, J. Pygopus encodes a nuclear protein essential for wingless/wnt signaling. *Development* **2002**, *129*, 4089–4101. [PubMed]
87. Hecht, A.; Vleminckx, K.; Stemmler, M.P.; van Roy, F.; Kemler, R. The P300/CBP acetyltransferases function as transcriptional coactivators of β-catenin in vertebrates. *EMBO J.* **2000**, *19*, 1839–1850. [CrossRef] [PubMed]
88. Wolf, D.; Rodova, M.; Miska, E.A.; Calvet, J.P.; Kouzarides, T. Acetylation of β-catenin by creb-binding protein (CBP). *J. Biol. Chem.* **2002**, *277*, 25562–25567. [CrossRef] [PubMed]
89. Mosimann, C.; Hausmann, G.; Basler, K. Parafibromin/hyrax activates wnt/wg target gene transcription by direct association with β-catenin/armadillo. *Cell* **2006**, *125*, 327–341. [CrossRef] [PubMed]
90. He, T.C.; Sparks, A.B.; Rago, C.; Hermeking, H.; Zawel, L.; da Costa, L.T.; Morin, P.J.; Vogelstein, B.; Kinzler, K.W. Identification of C-Myc as a target of the APC pathway. *Science* **1998**, *281*, 1509–1512. [CrossRef]
91. D'Amico, M.; Hulit, J.; Amanatullah, D.F.; Zafonte, B.T.; Albanese, C.; Bouzahzah, B.; Fu, M.; Augenlicht, L.H.; Donehower, L.A.; Takemaru, K.; et al. The integrin-linked kinase regulates the cyclin D1 gene through glycogen synthase kinase 3β and camp-responsive element-binding protein-dependent pathways. *J. Biol. Chem.* **2000**, *275*, 32649–32657. [CrossRef] [PubMed]
92. Shtutman, M.; Zhurinsky, J.; Simcha, I.; Albanese, C.; D'Amico, M.; Pestell, R.; Ben-Ze'ev, A. The cyclin d1 gene is a target of the β-catenin/LEF-1 pathway. *Proc. Natl. Acad. Sci. USA* **1999**, *96*, 5522–5527. [CrossRef] [PubMed]
93. Moreau, M.; Mourah, S.; Dosquet, C. Beta-Catenin and NF-KAPPAB cooperate to regulate the UPA/UPAR system in cancer cells. *Int. J. Cancer* **2011**, *128*, 1280–1292. [CrossRef] [PubMed]
94. Bisson, I.; Prowse, D.M. Wnt signaling regulates self-renewal and differentiation of prostate cancer cells with stem cell characteristics. *Cell Res.* **2009**, *19*, 683–697. [CrossRef] [PubMed]
95. Lu, W.; Tinsley, H.N.; Keeton, A.; Qu, Z.; Piazza, G.A.; Li, Y. Suppression of wnt/β-catenin signaling inhibits prostate cancer cell proliferation. *Eur. J. Pharmacol.* **2009**, *602*, 8–14. [CrossRef] [PubMed]
96. Lee, E.; Ha, S.; Logan, S.K. Divergent androgen receptor and beta-catenin signaling in prostate cancer cells. *PLoS ONE* **2015**, *10*, e0141589. [CrossRef] [PubMed]
97. Wan, X.; Liu, J.; Lu, J.F.; Tzelepi, V.; Yang, J.; Starbuck, M.W.; Diao, L.; Wang, J.; Efstathiou, E.; Vazquez, E.S.; et al. Activation of β-catenin signaling in androgen receptor-negative prostate cancer cells. *Clin. Cancer Res.: Off. J. Am. Assoc. Cancer Res.* **2012**, *18*, 726–736. [CrossRef] [PubMed]
98. Kazanskaya, O.; Glinka, A.; del Barco Barrantes, I.; Stannek, P.; Niehrs, C.; Wu, W. R-spondin2 is a secreted activator of wntβ-catenin signaling and is required for xenopus myogenesis. *Dev. Cell.* **2004**, *7*, 525–534. [CrossRef] [PubMed]
99. Barker, N.; van Es, J.H.; Kuipers, J.; Kujala, P.; van den Born, M.; Cozijnsen, M.; Haegebarth, A.; Korving, J.; Begthel, H.; Peters, P.J.; et al. Identification of stem cells in small intestine and colon by marker gene LGR5. *Nature* **2007**, *449*, 1003–1007. [CrossRef] [PubMed]
100. Haegebarth, A.; Clevers, H. Wnt signaling, LGR5, and stem cells in the intestine and skin. *Am. J. Pathol.* **2009**, *174*, 715–721. [CrossRef] [PubMed]
101. Grun, D.; Vaillant, M.; Pieri, V.; Diederich, N.J. Response to letter of the editor by tomoyuki kawada regarding the article "contributory factors to caregiver burden in parkinson disease" by grun et al. *J. Am. Med. Dir. Assoc.* **2016**, *17*, 1060–1061. [CrossRef] [PubMed]
102. De Lau, W.; Peng, W.C.; Gros, P.; Clevers, H. The r-spondin/LGR5/RNF43 module: Regulator of wnt signal strength. *Genes Dev.* **2014**, *28*, 305–316. [CrossRef] [PubMed]
103. Glinka, A.; Dolde, C.; Kirsch, N.; Huang, Y.L.; Kazanskaya, O.; Ingelfinger, D.; Boutros, M.; Cruciat, C.M.; Niehrs, C. LGR4 and LGR5 are R-spondin receptors mediating Wnt/β-catenin and Wnt/PCP signalling. *EMBO Rep.* **2011**, *12*, 1055–1061. [CrossRef] [PubMed]
104. Mii, Y.; Taira, M. Secreted wnt "inhibitors" are not just inhibitors: Regulation of extracellular Wnt by secreted frizzled-related proteins. *Dev. Growth Differ.* **2011**, *53*, 911–923. [CrossRef] [PubMed]
105. Bovolenta, P.; Esteve, P.; Ruiz, J.M.; Cisneros, E.; Lopez-Rios, J. Beyond Wnt inhibition: New functions of secreted frizzled-related proteins in development and disease. *J. Cell Sci.* **2008**, *121*, 737–746. [CrossRef] [PubMed]
106. Niehrs, C. Function and biological roles of the dickkopf family of wnt modulators. *Oncogene* **2006**, *25*, 7469–7481. [CrossRef] [PubMed]

107. Semenov, M.; Tamai, K.; He, X. Sost is a ligand for LRP5/LRP6 and a Wnt signaling inhibitor. *J. Biol. Chem.* **2005**, *280*, 26770–26775. [CrossRef] [PubMed]
108. Lintern, K.B.; Guidato, S.; Rowe, A.; Saldanha, J.W.; Itasaki, N. Characterization of wise protein and its molecular mechanism to interact with both Wnt and bmp signals. *J. Biol. Chem.* **2009**, *284*, 23159–23168. [CrossRef] [PubMed]
109. Herr, P.; Hausmann, G.; Basler, K. Wnt secretion and signalling in human disease. *Trends Mol. Med.* **2012**, *18*, 483–493. [CrossRef] [PubMed]
110. McEwen, D.G.; Peifer, M. Wnt signaling: Moving in a new direction. *Curr. Biol.: CB* **2000**, *10*, R562–R564. [CrossRef]
111. Veeman, M.T.; Axelrod, J.D.; Moon, R.T. A second canon. Functions and mechanisms of β-catenin-independent wnt signaling. *Dev. Cell* **2003**, *5*, 367–377. [CrossRef]
112. Sheldahl, L.C.; Slusarski, D.C.; Pandur, P.; Miller, J.R.; Kuhl, M.; Moon, R.T. Dishevelled activates Ca2+ FLUX, PKC, and CAMKII in vertebrate embryos. *J. Cell Biol.* **2003**, *161*, 769–777. [CrossRef] [PubMed]
113. Kohn, A.D.; Moon, R.T. Wnt and calcium signaling: β-catenin-independent pathways. *Cell Calcium* **2005**, *38*, 439–446. [CrossRef] [PubMed]
114. Ishitani, T.; Kishida, S.; Hyodo-Miura, J.; Ueno, N.; Yasuda, J.; Waterman, M.; Shibuya, H.; Moon, R.T.; Ninomiya-Tsuji, J.; Matsumoto, K. The TAK1-NLK mitogen-activated protein kinase cascade functions in the wnt-5a/Ca(2+) pathway to antagonize wnt/β-catenin signaling. *Mol. Cell. Biol.* **2003**, *23*, 131–139. [CrossRef] [PubMed]
115. Rao, T.P.; Kuhl, M. An updated overview on wnt signaling pathways: A prelude for more. *Circ. Res.* **2010**, *106*, 1798–1806. [CrossRef] [PubMed]
116. Hogan, P.G.; Chen, L.; Nardone, J.; Rao, A. Transcriptional regulation by calcium, calcineurin, and NFAT. *Genes Dev.* **2003**, *17*, 2205–2232. [CrossRef] [PubMed]
117. Feske, S.; Okamura, H.; Hogan, P.G.; Rao, A. Ca2+/calcineurin signalling in cells of the immune system. *Biochem. Biophys. Res. Commun.* **2003**, *311*, 1117–1132. [CrossRef] [PubMed]
118. Manda, K.R.; Tripathi, P.; Hsi, A.C.; Ning, J.; Ruzinova, M.B.; Liapis, H.; Bailey, M.; Zhang, H.; Maher, C.A.; Humphrey, P.A.; et al. NFATC1 promotes prostate tumorigenesis and overcomes pten loss-induced senescence. *Oncogene* **2016**, *35*, 3282–3292. [CrossRef] [PubMed]
119. Bengoa-Vergniory, N.; Kypta, R.M. Canonical and noncanonical wnt signaling in neural stem/progenitor cells. *Cell. Mol. Life Sci.: CMLS* **2015**, *72*, 4157–4172. [CrossRef] [PubMed]
120. Acebron, S.P.; Karaulanov, E.; Berger, B.S.; Huang, Y.L.; Niehrs, C. Mitotic wnt signaling promotes protein stabilization and regulates cell size. *Mol. Cell* **2014**, *54*, 663–674. [CrossRef] [PubMed]
121. Gomez-Orte, E.; Saenz-Narciso, B.; Moreno, S.; Cabello, J. Multiple functions of the noncanonical wnt pathway. *Trends Genet.: TIG* **2013**, *29*, 545–553. [CrossRef] [PubMed]
122. Weidinger, G.; Moon, R.T. When wnts antagonize wnts. *J. Cell Biol.* **2003**, *162*, 753–755. [CrossRef] [PubMed]
123. Timms, B.G. Prostate development: A historical perspective. *Differ. Res. Biol. Divers.* **2008**, *76*, 565–577. [CrossRef] [PubMed]
124. Shen, M.M.; Abate-Shen, C. Molecular genetics of prostate cancer: New prospects for old challenges. *Genes Dev.* **2010**, *24*, 1967–2000. [CrossRef] [PubMed]
125. Sugimura, Y.; Cunha, G.R.; Donjacour, A.A. Morphogenesis of ductal networks in the mouse prostate. *Biol. Reprod.* **1986**, *34*, 961–971. [CrossRef] [PubMed]
126. Peng, Y.C.; Joyner, A.L. Hedgehog signaling in prostate epithelial-mesenchymal growth regulation. *Dev. Biol.* **2015**, *400*, 94–104. [CrossRef] [PubMed]
127. Abate-Shen, C.; Shen, M.M. Molecular genetics of prostate cancer. *Genes Dev.* **2000**, *14*, 2410–2434. [CrossRef] [PubMed]
128. Staack, A.; Donjacour, A.A.; Brody, J.; Cunha, G.R.; Carroll, P. Mouse urogenital development: A practical approach. *Differ. Res. Biol. Divers.* **2003**, *71*, 402–413. [CrossRef] [PubMed]
129. Takeda, H.; Nakamoto, T.; Kokontis, J.; Chodak, G.W.; Chang, C. Autoregulation of androgen receptor expression in rodent prostate: Immunohistochemical and in situ hybridization analysis. *Biochem. Biophys. Res. Commun.* **1991**, *177*, 488–496. [CrossRef]
130. Cooke, P.S.; Young, P.; Cunha, G.R. Androgen receptor expression in developing male reproductive organs. *Endocrinology* **1991**, *128*, 2867–2873. [CrossRef] [PubMed]

131. Cunha, G.R.; Ricke, W.; Thomson, A.; Marker, P.C.; Risbridger, G.; Hayward, S.W.; Wang, Y.Z.; Donjacour, A.A.; Kurita, T. Hormonal, cellular, and molecular regulation of normal and neoplastic prostatic development. *J. Steroid Biochem. Mol. Biol.* **2004**, *92*, 221–236. [CrossRef] [PubMed]
132. Cunha, G.R. The role of androgens in the epithelio-mesenchymal interactions involved in prostatic morphogenesis in embryonic mice. *Anat. Rec.* **1973**, *175*, 87–96. [CrossRef] [PubMed]
133. Cunha, G.R.; Donjacour, A.A.; Cooke, P.S.; Mee, S.; Bigsby, R.M.; Higgins, S.J.; Sugimura, Y. The endocrinology and developmental biology of the prostate. *Endocr. Rev.* **1987**, *8*, 338–362. [CrossRef] [PubMed]
134. Cunha, G.R. Mesenchymal-Epithelial interactions: Past, present, and future. *Differ. Res. Biol. Divers.* **2008**, *76*, 578–586. [CrossRef] [PubMed]
135. Marker, P.C.; Donjacour, A.A.; Dahiya, R.; Cunha, G.R. Hormonal, cellular, and molecular control of prostatic development. *Dev. Biol.* **2003**, *253*, 165–174. [CrossRef]
136. Mehta, V.; Abler, L.L.; Keil, K.P.; Schmitz, C.T.; Joshi, P.S.; Vezina, C.M. Atlas of wnt and R-spondin gene expression in the developing male mouse lower urogenital tract. *Dev. Dyn.: Off. Publ. Am. Assoc. Anat.* **2011**, *240*, 2548–2560. [CrossRef] [PubMed]
137. Wang, Y.; Hayward, S.; Cao, M.; Thayer, K.; Cunha, G. Cell differentiation lineage in the prostate. *Differ. Res. Biol. Divers.* **2001**, *68*, 270–279. [CrossRef]
138. Hayward, S.W.; Baskin, L.S.; Haughney, P.C.; Cunha, A.R.; Foster, B.A.; Dahiya, R.; Prins, G.S.; Cunha, G.R. Epithelial development in the rat ventral prostate, anterior prostate and seminal vesicle. *Acta Anat.* **1996**, *155*, 81–93. [CrossRef] [PubMed]
139. Rittenhouse, H.G.; Finlay, J.A.; Mikolajczyk, S.D.; Partin, A.W. Human kallikrein 2 (HK2) and prostate-specific antigen (PSA): Two closely related, but distinct, kallikreins in the prostate. *Crit. Rev. Clin. Lab. Sci.* **1998**, *35*, 275–368. [CrossRef] [PubMed]
140. Muniyan, S.; Chaturvedi, N.K.; Dwyer, J.G.; Lagrange, C.A.; Chaney, W.G.; Lin, M.F. Human prostatic acid phosphatase: Structure, function and regulation. *Int. J. Mol. Sci.* **2013**, *14*, 10438–10464. [CrossRef] [PubMed]
141. Xue, Y.; van der Laak, J.; Smedts, F.; Schoots, C.; Verhofstad, A.; de la Rosette, J.; Schalken, J. Neuroendocrine cells during human prostate development: Does neuroendocrine cell density remain constant during fetal as well as postnatal life? *Prostate* **2000**, *42*, 116–123. [CrossRef]
142. Cohen, R.J.; Glezerson, G.; Taylor, L.F.; Grundle, H.A.; Naude, J.H. The neuroendocrine cell population of the human prostate gland. *J. Urol.* **1993**, *150*, 365–368. [PubMed]
143. Van Leenders, G.; Dijkman, H.; Hulsbergen-van de Kaa, C.; Ruiter, D.; Schalken, J. Demonstration of intermediate cells during human prostate epithelial differentiation in situ and in vitro using triple-staining confocal scanning microscopy. *Lab. Investig. J. Tech. Methods Pathol.* **2000**, *80*, 1251–1258. [CrossRef]
144. Uzgare, A.R.; Isaacs, J.T. Enhanced redundancy in AKT and mitogen-activated protein kinase-induced survival of malignant versus normal prostate epithelial cells. *Cancer Res.* **2004**, *64*, 6190–6199. [CrossRef] [PubMed]
145. Xin, L.; Lukacs, R.U.; Lawson, D.A.; Cheng, D.; Witte, O.N. Self-renewal and multilineage differentiation in vitro from murine prostate stem cells. *Stem Cells* **2007**, *25*, 2760–2769. [CrossRef] [PubMed]
146. Kwon, O.J.; Xin, L. Prostate epithelial stem and progenitor cells. *Am. J. Clin. Exp. Urol.* **2014**, *2*, 209–218. [PubMed]
147. Prins, G.S.; Putz, O. Molecular signaling pathways that regulate prostate gland development. *Differ. Res. Biol. Divers.* **2008**, *76*, 641–659. [CrossRef] [PubMed]
148. Zhang, T.J.; Hoffman, B.G.; Ruiz de Algara, T.; Helgason, C.D. Sage reveals expression of wnt signalling pathway members during mouse prostate development. *Gene Exp. Patterns: GEP* **2006**, *6*, 310–324. [CrossRef] [PubMed]
149. Pritchard, C.C.; Nelson, P.S. Gene expression profiling in the developing prostate. *Differ. Res. Biol. Divers.* **2008**, *76*, 624–640. [CrossRef] [PubMed]
150. Joesting, M.S.; Cheever, T.R.; Volzing, K.G.; Yamaguchi, T.P.; Wolf, V.; Naf, D.; Rubin, J.S.; Marker, P.C. Secreted frizzled related protein 1 is a paracrine modulator of epithelial branching morphogenesis, proliferation, and secretory gene expression in the prostate. *Dev. Biol.* **2008**, *317*, 161–173. [CrossRef] [PubMed]
151. Wang, B.E.; Wang, X.D.; Ernst, J.A.; Polakis, P.; Gao, W.Q. Regulation of epithelial branching morphogenesis and cancer cell growth of the prostate by wnt signaling. *PLoS ONE* **2008**, *3*, e2186. [CrossRef] [PubMed]

152. Huang, L.; Pu, Y.; Hu, W.Y.; Birch, L.; Luccio-Camelo, D.; Yamaguchi, T.; Prins, G.S. The role of Wnt5a in prostate gland development. *Dev. Biol.* **2009**, *328*, 188–199. [CrossRef] [PubMed]
153. Allgeier, S.H.; Lin, T.M.; Vezina, C.M.; Moore, R.W.; Fritz, W.A.; Chiu, S.Y.; Zhang, C.; Peterson, R.E. Wnt5a selectively inhibits mouse ventral prostate development. *Dev. Biol.* **2008**, *324*, 10–17. [CrossRef] [PubMed]
154. Gat, U.; DasGupta, R.; Degenstein, L.; Fuchs, E. De novo hair follicle morphogenesis and hair tumors in mice expressing a truncated beta-catenin in skin. *Cell* **1998**, *95*, 605–614. [CrossRef]
155. Hatsell, S.; Rowlands, T.; Hiremath, M.; Cowin, P. β-Catenin and TCFS in mammary development and cancer. *J. Mammary Gland Biol. Neoplasia* **2003**, *8*, 145–158. [CrossRef] [PubMed]
156. Liu, F.; Chu, E.Y.; Watt, B.; Zhang, Y.; Gallant, N.M.; Andl, T.; Yang, S.H.; Lu, M.M.; Piccolo, S.; Schmidt-Ullrich, R.; et al. Wnt/β-Catenin signaling directs multiple stages of tooth morphogenesis. *Dev. Biol.* **2008**, *313*, 210–224. [CrossRef] [PubMed]
157. Yu, X.; Wang, Y.; Jiang, M.; Bierie, B.; Roy-Burman, P.; Shen, M.M.; Taketo, M.M.; Wills, M.; Matusik, R.J. Activation of β-catenin in mouse prostate causes hgpin and continuous prostate growth after castration. *Prostate* **2009**, *69*, 249–262. [CrossRef] [PubMed]
158. Simons, B.W.; Hurley, P.J.; Huang, Z.; Ross, A.E.; Miller, R.; Marchionni, L.; Berman, D.M.; Schaeffer, E.M. Wnt signaling though β-catenin is required for prostate lineage specification. *Dev. Biol.* **2012**, *371*, 246–255. [CrossRef] [PubMed]
159. English, H.F.; Santen, R.J.; Isaacs, J.T. Response of glandular versus basal rat ventral prostatic epithelial cells to androgen withdrawal and replacement. *Prostate* **1987**, *11*, 229–242. [CrossRef] [PubMed]
160. Xin, L.; Ide, H.; Kim, Y.; Dubey, P.; Witte, O.N. In vivo regeneration of murine prostate from dissociated cell populations of postnatal epithelia and urogenital sinus mesenchyme. *Proc. Natl. Acad. Sci. USA* **2003**, *100*, 11896–11903. [CrossRef] [PubMed]
161. Garraway, I.P.; Sun, W.; Tran, C.P.; Perner, S.; Zhang, B.; Goldstein, A.S.; Hahm, S.A.; Haider, M.; Head, C.S.; Reiter, R.E.; et al. Human prostate sphere-forming cells represent a subset of basal epithelial cells capable of glandular regeneration in vivo. *Prostate* **2010**, *70*, 491–501. [CrossRef] [PubMed]
162. Lawson, D.A.; Zong, Y.; Memarzadeh, S.; Xin, L.; Huang, J.; Witte, O.N. Basal epithelial stem cells are efficient targets for prostate cancer initiation. *Proc. Natl. Acad. Sci. USA* **2010**, *107*, 2610–2615. [CrossRef] [PubMed]
163. Xin, L.; Lawson, D.A.; Witte, O.N. The Sca-1 cell surface marker enriches for a prostate-regenerating cell subpopulation that can initiate prostate tumorigenesis. *Proc. Natl. Acad. Sci. USA* **2005**, *102*, 6942–6947. [CrossRef] [PubMed]
164. Burger, P.E.; Xiong, X.; Coetzee, S.; Salm, S.N.; Moscatelli, D.; Goto, K.; Wilson, E.L. Sca-1 expression identifies stem cells in the proximal region of prostatic ducts with high capacity to reconstitute prostatic tissue. *Proc. Natl. Acad. Sci. USA* **2005**, *102*, 7180–7185. [CrossRef] [PubMed]
165. Goldstein, A.S.; Lawson, D.A.; Cheng, D.; Sun, W.; Garraway, I.P.; Witte, O.N. Trop2 identifies a subpopulation of murine and human prostate basal cells with stem cell characteristics. *Proc. Natl. Acad. Sci. USA* **2008**, *105*, 20882–20887. [CrossRef] [PubMed]
166. Lawson, D.A.; Xin, L.; Lukacs, R.U.; Cheng, D.; Witte, O.N. Isolation and functional characterization of murine prostate stem cells. *Proc. Natl. Acad. Sci. USA* **2007**, *104*, 181–186. [CrossRef] [PubMed]
167. Jiao, J.; Hindoyan, A.; Wang, S.; Tran, L.M.; Goldstein, A.S.; Lawson, D.; Chen, D.; Li, Y.; Guo, C.; Zhang, B.; et al. Identification of CD166 as a surface marker for enriching prostate stem/progenitor and cancer initiating cells. *PLoS ONE* **2012**, *7*, e42564. [CrossRef] [PubMed]
168. Richardson, G.D.; Robson, C.N.; Lang, S.H.; Neal, D.E.; Maitland, N.J.; Collins, A.T. Cd133, a novel marker for human prostatic epithelial stem cells. *J. Cell Sci.* **2004**, *117*, 3539–3545. [CrossRef] [PubMed]
169. Leong, K.G.; Wang, B.E.; Johnson, L.; Gao, W.Q. Generation of a prostate from a single adult stem cell. *Nature* **2008**, *456*, 804–808. [CrossRef] [PubMed]
170. Wang, X.; Kruithof-de Julio, M.; Economides, K.D.; Walker, D.; Yu, H.; Halili, M.V.; Hu, Y.P.; Price, S.M.; Abate-Shen, C.; Shen, M.M. A luminal epithelial stem cell that is a cell of origin for prostate cancer. *Nature* **2009**, *461*, 495–500. [CrossRef] [PubMed]
171. Wang, Z.A.; Shen, M.M. Revisiting the concept of cancer stem cells in prostate cancer. *Oncogene* **2011**, *30*, 1261–1271. [CrossRef] [PubMed]
172. Drost, J.; Karthaus, W.R.; Gao, D.; Driehuis, E.; Sawyers, C.L.; Chen, Y.; Clevers, H. Organoid culture systems for prostate epithelial and cancer tissue. *Nat. Protocols* **2016**, *11*, 347–358. [CrossRef] [PubMed]

173. Karthaus, W.R.; Iaquinta, P.J.; Drost, J.; Gracanin, A.; van Boxtel, R.; Wongvipat, J.; Dowling, C.M.; Gao, D.; Begthel, H.; Sachs, N.; et al. Identification of multipotent luminal progenitor cells in human prostate organoid cultures. *Cell* **2014**, *159*, 163–175. [CrossRef] [PubMed]
174. Blum, R.; Gupta, R.; Burger, P.E.; Ontiveros, C.S.; Salm, S.N.; Xiong, X.; Kamb, A.; Wesche, H.; Marshall, L.; Cutler, G.; et al. Molecular signatures of prostate stem cells reveal novel signaling pathways and provide insights into prostate cancer. *PLoS ONE* **2009**, *4*, e5722. [CrossRef] [PubMed]
175. Blum, R.; Gupta, R.; Burger, P.E.; Ontiveros, C.S.; Salm, S.N.; Xiong, X.; Kamb, A.; Wesche, H.; Marshall, L.; Cutler, G.; et al. Molecular signatures of the primitive prostate stem cell niche reveal novel mesenchymal-epithelial signaling pathways. *PLoS ONE* **2010**, *5*, e13024. [CrossRef] [PubMed]
176. Nikolova, T.; Wu, M.; Brumbarov, K.; Alt, R.; Opitz, H.; Boheler, K.R.; Cross, M.; Wobus, A.M. Wnt-conditioned media differentially affect the proliferation and differentiation of cord blood-derived CD133+ cells in vitro. *Differ. Res. Biol. Divers.* **2007**, *75*, 100–111. [CrossRef] [PubMed]
177. Singla, D.K.; Schneider, D.J.; LeWinter, M.M.; Sobel, B.E. Wnt3a but not wnt11 supports self-renewal of embryonic stem cells. *Biochem. Biophys. Res. Commun.* **2006**, *345*, 789–795. [CrossRef] [PubMed]
178. Lukacs, R.U.; Memarzadeh, S.; Wu, H.; Witte, O.N. BMI-1 is a crucial regulator of prostate stem cell self-renewal and malignant transformation. *Cell Stem Cell* **2010**, *7*, 682–693. [CrossRef] [PubMed]
179. Heinlein, C.A.; Chang, C. Androgen receptor in prostate cancer. *Endocr. Rev.* **2004**, *25*, 276–308. [CrossRef] [PubMed]
180. Heinlein, C.A.; Chang, C. Androgen receptor (AR) coregulators: An overview. *Endocr. Rev.* **2002**, *23*, 175–200. [CrossRef] [PubMed]
181. Jenster, G.; van der Korput, H.A.; van Vroonhoven, C.; van der Kwast, T.H.; Trapman, J.; Brinkmann, A.O. Domains of the human androgen receptor involved in steroid binding, transcriptional activation, and subcellular localization. *Mol. Endocrinol.* **1991**, *5*, 1396–1404. [CrossRef] [PubMed]
182. MacLean, H.E.; Warne, G.L.; Zajac, J.D. Localization of functional domains in the androgen receptor. *J. Steroid Biochem. Mol. Biol.* **1997**, *62*, 233–242. [CrossRef]
183. Ferraldeschi, R.; Welti, J.; Luo, J.; Attard, G.; de Bono, J.S. Targeting the androgen receptor pathway in castration-resistant prostate cancer: Progresses and prospects. *Oncogene* **2015**, *34*, 1745–1757. [CrossRef] [PubMed]
184. Helsen, C.; Kerkhofs, S.; Clinckemalie, L.; Spans, L.; Laurent, M.; Boonen, S.; Vanderschueren, D.; Claessens, F. Structural basis for nuclear hormone receptor DNA binding. *Mol. Cell. Endocrinol.* **2012**, *348*, 411–417. [CrossRef] [PubMed]
185. Clinckemalie, L.; Vanderschueren, D.; Boonen, S.; Claessens, F. The hinge region in androgen receptor control. *Mol. Cell. Endocrinol.* **2012**, *358*, 1–8. [CrossRef] [PubMed]
186. Dittmar, K.D.; Banach, M.; Galigniana, M.D.; Pratt, W.B. The role of DNAJ-like proteins in glucocorticoid receptor.HSP90 heterocomplex assembly by the reconstituted HSP90.P60.Hsp70 foldosome complex. *J. Biol. Chem.* **1998**, *273*, 7358–7366. [CrossRef] [PubMed]
187. Prescott, J.; Coetzee, G.A. Molecular chaperones throughout the life cycle of the androgen receptor. *Cancer Lett.* **2006**, *231*, 12–19. [CrossRef] [PubMed]
188. Chmelar, R.; Buchanan, G.; Need, E.F.; Tilley, W.; Greenberg, N.M. Androgen receptor coregulators and their involvement in the development and progression of prostate cancer. *Int. J. Cancer* **2007**, *120*, 719–733. [CrossRef] [PubMed]
189. Roy, A.K.; Lavrovsky, Y.; Song, C.S.; Chen, S.; Jung, M.H.; Velu, N.K.; Bi, B.Y.; Chatterjee, B. Regulation of androgen action. *Vitam. Horm.* **1999**, *55*, 309–352. [PubMed]
190. Lee, D.K.; Chang, C. Molecular communication between androgen receptor and general transcription machinery. *J. Steroid Biochem. Mol. Biol.* **2003**, *84*, 41–49. [CrossRef]
191. Lee, D.K.; Chang, C. Endocrine mechanisms of disease: Expression and degradation of androgen receptor: Mechanism and clinical implication. *J. Clin. Endocrinol. Metab.* **2003**, *88*, 4043–4054. [CrossRef] [PubMed]
192. Simental, J.A.; Sar, M.; Lane, M.V.; French, F.S.; Wilson, E.M. Transcriptional activation and nuclear targeting signals of the human androgen receptor. *J. Biol. Chem.* **1991**, *266*, 510–518. [PubMed]
193. Zhou, Z.X.; Sar, M.; Simental, J.A.; Lane, M.V.; Wilson, E.M. A ligand-dependent bipartite nuclear targeting signal in the human androgen receptor. Requirement for the DNA-binding domain and modulation by NH2-terminal and carboxyl-terminal sequences. *J. Biol. Chem.* **1994**, *269*, 13115–13123. [PubMed]

194. Gelmann, E.P. Molecular biology of the androgen receptor. *J. Clin. Oncol.: Off. J. Am. Soc. Clin. Oncol.* **2002**, *20*, 3001–3015. [CrossRef] [PubMed]
195. He, B.; Lee, L.W.; Minges, J.T.; Wilson, E.M. Dependence of selective gene activation on the androgen receptor NH2- and COOH-terminal interaction. *J. Biol. Chem.* **2002**, *277*, 25631–25639. [CrossRef] [PubMed]
196. Bennett, N.C.; Gardiner, R.A.; Hooper, J.D.; Johnson, D.W.; Gobe, G.C. Molecular cell biology of androgen receptor signalling. *Int. J. Biochem. Cell Biol.* **2010**, *42*, 813–827. [CrossRef] [PubMed]
197. Gioeli, D.; Ficarro, S.B.; Kwiek, J.J.; Aaronson, D.; Hancock, M.; Catling, A.D.; White, F.M.; Christian, R.E.; Settlage, R.E.; Shabanowitz, J.; et al. Androgen receptor phosphorylation. Regulation and identification of the phosphorylation sites. *J. Biol. Chem.* **2002**, *277*, 29304–29314. [CrossRef] [PubMed]
198. Blok, L.J.; de Ruiter, P.E.; Brinkmann, A.O. Forskolin-Induced dephosphorylation of the androgen receptor impairs ligand binding. *Biochemistry* **1998**, *37*, 3850–3857. [CrossRef] [PubMed]
199. Gaughan, L.; Logan, I.R.; Neal, D.E.; Robson, C.N. Regulation of androgen receptor and histone deacetylase 1 by MDM2-mediated ubiquitylation. *Nucleic Acids Res.* **2005**, *33*, 13–26. [CrossRef] [PubMed]
200. Xu, L.L.; Shi, Y.; Petrovics, G.; Sun, C.; Makarem, M.; Zhang, W.; Sesterhenn, I.A.; McLeod, D.G.; Sun, L.; Moul, J.W.; et al. PMEPA1, an androgen-regulated NEDD4-binding protein, exhibits cell growth inhibitory function and decreased expression during prostate cancer progression. *Cancer Res.* **2003**, *63*, 4299–4304. [PubMed]
201. Richter, E.; Srivastava, S.; Dobi, A. Androgen receptor and prostate cancer. *Prostate Cancer Prostatic Dis.* **2007**, *10*, 114–118. [CrossRef] [PubMed]
202. Terry, S.; Yang, X.; Chen, M.W.; Vacherot, F.; Buttyan, R. Multifaceted interaction between the androgen and wnt signaling pathways and the implication for prostate cancer. *J. Cell. Biochem.* **2006**, *99*, 402–410. [CrossRef] [PubMed]
203. Brinkmann, A.O.; Blok, L.J.; de Ruiter, P.E.; Doesburg, P.; Steketee, K.; Berrevoets, C.A.; Trapman, J. Mechanisms of androgen receptor activation and function. *J. Steroid Biochem. Mol. Biol.* **1999**, *69*, 307–313. [CrossRef]
204. Tomlins, S.A.; Rhodes, D.R.; Perner, S.; Dhanasekaran, S.M.; Mehra, R.; Sun, X.W.; Varambally, S.; Cao, X.; Tchinda, J.; Kuefer, R.; et al. Recurrent fusion of TMPRSS2 and ETS transcription factor genes in prostate cancer. *Science* **2005**, *310*, 644–648. [CrossRef] [PubMed]
205. Iljin, K.; Wolf, M.; Edgren, H.; Gupta, S.; Kilpinen, S.; Skotheim, R.I.; Peltola, M.; Smit, F.; Verhaegh, G.; Schalken, J.; et al. TMPRSS2 fusions with oncogenic ETS factors in prostate cancer involve unbalanced genomic rearrangements and are associated with HDAC1 and epigenetic reprogramming. *Cancer Res.* **2006**, *66*, 10242–10246. [CrossRef] [PubMed]
206. Yu, J.; Mani, R.S.; Cao, Q.; Brenner, C.J.; Cao, X.; Wang, X.; Wu, L.; Li, J.; Hu, M.; Gong, Y.; et al. An integrated network of androgen receptor, polycomb, and TMPRSS2-ERG gene fusions in prostate cancer progression. *Cancer Cell* **2010**, *17*, 443–454. [CrossRef] [PubMed]
207. Baena, E.; Shao, Z.; Linn, D.E.; Glass, K.; Hamblen, M.J.; Fujiwara, Y.; Kim, J.; Nguyen, M.; Zhang, X.; Godinho, F.J.; et al. ETV1 directs androgen metabolism and confers aggressive prostate cancer in targeted mice and patients. *Genes Dev.* **2013**, *27*, 683–698. [CrossRef] [PubMed]
208. Kyprianou, N.; Isaacs, J.T. Activation of programmed cell death in the rat ventral prostate after castration. *Endocrinology* **1988**, *122*, 552–562. [CrossRef] [PubMed]
209. Prins, G.S.; Birch, L. Immunocytochemical analysis of androgen receptor along the ducts of the separate rat prostate lobes after androgen withdrawal and replacement. *Endocrinology* **1993**, *132*, 169–178. [PubMed]
210. Kim, D.; Gregory, C.W.; French, F.S.; Smith, G.J.; Mohler, J.L. Androgen receptor expression and cellular proliferation during transition from androgen-dependent to recurrent growth after castration in the cwr22 prostate cancer xenograft. *Am. J. Pathol.* **2002**, *160*, 219–226. [CrossRef]
211. Titus, M.A.; Schell, M.J.; Lih, F.B.; Tomer, K.B.; Mohler, J.L. Testosterone and dihydrotestosterone tissue levels in recurrent prostate cancer. *Clin. Cancer Res.: Off. J. Am. Assoc. Cancer Res.* **2005**, *11*, 4653–4657. [CrossRef]
212. Stanbrough, M.; Bubley, G.J.; Ross, K.; Golub, T.R.; Rubin, M.A.; Penning, T.M.; Febbo, P.G.; Balk, S.P. Increased expression of genes converting adrenal androgens to testosterone in androgen-independent prostate cancer. *Cancer Res.* **2006**, *66*, 2815–2825. [CrossRef] [PubMed]
213. Locke, J.A.; Guns, E.S.; Lubik, A.A.; Adomat, H.H.; Hendy, S.C.; Wood, C.A.; Ettinger, S.L.; Gleave, M.E.; Nelson, C.C. Androgen levels increase by intratumoral de novo steroidogenesis during progression of castration-resistant prostate cancer. *Cancer Res.* **2008**, *68*, 6407–6415. [CrossRef] [PubMed]

214. Montgomery, R.L.; Potthoff, M.J.; Haberland, M.; Qi, X.; Matsuzaki, S.; Humphries, K.M.; Richardson, J.A.; Bassel-Duby, R.; Olson, E.N. Maintenance of cardiac energy metabolism by histone deacetylase 3 in mice. *J. Clin. Investig.* **2008**, *118*, 3588–3597. [CrossRef] [PubMed]
215. Bubendorf, L.; Kononen, J.; Koivisto, P.; Schraml, P.; Moch, H.; Gasser, T.C.; Willi, N.; Mihatsch, M.J.; Sauter, G.; Kallioniemi, O.P. Survey of gene amplifications during prostate cancer progression by high-throughout fluorescence in situ hybridization on tissue microarrays. *Cancer Res.* **1999**, *59*, 803–806. [PubMed]
216. Haapala, K.; Kuukasjarvi, T.; Hyytinen, E.; Rantala, I.; Helin, H.J.; Koivisto, P.A. Androgen receptor amplification is associated with increased cell proliferation in prostate cancer. *Hum. Pathol.* **2007**, *38*, 474–478. [CrossRef] [PubMed]
217. Linja, M.J.; Savinainen, K.J.; Saramaki, O.R.; Tammela, T.L.; Vessella, R.L.; Visakorpi, T. Amplification and overexpression of androgen receptor gene in hormone-refractory prostate cancer. *Cancer Res.* **2001**, *61*, 3550–3555. [PubMed]
218. Taylor, B.S.; Schultz, N.; Hieronymus, H.; Gopalan, A.; Xiao, Y.; Carver, B.S.; Arora, V.K.; Kaushik, P.; Cerami, E.; Reva, B.; et al. Integrative genomic profiling of human prostate cancer. *Cancer Cell* **2010**, *18*, 11–22. [CrossRef] [PubMed]
219. Visakorpi, T.; Hyytinen, E.; Koivisto, P.; Tanner, M.; Keinanen, R.; Palmberg, C.; Palotie, A.; Tammela, T.; Isola, J.; Kallioniemi, O.P. In vivo amplification of the androgen receptor gene and progression of human prostate cancer. *Nat. Genet.* **1995**, *9*, 401–406. [CrossRef] [PubMed]
220. Koivisto, P.; Kononen, J.; Palmberg, C.; Tammela, T.; Hyytinen, E.; Isola, J.; Trapman, J.; Cleutjens, K.; Noordzij, A.; Visakorpi, T.; et al. Androgen receptor gene amplification: A possible molecular mechanism for androgen deprivation therapy failure in prostate cancer. *Cancer Res.* **1997**, *57*, 314–319. [PubMed]
221. Miyoshi, Y.; Uemura, H.; Fujinami, K.; Mikata, K.; Harada, M.; Kitamura, H.; Koizumi, Y.; Kubota, Y. Fluorescence in situ hybridization evaluation of C-Myc and androgen receptor gene amplification and chromosomal anomalies in prostate cancer in japanese patients. *Prostate* **2000**, *43*, 225–232. [CrossRef]
222. Robinson, D.; Van Allen, E.M.; Wu, Y.M.; Schultz, N.; Lonigro, R.J.; Mosquera, J.M.; Montgomery, B.; Taplin, M.E.; Pritchard, C.C.; Attard, G.; et al. Integrative clinical genomics of advanced prostate cancer. *Cell* **2015**, *161*, 1215–1228. [CrossRef] [PubMed]
223. Watson, P.A.; Chen, Y.F.; Balbas, M.D.; Wongvipat, J.; Socci, N.D.; Viale, A.; Kim, K.; Sawyers, C.L. Constitutively active androgen receptor splice variants expressed in castration-resistant prostate cancer require full-length androgen receptor. *Proc. Natl. Acad. Sci. USA* **2010**, *107*, 16759–16765. [CrossRef] [PubMed]
224. Dehm, S.M.; Tindall, D.J. Alternatively spliced androgen receptor variants. *Endocr.-Relat. Cancer* **2011**, *18*, R183–R196. [CrossRef] [PubMed]
225. Hu, R.; Lu, C.; Mostaghel, E.A.; Yegnasubramanian, S.; Gurel, M.; Tannahill, C.; Edwards, J.; Isaacs, W.B.; Nelson, P.S.; Bluemn, E.; et al. Distinct transcriptional programs mediated by the ligand-dependent full-length androgen receptor and its splice variants in castration-resistant prostate cancer. *Cancer Res.* **2012**, *72*, 3457–3462. [CrossRef]
226. Antonarakis, E.S.; Lu, C.; Wang, H.; Luber, B.; Nakazawa, M.; Roeser, J.C.; Chen, Y.; Mohammad, T.A.; Fedor, H.L.; Lotan, T.L.; et al. AR-V7 and resistance to enzalutamide and abiraterone in prostate cancer. *N. Engl. J. Med.* **2014**, *371*, 1028–1038. [CrossRef] [PubMed]
227. Schaeffer, E.M.; Marchionni, L.; Huang, Z.; Simons, B.; Blackman, A.; Yu, W.; Parmigiani, G.; Berman, D.M. Androgen-induced programs for prostate epithelial growth and invasion arise in embryogenesis and are reactivated in cancer. *Oncogene* **2008**, *27*, 7180–7191. [CrossRef] [PubMed]
228. Mulholland, D.J.; Dedhar, S.; Coetzee, G.A.; Nelson, C.C. Interaction of nuclear receptors with the wnt/β-catenin/TCF signaling axis: Wnt you like to know? *Endocr. Rev.* **2005**, *26*, 898–915. [CrossRef] [PubMed]
229. Rubinfeld, B.; Souza, B.; Albert, I.; Muller, O.; Chamberlain, S.H.; Masiarz, F.R.; Munemitsu, S.; Polakis, P. Association of the apc gene product with β-catenin. *Science* **1993**, *262*, 1731–1734. [CrossRef] [PubMed]
230. Kharaishvili, G.; Simkova, D.; Makharoblidze, E.; Trtkova, K.; Kolar, Z.; Bouchal, J. Wnt signaling in prostate development and carcinogenesis. *Biomed. Papers Med. Fac. Univ. Palacky Olomouc Czechoslov.* **2011**, *155*, 11–18. [CrossRef]
231. Polakis, P. Wnt signaling in cancer. *Cold Spring Harb. Perspect. Biol.* **2012**. [CrossRef] [PubMed]

232. Polakis, P. Wnt signaling and cancer. *Genes Dev.* **2000**, *14*, 1837–1851. [CrossRef] [PubMed]
233. Voeller, H.J.; Truica, C.I.; Gelmann, E.P. β-catenin mutations in human prostate cancer. *Cancer Res.* **1998**, *58*, 2520–2523. [PubMed]
234. Chesire, D.R.; Ewing, C.M.; Sauvageot, J.; Bova, G.S.; Isaacs, W.B. Detection and analysis of β-catenin mutations in prostate cancer. *Prostate* **2000**, *45*, 323–334. [CrossRef]
235. de la Taille, A.; Rubin, M.A.; Chen, M.W.; Vacherot, F.; de Medina, S.G.; Burchardt, M.; Buttyan, R.; Chopin, D. β-catenin-related anomalies in apoptosis-resistant and hormone-refractory prostate cancer cells. *Clin. Cancer Res.: Off. J. Am. Assoc. Cancer Res.* **2003**, *9*, 1801–1807.
236. Chen, G.; Shukeir, N.; Potti, A.; Sircar, K.; Aprikian, A.; Goltzman, D.; Rabbani, S.A. Up-regulation of wnt-1 and β-catenin production in patients with advanced metastatic prostate carcinoma: Potential pathogenetic and prognostic implications. *Cancer* **2004**, *101*, 1345–1356. [CrossRef] [PubMed]
237. Wang, G.; Wang, J.; Sadar, M.D. Crosstalk between the androgen receptor and beta-catenin in castrate-resistant prostate cancer. *Cancer Res.* **2008**, *68*, 9918–9927. [CrossRef] [PubMed]
238. Schweizer, L.; Rizzo, C.A.; Spires, T.E.; Platero, J.S.; Wu, Q.; Lin, T.A.; Gottardis, M.M.; Attar, R.M. The androgen receptor can signal through wnt/β-catenin in prostate cancer cells as an adaptation mechanism to castration levels of androgens. *BMC Cell Biol.* **2008**, *9*, 4. [CrossRef] [PubMed]
239. Yokoyama, N.N.; Shao, S.; Hoang, B.H.; Mercola, D.; Zi, X. Wnt signaling in castration-resistant prostate cancer: Implications for therapy. *Am. J. Clin. Exp. Urol.* **2014**, *2*, 27–44. [PubMed]
240. Truica, C.I.; Byers, S.; Gelmann, E.P. β-Catenin affects androgen receptor transcriptional activity and ligand specificity. *Cancer Res.* **2000**, *60*, 4709–4713. [PubMed]
241. Yang, F.; Li, X.; Sharma, M.; Sasaki, C.Y.; Longo, D.L.; Lim, B.; Sun, Z. Linking β-catenin to androgen-signaling pathway. *J. Biol. Chem.* **2002**, *277*, 11336–11344. [CrossRef] [PubMed]
242. Song, L.N.; Herrell, R.; Byers, S.; Shah, S.; Wilson, E.M.; Gelmann, E.P. β-Catenin binds to the activation function 2 region of the androgen receptor and modulates the effects of the n-terminal domain and TIF2 on ligand-dependent transcription. *Mol. Cell. Biol.* **2003**, *23*, 1674–1687. [CrossRef] [PubMed]
243. Masiello, D.; Chen, S.Y.; Xu, Y.; Verhoeven, M.C.; Choi, E.; Hollenberg, A.N.; Balk, S.P. Recruitment of beta-catenin by wild-type or mutant androgen receptors correlates with ligand-stimulated growth of prostate cancer cells. *Mol. Endocrinol.* **2004**, *18*, 2388–2401. [CrossRef] [PubMed]
244. Chesire, D.R.; Ewing, C.M.; Gage, W.R.; Isaacs, W.B. In vitro evidence for complex modes of nuclear β-catenin signaling during prostate growth and tumorigenesis. *Oncogene* **2002**, *21*, 2679–2694. [CrossRef] [PubMed]
245. Mulholland, D.J.; Cheng, H.; Reid, K.; Rennie, P.S.; Nelson, C.C. The androgen receptor can promote β-catenin nuclear translocation independently of adenomatous polyposis coli. *J. Biol. Chem.* **2002**, *277*, 17933–17943. [CrossRef] [PubMed]
246. Li, Y.; Wang, L.; Zhang, M.; Melamed, J.; Liu, X.; Reiter, R.; Wei, J.; Peng, Y.; Zou, X.; Pellicer, A.; et al. LEF1 in androgen-independent prostate cancer: Regulation of androgen receptor expression, prostate cancer growth, and invasion. *Cancer Res.* **2009**, *69*, 3332–3338. [CrossRef] [PubMed]
247. Pawlowski, J.E.; Ertel, J.R.; Allen, M.P.; Xu, M.; Butler, C.; Wilson, E.M.; Wierman, M.E. Liganded androgen receptor interaction with β-catenin: Nuclear co-localization and modulation of transcriptional activity in neuronal cells. *J. Biol. Chem.* **2002**, *277*, 20702–20710. [CrossRef] [PubMed]
248. Wang, Q.; Li, W.; Zhang, Y.; Yuan, X.; Xu, K.; Yu, J.; Chen, Z.; Beroukhim, R.; Wang, H.; Lupien, M.; et al. Androgen receptor regulates a distinct transcription program in androgen-independent prostate cancer. *Cell* **2009**, *138*, 245–256. [CrossRef] [PubMed]
249. Chesire, D.R.; Dunn, T.A.; Ewing, C.M.; Luo, J.; Isaacs, W.B. Identification of aryl hydrocarbon receptor as a putative wnt/β-catenin pathway target gene in prostate cancer cells. *Cancer Res.* **2004**, *64*, 2523–2533. [CrossRef] [PubMed]
250. Wang, Q.; Symes, A.J.; Kane, C.A.; Freeman, A.; Nariculam, J.; Munson, P.; Thrasivoulou, C.; Masters, J.R.; Ahmed, A. A novel role for wnt/Ca2+ signaling in actin cytoskeleton remodeling and cell motility in prostate cancer. *PLoS ONE* **2010**, *5*, e10456. [CrossRef] [PubMed]
251. Yamamoto, H.; Oue, N.; Sato, A.; Hasegawa, Y.; Matsubara, A.; Yasui, W.; Kikuchi, A. Wnt5a signaling is involved in the aggressiveness of prostate cancer and expression of metalloproteinase. *Oncogene* **2010**, *29*, 2036–2046. [CrossRef] [PubMed]

252. Miyamoto, D.T.; Zheng, Y.; Wittner, B.S.; Lee, R.J.; Zhu, H.; Broderick, K.T.; Desai, R.; Fox, D.B.; Brannigan, B.W.; Trautwein, J.; et al. RNA-seq of single prostate CTCS implicates noncanonical wnt signaling in antiandrogen resistance. *Science* **2015**, *349*, 1351–1356. [CrossRef] [PubMed]
253. Hsieh, J.C.; Kodjabachian, L.; Rebbert, M.L.; Rattner, A.; Smallwood, P.M.; Samos, C.H.; Nusse, R.; Dawid, I.B.; Nathans, J. A new secreted protein that binds to wnt proteins and inhibits their activities. *Nature* **1999**, *398*, 431–436. [PubMed]
254. Jones, S.E.; Jomary, C. Secreted frizzled-related proteins: Searching for relationships and patterns. *BioEssays* **2002**, *24*, 811–820. [CrossRef] [PubMed]
255. Kawano, Y.; Kypta, R. Secreted antagonists of the wnt signalling pathway. *J. Cell Sci.* **2003**, *116*, 2627–2634. [CrossRef] [PubMed]
256. O'Hurley, G.; Perry, A.S.; O'Grady, A.; Loftus, B.; Smyth, P.; O'Leary, J.J.; Sheils, O.; Fitzpatrick, J.M.; Hewitt, S.M.; Lawler, M.; et al. The role of secreted frizzled-related protein 2 expression in prostate cancer. *Histopathology* **2011**, *59*, 1240–1248. [CrossRef] [PubMed]
257. Wissmann, C.; Wild, P.J.; Kaiser, S.; Roepcke, S.; Stoehr, R.; Woenckhaus, M.; Kristiansen, G.; Hsieh, J.C.; Hofstaedter, F.; Hartmann, A.; et al. WIF1, a component of the wnt pathway, is down-regulated in prostate, breast, lung, and bladder cancer. *J. Pathol.* **2003**, *201*, 204–212. [CrossRef] [PubMed]
258. Zi, X.; Guo, Y.; Simoneau, A.R.; Hope, C.; Xie, J.; Holcombe, R.F.; Hoang, B.H. Expression of FRZB/secreted frizzled-related protein 3, a secreted wnt antagonist, in human androgen-independent prostate cancer PC-3 cells suppresses tumor growth and cellular invasiveness. *Cancer Res.* **2005**, *65*, 9762–9770. [CrossRef] [PubMed]
259. Yee, D.S.; Tang, Y.; Li, X.; Liu, Z.; Guo, Y.; Ghaffar, S.; McQueen, P.; Atreya, D.; Xie, J.; Simoneau, A.R.; et al. The wnt inhibitory factor 1 restoration in prostate cancer cells was associated with reduced tumor growth, decreased capacity of cell migration and invasion and a reversal of epithelial to mesenchymal transition. *Mol. Cancer* **2010**. [CrossRef] [PubMed]
260. Thiele, S.; Rauner, M.; Goettsch, C.; Rachner, T.D.; Benad, P.; Fuessel, S.; Erdmann, K.; Hamann, C.; Baretton, G.B.; Wirth, M.P.; et al. Expression profile of wnt molecules in prostate cancer and its regulation by aminobisphosphonates. *J. Cell. Biochem.* **2011**, *112*, 1593–1600. [CrossRef] [PubMed]
261. Hall, C.L.; Daignault, S.D.; Shah, R.B.; Pienta, K.J.; Keller, E.T. Dickkopf-1 expression increases early in prostate cancer development and decreases during progression from primary tumor to metastasis. *Prostate* **2008**, *68*, 1396–1404. [CrossRef] [PubMed]
262. Lawson, D.A.; Witte, O.N. Stem cells in prostate cancer initiation and progression. *J. Clin. Investig.* **2007**, *117*, 2044–2050. [CrossRef] [PubMed]
263. Jiang, Y.; Dai, J.; Zhang, H.; Sottnik, J.L.; Keller, J.M.; Escott, K.J.; Sanganee, H.J.; Yao, Z.; McCauley, L.K.; Keller, E.T. Activation of the wnt pathway through AR79, a GSK3BETA inhibitor, promotes prostate cancer growth in soft tissue and bone. *Mol. Cancer Res.: MCR* **2013**, *11*, 1597–1610. [CrossRef] [PubMed]
264. Van den Hoogen, C.; van der Horst, G.; Cheung, H.; Buijs, J.T.; Lippitt, J.M.; Guzman-Ramirez, N.; Hamdy, F.C.; Eaton, C.L.; Thalmann, G.N.; Cecchini, M.G.; et al. High aldehyde dehydrogenase activity identifies tumor-initiating and metastasis-initiating cells in human prostate cancer. *Cancer Res.* **2010**, *70*, 5163–5173. [CrossRef] [PubMed]
265. Trerotola, M.; Rathore, S.; Goel, H.L.; Li, J.; Alberti, S.; Piantelli, M.; Adams, D.; Jiang, Z.; Languino, L.R. CD133, trop-2 and alpha2beta1 integrin surface receptors as markers of putative human prostate cancer stem cells. *Am. J. Transl. Res.* **2010**, *2*, 135–144. [PubMed]
266. Yun, E.J.; Zhou, J.; Lin, C.J.; Hernandez, E.; Fazli, L.; Gleave, M.; Hsieh, J.T. Targeting cancer stem cells in castration-resistant prostate cancer. *Clin. Cancer Res.* **2016**, *22*, 670–679. [CrossRef] [PubMed]
267. Rajan, P.; Sudbery, I.M.; Villasevil, M.E.; Mui, E.; Fleming, J.; Davis, M.; Ahmad, I.; Edwards, J.; Sansom, O.J.; Sims, D.; et al. Next-generation sequencing of advanced prostate cancer treated with androgen-deprivation therapy. *Eur. Urol.* **2014**, *66*, 32–39. [CrossRef] [PubMed]
268. Lee, E.; Madar, A.; David, G.; Garabedian, M.J.; Dasgupta, R.; Logan, S.K. Inhibition of androgen receptor and beta-catenin activity in prostate cancer. *Proc. Natl. Acad. Sci. USA* **2013**, *110*, 15710–15715. [CrossRef] [PubMed]
269. Panet-Raymond, V.; Gottlieb, B.; Beitel, L.K.; Pinsky, L.; Trifiro, M.A. Interactions between androgen and estrogen receptors and the effects on their transactivational properties. *Mol. Cell. Endocrinol.* **2000**, *167*, 139–150. [CrossRef]

270. Hickey, T.E.; Robinson, J.L.; Carroll, J.S.; Tilley, W.D. Minireview: The androgen receptor in breast tissues: Growth inhibitor, tumor suppressor, oncogene? *Mol. Endocrinol.* **2012**, *26*, 1252–1267. [CrossRef] [PubMed]
271. Peters, A.A.; Ingman, W.V.; Tilley, W.D.; Butler, L.M. Differential effects of exogenous androgen and an androgen receptor antagonist in the peri- and postpubertal murine mammary gland. *Endocrinology* **2011**, *152*, 3728–3737. [CrossRef] [PubMed]
272. Zhou, J.; Ng, S.; Adesanya-Famuiya, O.; Anderson, K.; Bondy, C.A. Testosterone inhibits estrogen-induced mammary epithelial proliferation and suppresses estrogen receptor expression. *FASEB J.* **2000**, *14*, 1725–1730. [CrossRef] [PubMed]
273. Gao, Y.R.; Walters, K.A.; Desai, R.; Zhou, H.; Handelsman, D.J.; Simanainen, U. Androgen receptor inactivation resulted in acceleration in pubertal mammary gland growth, upregulation of eralpha expression, and wnt/β-catenin signaling in female mice. *Endocrinology* **2014**, *155*, 4951–4963. [CrossRef] [PubMed]
274. Peters, A.A.; Buchanan, G.; Ricciardelli, C.; Bianco-Miotto, T.; Centenera, M.M.; Harris, J.M.; Jindal, S.; Segara, D.; Jia, L.; Moore, N.L.; et al. Androgen receptor inhibits estrogen receptor-alpha activity and is prognostic in breast cancer. *Cancer Res.* **2009**, *69*, 6131–6140. [CrossRef] [PubMed]
275. Park, S.; Koo, J.; Park, H.S.; Kim, J.H.; Choi, S.Y.; Lee, J.H.; Park, B.W.; Lee, K.S. Expression of androgen receptors in primary breast cancer. *Ann. Oncol.* **2010**, *21*, 488–492. [CrossRef] [PubMed]
276. Dorgan, J.F.; Stanczyk, F.Z.; Kahle, L.L.; Brinton, L.A. Prospective case-control study of premenopausal serum estradiol and testosterone levels and breast cancer risk. *Breast Cancer Res.* **2010**. [CrossRef] [PubMed]
277. Zeleniuch-Jacquotte, A.; Shore, R.E.; Koenig, K.L.; Akhmedkhanov, A.; Afanasyeva, Y.; Kato, I.; Kim, M.Y.; Rinaldi, S.; Kaaks, R.; Toniolo, P. Postmenopausal levels of oestrogen, androgen, and SHBG and breast cancer: Long-term results of a prospective study. *Br. J. Cancer* **2004**, *90*, 153–159. [CrossRef] [PubMed]
278. Gonzalez, L.O.; Corte, M.D.; Vazquez, J.; Junquera, S.; Sanchez, R.; Alvarez, A.C.; Rodriguez, J.C.; Lamelas, M.L.; Vizoso, F.J. Androgen receptor expresion in breast cancer: Relationship with clinicopathological characteristics of the tumors, prognosis, and expression of metalloproteases and their inhibitors. *BMC Cancer* **2008**. [CrossRef] [PubMed]
279. Vera-Badillo, F.E.; Templeton, A.J.; de Gouveia, P.; Diaz-Padilla, I.; Bedard, P.L.; Al-Mubarak, M.; Seruga, B.; Tannock, I.F.; Ocana, A.; Amir, E. Androgen receptor expression and outcomes in early breast cancer: A systematic review and meta-analysis. *J. Natl. Cancer Inst.* **2014**. [CrossRef] [PubMed]
280. Proverbs-Singh, T.; Feldman, J.L.; Morris, M.J.; Autio, K.A.; Traina, T.A. Targeting the androgen receptor in prostate and breast cancer: Several new agents in development. *Endocr. Relat. Cancer* **2015**, *22*, R87–R106. [CrossRef] [PubMed]
281. Safarpour, D.; Pakneshan, S.; Tavassoli, F.A. Androgen receptor (ar) expression in 400 breast carcinomas: Is routine ar assessment justified? *Am. J. Cancer Res.* **2014**, *4*, 353–368. [PubMed]
282. Micello, D.; Marando, A.; Sahnane, N.; Riva, C.; Capella, C.; Sessa, F. Androgen receptor is frequently expressed in HER2-positive, ER/PR-negative breast cancers. *Virchows Arch.* **2010**, *457*, 467–476. [CrossRef] [PubMed]
283. McNamara, K.M.; Moore, N.L.; Hickey, T.E.; Sasano, H.; Tilley, W.D. Complexities of androgen receptor signalling in breast cancer. *Endocr. Relat. Cancer* **2014**, *21*, T161–T181. [CrossRef] [PubMed]
284. Kennedy, B.J. Fluoxymesterone therapy in advanced breast cancer. *N. Engl. J. Med.* **1958**, *259*, 673–675. [CrossRef] [PubMed]
285. Narayanan, R.; Ahn, S.; Cheney, M.D.; Yepuru, M.; Miller, D.D.; Steiner, M.S.; Dalton, J.T. Selective androgen receptor modulators (SARMS) negatively regulate triple-negative breast cancer growth and epithelial:Mesenchymal stem cell signaling. *PLoS ONE* **2014**, *9*, e103202. [CrossRef] [PubMed]
286. Santagata, S.; Thakkar, A.; Ergonul, A.; Wang, B.; Woo, T.; Hu, R.; Harrell, J.C.; McNamara, G.; Schwede, M.; Culhane, A.C.; et al. Taxonomy of breast cancer based on normal cell phenotype predicts outcome. *J. Clin. Invest.* **2014**, *124*, 859–870. [CrossRef] [PubMed]
287. Peters, K.M.; Edwards, S.L.; Nair, S.S.; French, J.D.; Bailey, P.J.; Salkield, K.; Stein, S.; Wagner, S.; Francis, G.D.; Clark, S.J.; et al. Androgen receptor expression predicts breast cancer survival: The role of genetic and epigenetic events. *BMC Cancer* **2012**. [CrossRef] [PubMed]
288. Chia, K.; O'Brien, M.; Brown, M.; Lim, E. Targeting the androgen receptor in breast cancer. *Curr. Oncol. Rep.* **2015**. [CrossRef] [PubMed]

289. Feng, J.; Li, L.; Zhang, N.; Liu, J.; Zhang, L.; Gao, H.; Wang, G.; Li, Y.; Zhang, Y.; Li, X.; et al. Androgen and AR contribute to breast cancer development and metastasis: An insight of mechanisms. *Oncogene* **2016**. [CrossRef]
290. Gucalp, A.; Tolaney, S.; Isakoff, S.J.; Ingle, J.N.; Liu, M.C.; Carey, L.A.; Blackwell, K.; Rugo, H.; Nabell, L.; Forero, A.; et al. Phase II trial of bicalutamide in patients with androgen receptor-positive, estrogen receptor-negative metastatic breast cancer. *Clin. Cancer Res.* **2013**, *19*, 5505–5512. [CrossRef] [PubMed]
291. Tang, D.; Xu, S.; Zhang, Q.; Zhao, W. The expression and clinical significance of the androgen receptor and E-cadherin in triple-negative breast cancer. *Med. Oncol.* **2012**, *29*, 526–533. [CrossRef] [PubMed]
292. Ogawa, Y.; Hai, E.; Matsumoto, K.; Ikeda, K.; Tokunaga, S.; Nagahara, H.; Sakurai, K.; Inoue, T.; Nishiguchi, Y. Androgen receptor expression in breast cancer: Relationship with clinicopathological factors and biomarkers. *Int. J. Clin. Oncol.* **2008**, *13*, 431–435. [CrossRef] [PubMed]
293. Choi, J.E.; Kang, S.H.; Lee, S.J.; Bae, Y.K. Androgen receptor expression predicts decreased survival in early stage triple-negative breast cancer. *Ann. Surg. Oncol.* **2015**, *22*, 82–89. [CrossRef] [PubMed]
294. Cochrane, D.R.; Bernales, S.; Jacobsen, B.M.; Cittelly, D.M.; Howe, E.N.; D'Amato, N.C.; Spoelstra, N.S.; Edgerton, S.M.; Jean, A.; Guerrero, J.; et al. Role of the androgen receptor in breast cancer and preclinical analysis of enzalutamide. *Breast Cancer Res.* **2014**. [CrossRef] [PubMed]
295. Niemeier, L.A.; Dabbs, D.J.; Beriwal, S.; Striebel, J.M.; Bhargava, R. Androgen receptor in breast cancer: Expression in estrogen receptor-positive tumors and in estrogen receptor-negative tumors with apocrine differentiation. *Mod. Pathol.* **2010**, *23*, 205–212. [CrossRef] [PubMed]
296. Qi, J.P.; Yang, Y.L.; Zhu, H.; Wang, J.; Jia, Y.; Liu, N.; Song, Y.J.; Zan, L.K.; Zhang, X.; Zhou, M.; et al. Expression of the androgen receptor and its correlation with molecular subtypes in 980 chinese breast cancer patients. *Breast Cancer* **2012**, *6*, 1–8. [PubMed]
297. Ni, M.; Chen, Y.; Lim, E.; Wimberly, H.; Bailey, S.T.; Imai, Y.; Rimm, D.L.; Liu, X.S.; Brown, M. Targeting androgen receptor in estrogen receptor-negative breast cancer. *Cancer Cell* **2011**, *20*, 119–131. [CrossRef] [PubMed]
298. Lehmann, B.D.; Bauer, J.A.; Chen, X.; Sanders, M.E.; Chakravarthy, A.B.; Shyr, Y.; Pietenpol, J.A. Identification of human triple-negative breast cancer subtypes and preclinical models for selection of targeted therapies. *J. Clin. Investig.* **2011**, *121*, 2750–2767. [CrossRef] [PubMed]
299. Higa, G.M.; Fell, R.G. Sex hormone receptor repertoire in breast cancer. *Int. J. Breast Cancer* **2013**. [CrossRef] [PubMed]
300. Leung, B.S.; Fletcher, W.S.; Lindell, T.D.; Wood, D.C.; Krippaechne, W.W. Predictability of response to endocrine ablation in advanced breast carcinoma. A correlation to estrogen receptor and steroid sulfurylation. *Arch. Surg.* **1973**, *106*, 515–519. [CrossRef] [PubMed]
301. Kennedy, B.J. Systemic effects of androgenic and estrogenic hormones in advanced breast cancer. *J. Am. Geriatr. Soc.* **1965**, *13*, 230–235. [CrossRef] [PubMed]
302. Pietri, E.; Conteduca, V.; Andreis, D.; Massa, I.; Melegari, E.; Sarti, S.; Cecconetto, L.; Schirone, A.; Bravaccini, S.; Serra, P.; et al. Androgen receptor signaling pathways as a target for breast cancer treatment. *Endocr. Relat. Cancer* **2016**, *23*, R485–R498. [CrossRef] [PubMed]
303. Jordan, V.C.; Robinson, S.P. Species-specific pharmacology of antiestrogens: Role of metabolism. *Fed. Proc.* **1987**, *46*, 1870–1874. [PubMed]
304. Boni, C.; Pagano, M.; Panebianco, M.; Bologna, A.; Sierra, N.M.; Gnoni, R.; Formisano, D.; Bisagni, G. Therapeutic activity of testosterone in metastatic breast cancer. *Anticancer Res.* **2014**, *34*, 1287–1290. [PubMed]
305. Ingle, J.N.; Twito, D.I.; Schaid, D.J.; Cullinan, S.A.; Krook, J.E.; Mailliard, J.A.; Tschetter, L.K.; Long, H.J.; Gerstner, J.G.; Windschitl, H.E.; et al. Combination hormonal therapy with tamoxifen plus fluoxymesterone versus tamoxifen alone in postmenopausal women with metastatic breast cancer. An updated analysis. *Cancer* **1991**, *67*, 886–891. [CrossRef]
306. Perrault, D.J.; Logan, D.M.; Stewart, D.J.; Bramwell, V.H.; Paterson, A.H.; Eisenhauer, E.A. Phase ii study of flutamide in patients with metastatic breast cancer. A National Cancer Institute of Canada Clinical Trials Group Study. *Invest. New Drugs* **1988**, *6*, 207–210. [CrossRef] [PubMed]
307. Anestis, A.; Karamouzis, M.V.; Dalagiorgou, G.; Papavassiliou, A.G. Is androgen receptor targeting an emerging treatment strategy for triple negative breast cancer? *Cancer Treat. Rev.* **2015**, *41*, 547–553. [CrossRef] [PubMed]

308. Collins, L.C.; Cole, K.S.; Marotti, J.D.; Hu, R.; Schnitt, S.J.; Tamimi, R.M. Androgen receptor expression in breast cancer in relation to molecular phenotype: Results from the nurses' health study. *Mod. Pathol.* **2011**, *24*, 924–931. [CrossRef] [PubMed]
309. Fioretti, F.M.; Sita-Lumsden, A.; Bevan, C.L.; Brooke, G.N. Revising the role of the androgen receptor in breast cancer. *J. Mol. Endocrinol.* **2014**, *52*, R257–R265. [CrossRef] [PubMed]
310. Lanzino, M.; De Amicis, F.; McPhaul, M.J.; Marsico, S.; Panno, M.L.; Ando, S. Endogenous coactivator ARA70 interacts with estrogen receptor alpha (eralpha) and modulates the functional eralpha/androgen receptor interplay in mcf-7 cells. *J. Biol. Chem.* **2005**, *280*, 20421–20430. [CrossRef] [PubMed]
311. Hu, R.; Dawood, S.; Holmes, M.D.; Collins, L.C.; Schnitt, S.J.; Cole, K.; Marotti, J.D.; Hankinson, S.E.; Colditz, G.A.; Tamimi, R.M. Androgen receptor expression and breast cancer survival in postmenopausal women. *Clin. Cancer Res.* **2011**, *17*, 1867–1874. [CrossRef] [PubMed]
312. Castellano, I.; Allia, E.; Accortanzo, V.; Vandone, A.M.; Chiusa, L.; Arisio, R.; Durando, A.; Donadio, M.; Bussolati, G.; Coates, A.S.; et al. Androgen receptor expression is a significant prognostic factor in estrogen receptor positive breast cancers. *Breast Cancer Res. Treat.* **2010**, *124*, 607–617. [CrossRef] [PubMed]
313. Gonzalez-Angulo, A.M.; Stemke-Hale, K.; Palla, S.L.; Carey, M.; Agarwal, R.; Meric-Berstam, F.; Traina, T.A.; Hudis, C.; Hortobagyi, G.N.; Gerald, W.L.; et al. Androgen receptor levels and association with pik3ca mutations and prognosis in breast cancer. *Clin. Cancer Res.* **2009**, *15*, 2472–2478. [CrossRef] [PubMed]
314. Tokunaga, E.; Hisamatsu, Y.; Taketani, K.; Yamashita, N.; Akiyoshi, S.; Okada, S.; Tanaka, K.; Saeki, H.; Oki, E.; Aishima, S.; et al. Differential impact of the expression of the androgen receptor by age in estrogen receptor-positive breast cancer. *Cancer Med.* **2013**, *2*, 763–773. [CrossRef] [PubMed]
315. Park, S.; Koo, J.S.; Kim, M.S.; Park, H.S.; Lee, J.S.; Lee, J.S.; Kim, S.I.; Park, B.W.; Lee, K.S. Androgen receptor expression is significantly associated with better outcomes in estrogen receptor-positive breast cancers. *Ann. Oncol.* **2011**, *22*, 1755–1762. [CrossRef] [PubMed]
316. Chia, K.M.; Liu, J.; Francis, G.D.; Naderi, A. A feedback loop between androgen receptor and ERK signaling in estrogen receptor-negative breast cancer. *Neoplasia* **2011**, *13*, 154–166. [CrossRef] [PubMed]
317. Ni, M.; Chen, Y.; Fei, T.; Li, D.; Lim, E.; Liu, X.S.; Brown, M. Amplitude modulation of androgen signaling by C-Myc. *Genes Dev.* **2013**, *27*, 734–748. [CrossRef] [PubMed]
318. Naderi, A.; Chia, K.M.; Liu, J. Synergy between inhibitors of androgen receptor and mek has therapeutic implications in estrogen receptor-negative breast cancer. *Breast Cancer Res.* **2011**, *13*. [CrossRef] [PubMed]
319. Farmer, P.; Bonnefoi, H.; Becette, V.; Tubiana-Hulin, M.; Fumoleau, P.; Larsimont, D.; Macgrogan, G.; Bergh, J.; Cameron, D.; Goldstein, D.; et al. Identification of molecular apocrine breast tumours by microarray analysis. *Oncogene* **2005**, *24*, 4660–4671. [CrossRef] [PubMed]
320. Doane, A.S.; Danso, M.; Lal, P.; Donaton, M.; Zhang, L.; Hudis, C.; Gerald, W.L. An estrogen receptor-negative breast cancer subset characterized by a hormonally regulated transcriptional program and response to androgen. *Oncogene* **2006**, *25*, 3994–4008. [CrossRef] [PubMed]
321. Cuenca-Lopez, M.D.; Montero, J.C.; Morales, J.C.; Prat, A.; Pandiella, A.; Ocana, A. Phospho-kinase profile of triple negative breast cancer and androgen receptor signaling. *BMC Cancer* **2014**. [CrossRef] [PubMed]
322. Lehmann, B.D.; Bauer, J.A.; Schafer, J.M.; Pendleton, C.S.; Tang, L.; Johnson, K.C.; Chen, X.; Balko, J.M.; Gomez, H.; Arteaga, C.L.; et al. PIK3CA mutations in androgen receptor-positive triple negative breast cancer confer sensitivity to the combination of PI3K and androgen receptor inhibitors. *Breast Cancer Res.* **2014**. [CrossRef] [PubMed]
323. Arce-Salinas, C.; Riesco-Martinez, M.C.; Hanna, W.; Bedard, P.; Warner, E. Complete response of metastatic androgen receptor-positive breast cancer to bicalutamide: Case report and review of the literature. *J. Clin. Oncol.* **2016**, *34*, e21–e24. [CrossRef] [PubMed]
324. Lim, S.K.; Lu, S.Y.; Kang, S.A.; Tan, H.J.; Li, Z.; Adrian Wee, Z.N.; Guan, J.S.; Reddy Chichili, V.P.; Sivaraman, J.; Putti, T.; et al. Wnt signaling promotes breast cancer by blocking itch-mediated degradation of yap/taz transcriptional coactivator wbp2. *Cancer Res.* **2016**, *76*, 6278–6289. [CrossRef] [PubMed]
325. Turashvili, G.; Bouchal, J.; Burkadze, G.; Kolar, Z. Wnt signaling pathway in mammary gland development and carcinogenesis. *Pathobiology* **2006**, *73*, 213–223. [CrossRef] [PubMed]
326. Gavin, B.J.; McMahon, A.P. Differential regulation of the wnt gene family during pregnancy and lactation suggests a role in postnatal development of the mammary gland. *Mol. Cell Biol.* **1992**, *12*, 2418–2423. [CrossRef] [PubMed]

327. Weber-Hall, S.J.; Phippard, D.J.; Niemeyer, C.C.; Dale, T.C. Developmental and hormonal regulation of wnt gene expression in the mouse mammary gland. *Differentiation* **1994**, *57*, 205–214. [CrossRef] [PubMed]
328. Huguet, E.L.; McMahon, J.A.; McMahon, A.P.; Bicknell, R.; Harris, A.L. Differential expression of human wnt genes 2, 3, 4, and 7b in human breast cell lines and normal and disease states of human breast tissue. *Cancer Res.* **1994**, *54*, 2615–2621. [PubMed]

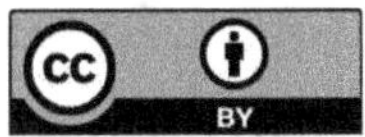

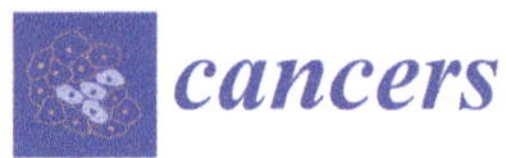 MDPI

Review

AR Signaling in Breast Cancer

Bilal Rahim and Ruth O'Regan *

Department of Medicine, Division of Hematology & Oncology, University of Wisconsin School of Medicine and Public Health, Madison, WI 53792, USA; brahim@uwhealth.org

* Correspondence: roregan@medicine.wisc.edu; Tel.: +1-608-262-9368

Academic Editor: Emmanuel S. Antonarakis

Received: 5 December 2016; Accepted: 18 February 2017; Published: 24 February 2017

Abstract: Androgen receptor (AR, a member of the steroid hormone receptor family) status has become increasingly important as both a prognostic marker and potential therapeutic target in breast cancer. AR is expressed in up to 90% of estrogen receptor (ER) positive breast cancer, and to a lesser degree, human epidermal growth factor 2 (HER2) amplified tumors. In the former, AR signaling has been correlated with a better prognosis given its inhibitory activity in estrogen dependent disease, though conversely has also been shown to increase resistance to anti-estrogen therapies such as tamoxifen. AR blockade can mitigate this resistance, and thus serves as a potential target in ER-positive breast cancer. In HER2 amplified breast cancer, studies are somewhat conflicting, though most show either no effect or are associated with poorer survival. Much of the available data on AR signaling is in triple-negative breast cancer (TNBC), which is an aggressive disease with inferior outcomes comparative to other breast cancer subtypes. At present, there are no approved targeted therapies in TNBC, making study of the AR signaling pathway compelling. Gene expression profiling studies have also identified a luminal androgen receptor (LAR) subtype that is dependent on AR signaling in TNBC. Regardless, there seems to be an association between AR expression and improved outcomes in TNBC. Despite lower pathologic complete response (pCR) rates with neoadjuvant therapy, patients with AR-expressing TNBC have been shown to have a better prognosis than those that are AR-negative. Clinical studies targeting AR have shown somewhat promising results. In this paper we review the literature on the biology of AR in breast cancer and its prognostic and predictive roles. We also present our thoughts on therapeutic strategies.

Keywords: AR signaling; AR/PARP interplay; AR/BET interplay; breast cancer

---

1. Introduction

Androgen receptor (AR) signaling has become increasingly important in understanding the biology of breast cancer, and serves as a potential therapeutic target in the era of precision medicine. Previously, breast cancer has been categorized based on hormone receptor (HR) status, and the presence or absence of human epidermal growth factor 2 (HER2) amplification. More recently, it has become apparent that the AR pathway is associated with breast tumor carcinogenesis, with differing mechanisms dependent on co-expression of HR or HER2 amplification [1,2] Although our understanding is still early, this signaling pathway has important prognostic and therapeutic implications. This review will aim to further clarify the complexities of the AR pathway in relation to breast cancer tumorigenesis, prognostic associations in relation to HR expression and HER2 amplification and potential therapeutic options.

2. AR Pathway in Breast Cancer

The AR is a steroid-hormone activated transcription factor belonging to the nuclear receptor superfamily, a group that also includes the estrogen receptor (ER) and progesterone receptor (PR).

Upon binding of its androgen ligand, the protein translocates to the nucleus where it stimulates transcription of androgen-responsive genes [2,3]. More recently, non-genomic actions of the AR signaling pathway have been described and are still being investigated in both normal female tissue and in tumor carcinogenesis [4]. AR binds androgens that are produced in a normal physiological manner from the female adrenal glands and ovaries, and in descending order of concentration include dehydroepiandrosterone sulphate (DHEAS), dehydroepiandsoterone (DHEA), androstenedione (A), testosterone (T), and dihydrotestosterone (DHT) (Figure 1) [5,6]. Only testosterone and DHT bind directly to AR, and are primarily formed by peripheral conversion of DHEAS, DHEA, and A in adipose tissue, liver and skin [5,7]. It is important to note that although testosterone can itself bind to AR, or be converted to the more potent DHT via 5α reductase, it can also be converted to estradiol (E2) via the aromatase enzyme that is found in numerous tissues including the breast [8–10]. This conversion to estradiol is important, as estradiol serves as the primary ER ligand for both ERα and ERβ receptors in breast cancer. ERα has been shown to have proliferative effect on tumors, while ERβ has been associated with anti-proliferative effect, though these mechanisms are complex and our understanding remains limited [11–14].

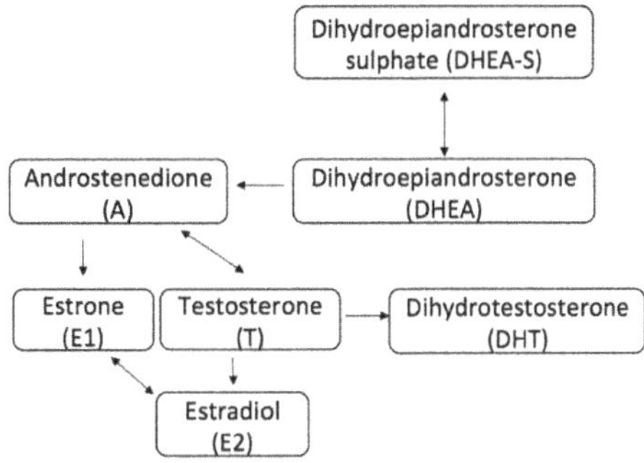

Figure 1. Abbreviated androgen and estrogen pathway. Arrows represent direction of enzymatic conversion.

AR is found in up to 70%–90% of all breast cancers, making it more abundant than ER or PR activity [15–19]. However, identifying exact percentages of AR expression among the various breast cancers—HR-positive, HER2-positive, or triple negative breast cancer (TNBC)—is somewhat challenging due to considerable variability in methodology, including differing locations of expression (cytoplasmic versus nuclear), cut off points for immunohistochemical (IHC) receptor expression ($\geq$1%, $\geq$5% or $\geq$10%), and the antibody used in staining. One very large systematic review aimed to address AR expression in ER-positive versus ER-negative breast cancers by analyzing 19 studies, including 7693 patients, and found AR co-expression with ER-positive disease to be 74.8% [20]. AR was also found in ER-negative tumors at a lower rate of 31.8% from the same study, although other studies show significant variability in this percentage depending on HER2 or TNBC status [20]. For example, HR-negative and HER2-positive breast cancers seem to express AR in the range of 50%–60%; TNBC is generally between 20% and 40% [15,16,21–28]. AR is also variably expressed in certain histologically distinct subsets of mammary epithelial cells, including invasive apocrine carcinomas, with molecular apocrine cells uniformly expressing AR but not ER or PR [29,30]. Luminal epithelial cells have also been found to express AR in up to 30%, often with co-expression of ER and PR [31].

Gene expression profiling has also led to distinct molecular subtyping that is sometimes used to classify breast cancer, and these tumors seem to show variable rates of AR expression [32,33]. For example, the luminal A and luminal B subtypes, as defined by ER positivity seem to express AR anywhere from 50% to 90% depending on the study. The HER2-positive molecular subtype expresses AR between approximately 20%–60%, and TNBC molecular subtype between 20% and 50% [34,35].

In regards to AR activity in breast cancer carcinogenesis, multiple in vitro studies using several laboratory breast cancer cell lines (i.e., MCF-7, T47-D, and BT20) have shown an anti-proliferative effect of AR antagonism [1,36–39]. Interestingly, in the presence of ERα, the AR pathway can be either antagonistic or agonistic to tumorigenesis, and at least partially is influenced by the level of receptor expression and availability of their respective ligands [40–43]. Alternatively, ERα-negative and AR-positive breast cancers fall into a category termed the "molecular apocrine" subtype, with typically distinct histological features of eosinophilic and granular cytoplasm [44]. Within this subtype, a preclinical study by Doane and colleagues utilizing the cell line MDA-MB-453 found the absence of ER but continued dependence on hormonally regulated transcription, which was previously thought to be solely the product of ER activation. Further gene expression profiling revealed the presence of AR, and incubation of the cell line with synthetic androgen led to proliferation that could be blocked by the anti-androgen flutamide [45]. The proliferative activity of AR seems to be consistent in the presence of HER2, with at least partial "cross-talk" between the receptor pathways, and in TNBC as well [46–48]. This heterogeneity of AR signaling in relation to co-expression of ERα, HER2 and in TNBC will be discussed in further detail in their respective sections of this paper.

3. AR Pathway in ER+ Breast Cancer

Like AR, ER is a steroid hormone receptor. There are naturally two receptors expressed in normal breast tissue, ERα and ERβ, which are involved in the development of reproductive organs, bone density, cell cycle regulation, DNA replication and variety of other processes that occur through both genomic and non-genomic mechanisms. Its ligand is estradiol, and in normal breast tissue ERβ is the dominant receptor. In breast cancer, ERα expression increases and is implicated in tumorigenesis [49]. The function of AR depends largely on the level of co-expression of ERα in HR-positive breast cancer (i.e., luminal breast cancer). Interestingly, many pre-clinical studies show differing proliferative versus anti-proliferative effects in ERα and AR-positive breast cancer that correlates with variation in the ratio of these steroid receptors and the availability of their respective ligands (i.e., estradiol and DHT). As noted earlier in this paper, androgens can be peripherally converted to estradiol (Figure 1), making the interplay between androgens and estrogens in patients expressing both AR and ER quite complex. Early in vitro studies have tried to elucidate the complex relationship between AR and ER expression and the variable responses to hormones and their antagonists in breast cancer cells.

Some studies show AR agonists to actually have anti-tumor effect in the setting of ERα. This has been demonstrated through in vitro modeling in which higher levels of AR confer anti-proliferative effects in the MCF-7 cell line [41]. Some older in vitro studies show increased apoptotic activity with the use of androgens, as well as down regulation of the *bcl-2* proto-oncogene, which could be reversed with the addition of the anti-androgen hydroxyflutamide [50,51]. There are even some older clinical trials that have demonstrated that treatments with exogenous androgens can successfully treat certain breast cancers, with regression rates of approximately 20% [42]. These early clinical studies, though, did not categorize the receptor status of treated patients.

Overexpression of AR in the MCF-7 breast cancer cell line, as postulated by Britton and colleagues, is thought to be due to cross talk between ERα and the EGFR/MAPK pathway, which leads to a self-propogating autocrine growth-regulatory loop through ERα mediated development of AR [52]. Yeast and mammalian two-hybrid systems found ER and AR co-expression led to ER-AR heterodimerization, rather than ER-ER or AR-AR homodimerization, and thus a decrease in AR transactivation by 35% [43]. This fell in line with other older studies, which showed a dose-dependent decrease in AR transcriptional activity in the presence of ER co-expression and estradiol [53]. Another potential way AR down-regulates ERα activity is by competing for and binding to estrogen response elements (EREs) on DNA [54]. Chromatin immunoprecipitation sequencing (ChIP-seq) and gene microarray analysis of the ZR-75-1 luminal breast cancer cell line identified that increased presence of one respective steroid hormone ligand (DHT versus estradiol) over the other leads to antagonism of the other pathway, specifically at the level of transcription by binding to DNA response elements [40].

For example, if AR binds to EREs it leads to an anti-proliferative effect rather than the proliferative effect of ERα binding to ERE and vice versa for ERα binding to androgen response elements (AREs). In certain studies, ER and AR interplay actually leads to increased resistance to traditional endocrine targeted therapies [55,56].

ER expression serves as a primary target for therapy and one of the first treatments targeting this pathway was the anti-estrogen tamoxifen, which was FDA approved in 1998. It is a selective estrogen receptor modulator (SERM) that has differential ER agonist and antagonist activity depending on the target tissue, and acts as a competitive inhibitor of estradiol [57]. Tamoxifen-resistance can occur in HR-positive breast cancers and AR signaling has been implicated in this process, leading to some clinical insight into the relationship between ER and AR signaling pathways. Toth-Fejel and colleagues noted the androgen DHEA-S induced growth in the AR and ER-positive cell line T-47D by 43.4%, but inhibited the AR-positive and ER-negative cell line HCC1937 by 22% [58]. They also found that pre-treatment of the cell lines with tamoxifen in T-47D cells could increase the inhibitory activity of DHEA-S, presumably though increased activity at the level of the AR receptor.

A somewhat conflicting pre-clinical model to that of Toth-Fejel and colleagues noted in the MCF-7 cell line that overexpression of AR made ERα-positive breast cancer cells resistant to the inhibitory effects of tamoxifen in xenograft and nude mice studies, and that treatment with anti-androgen therapy could overcome this resistance [59]. The postulated mechanism was an AR-associated increase in tamoxifen agonist activity on ER, rather than an antagonistic effect [58,59]. A more recent preclinical study found that the agonist activity of tamoxifen on ER signaling in the presence of high levels of AR leads to activation of epidermal growth factor receptor (EGFR), which could be blocked by use of the non-steroidal anti-androgen enzalutamide and/or the anti-EGFR therapy gefitinib [60]. Additionally, tamoxifen-resistant cancers in which AR is present tend to have both higher levels of AR expression and in one study, higher AR to ER nuclear expression [56].

4. Prognostic Implications of AR in ER+ Breast Cancer

Several larger studies and meta-analyses reviewing the prognostic implications of AR-positive breast cancer report their findings without discussion of AR in relation to co-receptor status, or male breast cancer. Given the size of these studies, and the unique look into male breast cancer, they remain important and will be discussed briefly here prior to reviewing the significance of AR in relation to ER in this section, and HER2 co-expression versus TNBC in later sections. The largest meta-analysis to date presented by Vera-Badillo and colleagues encompassed 19 studies and 7693 patients with stage I-III disease [20]. Specifically, this study looked at the odds ratios for overall survival (OS) and disease free survival (DFS) at 3 and 5 years for patients with AR expression, in which 4658 patients (60.5%) had breast cancers that were notably AR-positive. Independent of ER expression, patients with AR-positive breast cancers were found to have statistically significant improvements in OS and DFS at both 3 year and 5 year time points, including a 13.5% absolute improvement in 5 year OS and 20.7% in DFS [20]. Another meta-analysis reviewing DFS and OS by Qu et al. evaluated 12 studies and 5270 patients that met their criteria. The combined hazard ratio for DFS of all included studies was 0.52, which was statistically significant, indicating a lower risk of recurrence for patients with AR-positive breast cancers. However, although showing a trend toward improvement, the difference in OS was not statistically significant [61]. Aleskandarany et al. performed a retrospective cohort study of stage I-III patients (n = 1141) with tumors $\leq$5 cm from 1987 to 1997 [62]. High AR expression was associated with longer breast cancer specific survival (BCSS) and was an independent predictor of better outcome regardless of tumor size, grade and nodal stage. Moreover, low AR expression was associated with increased risk of distant metastasis [62]. The Nurses' Health Study (NHS) showed similar results in a prospective analysis of stage I-III patients conducted from 1976 to 2008 of postmenopausal women. AR-positive tumors were associated with small tumor size ($\leq$2 cm), lower histologic grade, and stage. Breast cancer survival rates at 5 and 10 years were 88% and 82% for AR-negative patients, and 95% and 88% for AR-positive patients [63].

Regarding male breast cancer, these cases comprise only approximately 1% of all breast cancer. In a Chinese study analyzing 116 patients from 1995 to 2008, men were found to have poorer outcomes if their breast cancers were AR-positive [64]. Unlike comparable studies in female breast cancer, AR expression was not correlated with pathologic T stage, histologic grade, or HR expression. Likewise, in contrast to the studies outlined above, OS and DFS rates were significantly shorter with 5 year OS at 54% versus 72%, and 5 year DFS at 39% versus 61%, for AR-positive versus AR-negative cancers respectively, echoing the results of an earlier Polish study [65,66]. However, AR signaling in male breast cancer remains poorly understood with conflicting results, largely due to the relatively small series available. Where one study indicates a lack of correlation between AR expression and male breast cancer, another indicates decreased AR expression is correlated with earlier development of cancer [67,68]. Further studies are necessary to help clarify this patient population further.

In relation to ER-positive breast cancer, several studies have established that AR positivity has prognostic value. AR and ER co-expressing breast cancers generally have better outcomes in terms of time to relapse (TTR), as well as disease specific survival (DSS) as noted from a study by Castellano and colleagues [69]. The study analyzed 953 ER-positive patients from 1998 to 2003 treated with chemotherapy, hormone therapy or both, of which 859 were evaluable for AR expression and 609 were positive (70.9%). The median TTR was 11.72 years versus 13.22 years and the DSS was 12.33 and 13.91 respectively. Regarding clinical and pathologic features, the study established a correlation with AR positivity and smaller tumor size (<2 cm), absence of lymph node metastases and PR expression [69].

A Swedish population-based prospective cohort study assessing patients from 2002 to 2012 also showed a statistically significant improvement in DFS (at 6 years, approximately 90% versus 78%) in breast cancers co-expressing AR and ER [70]. Tsang et al. reviewed data from 3 Chinese institutions from the years 2002 to 2009 and showed AR and ER co-expression to be associated with lower pathologic T stage, lower tumor grade, PR positivity and better outcomes, and postulated that the favorable result could be due to the inhibitory effect of the AR signaling [34,58]. The Nurses' Health Study noted the best survival rates in AR and ER co-expressing breast cancers were in postmenopausal women with stage I-III breast cancer, with an overall 30% reduction in breast cancer mortality [63]. Jiang and colleagues also noted a significantly better DFS in the ER-positive molecular luminal (A and B) subtypes [71].

Reduced AR expression in ER-positive disease can predict for an increased risk of relapse, breast-cancer associated death and worse DFS as well [71]. A study of 215 invasive ductal carcinoma samples noted that breast cancers with higher expression (median of 75% nuclear positivity by the AR-U407 IHC assay), was associated with a 3 fold increased risk of relapse and 4.6 fold increased risk in breast cancer related death, as well as a statistically significant decrease in OS [54].

5. AR Pathway in HER2 Amplified Breast Cancer

The HER2 receptor in breast cancer was first noted in the late 1980s. Historically, it has been associated with poorer outcomes and is amplified in approximately 15%–25% of invasive breast cancers [72,73]. HER2 amplified breast cancers have lower rates of ER co-expression, ranging from 28% to 49%, with typically better outcomes when ER is present [73,74]. Previous molecular studies have distinguished a group of patients with ER-negative but HER2-positive disease that did not easily fall into a pre-defined category. An important study by Farmer et al. in 2005 aimed to better define ER-negative, HER2-positive disease by tissue microarray and found an increase in AR signaling [44]. These cells in further review were notable for apocrine differentiation when exposed to high amounts of androgens in the in vitro setting, and became known as molecular apocrine with separate distinct characteristics than traditional apocrine tumors [44,75]. One early pre-clinical study postulated that the molecular apocrine subtype was associated with cell proliferation in the presence of androgen due to complex interactions between AR and the HER2 signal transduction pathway in the absence of interference by the ER pathway [45]. A related investigation in prostate cancer found that HER2 kinase signaling is required for full activity of AR at low androgen concentration. In particular, HER2 signaling led to increased binding of AR to the appropriate DNA targets to promote transcription, and protected AR from ubiquitin associated degradation [76].

This interplay was further elucidated by Naderi and Hughes-Davies, who showed in the cell lines MDA-MB-453 and MDA-MB-361, and in fresh tumor samples, that there is cross-regulation of certain genes between AR and HER2. In particular, there was increased expression of steroid response genes FOXA1, XBP1 and TFF3, as well as, increased cell proliferation when either AR or HER2 were stimulated. When exposed to the anti-androgen flutamide, or HER2 inhibition there were pro-apoptotic effects, which was notably additive when given in combination [46]. Later, the same group in a study by Chia et al., further identified a positive feedback loop between the AR and extracellular signal-regulated kinase (ERK) signaling pathways, in which HER2 is a transcriptional target of AR, and leads to increased ERK activity [77]. The ERK pathway was also found to increase AR expression, which could be down-regulated both with the androgen targeting flutamide, or the ERK pathway targeting MEK inhibitor in an in vivo mouse model [77]. Similar models have been described in prostate cancer, and serve as potential therapeutic targets [78].

To further add to the complexity of AR in HER2 amplified disease, a study by Ni and colleagues looking at the AR cistrome in the MDA-MB-453 breast cancer cell line, had several interesting findings. They noted that forkhead factor binding motif FOXA1, was highly expressed in HER2 and AR-positive breast tumors, which is similar to AR-positive prostate cancers and seems to be involved in recruitment of ER and AR to their transcription regulatory elements [28,79,80]. AR mediated activation of HER2/HER3 signaling led to increased activity of MYC gene activity, which increased transcriptional activity of androgen-response genes in ER-negative and AR-positive molecular apocrine breast cancers [81]. In an earlier study, this same group showed DHT stimulation, likely through AR promotion of FOXA1 and wnt/B-catenin pathway led to up-regulation of HER2 and HER3 phosphorylation and activation of the phosphoinositide 3-kinse (PI3K) pathway in the MDA-MB-453 cell line.

Also identified by another group is that AR activates the Wnt/β-catenin pathway, which leads to upregulation of HER3 and has been previously implicated in breast oncogenesis [82]. Exposure to the androgen DHT led to increased growth signaling activity of AR, HER2/HER3 and as a downstream event, and activation of PI3K/AKT pathway and these events could be blocked with the addition of the anti-androgen bicalutamide in an in vivo mouse model [28]. It should be noted that the cell line used in this study has been found to have a homozygous deletion of TP53, a homozygous PTEN missense mutation, and an oncogenic mutation in PI3K that might confound this data [83–85].

6. Prognostic Implications of AR in HER2 Amplified Breast Cancer

The prognostic significance of AR in HER2 amplified breast cancer seems to either show no association with survival, or indicate poorer outcomes. However, many of these studies are limited by smaller sample sizes. One analysis looking at prognostic variables in AR expressing breast cancer showed no association with BCSS or distant metastasis free interval, though this only comprised a sample of 59 patients [62]. A large prospective study assessing postmenopausal women notably had 1154 samples with AR-positive disease, but only 81 patients with HER2 amplification and noted no differences in survival [63].

Other studies, including a retrospective analysis by Park et al. analyzed 931 breast cancer tissue samples in stage I–III disease without prior therapy. Forty-nine patients with AR-positive, HER2 amplified breast cancer were categorized as molecular apocrine subtype, and survival analysis revealed a trend toward poorer OS, though this did not reach statistical significance [23]. Along these lines, Schippinger and colleagues in a study looking at 232 specimens of metastatic breast cancer noted that DFS in patients with AR expression and HER2-amplification was 9.07 months compared to 17.51 in all patients with AR expressed disease, though again not statistically significant. Moreover, the median survival after recurrence (SAR) in this population was only 10.89 months, which was similar to the 11.99 months in patients with AR-negative disease [86].

7. AR Pathway in TNBC

TNBC, as defined by lack of expression of ER and PR and a lack of HER2 amplification, comprises between 10% and 20% of all breast cancers [48,87,88]. Traditionally, outcomes in TNBC have been poor with a median overall survival in metastatic disease of approximately 13 months, as well as a shorter time from recurrent disease until death compared to other breast cancers [89,90]. Pathologic features include higher mitotic indices and an increase in BRCA1 mutations [91]. Demographically, TNBC has been associated with higher proportion of African American and Hispanic patients based on population studies and tend to occur at a higher frequency in younger patients [92–95]. Despite these common characteristics, TNBC remains a biologically variable disease and thus a common signaling pathway that could serve as a target for therapy has proven elusive [96]. Traditional cytotoxic chemotherapy remains the main approach to treatment in these patients, but significant research at the molecular level is being conducted to identify at least subsets of TNBC that might benefit from treatments focused on driver pathways such as AR signaling.

Gene expression profiling has increasingly been used to classify invasive cancer subtypes over the last 15 years. In TNBC, the majority of cases fall into a category of basal-like subtype, first described by Perou, et al. in 2000 [32]. Expanded studies on the basal-like subtype have identified that this heterogeneous group comprises approximately 16% of all breast cancers [97]. The basal-like subtype has several common and more aggressive clinical features, including higher histologic grade and mitotic indices, as well as earlier disease recurrence that lead to poorer outcomes [33,98–100]. Many of these features have clinical overlap with the broader category of TNBC. Depending on the study, the basal-like subtype is found in anywhere from 56% to 95% of cases and has sometimes been used synonymously with the term TNBC [101–104]. With improved methods in molecular biology and gene expression profiling, the heterogeneity of TNBC is becoming increasingly understood.

Lehmann et al. initially categorized TNBC into 6 separate subtypes, including basal-like 1 (BL1), basal-like 2 (BL2), immunomodulatory (IM), mesenchymal (M), mesenchymal stem-like (MSL), and luminal androgen receptor (LAR), each with distinct gene signatures predicting for driver signaling pathways that could potentially serve as therapeutic targets [48]. Specifically, the LAR subtype was found to be enriched in mRNA expression of AR signaling, as well as multiple downstream AR targets with in vitro studies showing increased sensitivity to the AR antagonist bicalutamide [48]. Lehmann and colleagues later adjusted their classification in 2016, utilizing more refined techniques, to include only 4 subtypes with the omission of the IM and MSL categories [105]. Regardless, the LAR subtype remains validated within the Lehmann lab and among other research groups, including Yu et al., and more recently Jezequel and colleagues who found the subtype to account for approximately 22% of TNBC [106,107]. Moreover, Lehmann's group later noted that all commercially available AR expressing TNBC cell lines also had PIK3CA mutations. They performed Sanger sequencing on 26 AR-positive and 26 AR-negative TNBC clinical cases, and found clonal PIK3CA mutations were significantly higher in AR-positive (40%) versus AR-negative (4%) tumors [108]. Further analysis of 5 LAR cell lines revealed activating PIK3CA mutations and sensitivity to PI3K inhibition suggesting interplay between these pathways as well [48,108].

Even non-LAR TNBC cell lines SUM159PT, HCC1806, BT549, and MDA-MB-231 seem to have a role for AR signaling. Gene microarray and ChIP-seq analysis shows AR mediated up-regulation of the EGFR ligand amphiregulin, which promotes proliferation via the EGFR pathway. This proliferative activity appeared to be blocked with the anti-androgen enzalutamide [47].

8. Prognostic Implications of AR in TNBC Breast Cancer

AR positivity has been associated with more favorable prognoses in TNBC. There are several studies that show AR is associated with lower Ki-67 proliferative marker, lower mitotic score, lower histologic grade and lower clinical stage [23,27,63,109–112]. Interestingly, TNBC has been associated with the poor prognostic TP53 mutation in up to 80% of patients, but at least one study has shown that patients with AR-positive TNBC have a lower rate of TP53 mutations as well [109,113]. This improvement in histological and genetic features seems to translate to clinical benefit and AR-positive TNBC have both improved DFS and OS versus AR-negative [110,114,115] One retrospective study analyzing tissue microarrays from 287 patients with operable TNBC breast cancer found a statistically significant decrease in lymph node positivity in AR-positive disease. The same study showed a significant difference between AR-positive and AR-negative disease in which 5 year DFS was 87% versus 74.2% and 5 year OS was 94.2% versus 82.3% [114]. A prospective study by Loibl and colleagues that was linked to the German GeparTrio trial noted AR expression predicted a significantly better 5 year DFS of 85.7% compared to 65.5% and 5 year OS of 95.2% compared to 76.2% [116]. Other studies have also shown that lack of AR expression is associated with an increased risk of recurrence and distant metastases, especially in patients with lymph node positive disease [111,112].

Other analyses have shown either no difference or worse outcomes for AR-positive TNBC. McGhan et al., looking at 119 patients with resectable disease, found patients with AR-positive cancers trended toward more advanced stages (stage II and III) breast cancer, with no differences in DSS or OS [21]. Mrklic in a retrospective study analyzing 83 patients with TNBC found no difference in DFS and OS in patients with AR-positive disease versus AR-negative, though only 27 cancers were AR-positive [27]. Pistelli in a similar study analyzing 81 cancers with only 15 positive for AR showed no difference in DFS and OS, and the same was the case for Park and colleagues, in which 21 of 156 TNBC samples expressed AR and no survival differences were noted [117,118]. Another study with 97 AR-positive TNBC cases failed to find a difference in relapse free survival (RFS) or OS compared to AR-negative disease [119]. The large prospective NHS study previously referenced was also evaluated for the prognostic significance of AR in TNBC and found that in 78 out of 211 AR-positive TNBC there was a statistically significant 83% increase in overall mortality compared to AR-negative in a multivariate model [63]. This data conflicts with most other studies as noted above, which generally show improved to no differences in outcomes.

More recently, pathological complete response (pCR) has become a surrogate marker for outcome in patients treated with neoadjuvant therapies [120]. In terms of chemosensitivity in AR-positive TNBC, a limited number of studies have shown a lower rate of pCR. Loibl and colleagues in the GeparTrio trial showed AR-positive disease to have a pCR of 12.85% (n = 358), compared to AR-negative tumors at 25.4% (n = 315). In multivariate analysis, AR independently predicted pCR. Interestingly, though patients with AR-negative disease had a higher chance of achieving pCR, those with AR-positive disease had similar DFS and OS whether or not pCR was achieved [116]. Specifically, patients who achieved a pCR and had AR-negative cancers had a 5 year DFS of 77.9% and 5 year OS of 87% compared to patients who did not achieve a pCR and were AR-positive in which DFS was 77.5% and OS 88.6% [116]. The patients in the GeparTrio trial received a regimen of doxorubicin, cyclophosphamide and docetaxel (TAC), and if considered a non-responder, went on to receive either more TAC or vinorelbine and capecitabine prior to surgical intervention [116]. Another retrospective study by Asano and colleagues examined 177 patients with resectable early stage breast cancer treated with neoadjuvant fluorouracil, epirubicin, and cyclophosphamide (FEC100) followed by paclitaxel. Sixty-one patients were found to have TNBC, with 23 (37.7%) of these with AR positivity. Though the numbers were quite small, the pCR rates were lower in AR-positive versus negative disease at 17.4% (n = 4) compared to 63.2% (n = 24) [121]. Notably, the latter AR-negative pCR response was particularly robust in comparison to the Loibl study, and likely contributed to improved OS and non-recurrence free survival in AR-negative TNBC in their population [121].

Also, of interest and somewhat opposite to the above studies looking at pCR is a recent article by Jiang and colleagues in which whole exome sequencing was performed on 29 biopsy samples obtained prior to treatment of patients who were found to have either a pCR (n = 18) or extensive residual disease (n = 11) after neoadjuvant chemotherapy with adriamycin, cyclophosphamide and paclitaxel (ACT). Pathway databases were used to predict the impact of somatic mutations on certain pathways associated with cancer. Though no single mutation was found to be predictive of response to chemotherapy in TNBC, they did find tumors with mutations in the AR pathway and FOXA1 transcription factor networks had a significantly higher pCR (94.1% vs. 16.6%) compared to those that did not carry such mutations [122]. The FOXA1 transcription factor is thought to be activated by AR signaling [123]. It should be noted that the study did not designate if the samples with somatic mutations in the AR or FOXA1 pathways expressed AR by IHC, which is the surrogate marker of AR pathway activity in most studies.

9. Treatment Options in AR+ Breast Cancer

9.1. Bicalutamide

As previously described, the mechanism of AR-signaling in breast cancer is quite complex and depends on the presence or absence of other signaling mechanisms in concert (Figure 2). Early pre- clinical models have shown both a proliferative effect of androgens on cell activity and an anti-proliferative effect, leading to studying the therapeutic effects of anti-androgen medications. Bicalutamide is a non-steroidal peripherally selective anti-androgen that binds AR as an antagonist [124]. One study showed that in MCF-7 cells transfected with an AR vector, androgens prevented the cells from proliferating, while the addition of the synthetic anti-androgen bicalutamide actually reversed this effect, leading to continued proliferation [41]. Another study by Toth-Fejel and colleagues further differentiated cell lines into ER and AR-positive versus ER-negative and AR-positive disease. They found ER-negative and AR-positive cells were inhibited by 22% with the addition of androgen, but that this could be reversed with pre-treatment with bicalutamide. However, bicalutamide was not studied in the cell line that was ER and AR-positive, thus it was unclear what effect it might have on cell proliferation (i.e., inhibition of cell proliferation?) [58]. De Amicis and colleagues studied the interplay between AR expression and response to the anti-estrogen tamoxifen in the ER and AR-positive MCF-7 cell line. They found in tamoxifen-resistant cells an elevated level of AR and reduced ER mRNA, essentially showing that AR overexpression was associated with tamoxifen resistance, possibly by enhancing its agonistic effects rather than antagonist. This resistance could be overcome with the addition of bicalutamide, which offers interesting therapeutic implications in tamoxifen resistance cancers in which AR is expressed [59]. Further studies assessing bicalutamide in treatment of tamoxifen resistance, or as prophylaxis to resistance, in ER and AR-positive disease are certainly warranted.

There are not many studies that have assessed the role of bicalutamide activity in HER2 amplified disease. Ni and colleagues though, did show an in vivo ability to block stimulation by androgen and induce apoptosis with the use of bicalutamide in ER-negative, AR and HER2-positive breast cancer, giving further evidence of the possible therapeutic effects of anti-androgens in certain AR-positive breast cancers [28].

Bicalutamide has been studied in TNBC. In addition to identifying the molecular LAR subtype, Lehmann and colleagues found this subtype to be quite sensitive to bicalutamide [48]. Zhu and colleagues showed in MSL TNBC cell lines MDA-MB-231 and Hs578T that androgens induce cell proliferation and inhibits apoptosis in vitro and in vivo and that bicalutamide promotes apoptosis, as well as other inhibitory effects [125]. Another study aimed at understanding the interplay between the transcription factor ZEB1, which plays a role in cancer progression by regulating the epithelial to mesenchymal transition (i.e., increased tumor migration and invasion) in breast cancer, and AR signaling in TNBC noted that by inhibiting ZEB1, AR expression was decreased and perhaps more importantly, inhibition of AR signaling with bicalutamide suppressed ZEB1 expression [126]. Mehta and colleagues analyzed the TNBC cell line MDA-MB-453, which in addition to AR positivity, also has PTEN and p53 mutations [127]. They identified 10 genes as AR targets using RT-qPCR and ChIP sequencing techniques and found that androgens promote cell proliferation and decrease apoptosis via these gene targets. They found that the addition of the anti-androgen bicalutamide could reverse this effect. Additionally, they hypothesized that the reason for poorer response to adjuvant or neoadjuvant chemotherapy in AR-positive TNBC was due to an AR-mediated resistance to apoptosis. The effects of paclitaxel, 5-fluorouracil and cyclophosphamide in AR-positive TNBC were studied and cells were found to have significant increases in cell survival and decreased apoptosis in the presence of androgen and that this could be reversed with the addition of bicalutamide [127]. As previously noted, patients with TNBC receiving neoadjuvant chemotherapy have been found to have lower pCR rates when AR-positive and this study provides rationale that perhaps targeting the AR pathway may help improve pCR rates [116].

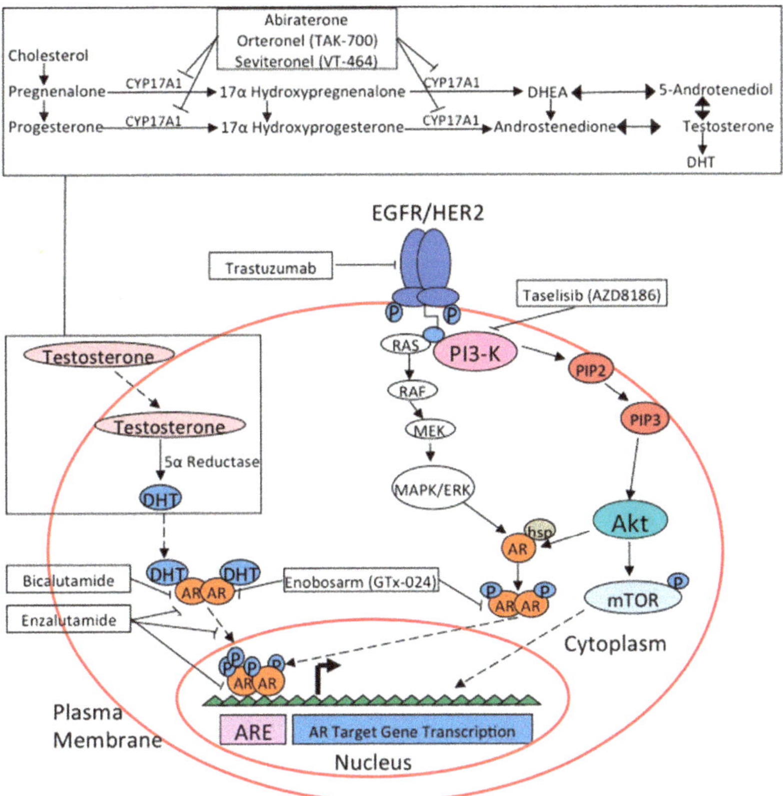

Figure 2. Drug targets in AR signaling pathway.

Evaluation of the correlation between membrane tyrosine kinase receptors and expression of AR in TNBC has shown a positive correlation with EGFR, and platelet derived growth factor beta (PDGFRβ) [128]. The same study found increased PI3K/Akt activity in AR-positive TNBC and found that co administration of bicalutamide with agents targeting EGFR, PDGFRβ, PI3K/ mammalian target of rapamycin (mTOR), and ERK pathways led to synergistic activity and provides some rationale to further evaluate combination therapy in AR-positive TNBC [128]. To further the argument that dual blockade of AR and PI3K/mTOR inhibition can lead to synergistic effects, is a study by Lehmann and colleagues. They noted a much higher rate of concurrent clonal phosphatidylinositol-4,5-bisphosphate 3-kinase, catalytic subunit alpha gene (PIK3CA) mutations (40%) in AR-positive TNBC versus AR-negative (4%), and also that targeting dual targeting of PI3K and AR had an additive inhibitory effect on tumor growth [108].

An alternative combination target may include the use of cyclin-dependent kinases 4 and 6 (CDK4 and CDK6). These kinases are activated by cyclin D, and promote cell cycle entry by phosphorylating proteins that drive the transition from G1 to the S1 phase and when disrupted can lead to unrestricted cell proliferation in breast cancer [129,130]. Certain preclinical models have shown that resistance to anti-androgen therapy is linked to a F876L mutation in AR, leading to a change from antagonist activity to agonist. CDK4/6 inhibitors have been shown to restore activity of anti-androgen treatment by antagonizing AR F876L [131]. There is currently a phase I/II trial of palbociclib in combination with bicalutamide for the treatment of metastatic AR-positive TNBC which is accruing (NCT02605486) (Table 1) [132].

Table 1. Ongoing breast cancer clinical trials.

Trial ID	Agent(s)	Mechanism(s) of Action	Patient Population	Study Design
NCT02605486	Palbociclib & Bicalutamide	CD4/CD6 Inhibitor & Androgen Receptor Inhibitor	AR-positive metastatic breast cancer	Non-randomized, open-label, phase I/II
NCT02457910	Taselisib & Enzalutamide	PI3K Inhibitor & Androgen Receptor Inhibitor	AR-positive metastatic TNBC	Partially-randomized, open-label phase IB/II
NCT02091960	Enzalutamide & Trastuzumab	Androgen Receptor Inhibitor & HER2 Targeted Monoclonal Antibody	AR-positive, HER2 amplified metastatic or locally advanced breast cancer	Non-randomized, open label, phase II
NCT02689427	Enzalutamide & Paclitaxel	Androgen Receptor Inhibitor & Microtubule Stabilizer	AR-positive TNBC, stage I–III breast cancer (neoadjuvant therapy)	Non-randomized, open label, phase IIB
NCT02750358	Enzalutamide	Androgen Receptor Inhibitor	AR-positive TNBC, stage I–III breast cancer (adjuvant therapy)	Non-randomized, open-label, feasibility study
NCT00755885	Abiraterone Acetate	CYP17 Inhibitor	ER or AR-positive postmenopausal metastatic or locally advanced breast cancer	Non-randomized, open-label, phase I/II
NCT01884285	AZD8186 +/− Abiraterone Acetate or AZD2014	PI3K Inhibitor +/− CYP17 Inhibitor or mTOR Inhibitor	Advanced TNBC	Non-randomized, open-label, phase I
NCT01990209	Orteronel	CYP17 Inhibitor	AR-positive metastatic breast cancer	Non-randomized, open-label, phase II
NCT02580448	VT-464	CYP17 Inhibitor	Advanced breast cancer. Phase I: TNBC or ER-positive, HER2 negative Phase II: AR-positive TNBC or ER-positive, HER2 negative	Non-randomized, open-label, phase I/II
NCT02368691	GTx-024	Selective Androgen Receptor Modulator	AR-positive advanced TNBC	Non-randomized, open-label, phase II

Preclinical studies led to a phase II clinical trial evaluating bicalutamide in metastatic ER-negative and AR-positive cancers as a proof of concept study led by Gucalp and colleagues. Patients with >10% nuclear expression of AR by IHC were included and treated with bicalutamide 150 mg daily, with the primary endpoint being clinical benefit rate (CBR) defined as the total number of patients who showed a complete response (CR), partial response (PR) or stable disease (SD) > 6 months. The study found the CBR to be 19% for the 26 study participants, driven by SD as there were no CRs or PRs, and a median progression free survival (PFS) of 12 weeks. Though HER2 status was not an exclusion criteria, only 1 of the 26 patients had HER2 amplified cancers and 1 of the 5 patients with SD had initial negative HER2 status that was later considered positive after undergoing a curative intent mastectomy [133]. A more recent case reported by Arce-Salinas of a patient with recurrent AR-positive metastatic TNBC, molecular apocrine subtype, had a CR with use of bicalutamide despite heavy pretreatment with palliative chemotherapy, showing that a CR with anti-androgen therapy alone does seem to be possible [134]. Briefly, it should be noted that the older nonsteroidal anti-androgen flutamide, which is less potent than bicalutamide, was studied in two phase II clinical trials in 1988 in patients with metastatic breast cancer. Neither of these studies yielded promising results, though were conducted in a patient population unselected for AR, ER, PR or HER2 status [135,136].

9.2. Enzalutamide

Enzalutamide is a newer generation nonsteroidal anti-androgen that binds the androgen receptor with greater affinity than bicalutamide, decreases nuclear translocation, and impairs binding to androgen response elements and co-activators [137]. An interesting study by Cochrane and colleagues examined the effects of enzalutamide in AR-positive breast cancer in both ER-positive and ER-negative tumors. The study found both in vitro and in vivo that enzalutamide inhibits androgen mediated growth in both ER-positive and ER-negative cancers expressing AR. Interestingly, enzalutamide also inhibited estrogen-mediated growth in ER-positive, AR-positive cells, whereas previous preclinical studies have shown bicalutamide to increase cell proliferation in this cell population [56]. A more recent study by D'Amato and colleagues had similar results, and found AR inhibition reduced estradiol mediated proliferation in ER-positive and AR-positive disease [138]. These studies suggest that the AR signaling pathway may be a potential target in ER-positive disease as well, which has not been shown with bicalutamide. Along these lines, a number of studies have shown that when ER is expressed in breast cancer, AR positivity is associated with tamoxifen-resistance. Ciupek and colleagues suggest that in the presence of AR, tamoxifen leads to AR-mediated EGFR activation as a mechanism of resistance. This could be blocked with the use of enzalutamide and the EGFR inhibitor gefitinib and may provide a viable preventive or salvage therapy in ER-positive, AR-positive disease treated with tamoxifen [60].

In TNBC, an in vivo study by Barton and colleagues analyzed 4 TNBC cell lines (SUM159PT, HC1806, BT549, and MDA-MB-231) and noted that the anti-androgen enzalutamide was not only active in the LAR molecular subtype, but also in the M, MSL and BL2 subtypes. They noted that AR activation up-regulates the EGFR pathway, as in ER-positive disease noted above, which could be blocked by enzalutamide and makes it potentially applicable to a broader range of TNBC [47]. Combination therapy with anti-androgens and mTOR inhibition has shown some promising results and Robles and colleagues found additive anti-proliferative effect in the LAR molecular subtype in the MDA-MB-453 cell line and LAR xenograft model [139]. Given that mTOR is downstream from PI3K, this further strengthens the rationale that the PI3K is important in TNBC and a possible target with concurrent enzalutamide as well. There is currently a phase IB/II clinical trial that is in process, which is assessing the CBR at 16 weeks of the PI3K inhibitor taselisib in combination with enzalutamide in advanced TNBC (NCT02457910) [140].

Also of importance is that enzalutamide has been associated with immunogenic modulation, which may increase the susceptibility of tumor cells to immune-mediated cell death [141]. A study by Kwilas et al. showed growth inhibition with enzalutamide and abiraterone in breast cancer cells, with improved immune mediated lysis. They found this increase in immune mediated activity to be associated with increased cell surface expression of tumor necrosis factor-related apoptosis-inducing ligand (TRAIL) and reduction in expression of osteoprotegerin (OPG) [142]. Enzalutamide and the anti-androgen abiraterone acetate, which inhibits the CYP17A1 enzyme involved in androgen biosynthesis, decreased cell proliferation and enhanced immune mediated lysis in AR-positive disease. Even more interesting, both of these medications enhanced immune mediated lysis even in AR-negative disease [142]. An earlier study by Kwilas and colleagues also showed increased immune activity when a pox viral based cancer vaccine was combined with enzalutamide in in vivo mice models, and furthers the idea that this medication increases immunogenic modulation and may have importance in newer immunotherapy trials [143]. There is currently an ongoing phase II clinical trial evaluating dual therapy with enzalutamide and the monoclonal antibody trastuzumab in HER2 amplified, AR-positive metastatic breast cancer with a primary endpoint of CBR at $\geq$24 weeks (NCT02091960) [144]. Although it would be difficult to tease out the immunogenic modulation of enzalutamide in this study, it may boost the effect of trastuzumab. Enzalutamide is also currently being assessed in several AR-positive TNBC clinical trials, either alone or in combination, which will be discussed below.

Traina and colleagues shared preliminary results of a phase II clinical trial assessing enzalutamide in AR-positive metastatic TNBC [145]. The single-arm, non-randomized phase II trial assessed patients with TNBC who screened for AR positivity as defined by AR expression greater than 0% by IHC. A total of 118 women were enrolled in the trial, with a majority of patients treated in the first or second line setting. The primary end point was CBR at 4 months, which was 35% at that time point, and 29% at 6 months. The median PFS was 14 weeks, and included 2 CRs and 5 PRs and the medication was well tolerated without any new safety concerns [145]. As a side benefit, the study also led to the development of a predictive assay termed PREDICT AR, in which they noted patients who responded to enzalutamide had a distinct gene expression profile, and had a better CBR of 36% at 24 weeks compared to 6% in patients who were PREDICT AR-negative [145,146].

As previously discussed, patients with AR-positive TNBC have a relatively low pCR rate of 12.85% [116]. Aimed at this group is a phase IIB clinical trial in the neoadjuvant setting looking at the use of enzalutamide with weekly paclitaxel with a primary endpoint of pCR that is meant to hopefully improve the response rate (NCT02689427) [147]. There is also a feasibility study accruing that is looking at the use of 1 year of adjuvant enzalutamide for the treatment of patients with early stage, AR-positive TNBC (NCT02750358) [148].

9.3. *Abiraterone*

Abiraterone acetate is a selective, irreversible and potent inhibitor of 17α-hydroxylase and 17,20-lyase (CYP17) enzymatic activity and is commonly used in castration-resistant prostate cancer (CRPC) [149]. It has also been studied in ER-positive metastatic breast cancer with at least part of the rationale being that CYP17 inhibition decrease the synthesis of both androgens and estrogens and may be more effective than an AI alone. A phase II, randomized open-label clinical trial assessing 297 patients with metastatic ER-positive breast cancer looked to clarify the role of abiraterone, though AR positivity was not a stratification factor. Eligibility required sensitivity to an aromatase inhibitor (AI) prior to disease progression and AR positivity was reportedly balanced between treatment arms, including abiraterone plus prednisone, versus abiraterone with exemestane versus exemestane alone with primary end point of PFS. Abiraterone either in combination with prednisone or with exemestane did not improve PFS, compared to exemestane [150,151]. Another phase II clinical trial assessed the safety and efficacy of abiraterone plus prednisone in molecular apocrine AR-positive metastatic breast cancer with a primary endpoint of CBR at 6 months. The CBR was found to be 20%, which included 1 CR and 5 SD, although the overall response rate was only 6.7% with a median PFS 2.8 months [152]. At the time of analysis, five patients remained on treatment with clinical benefit ranging between 6.4 and 24 months. There are currently two other clinical trials assessing abiraterone in breast cancer. A phase I/II UK study evaluated abiraterone in postmenopausal women with advanced metastatic ER or AR-positive breast cancer. This study is no longer recruiting, and results are awaited (NCT0075585) [153]. A phase I, open-label, multicenter trial evaluating abiraterone in combination with the PI3K inhibitor AZD8186 in a variety of solid malignancies, including TNBC, is still recruiting patients (NCT01884285) [154].

9.4. *Newer Anti-Androgens*

A number of other novel nonsteroidal anti-androgen agents are currently under analysis. Orteronel (TAK-700) is a reversible, selective CYP17 inhibitor, similar to abiraterone with a higher specificity for 17,20 lyase inhibition and known activity in CRPC [155,156]. This agent is being studied in a phase II clinical trial in patients with AR-positive metastatic breast cancer, with 2 separate cohorts assessing ER-positive disease and TNBC (NCT01990209) [157]. Seviteronel (VT-464) is a similar newer generation CYP17 inhibitor, with a current phase I/II study accruing patients with advanced breast cancer with separate cohorts for ER-positive disease and TNBC (NCT02580448) [158]. There are more potent and novel anti-androgens in development. A recent study by Kandil and colleagues showed up to 30 to 50 fold improvement in activity with the use of pure novel AR antagonists with 7-substituted umbelliferone derivatives over enzalutamide and bicalutamide respectively [159]. These agents clearly require further testing, but purer compounds may be important in AR-positive TNBC in the future if current clinical trials confirm a significant signal.

9.5. SARMs

Somewhat contradictory to other studies presenting therapeutic options, Narayanan and colleagues demonstrated in the MDA-MB-231 cell line that nonsteroidal, tissue selective androgen receptor modulators (SARMs), rather than anti-androgens could inhibit breast cancer growth [160]. They chose the genomically stable MDA-MB-231 TNBC cell line, in which they transfected an AR plasmid, over the often used MDA-MB-453 cell line as the latter is known to express mutated AR, PTEN and p53 that could potentially confound results. Both in vitro and in vivo, they found the addition of SARMs inhibited intratumoral expression of genetic pathways that promote breast cancer development, metastasis-promoting paracrine factors (i.e., IL6, MMP13) and cell proliferation [160]. Based largely on this study, a phase II, multicenter clinical trial investigating the efficacy and safety of the SARM enobosarm (GTx-024) in advanced AR-positive TNBC is currently underway (NCT02368691) [161].

9.6. Other Drugs

Poly ADP-ribose polymerase (PARP) inhibitors are a group of agents aimed at the PARP1 protein that acts to repair single strand breaks in DNA. These breaks occur frequently in the cell cycle, and rely on mechanisms such as PARP1 activity to resolve the errors via the base excision repair pathway. Patients with breast cancer susceptibility gene 1 (BRCA1) and 2 (BRCA2), as well as partner and localizer of BRCA2 (PALB2) mutations are susceptible to DNA double strand breaks, as these genes normally function to correct such breaks. In patients with these underlying mutations, the addition of a PARP inhibitor leads to cell death due to dysfunction of both repair pathways [162]. In regards to AR signaling and PARP inhibition, there is minimal data. However, Park and colleagues identified that BRCA1 increased ligand-dependent AR transactivation, as well as synergistically combined with co-activators of the AR pathway, leading to increased efficacy. They postulated that lack of the BRCA1 gene would reduce AR-dependent signaling [163]. Shin et al. found non-mutated BRCA2 synergizes with the co-activator p160 to enhance AR-mediated transcription, similar to BRCA1, and was associated with an anti-proliferative effect [164]. A small study evaluated 41 patients with BRCA1 mutations and 14 with BRCA2 mutations and analyzed AR status by IHC and found only 12% of BRCA1, and 50% of BRCA2 mutated tumors expressed AR [165]. Another study found AR positivity in 13 of 43 (30%) BRCA1 and 14 of 18 (78%) of BRCA2 mutated tumors [166]. At present, there have been no preclinical or clinical studies looking at PARP inhibition specifically in AR-positive disease. Although PARP inhibition has become an important tool in breast cancer treatment, especially in BRCA1, BRCA2 or PALB2 mutated cells, its activity needs to be better defined in relation to the AR pathway in preclinical models before we can identify if there is significant rationale for their use in AR-positive disease.

Bromodomain and extraterminal (BET) signaling has emerged recently as an important pathway in AR signaling. These proteins, which are expressed by the majority of cancer cells, are involved in epigenetic activity and chromatin "reading" and include BRD2, BRD3, BRD4 and BRDT [167]. BRD4 has a significant role in RNA polymerase II transcription by helping to recruit the positive transcription elongation factor P-TEFb [168,169]. Previous studies established the anti-cancer activity of BET inhibitors that target BRD4, which was further evaluated in CRPC by Asangani and colleagues [167]. They found BET inhibition with the small molecule JQ1 to induce G0-G1 cell cycle arrest, apoptosis and transcriptional down-regulation of anti-apoptotic BCL-xl in AR-positive cells. Moreover, they noted a direct AR-BRD4 interaction, which was inhibited by JQ1 leading to a more robust anti-proliferative effect than enzalutamide [167].

BET signaling has been studied in breast cancer as well. The ER-positive MCF-7 breast cancer cell was noted to have increased T-bet activity associated with insulin exposure, which also was associated with tamoxifen-resistance [170]. Feng and colleagues furthered this understanding by noting that ER signaling was positively associated with WHSC1, a histone methyltransferase recruited to the ERα gene by BET proteins. They found this pathway could be blocked with BET inhibition with JQ1 and overcome tamoxifen-resistance in cell culture and xenograft models [171]. Further, Sengupta et al. noted JQ1 suppression of estrogen-induced growth and transcription in MCF7 and T47D cell lines [172]. BET signaling has been studied in HER2 amplified breast cancer, using the cell lines HCC1954 and MD-MBA-361 in which it was shown that BET inhibition could overcome lapatinib resistance associated with kinome reprogramming [173]. Other studies have found that resistance to PI3K inhibitors and mTOR inhibitors is associated with feedback activation of tyrosine kinase receptors in metastatic breast cancer and can be overcome with dual use of PI3K and BET inhibition or mTOR and BET inhibition [174,175]. Borbely and colleagues noted activity of combination therapy with a histone deacetylase (HDAC) inhibitor and BET inhibitor JQ1 by increasing activity of ubiquitin-specific protease 17 (USP17), which down-regulated the Ras/MAPK pathway and thus reduced cell proliferation in 2 separate TNBC (MDA-MB-231 and BT549) and 2 ER-positive (MCF7 and T47D) cell lines [176]. Synergy with the chemotherapeutic agents docetaxel, vinorelbine, cisplatin and carboplatin has been shown with JQ1 in preclinical evaluation of several breast cancer cell lines [177]. An association with hypoxia responsive genes and angiogenesis has been noted, which can be down-regulated with BET inhibition in cell culture and xenograft models [178]. Finally, Sahini and colleagues noted that BET inhibition results in growth suppression of TNBC independent of their intrinsic molecular subtype [179]. BET signaling certainly is an exciting area in breast cancer. However, a limitation to all the above mentioned studies regarding BET and breast cancer is that none of them further clarify the role of AR signaling in the effects that are being described. Given the findings in prostate cancer showing clear activity with AR signaling and the BET pathway, it is important to clarify the role of AR and BET signaling in breast cancer in order to identify its role as a therapeutic target. Currently, there are three early phase clinical trials assessing BET inhibitors in TNBC along with other malignancies [180–182].

10. Discussion

Our study aimed to describe advances in understanding of the complex AR signaling pathways in relation to co-receptor signaling, as well as prognostic and therapeutic implications. However, there are some inherent limitations to the data presented. In particular, several of the above-mentioned pre-clinical studies utilize commercially available breast cancer cell lines. Though there are advantages to the use of these classic cell line models, over time multiple cycles of cell cultures can select for certain subclones that can create variability in genetic and phenotypic expression across labs [183]. For example, in one study the cell line MDA-MB-453 notably had a homozygous deletion in TP53, a homozygous PTEN missense mutation and a PI3K mutation and it is unclear if these are preserved changes in the cell line or unique to the specific version from that particular lab [127]. Several studies do utilize cells fresh tumor samples to help corroborate their findings, but many do not and thus reproducibility of the findings is a question.

Additionally, most in vitro studies do not distinguish whether the cell line, or cells from fresh biopsy material are early stage or metastatic in origin. Independent review of commercially available cell lines reveals that most are metastatic in origin, and often from malignant pleural fluid, which some might argue indicates particularly aggressive biology that does not reflect the general population [183]. Lobular carcinoma represents approximately 10% of all invasive breast cancer, and none of the above studies looking at AR signaling studied these tumors, raising concerns of the generalizability of findings in these patients. In terms of co-receptor expression, ERα is known to be proliferative in breast cancer but ERβ is less understood, especially in relation to AR. It is possible that ERβ, as another steroid receptor, might have importance given the competitive activity between AR and ER as steroid hormones. There is also controversy over what constitutes IHC positivity of AR expression, with cut off values of $\geq$1%, $\geq$5% or $\geq$10% depending on the study. This lack of consensus guidelines makes it difficult to interpret prognostic value of AR expression in comparison between studies. Lastly, several of the larger studies and meta-analyses do not distinguish differences in prognostic value of AR in relation to co-receptor expression of ER, HER2 or in TNBC. These are somewhat offset by the multiple studies reviewed that do distinguish between these different subtypes of breast cancer.

AR remains an area of study that is rapidly evolving. The current study is a comprehensive review of the available data regarding the pathophysiology of AR-positive breast cancer, and makes important efforts to discuss the nuanced differences between AR-positive breast cancers in relation to co-receptor status. Also, prognostic implications of AR are discussed in the same manner, noting clear differences in ER-positive, HER2 amplified and TNBC. Therapeutic targets along the AR pathway are discussed with emphasis on novel agents and combination therapy with promising results. As our understanding of the complexities of AR signaling in regards to tumorigenesis becomes more refined, we will better be able to use AR expression as a prognostic marker and therapeutic target.

11. Conclusions

The identification of the AR signaling pathway in breast cancer has led to an interesting and growing field, especially in regards to basic and translational research. Not only have we identified important prognostic associations with ER-positive, HER2 amplified and TNBC, but also potential therapeutic targets either with monotherapy or in unique combinations. Clearly, there is still significant room to expand the field and grow our understanding of these complex pathways, but early work is encouraging regarding the ability to use targeted therapies in new and exciting ways and we look forward to future of the field.

Conflicts of Interest: The authors declare no conflict of interest.

References

1. Birrell, S.N.; Bentel, J.M.; Hickey, T.E.; Ricciardelli, C.; Weger, M.A.; Horsfall, D.J.; Tilley, W.D. Androgens induce divergent proliferative responses in human breast cancer cell lines. *J. Steroid Biochem. Mol. Biol.* **1995**, *52*, 459–467. [CrossRef]
2. Zhu, X.; Li, H.; Liu, J.P.; Funder, J.W. Androgen stimulates mitogen-activated protein kinase in human breast cancer cells. *Mol. Cell. Endocrinol.* **1999**, *152*, 199–206. [CrossRef]
3. Quigley, C.A.; De Bellis, A.; Marschke, K.B.; el-Awady, M.K.; Wilson, E.M.; French, F.S. Androgen receptor defects: Historical, clinical, and molecular perspectives. *Endocr. Rev.* **1995**, *16*, 271–321. [CrossRef] [PubMed]
4. Foradori, C.D.; Weiser, M.J.; Handa, R.J. Non-genomic actions of androgens. *Front. Neuroendocrinol.* **2008**, *29*, 169–181. [CrossRef] [PubMed]
5. Burger, H.G. Androgen production in women. *Fertil. Steril.* **2002**, *77* (Suppl. S4), S3–S5. [CrossRef]
6. Davison, S.L.; Davis, S.R. Androgens in women. *J. Steroid Biochem. Mol. Biol.* **2003**, *85*, 363–366. [CrossRef]
7. Walters, K.A. Role of androgens in normal and pathological ovarian function. *Reproduction* **2015**, *149*, R193–R218. [CrossRef] [PubMed]
8. Labrie, F.; Luu-The, V.; Labrie, C.; Belanger, A.; Simard, J.; Lin, S.X.; Pelletier, G. Endocrine and intracrine sources of androgens in women: Inhibition of breast cancer and other roles of androgens and their precursor dehydroepiandrosterone. *Endocr. Rev.* **2003**, *24*, 152–182. [CrossRef] [PubMed]
9. Birrell, S.N.; Butler, L.M.; Harris, J.M.; Buchanan, G.; Tilley, W.D. Disruption of androgen receptor signaling by synthetic progestins may increase risk of developing breast cancer. *FASEB J.* **2007**, *21*, 2285–2293. [CrossRef] [PubMed]
10. Wilson, J.D.; Griffin, J.E.; Leshin, M.; George, F.W. Role of gonadal hormones in development of the sexual phenotypes. *Hum. Genet.* **1981**, *58*, 78–84. [CrossRef] [PubMed]
11. Shaaban, A.M.; O'Neill, P.A.; Davies, M.P.; Sibson, R.; West, C.R.; Smith, P.H.; Foster, C.S. Declining estrogen receptor-beta expression defines malignant progression of human breast neoplasia. *Am. J. Surg. Pathol.* **2003**, *27*, 1502–1512. [CrossRef] [PubMed]

12. Skliris, G.P.; Munot, K.; Bell, S.M.; Carder, P.J.; Lane, S.; Horgan, K.; Lansdown, M.R.; Parkes, A.T.; Hanby, A.M.; Markham, A.F.; et al. Reduced expression of oestrogen receptor beta in invasive breast cancer and its re-expression using DNA methyl transferase inhibitors in a cell line model. *J. Pathol.* **2003**, *201*, 213–220. [CrossRef] [PubMed]
13. Roger, P.; Sahla, M.E.; Makela, S.; Gustafsson, J.A.; Baldet, P.; Rochefort, H. Decreased expression of estrogen receptor beta protein in proliferative preinvasive mammary tumors. *Cancer Res.* **2001**, *61*, 2537–2541. [PubMed]
14. Marotti, J.D.; Collins, L.C.; Hu, R.; Tamimi, R.M. Estrogen receptor-beta expression in invasive breast cancer in relation to molecular phenotype: results from the Nurses' Health Study. *Mod. Pathol.* **2010**, *23*, 197–204. [CrossRef] [PubMed]
15. Collins, L.C.; Cole, K.S.; Marotti, J.D.; Hu, R.; Schnitt, S.J.; Tamimi, R.M. Androgen receptor expression in breast cancer in relation to molecular phenotype: Results from the Nurses' Health Study. *Mod. Pathol.* **2011**, *24*, 924–931. [CrossRef] [PubMed]
16. Niemeier, L.A.; Dabbs, D.J.; Beriwal, S.; Striebel, J.M.; Bhargava, R. Androgen receptor in breast cancer: Expression in estrogen receptor-positive tumors and in estrogen receptor-negative tumors with apocrine differentiation. *Mod. Pathol.* **2010**, *23*, 205–212. [CrossRef] [PubMed]
17. Guedj, M.; Marisa, L.; de Reynies, A.; Orsetti, B.; Schiappa, R.; Bibeau, F.; MacGrogan, G.; Lerebours, F.; Finetti, P.; Longy, M.; et al. A refined molecular taxonomy of breast cancer. *Oncogene* **2012**, *31*, 1196–1206. [CrossRef] [PubMed]
18. Kuenen-Boumeester, V.; Van der Kwast, T.H.; Claassen, C.C.; Look, M.P.; Liem, G.S.; Klijn, J.G.; Henzen-Logmans, S.C. The clinical significance of androgen receptors in breast cancer and their relation to histological and cell biological parameters. *Eur. J. Cancer* **1996**, *32*, 1560–1565. [CrossRef]
19. Moinfar, F.; Okcu, M.; Tsybrovskyy, O.; Regitnig, P.; Lax, S.F.; Weybora, W.; Ratschek, M.; Tavassoli, F.A.; Denk, H. Androgen receptors frequently are expressed in breast carcinomas: Potential relevance to new therapeutic strategies. *Cancer* **2003**, *98*, 703–711. [CrossRef] [PubMed]
20. Vera-Badillo, F.E.; Templeton, A.J.; de Gouveia, P.; Diaz-Padilla, I.; Bedard, P.L.; Al-Mubarak, M.; Seruga, B.; Tannock, I.F.; Ocana, A.; Amir, E. Androgen receptor expression and outcomes in early breast cancer: A systematic review and meta-analysis. *J. Natl. Cancer Inst.* **2014**. [CrossRef] [PubMed]
21. McGhan, L.J.; McCullough, A.E.; Protheroe, C.A.; Dueck, A.C.; Lee, J.J.; Nunez-Nateras, R.; Castle, E.P.; Gray, R.J.; Wasif, N.; Goetz, M.P.; et al. Androgen receptor-positive triple negative breast cancer: A unique breast cancer subtype. *Ann. Surg. Oncol.* **2014**, *21*, 361–367. [CrossRef] [PubMed]
22. Gucalp, A.; Traina, T.A. Triple-negative breast cancer: Role of the androgen receptor. *Cancer J.* **2010**, *16*, 62–65. [CrossRef] [PubMed]
23. Park, S.; Koo, J.; Park, H.S.; Kim, J.H.; Choi, S.Y.; Lee, J.H.; Park, B.W.; Lee, K.S. Expression of androgen receptors in primary breast cancer. *Ann. Oncol.* **2010**, *21*, 488–492. [CrossRef] [PubMed]
24. Chia, K.; O'Brien, M.; Brown, M.; Lim, E. Targeting the androgen receptor in breast cancer. *Curr. Oncol. Rep.* **2015**. [CrossRef] [PubMed]
25. McNamara, K.M.; Yoda, T.; Takagi, K.; Miki, Y.; Suzuki, T.; Sasano, H. Androgen receptor in triple negative breast cancer. *J. Steroid Biochem. Mol. Biol.* **2013**, *133*, 66–76. [CrossRef] [PubMed]
26. Gasparini, P.; Fassan, M.; Cascione, L.; Guler, G.; Balci, S.; Irkkan, C.; Paisie, C.; Lovat, F.; Morrison, C.; Zhang, J.; et al. Androgen receptor status is a prognostic marker in non-basal triple negative breast cancers and determines novel therapeutic options. *PLoS ONE* **2014**, *9*, e88525. [CrossRef] [PubMed]
27. Mrklic, I.; Pogorelic, Z.; Capkun, V.; Tomic, S. Expression of androgen receptors in triple negative breast carcinomas. *Acta Histochem.* **2013**, *115*, 344–348. [CrossRef] [PubMed]
28. Ni, M.; Chen, Y.; Lim, E.; Wimberly, H.; Bailey, S.T.; Imai, Y.; Rimm, D.L.; Liu, X.S.; Brown, M. Targeting androgen receptor in estrogen receptor-negative breast cancer. *Cancer Cell* **2011**, *20*, 119–131. [CrossRef] [PubMed]
29. Wells, C.A.; El-Ayat, G.A. Non-operative breast pathology: Apocrine lesions. *J. Clin. Pathol.* **2007**, *60*, 1313–1320. [CrossRef] [PubMed]
30. Selim, A.G.; Wells, C.A. Immunohistochemical localisation of androgen receptor in apocrine metaplasia and apocrine adenosis of the breast: Relation to oestrogen and progesterone receptors. *J. Clin. Pathol.* **1999**, *52*, 838–841. [CrossRef] [PubMed]

31. Safarpour, D.; Pakneshan, S.; Tavassoli, F.A. Androgen receptor (AR) expression in 400 breast carcinomas: Is routine AR assessment justified? *Am. J. Cancer Res.* **2014**, *4*, 353–368. [PubMed]
32. Perou, C.M.; Sorlie, T.; Eisen, M.B.; van de Rijn, M.; Jeffrey, S.S.; Rees, C.A.; Pollack, J.R.; Ross, D.T.; Johnsen, H.; Akslen, L.A.; et al. Molecular portraits of human breast tumours. *Nature* **2000**, *406*, 747–752. [CrossRef] [PubMed]
33. Sorlie, T.; Tibshirani, R.; Parker, J.; Hastie, T.; Marron, J.S.; Nobel, A.; Deng, S.; Johnsen, H.; Pesich, R.; Geisler, S.; et al. Repeated observation of breast tumor subtypes in independent gene expression data sets. *Proc. Natl. Acad. Sci. USA* **2003**, *100*, 8418–8423. [CrossRef] [PubMed]
34. Tsang, J.Y.; Ni, Y.B.; Chan, S.K.; Shao, M.M.; Law, B.K.; Tan, P.H.; Tse, G.M. Androgen receptor expression shows distinctive significance in ER positive and negative breast cancers. *Ann. Surg. Oncol.* **2014**, *21*, 2218–2228. [CrossRef] [PubMed]
35. Qi, J.P.; Yang, Y.L.; Zhu, H.; Wang, J.; Jia, Y.; Liu, N.; Song, Y.J.; Zan, L.K.; Zhang, X.; Zhou, M.; et al. Expression of the androgen receptor and its correlation with molecular subtypes in 980 chinese breast cancer patients. *Breast Cancer* **2012**, *6*, 1–8. [PubMed]
36. Cops, E.J.; Bianco-Miotto, T.; Moore, N.L.; Clarke, C.L.; Birrell, S.N.; Butler, L.M.; Tilley, W.D. Antiproliferative actions of the synthetic androgen, mibolerone, in breast cancer cells are mediated by both androgen and progesterone receptors. *J. Steroid Biochem. Mol. Biol.* **2008**, *110*, 236–243. [CrossRef] [PubMed]
37. Hackenberg, R.; Luttchens, S.; Hofmann, J.; Kunzmann, R.; Holzel, F.; Schulz, K.D. Androgen sensitivity of the new human breast cancer cell line MFM-223. *Cancer Res.* **1991**, *51*, 5722–5727. [PubMed]
38. Poulin, R.; Baker, D.; Labrie, F. Androgens inhibit basal and estrogen-induced cell proliferation in the ZR-75-1 human breast cancer cell line. *Breast Cancer Res. Treat.* **1988**, *12*, 213–225. [CrossRef] [PubMed]
39. Ando, S.; De Amicis, F.; Rago, V.; Carpino, A.; Maggiolini, M.; Panno, M.L.; Lanzino, M. Breast cancer: From estrogen to androgen receptor. *Mol. Cell. Endocrinol.* **2002**, *193*, 121–128. [CrossRef]
40. Need, E.F.; Selth, L.A.; Harris, T.J.; Birrell, S.N.; Tilley, W.D.; Buchanan, G. Research resource: Interplay between the genomic and transcriptional networks of androgen receptor and estrogen receptor alpha in luminal breast cancer cells. *Mol. Endocrinol.* **2012**, *26*, 1941–1952. [CrossRef] [PubMed]
41. Szelei, J.; Jimenez, J.; Soto, A.M.; Luizzi, M.F.; Sonnenschein, C. Androgen-induced inhibition of proliferation in human breast cancer MCF7 cells transfected with androgen receptor. *Endocrinology* **1997**, *138*, 1406–1412. [CrossRef] [PubMed]
42. Goldenberg, I.S.; Sedransk, N.; Volk, H.; Segaloff, A.; Kelley, R.M.; Haines, C.R. Combined androgen and antimetabolite therapy of advanced female breast cancer. A report of the cooperative breast cancer group. *Cancer* **1975**, *36*, 308–310. [CrossRef]
43. Panet-Raymond, V.; Gottlieb, B.; Beitel, L.K.; Pinsky, L.; Trifiro, M.A. Interactions between androgen and estrogen receptors and the effects on their transactivational properties. *Mol. Cell. Endocrinol.* **2000**, *167*, 139–150. [CrossRef]
44. Farmer, P.; Bonnefoi, H.; Becette, V.; Tubiana-Hulin, M.; Fumoleau, P.; Larsimont, D.; Macgrogan, G.; Bergh, J.; Cameron, D.; Goldstein, D.; et al. Identification of molecular apocrine breast tumours by microarray analysis. *Oncogene* **2005**, *24*, 4660–4671. [CrossRef] [PubMed]
45. Doane, A.S.; Danso, M.; Lal, P.; Donaton, M.; Zhang, L.; Hudis, C.; Gerald, W.L. An estrogen receptor-negative breast cancer subset characterized by a hormonally regulated transcriptional program and response to androgen. *Oncogene* **2006**, *25*, 3994–4008. [CrossRef] [PubMed]
46. Naderi, A.; Hughes-Davies, L. A functionally significant cross-talk between androgen receptor and ErbB2 pathways in estrogen receptor negative breast cancer. *Neoplasia* **2008**, *10*, 542–548. [CrossRef] [PubMed]
47. Barton, V.N.; D'Amato, N.C.; Gordon, M.A.; Lind, H.T.; Spoelstra, N.S.; Babbs, B.L.; Heinz, R.E.; Elias, A.; Jedlicka, P.; Jacobsen, B.M.; et al. Multiple molecular subtypes of triple-negative breast cancer critically rely on androgen receptor and respond to enzalutamide in vivo. *Mol. Cancer Ther.* **2015**, *14*, 769–778. [CrossRef] [PubMed]
48. Lehmann, B.D.; Bauer, J.A.; Chen, X.; Sanders, M.E.; Chakravarthy, A.B.; Shyr, Y.; Pietenpol, J.A. Identification of human triple-negative breast cancer subtypes and preclinical models for selection of targeted therapies. *J. Clin. Investig.* **2011**, *121*, 2750–2767. [CrossRef] [PubMed]
49. Rondon-Lagos, M.; Villegas, V.E.; Rangel, N.; Sanchez, M.C.; Zaphiropoulos, P.G. Tamoxifen Resistance: Emerging Molecular Targets. *Int. J. Mol. Sci.* **2016**, *17*, 1357. [CrossRef] [PubMed]

50. Kandouz, M.; Lombet, A.; Perrot, J.Y.; Jacob, D.; Carvajal, S.; Kazem, A.; Rostene, W.; Therwath, A.; Gompel, A. Proapoptotic effects of antiestrogens, progestins and androgen in breast cancer cells. *J. Steroid Biochem. Mol. Biol.* **1999**, *69*, 463–471. [CrossRef]
51. Lapointe, J.; Fournier, A.; Richard, V.; Labrie, C. Androgens down-regulate bcl-2 protooncogene expression in ZR-75-1 human breast cancer cells. *Endocrinology* **1999**, *140*, 416–421. [CrossRef] [PubMed]
52. Britton, D.J.; Hutcheson, I.R.; Knowlden, J.M.; Barrow, D.; Giles, M.; McClelland, R.A.; Gee, J.M.; Nicholson, R.I. Bidirectional cross talk between ERalpha and EGFR signalling pathways regulates tamoxifen-resistant growth. *Breast Cancer Res. Treat.* **2006**, *96*, 131–146. [CrossRef] [PubMed]
53. Kumar, M.V.; Leo, M.E.; Tindall, D.J. Modulation of androgen receptor transcriptional activity by the estrogen receptor. *J. Androl.* **1994**, *15*, 534–542. [PubMed]
54. Peters, A.A.; Buchanan, G.; Ricciardelli, C.; Bianco-Miotto, T.; Centenera, M.M.; Harris, J.M.; Jindal, S.; Segara, D.; Jia, L.; Moore, N.L.; et al. Androgen receptor inhibits estrogen receptor-alpha activity and is prognostic in breast cancer. *Cancer Res.* **2009**, *69*, 6131–6140. [CrossRef] [PubMed]
55. Rechoum, Y.; Rovito, D.; Iacopetta, D.; Barone, I.; Ando, S.; Weigel, N.L.; O'Malley, B.W.; Brown, P.H.; Fuqua, S.A. AR collaborates with ERalpha in aromatase inhibitor-resistant breast cancer. *Breast Cancer Res. Treat.* **2014**, *147*, 473–485. [CrossRef] [PubMed]
56. Cochrane, D.R.; Bernales, S.; Jacobsen, B.M.; Cittelly, D.M.; Howe, E.N.; D'Amato, N.C.; Spoelstra, N.S.; Edgerton, S.M.; Jean, A.; Guerrero, J.; et al. Role of the androgen receptor in breast cancer and preclinical analysis of enzalutamide. *Breast Cancer Res.* **2014**. [CrossRef] [PubMed]
57. Osborne, C.K. Tamoxifen in the treatment of breast cancer. *N. Engl. J. Med.* **1998**, *339*, 1609–1618. [PubMed]
58. Toth-Fejel, S.; Cheek, J.; Calhoun, K.; Muller, P.; Pommier, R.F. Estrogen and androgen receptors as comediators of breast cancer cell proliferation: Providing a new therapeutic tool. *Arch. Surg.* **2004**, *139*, 50–54. [CrossRef] [PubMed]
59. De Amicis, F.; Thirugnansampanthan, J.; Cui, Y.; Selever, J.; Beyer, A.; Parra, I.; Weigel, N.L.; Herynk, M.H.; Tsimelzon, A.; Lewis, M.T.; et al. Androgen receptor overexpression induces tamoxifen resistance in human breast cancer cells. *Breast Cancer Res. Treat.* **2010**, *121*, 1–11. [CrossRef] [PubMed]
60. Ciupek, A.; Rechoum, Y.; Gu, G.; Gelsomino, L.; Beyer, A.R.; Brusco, L.; Covington, K.R.; Tsimelzon, A.; Fuqua, S.A. Androgen receptor promotes tamoxifen agonist activity by activation of EGFR in ERalpha-positive breast cancer. *Breast Cancer Res. Treat.* **2015**, *154*, 225–237. [CrossRef] [PubMed]
61. Qu, Q.; Mao, Y.; Fei, X.C.; Shen, K.W. The impact of androgen receptor expression on breast cancer survival: A retrospective study and meta-analysis. *PLoS ONE* **2013**, *8*, e82650. [CrossRef] [PubMed]
62. Aleskandarany, M.A.; Abduljabbar, R.; Ashankyty, I.; Elmouna, A.; Jerjees, D.; Ali, S.; Buluwela, L.; Diez-Rodriguez, M.; Caldas, C.; Green, A.R.; et al. Prognostic significance of androgen receptor expression in invasive breast cancer: Transcriptomic and protein expression analysis. *Breast Cancer Res. Treat.* **2016**, *159*, 215–227. [CrossRef] [PubMed]
63. Hu, R.; Dawood, S.; Holmes, M.D.; Collins, L.C.; Schnitt, S.J.; Cole, K.; Marotti, J.D.; Hankinson, S.E.; Colditz, G.A.; Tamimi, R.M. Androgen receptor expression and breast cancer survival in postmenopausal women. *Clin. Cancer Res.* **2011**, *17*, 1867–1874. [CrossRef] [PubMed]
64. Siegel, R.L.; Miller, K.D.; Jemal, A. Cancer statistics, 2016. *CA Cancer J. Clin.* **2016**, *66*, 7–30. [CrossRef] [PubMed]
65. Wenhui, Z.; Shuo, L.; Dabei, T.; Ying, P.; Zhipeng, W.; Lei, Z.; Xiaohui, H.; Jingshu, G.; Hongtao, S.; Qingyuan, Z. Androgen receptor expression in male breast cancer predicts inferior outcome and poor response to tamoxifen treatment. *Eur. J. Endocrinol.* **2014**, *171*, 527–533. [CrossRef] [PubMed]
66. Kwiatkowska, E.; Teresiak, M.; Filas, V.; Karczewska, A.; Breborowicz, D.; Mackiewicz, A. BRCA2 mutations and androgen receptor expression as independent predictors of outcome of male breast cancer patients. *Clin. Cancer Res.* **2003**, *9*, 4452–4459. [PubMed]
67. Pich, A.; Margaria, E.; Chiusa, L.; Candelaresi, G.; Dal Canton, O. Androgen receptor expression in male breast carcinoma: Lack of clinicopathological association. *Br. J. Cancer.* **1999**, *79*, 959–964. [CrossRef] [PubMed]
68. Munoz, F.; Quevedo, C.; Martin, M.E.; Alcazar, A.; Salinas, M.; Fando, J.L. Increased activity of eukaryotic initiation factor 2B in PC12 cells in response to differentiation by nerve growth factor. *J. Neurochem.* **1998**, *71*, 1905–1911. [CrossRef] [PubMed]

69. Castellano, I.; Allia, E.; Accortanzo, V.; Vandone, A.M.; Chiusa, L.; Arisio, R.; Durando, A.; Donadio, M.; Bussolati, G.; Coates, A.S.; et al. Androgen receptor expression is a significant prognostic factor in estrogen receptor positive breast cancers. *Breast Cancer Res. Treat.* **2010**, *124*, 607–617. [CrossRef] [PubMed]
70. Elebro, K.; Borgquist, S.; Simonsson, M.; Markkula, A.; Jirstrom, K.; Ingvar, C.; Rose, C.; Jernstrom, H. Combined Androgen and Estrogen Receptor Status in Breast Cancer: Treatment Prediction and Prognosis in a Population-Based Prospective Cohort. *Clin. Cancer Res.* **2015**, *21*, 3640–3650. [CrossRef] [PubMed]
71. Jiang, H.S.; Kuang, X.Y.; Sun, W.L.; Xu, Y.; Zheng, Y.Z.; Liu, Y.R.; Lang, G.T.; Qiao, F.; Hu, X.; Shao, Z.M. Androgen receptor expression predicts different clinical outcomes for breast cancer patients stratified by hormone receptor status. *Oncotarget.* **2016**, *7*, 41285–41293. [CrossRef] [PubMed]
72. Slamon, D.J.; Clark, G.M.; Wong, S.G.; Levin, W.J.; Ullrich, A.; McGuire, W.L. Human breast cancer: Correlation of relapse and survival with amplification of the HER-2/neu oncogene. *Science* **1987**, *235*, 177–182. [CrossRef] [PubMed]
73. Lal, P.; Tan, L.K.; Chen, B. Correlation of HER-2 status with estrogen and progesterone receptors and histologic features in 3,655 invasive breast carcinomas. *Am. J. Clin. Pathol.* **2005**, *123*, 541–546. [CrossRef] [PubMed]
74. Horiguchi, J.; Koibuchi, Y.; Iijima, K.; Yoshida, T.; Yoshida, M.; Takata, D.; Oyama, T.; Iino, Y.; Morishita, Y. Immunohistochemical double staining with estrogen receptor and HER2 on primary breast cancer. *Int. J. Mol. Med.* **2003**, *12*, 855–859. [CrossRef] [PubMed]
75. Sanga, S.; Broom, B.M.; Cristini, V.; Edgerton, M.E. Gene expression meta-analysis supports existence of molecular apocrine breast cancer with a role for androgen receptor and implies interactions with ErbB family. *BMC Med. Genom.* **2009**. [CrossRef] [PubMed]
76. Mellinghoff, I.K.; Vivanco, I.; Kwon, A.; Tran, C.; Wongvipat, J.; Sawyers, C.L. HER2/neu kinase-dependent modulation of androgen receptor function through effects on DNA binding and stability. *Cancer Cell* **2004**, *6*, 517–527. [CrossRef] [PubMed]
77. Chia, K.M.; Liu, J.; Francis, G.D.; Naderi, A. A feedback loop between androgen receptor and ERK signaling in estrogen receptor-negative breast cancer. *Neoplasia* **2011**, *13*, 154–166. [CrossRef] [PubMed]
78. Shigemura, K.; Isotani, S.; Wang, R.; Fujisawa, M.; Gotoh, A.; Marshall, F.F.; Zhau, H.E.; Chung, L.W. Soluble factors derived from stroma activated androgen receptor phosphorylation in human prostate LNCaP cells: Roles of ERK/MAP kinase. *Prostate* **2009**, *69*, 949–955. [CrossRef] [PubMed]
79. Mirosevich, J.; Gao, N.; Gupta, A.; Shappell, S.B.; Jove, R.; Matusik, R.J. Expression and role of Foxa proteins in prostate cancer. *Prostate* **2006**, *66*, 1013–1028. [CrossRef] [PubMed]
80. Lupien, M.; Eeckhoute, J.; Meyer, C.A.; Wang, Q.; Zhang, Y.; Li, W.; Carroll, J.S.; Liu, X.S.; Brown, M. FoxA1 translates epigenetic signatures into enhancer-driven lineage-specific transcription. *Cell* **2008**, *132*, 958–970. [CrossRef] [PubMed]
81. Ni, M.; Chen, Y.; Fei, T.; Li, D.; Lim, E.; Liu, X.S.; Brown, M. Amplitude modulation of androgen signaling by c-MYC. *Genes Dev.* **2013**, *27*, 734–748. [CrossRef] [PubMed]
82. Turashvili, G.; Bouchal, J.; Burkadze, G.; Kolar, Z. Wnt signaling pathway in mammary gland development and carcinogenesis. *Pathobiology* **2006**, *73*, 213–223. [CrossRef] [PubMed]
83. Garay, J.P.; Karakas, B.; Abukhdeir, A.M.; Cosgrove, D.P.; Gustin, J.P.; Higgins, M.J.; Konishi, H.; Konishi, Y.; Lauring, J.; Mohseni, M.; et al. The growth response to androgen receptor signaling in ERalpha-negative human breast cells is dependent on p21 and mediated by MAPK activation. *Breast Cancer Res.* **2012**. [CrossRef] [PubMed]
84. Wasielewski, M.; Elstrodt, F.; Klijn, J.G.; Berns, E.M.; Schutte, M. Thirteen new p53 gene mutants identified among 41 human breast cancer cell lines. *Breast Cancer Res. Treat.* **2006**, *99*, 97–101. [CrossRef] [PubMed]
85. She, Q.B.; Chandarlapaty, S.; Ye, Q.; Lobo, J.; Haskell, K.M.; Leander, K.R.; DeFeo-Jones, D.; Huber, H.E.; Rosen, N. Breast tumor cells with PI3K mutation or HER2 amplification are selectively addicted to Akt signaling. *PLoS ONE* **2008**, *3*, e3065. [CrossRef] [PubMed]
86. Schippinger, W.; Regitnig, P.; Dandachi, N.; Wernecke, K.D.; Bauernhofer, T.; Samonigg, H.; Moinfar, F. Evaluation of the prognostic significance of androgen receptor expression in metastatic breast cancer. *Virchows Arch.* **2006**, *449*, 24–30. [CrossRef] [PubMed]
87. Howlader, N.; Altekruse, S.F.; Li, C.I.; Chen, V.W.; Clarke, C.A.; Ries, L.A.; Cronin, K.A. US incidence of breast cancer subtypes defined by joint hormone receptor and HER2 status. *J. Natl. Cancer Inst.* **2014**. [CrossRef] [PubMed]

88. Rakha, E.A.; Elsheikh, S.E.; Aleskandarany, M.A.; Habashi, H.O.; Green, A.R.; Powe, D.G.; El-Sayed, M.E.; Benhasouna, A.; Brunet, J.S.; Akslen, L.A.; et al. Triple-negative breast cancer: Distinguishing between basal and nonbasal subtypes. *Clin. Cancer Res.* **2009**, *15*, 2302–2310. [CrossRef] [PubMed]
89. Kassam, F.; Enright, K.; Dent, R.; Dranitsaris, G.; Myers, J.; Flynn, C.; Fralick, M.; Kumar, R.; Clemons, M. Survival outcomes for patients with metastatic triple-negative breast cancer: Implications for clinical practice and trial design. *Clin. Breast Cancer* **2009**, *9*, 29–33. [CrossRef] [PubMed]
90. Dent, R.; Trudeau, M.; Pritchard, K.I.; Hanna, W.M.; Kahn, H.K.; Sawka, C.A.; Lickley, L.A.; Rawlinson, E.; Sun, P.; Narod, S.A. Triple-negative breast cancer: Clinical features and patterns of recurrence. *Clin. Cancer Res.* **2007**, *13*, 4429–4434. [CrossRef] [PubMed]
91. Boyle, P. Triple-negative breast cancer: Epidemiological considerations and recommendations. *Ann. Oncol.* **2012**, *23* (Suppl. S6), vi7–vi12. [CrossRef] [PubMed]
92. Bauer, K.R.; Brown, M.; Cress, R.D.; Parise, C.A.; Caggiano, V. Descriptive analysis of estrogen receptor (ER)-negative, progesterone receptor (PR)-negative, and HER2-negative invasive breast cancer, the so-called triple-negative phenotype: A population-based study from the California cancer Registry. *Cancer* **2007**, *109*, 1721–1728. [CrossRef] [PubMed]
93. Carey, L.A.; Perou, C.M.; Livasy, C.A.; Dressler, L.G.; Cowan, D.; Conway, K.; Karaca, G.; Troester, M.A.; Tse, C.K.; Edmiston, S.; et al. Race, breast cancer subtypes, and survival in the Carolina Breast Cancer Study. *JAMA* **2006**, *295*, 2492–2502. [CrossRef] [PubMed]
94. Lara-Medina, F.; Perez-Sanchez, V.; Saavedra-Perez, D.; Blake-Cerda, M.; Arce, C.; Motola-Kuba, D.; Villarreal-Garza, C.; Gonzalez-Angulo, A.M.; Bargallo, E.; Aguilar, J.L.; et al. Triple-negative breast cancer in Hispanic patients: High prevalence, poor prognosis, and association with menopausal status, body mass index, and parity. *Cancer* **2011**, *117*, 3658–3669. [CrossRef] [PubMed]
95. Kwan, M.L.; Kushi, L.H.; Weltzien, E.; Maring, B.; Kutner, S.E.; Fulton, R.S.; Lee, M.M.; Ambrosone, C.B.; Caan, B.J. Epidemiology of breast cancer subtypes in two prospective cohort studies of breast cancer survivors. *Breast Cancer Res.* **2009**. [CrossRef] [PubMed]
96. Metzger-Filho, O.; Tutt, A.; de Azambuja, E.; Saini, K.S.; Viale, G.; Loi, S.; Bradbury, I.; Bliss, J.M.; Azim, H.A., Jr.; Ellis, P.; et al. Dissecting the heterogeneity of triple-negative breast cancer. *J. Clin. Oncol.* **2012**, *30*, 1879–1887. [CrossRef] [PubMed]
97. Millikan, R.C.; Newman, B.; Tse, C.K.; Moorman, P.G.; Conway, K.; Dressler, L.G.; Smith, L.V.; Labbok, M.H.; Geradts, J.; Bensen, J.T.; et al. Epidemiology of basal-like breast cancer. *Breast Cancer Res. Treat.* **2008**, *109*, 123–139. [CrossRef] [PubMed]
98. Livasy, C.A.; Karaca, G.; Nanda, R.; Tretiakova, M.S.; Olopade, O.I.; Moore, D.T.; Perou, C.M. Phenotypic evaluation of the basal-like subtype of invasive breast carcinoma. *Mod. Pathol.* **2006**, *19*, 264–271. [CrossRef] [PubMed]
99. Nielsen, T.O.; Hsu, F.D.; Jensen, K.; Cheang, M.; Karaca, G.; Hu, Z.; Hernandez-Boussard, T.; Livasy, C.; Cowan, D.; Dressler, L.; et al. Immunohistochemical and clinical characterization of the basal-like subtype of invasive breast carcinoma. *Clin. Cancer Res.* **2004**, *10*, 5367–5374. [CrossRef] [PubMed]
100. Kennecke, H.; Yerushalmi, R.; Woods, R.; Cheang, M.C.; Voduc, D.; Speers, C.H.; Nielsen, T.O.; Gelmon, K. Metastatic behavior of breast cancer subtypes. *J. Clin. Oncol.* **2010**, *28*, 3271–3277. [CrossRef] [PubMed]
101. Prat, A.; Lluch, A.; Albanell, J.; Barry, W.T.; Fan, C.; Chacon, J.I.; Parker, J.S.; Calvo, L.; Plazaola, A.; Arcusa, A.; et al. Predicting response and survival in chemotherapy-treated triple-negative breast cancer. *Br. J. Cancer.* **2014**, *111*, 1532–1541. [CrossRef] [PubMed]
102. Sikov, W.M.; Berry, D.A.; Perou, C.M.; Singh, B.; Cirrincione, C.T.; Tolaney, S.M.; Kuzma, C.S.; Pluard, T.J.; Somlo, G.; Port, E.R.; et al. Impact of the addition of carboplatin and/or bevacizumab to neoadjuvant once-per-week paclitaxel followed by dose-dense doxorubicin and cyclophosphamide on pathologic complete response rates in stage II to III triple-negative breast cancer: CALGB 40603 (Alliance). *J. Clin. Oncol.* **2015**, *33*, 13–21. [PubMed]
103. Bastien, R.R.; Rodriguez-Lescure, A.; Ebbert, M.T.; Prat, A.; Munarriz, B.; Rowe, L.; Miller, P.; Ruiz-Borrego, M.; Anderson, D.; Lyons, B.; et al. PAM50 breast cancer subtyping by RT-qPCR and concordance with standard clinical molecular markers. *BMC Med. Genom.* **2012**. [CrossRef] [PubMed]

104. Prat, A.; Adamo, B.; Cheang, M.C.; Anders, C.K.; Carey, L.A.; Perou, C.M. Molecular characterization of basal-like and non-basal-like triple-negative breast cancer. *Oncologist* **2013**, *18*, 123–133. [CrossRef] [PubMed]
105. Lehmann, B.D.; Jovanovic, B.; Chen, X.; Estrada, M.V.; Johnson, K.N.; Shyr, Y.; Moses, H.L.; Sanders, M.E.; Pietenpol, J.A. Refinement of Triple-Negative Breast Cancer Molecular Subtypes: Implications for Neoadjuvant Chemotherapy Selection. *PLoS ONE* **2016**, *11*, e0157368. [CrossRef] [PubMed]
106. Yu, K.D.; Zhu, R.; Zhan, M.; Rodriguez, A.A.; Yang, W.; Wong, S.; Makris, A.; Lehmann, B.D.; Chen, X.; Mayer, I.; et al. Identification of prognosis-relevant subgroups in patients with chemoresistant triple-negative breast cancer. *Clin. Cancer Res.* **2013**, *19*, 2723–2733. [CrossRef] [PubMed]
107. Jezequel, P.; Loussouarn, D.; Guerin-Charbonnel, C.; Campion, L.; Vanier, A.; Gouraud, W.; Lasla, H.; Guette, C.; Valo, I.; Verriele, V.; et al. Gene-expression molecular subtyping of triple-negative breast cancer tumours: Importance of immune response. *Breast Cancer Res.* **2015**. [CrossRef] [PubMed]
108. Lehmann, B.D.; Bauer, J.A.; Schafer, J.M.; Pendleton, C.S.; Tang, L.; Johnson, K.C.; Chen, X.; Balko, J.M.; Gomez, H.; Arteaga, C.L.; et al. PIK3CA mutations in androgen receptor-positive triple negative breast cancer confer sensitivity to the combination of PI3K and androgen receptor inhibitors. *Breast Cancer Res.* **2014**. [CrossRef] [PubMed]
109. Ogawa, Y.; Hai, E.; Matsumoto, K.; Ikeda, K.; Tokunaga, S.; Nagahara, H.; Sakurai, K.; Inoue, T.; Nishiguchi, Y. Androgen receptor expression in breast cancer: Relationship with clinicopathological factors and biomarkers. *Int. J. Clin. Oncol.* **2008**, *13*, 431–435. [CrossRef] [PubMed]
110. Luo, X.; Shi, Y.X.; Li, Z.M.; Jiang, W.Q. Expression and clinical significance of androgen receptor in triple negative breast cancer. *Chin. J. Cancer* **2010**, *29*, 585–590. [CrossRef] [PubMed]
111. Rakha, E.A.; El-Sayed, M.E.; Green, A.R.; Lee, A.H.; Robertson, J.F.; Ellis, I.O. Prognostic markers in triple-negative breast cancer. *Cancer* **2007**, *109*, 25–32. [CrossRef] [PubMed]
112. Sutton, L.M.; Cao, D.; Sarode, V.; Molberg, K.H.; Torgbe, K.; Haley, B.; Peng, Y. Decreased androgen receptor expression is associated with distant metastases in patients with androgen receptor-expressing triple-negative breast carcinoma. *Am. J. Clin. Pathol.* **2012**, *138*, 511–516. [CrossRef] [PubMed]
113. Darb-Esfahani, S.; Denkert, C.; Stenzinger, A.; Salat, C.; Sinn, B.; Schem, C.; Endris, V.; Klare, P.; Schmitt, W.; Blohmer, J.U.; et al. Role of TP53 mutations in triple negative and HER2-positive breast cancer treated with neoadjuvant anthracycline/taxane-based chemotherapy. *Oncotarget* **2016**. [CrossRef] [PubMed]
114. He, J.; Peng, R.; Yuan, Z.; Wang, S.; Peng, J.; Lin, G.; Jiang, X.; Qin, T. Prognostic value of androgen receptor expression in operable triple-negative breast cancer: A retrospective analysis based on a tissue microarray. *Med. Oncol.* **2012**, *29*, 406–410. [CrossRef] [PubMed]
115. Tang, D.; Xu, S.; Zhang, Q.; Zhao, W. The expression and clinical significance of the androgen receptor and E-cadherin in triple-negative breast cancer. *Med. Oncol.* **2012**, *29*, 526–533. [CrossRef] [PubMed]
116. Loibl, S.; Muller, B.M.; von Minckwitz, G.; Schwabe, M.; Roller, M.; Darb-Esfahani, S.; Ataseven, B.; du Bois, A.; Fissler-Eckhoff, A.; Gerber, B.; et al. Androgen receptor expression in primary breast cancer and its predictive and prognostic value in patients treated with neoadjuvant chemotherapy. *Breast Cancer Res. Treat.* **2011**, *130*, 477–487. [CrossRef] [PubMed]
117. Pistelli, M.; Caramanti, M.; Biscotti, T.; Santinelli, A.; Pagliacci, A.; De Lisa, M.; Ballatore, Z.; Ridolfi, F.; Maccaroni, E.; Bracci, R.; et al. Androgen receptor expression in early triple-negative breast cancer: Clinical significance and prognostic associations. *Cancers* **2014**, *6*, 1351–1362. [CrossRef] [PubMed]
118. Park, S.; Koo, J.S.; Kim, M.S.; Park, H.S.; Lee, J.S.; Lee, J.S.; Kim, S.I.; Park, B.W.; Lee, K.S. Androgen receptor expression is significantly associated with better outcomes in estrogen receptor-positive breast cancers. *Ann. Oncol.* **2011**, *22*, 1755–1762. [CrossRef] [PubMed]
119. Gonzalez-Angulo, A.M.; Stemke-Hale, K.; Palla, S.L.; Carey, M.; Agarwal, R.; Meric-Berstam, F.; Traina, T.A.; Hudis, C.; Hortobagyi, G.N.; Gerald, W.L.; et al. Androgen receptor levels and association with PIK3CA mutations and prognosis in breast cancer. *Clin. Cancer Res.* **2009**, *15*, 2472–2478. [CrossRef] [PubMed]
120. Von Minckwitz, G.; Untch, M.; Blohmer, J.U.; Costa, S.D.; Eidtmann, H.; Fasching, P.A.; Gerber, B.; Eiermann, W.; Hilfrich, J.; Huober, J.; et al. Definition and impact of pathologic complete response on prognosis after neoadjuvant chemotherapy in various intrinsic breast cancer subtypes. *J. Clin. Oncol.* **2012**, *30*, 1796–1804. [CrossRef] [PubMed]
121. Asano, Y.; Kashiwagi, S.; Onoda, N.; Kurata, K.; Morisaki, T.; Noda, S.; Takashima, T.; Ohsawa, M.; Kitagawa, S.; Hirakawa, K. Clinical verification of sensitivity to preoperative chemotherapy in cases of androgen receptor-expressing positive breast cancer. *Br. J. Cancer* **2016**, *114*, 14–20. [CrossRef] [PubMed]

122. Jiang, T.; Shi, W.; Wali, V.B.; Pongor, L.S.; Li, C.; Lau, R.; Gyorffy, B.; Lifton, R.P.; Symmans, W.F.; Pusztai, L.; et al. Predictors of Chemosensitivity in Triple Negative Breast Cancer: An Integrated Genomic Analysis. *PLoS Med.* **2016**, *13*, e1002193. [CrossRef] [PubMed]
123. Robinson, J.L.; Macarthur, S.; Ross-Innes, C.S.; Tilley, W.D.; Neal, D.E.; Mills, I.G.; Carroll, J.S. Androgen receptor driven transcription in molecular apocrine breast cancer is mediated by FoxA1. *EMBO J.* **2011**, *30*, 3019–3027. [CrossRef] [PubMed]
124. Furr, B.J.; Valcaccia, B.; Curry, B.; Woodburn, J.R.; Chesterson, G.; Tucker, H. ICI 176,334: A novel non-steroidal, peripherally selective antiandrogen. *J. Endocrinol.* **1987**, *113*, R7–R9. [CrossRef] [PubMed]
125. Zhu, A.; Li, Y.; Song, W.; Xu, Y.; Yang, F.; Zhang, W.; Yin, Y.; Guan, X. Antiproliferative Effect of Androgen Receptor Inhibition in Mesenchymal Stem-Like Triple-Negative Breast Cancer. *Cell. Physiol. Biochem.* **2016**, *38*, 1003–1014. [CrossRef] [PubMed]
126. Graham, T.R.; Yacoub, R.; Taliaferro-Smith, L.; Osunkoya, A.O.; Odero-Marah, V.A.; Liu, T.; Kimbro, K.S.; Sharma, D.; O'Regan, R.M. Reciprocal regulation of ZEB1 and AR in triple negative breast cancer cells. *Breast Cancer Res. Treat.* **2010**, *123*, 139–147. [CrossRef] [PubMed]
127. Mehta, J.; Asthana, S.; Mandal, C.C.; Saxena, S. A molecular analysis provides novel insights into androgen receptor signalling in breast cancer. *PLoS ONE* **2015**, *10*, e0120622. [CrossRef] [PubMed]
128. Cuenca-Lopez, M.D.; Montero, J.C.; Morales, J.C.; Prat, A.; Pandiella, A.; Ocana, A. Phospho-kinase profile of triple negative breast cancer and androgen receptor signaling. *BMC Cancer* **2014**. [CrossRef] [PubMed]
129. Asghar, U.; Witkiewicz, A.K.; Turner, N.C.; Knudsen, E.S. The history and future of targeting cyclin-dependent kinases in cancer therapy. *Nat. Rev. Drug Discov.* **2015**, *14*, 130–146. [CrossRef] [PubMed]
130. Dickson, C.; Fantl, V.; Gillett, C.; Brookes, S.; Bartek, J.; Smith, R.; Fisher, C.; Barnes, D.; Peters, G. Amplification of chromosome band 11q13 and a role for cyclin D1 in human breast cancer. *Cancer Lett.* **1995**, *90*, 43–50. [CrossRef]
131. Korpal, M.; Korn, J.M.; Gao, X.; Rakiec, D.P.; Ruddy, D.A.; Doshi, S.; Yuan, J.; Kovats, S.G.; Kim, S.; Cooke, V.G.; et al. An F876L mutation in androgen receptor confers genetic and phenotypic resistance to MDV3100 (enzalutamide). *Cancer Discov.* **2013**, *3*, 1030–1043. [CrossRef] [PubMed]
132. National Cancer Institute (NCI). Palbociclib in Combination with Bicalutamide for the Treatment of AR+ Metastatic Breast Cancer. NCT02605486. Available online: https://clinicaltrials.gov/ct2/show/NCT02605486 (accessed on 9 November 2016).
133. Gucalp, A.; Tolaney, S.; Isakoff, S.J.; Ingle, J.N.; Liu, M.C.; Carey, L.A.; Blackwell, K.; Rugo, H.; Nabell, L.; Forero, A.; et al. Phase II trial of bicalutamide in patients with androgen receptor-positive, estrogen receptor-negative metastatic Breast Cancer. *Clin. Cancer Res.* **2013**, *19*, 5505–5512. [CrossRef] [PubMed]
134. Arce-Salinas, C.; Riesco-Martinez, M.C.; Hanna, W.; Bedard, P.; Warner, E. Complete Response of Metastatic Androgen Receptor-Positive Breast Cancer to Bicalutamide: Case Report and Review of the Literature. *J. Clin. Oncol.* **2016**, *34*, e21–e24. [CrossRef] [PubMed]
135. Zhao, T.P.; He, G.F. A phase II clinical trial of flutamide in the treatment of advanced breast cancer. *Tumori* **1988**, *74*, 53–56. [PubMed]
136. Perrault, D.J.; Logan, D.M.; Stewart, D.J.; Bramwell, V.H.; Paterson, A.H.; Eisenhauer, E.A. Phase II study of flutamide in patients with metastatic breast cancer. A National Cancer Institute of Canada Clinical Trials Group study. *Investig. New Drugs* **1988**, *6*, 207–210. [CrossRef]
137. Tran, C.; Ouk, S.; Clegg, N.J.; Chen, Y.; Watson, P.A.; Arora, V.; Wongvipat, J.; Smith-Jones, P.M.; Yoo, D.; Kwon, A.; et al. Development of a second-generation antiandrogen for treatment of advanced prostate cancer. *Science* **2009**, *324*, 787–790. [CrossRef] [PubMed]
138. D'Amato, N.C.; Gordon, M.A.; Babbs, B.; Spoelstra, N.S.; Carson Butterfield, K.T.; Torkko, K.C.; Phan, V.T.; Barton, V.N.; Rogers, T.J.; Sartorius, C.A.; et al. Cooperative Dynamics of AR and ER Activity in Breast Cancer. *Mol. Cancer Res.* **2016**, *14*, 154–1067. [CrossRef] [PubMed]
139. Robles, A.J.; Cai, S.; Cichewicz, R.H.; Mooberry, S.L. Selective activity of deguelin identifies therapeutic targets for androgen receptor-positive breast cancer. *Breast Cancer Res. Treat.* **2016**, *157*, 475–488. [CrossRef] [PubMed]
140. National Cancer Institute (NCI). Taselisib and Enzalutamide in Treating Patients with Androgen Receptor Positive Triple-Negative Metastatic Breast Cancer. NCT 02457910. Available online: https://clinicaltrials.gov/ct2/show/NCT02457910 (accessed on 9 November 2016).

141. Ardiani, A.; Farsaci, B.; Rogers, C.J.; Protter, A.; Guo, Z.; King, T.H.; Apelian, D.; Hodge, J.W. Combination therapy with a second-generation androgen receptor antagonist and a metastasis vaccine improves survival in a spontaneous prostate cancer model. *Clin. Cancer Res.* **2013**, *19*, 6205–6218. [CrossRef] [PubMed]
142. Kwilas, A.R.; Ardiani, A.; Gameiro, S.R.; Richards, J.; Hall, A.B.; Hodge, J.W. Androgen deprivation therapy sensitizes triple negative breast cancer cells to immune-mediated lysis through androgen receptor independent modulation of osteoprotegerin. *Oncotarget* **2016**, *7*, 23498–23511. [CrossRef] [PubMed]
143. Kwilas, A.R.; Ardiani, A.; Dirmeier, U.; Wottawah, C.; Schlom, J.; Hodge, J.W. A poxviral-based cancer vaccine the transcription factor twist inhibits primary tumor growth and metastases in a model of metastatic breast cancer and improves survival in a spontaneous prostate cancer model. *Oncotarget* **2015**, *6*, 28194–28210. [CrossRef] [PubMed]
144. National Cancer Institute (NCI). A Study to Assess the Efficacy and Safety of Enzalutamide with Trastuzumab in Subjects with Human Epidermal Growth Factor Receptor 2 Positive (HER2+), Androgen Receptor Positive (AR+) Metastatic or Locally Advanced Breast Cancer. NCT02091960. Available online: https://clinicaltrials.gov/ct2/show/NCT02091960 (accessed on 9 November 2016).
145. Traina, T.A. Results from a phase 2 study of enzalutamide (Enza), an androgen receptor (AR) inhibitor, in advanced AR+ triple-negative breast cancer. In Proceedings of the ASCO Annual Meeting, Chicago, IL, USA, 29 May–2 June 2015.
146. Parker, J.S.; Peterson, A.C.; Tudor, I.C.; Hoffman, J.; Uppal, H. A novel biomarker to predict sensitivity to enzalutamide in TNBC. In Proceedings of the ASCO Annual Meeting, Chicago, IL, USA, 29 May–2 June 2015.
147. National Cancer Institute (NCI). Phase IIB Neoadjuvant Enzalutamide (ZT) Plus Taxol for Androgen Receptor (AR)-Positive Triple-Negative Breast Cancer (AR+ TNBC). NCT02689427. Available online: https://clinicaltrials.gov/ct2/show/NCT02689427 (accessed on 9 November 2016).
148. National Cancer Institute (NCI). Feasibility Study of Adjuvant Enzalutamide for the Treatment of Early Stage AR (+) Triple Negative Breast Cancer. NCT02750358. Available online: https://clinicaltrials.gov/ct2/show/NCT02750358 (accessed on 9 November 2016).
149. Barrie, S.E.; Potter, G.A.; Goddard, P.M.; Haynes, B.P.; Dowsett, M.; Jarman, M. Pharmacology of novel steroidal inhibitors of cytochrome P450(17) alpha (17 alpha-hydroxylase/C17-20 lyase). *J. Steroid Biochem. Mol. Biol.* **1994**, *50*, 267–273. [CrossRef]
150. O'Shaughnessy, J.; Campone, M.; Brain, E.; Neven, P.; Hayes, D.; Bondarenko, I.; Griffin, T.W.; Martin, J.; De Porre, P.; Kheoh, T.; et al. Abiraterone acetate, exemestane or the combination in postmenopausal patients with estrogen receptor-positive metastatic breast cancer. *Ann. Oncol.* **2016**, *27*, 106–113. [CrossRef] [PubMed]
151. Li, W.; O'Shaughnessy, J.A.; Hayes, D.F.; Campone, M.; Bondarenko, I.; Zbarskaya, I.; Brain, E.; Stenina, M.; Ivanova, O.; Graas, M.P.; et al. Biomarker Associations with Efficacy of Abiraterone Acetate and Exemestane in Postmenopausal Patients with Estrogen Receptor-Positive Metastatic Breast Cancer. *Clin. Cancer Res.* **2016**, *22*, 6002–6009. [CrossRef] [PubMed]
152. Bonnefoi, H.; Grellety, T.; Tredan, O.; Saghatchian, M.; Dalenc, F.; Mailliez, A.; L'Haridon, T.; Cottu, P.; Abadie-Lacourtoisie, S.; You, B.; et al. A phase II trial of abiraterone acetate plus prednisone in patients with triple-negative androgen receptor positive locally advanced or metastatic breast cancer (UCBG 12-1). *Ann. Oncol.* **2016**, *27*, 812–818. [CrossRef] [PubMed]
153. National Cancer Institute (NCI). Abiraterone Acetate in Treating Postmenopausal Women with Advanced or Metastatic breast Cancer. NCT00755885. Available online: https://clinicaltrials.gov/ct2/show/NCT00755885 (accessed on 9 November 2016).
154. National Cancer Institute (NCI). AZD8186 First Time in Patient Ascending Dose Study. NCT01884285. Available online: https://clinicaltrials.gov/ct2/show/NCT01884285 (accessed on 9 November 2016).
155. Fizazi, K.; Jones, R.; Oudard, S.; Efstathiou, E.; Saad, F.; de Wit, R.; De Bono, J.; Cruz, F.M.; Fountzilas, G.; Ulys, A.; et al. Phase III, randomized, double-blind, multicenter trial comparing orteronel (TAK-700) plus prednisone with placebo plus prednisone in patients with metastatic castration-resistant prostate cancer that has progressed during or after docetaxel-based therapy: ELM-PC 5. *J. Clin. Oncol.* **2015**, *33*, 723–731. [PubMed]
156. Saad, F.; Fizazi, K.; Jinga, V.; Efstathiou, E.; Fong, P.C.; Hart, L.L.; Jones, R.; McDermott, R.; Wirth, M.; Suzuki, K.; et al. Orteronel plus prednisone in patients with chemotherapy-naive metastatic

castration-resistant prostate cancer (ELM-PC 4): A double-blind, multicentre, phase 3, randomised, placebo-controlled trial. *Lancet Oncol.* **2015**, *16*, 338–348. [CrossRef]

157. National Cancer Institute (NCI). Orteronel as Monotherapy in Patients with Metastatic Breast Cancer (MBC) that Expresses the Androgen Receptor *(AR)*. NCT01990209. Available online: https://clinicaltrials.gov/ct2/show/NCT01990209 (accessed on 9 November 2016).
158. National Cancer Institute (NCI). A Open-Label Study to Evaluate the Safety, Tolerability, Pharmacokinetics, Pharmacodynamics and Efficacy of VT-464 in Patients with Advanced Breast Cancer. NCT02580448. Available online: https://clinicaltrials.gov/ct2/show/NCT02580448 (accessed on 9 November 2016).
159. Kandil, S.; Westwell, A.D.; McGuigan, C. 7-Substituted umbelliferone derivatives as androgen receptor antagonists for the potential treatment of prostate and breast cancer. *Bioorg. Med. Chem. Lett.* **2016**, *26*, 2000–2004. [CrossRef] [PubMed]
160. Narayanan, R.; Ahn, S.; Cheney, M.D.; Yepuru, M.; Miller, D.D.; Steiner, M.S.; Dalton, J.T. Selective androgen receptor modulators (SARMs) negatively regulate triple-negative breast cancer growth and epithelial:mesenchymal stem cell signaling. *PLoS ONE* **2014**, *9*, e103202. [CrossRef] [PubMed]
161. National Cancer Institute (NCI). Efficacy and Safety of GTx-024 in Patients with Androgen Receptor-Positive Triple Negative Breast Cancer (AR+ TNBC). NCT02368691. Available online: https://clinicaltrials.gov/ct2/show/NCT02368691 (accessed on 9 November 2016).
162. Livraghi, L.; Garber, J.E. PARP inhibitors in the management of breast cancer: Current data and future prospects. *BMC Med.* **2015**. [CrossRef] [PubMed]
163. Park, J.J.; Irvine, R.A.; Buchanan, G.; Koh, S.S.; Park, J.M.; Tilley, W.D.; Stallcup, M.R.; Press, M.F.; Coetzee, G.A. Breast cancer susceptibility gene 1 (BRCAI) is a coactivator of the androgen receptor. *Cancer Res.* **2000**, *60*, 5946–5949. [PubMed]
164. Shin, S.; Verma, I.M. BRCA2 cooperates with histone acetyltransferases in androgen receptor-mediated transcription. *Proc. Natl. Acad. Sci. USA* **2003**, *100*, 7201–7206. [CrossRef] [PubMed]
165. Berns, E.M.; Dirkzwager-Kiel, M.J.; Kuenen-Boumeester, V.; Timmermans, M.; Verhoog, L.C.; van den Ouweland, A.M.; Meijer-Heijboer, H.; Klijn, J.G.; van der Kwast, T.H. Androgen pathway dysregulation in BRCA1-mutated breast tumors. *Breast Cancer Res. Treat.* **2003**, *79*, 121–127. [CrossRef] [PubMed]
166. Pristauz, G.; Petru, E.; Stacher, E.; Geigl, J.B.; Schwarzbraun, T.; Tsybrovskyy, O.; Winter, R.; Moinfar, F. Androgen receptor expression in breast cancer patients tested for BRCA1 and BRCA2 mutations. *Histopathology* **2010**, *57*, 877–884. [CrossRef] [PubMed]
167. Asangani, I.A.; Dommeti, V.L.; Wang, X.; Malik, R.; Cieslik, M.; Yang, R.; Escara-Wilke, J.; Wilder-Romans, K.; Dhanireddy, S.; Engelke, C.; et al. Therapeutic targeting of BET bromodomain proteins in castration-resistant prostate cancer. *Nature* **2014**, *510*, 278–282. [CrossRef] [PubMed]
168. Jang, M.K.; Mochizuki, K.; Zhou, M.; Jeong, H.S.; Brady, J.N.; Ozato, K. The bromodomain protein Brd4 is a positive regulatory component of P-TEFb and stimulates RNA polymerase II-dependent transcription. *Mol. Cell* **2005**, *19*, 523–534. [CrossRef] [PubMed]
169. Yang, Z.; Yik, J.H.; Chen, R.; He, N.; Jang, M.K.; Ozato, K.; Zhou, Q. Recruitment of P-TEFb for stimulation of transcriptional elongation by the bromodomain protein Brd4. *Mol. Cell* **2005**, *19*, 535–545. [CrossRef] [PubMed]
170. McCune, K.; Bhat-Nakshatri, P.; Thorat, M.A.; Nephew, K.P.; Badve, S.; Nakshatri, H. Prognosis of hormone-dependent breast cancers: Implications of the presence of dysfunctional transcriptional networks activated by insulin via the immune transcription factor T-bet. *Cancer Res.* **2010**, *70*, 685–696. [CrossRef] [PubMed]
171. Feng, Q.; Zhang, Z.; Shea, M.J.; Creighton, C.J.; Coarfa, C.; Hilsenbeck, S.G.; Lanz, R.; He, B.; Wang, L.; Fu, X.; et al. An epigenomic approach to therapy for tamoxifen-resistant breast cancer. *Cell Res.* **2014**, *24*, 809–819. [CrossRef] [PubMed]
172. Sengupta, S.; Biarnes, M.C.; Clarke, R.; Jordan, V.C. Inhibition of BET proteins impairs estrogen-mediated growth and transcription in breast cancers by pausing RNA polymerase advancement. *Breast Cancer Res. Treat.* **2015**, *150*, 265–278. [CrossRef] [PubMed]
173. Stuhlmiller, T.J.; Miller, S.M.; Zawistowski, J.S.; Nakamura, K.; Beltran, A.S.; Duncan, J.S.; Angus, S.P.; Collins, K.A.; Granger, D.A.; Reuther, R.A.; et al. Inhibition of Lapatinib-Induced Kinome Reprogramming

in ERBB2-Positive Breast Cancer by Targeting BET Family Bromodomains. *Cell Rep.* **2015**, *11*, 390–404. [CrossRef] [PubMed]

174. Stratikopoulos, E.E.; Dendy, M.; Szabolcs, M.; Khaykin, A.J.; Lefebvre, C.; Zhou, M.M.; Parsons, R. Kinase and BET Inhibitors Together Clamp Inhibition of PI3K Signaling and Overcome Resistance to Therapy. *Cancer Cell* **2015**, *27*, 837–851. [CrossRef] [PubMed]
175. Bihani, T.; Ezell, S.A.; Ladd, B.; Grosskurth, S.E.; Mazzola, A.M.; Pietras, M.; Reimer, C.; Zinda, M.; Fawell, S.; D'Cruz, C.M. Resistance to everolimus driven by epigenetic regulation of MYC in ER+ breast cancers. *Oncotarget* **2015**, *6*, 2407–2420. [CrossRef] [PubMed]
176. Borbely, G.; Haldosen, L.A.; Dahlman-Wright, K.; Zhao, C. Induction of USP17 by combining BET and HDAC inhibitors in breast cancer cells. *Oncotarget* **2015**, *6*, 33623–33635. [PubMed]
177. Perez-Pena, J.; Serrano-Heras, G.; Montero, J.C.; Corrales-Sanchez, V.; Pandiella, A.; Ocana, A. In Silico Analysis Guides Selection of BET Inhibitors for Triple-Negative Breast Cancer Treatment. *Mol. Cancer Ther.* **2016**, *15*, 1823–1833. [CrossRef] [PubMed]
178. Da Motta, L.L.; Ledaki, I.; Purshouse, K.; Haider, S.; De Bastiani, M.A.; Baban, D.; Morotti, M.; Steers, G.; Wigfield, S.; Bridges, E.; et al. The BET inhibitor JQ1 selectively impairs tumour response to hypoxia and downregulates CA9 and angiogenesis in triple negative breast cancer. *Oncogene* **2017**, *36*, 122–132. [CrossRef] [PubMed]
179. Sahni, J.M.; Gayle, S.S.; Bonk, K.L.; Vite, L.C.; Yori, J.L.; Webb, B.; Ramos, E.K.; Seachrist, D.D.; Landis, M.D.; Chang, J.C.; et al. Bromodomain and Extraterminal Protein Inhibition Blocks Growth of Triple-negative Breast Cancers through the Suppression of Aurora Kinases. *J. Biol. Chem.* **2016**, *291*, 23756–23768. [CrossRef] [PubMed]
180. National Cancer Institute (NCI). A Dose-Finding Study of OTX105/MK-8628, a Small Molecule Inhibitor of the Bromodomain and Extra-Terminal (BET) Proteins, in Adults with Selected Advanced Solid Tumors (MK-8628-003). NCT02259114. Available online: https://clinicaltrials.gov/ct2/show/NCT02259114 (accessed on 9 November 2016).
181. National Cancer Institute (NCI). A Dose Exploration Study with MK-8628 in Participants with Selected Advanced Solid Tumors (MK-8628-006). NCT02698176. Available online: https://clinicaltrials.gov/ct2/show/NCT02698176 (accessed on 9 November 2016).
182. National Cancer Institute (NCI). A Study to Investigate Safety, Pharmacokinetics, Pharmacodynamics, and Clinical Activity of GSK525762 in Subjects with NUT Midline Carcinoma (NMC) and Other Cancers. NCT01587703. Available online: https://clinicaltrials.gov/ct2/show/NCT01587703 (accessed on 9 November 2016).
183. Burdall, S.E.; Hanby, A.M.; Lansdown, M.R.; Speirs, V. Breast cancer cell lines: Friend or foe? *Breast Cancer Res.* **2003**, *5*, 89–95. [CrossRef] [PubMed]

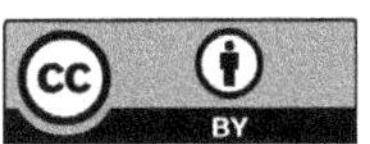

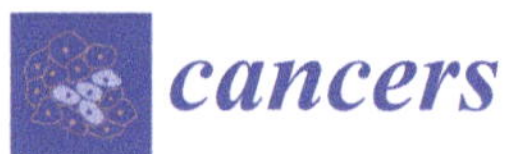 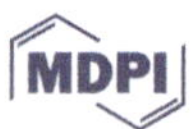

Review

Androgen Receptor: A Complex Therapeutic Target for Breast Cancer

Ramesh Narayanan [1] and James T. Dalton [2,*]

[1] Department of Medicine, University of Tennessee Health Science Center, Memphis, TN 38103, USA; rnaraya4@uthsc.edu
[2] College of Pharmacy, University of Michigan, Ann Arbor, MI 48109, USA
* Correspondence: daltonjt@umich.edu

Academic Editor: Emmanuel S. Antonarakis
Received: 28 September 2016; Accepted: 23 November 2016; Published: 2 December 2016

Abstract: Molecular and histopathological profiling have classified breast cancer into multiple sub-types empowering precision treatment. Although estrogen receptor (ER) and human epidermal growth factor receptor (HER2) are the mainstay therapeutic targets in breast cancer, the androgen receptor (AR) is evolving as a molecular target for cancers that have developed resistance to conventional treatments. The high expression of AR in breast cancer and recent discovery and development of new nonsteroidal drugs targeting the AR provide a strong rationale for exploring it again as a therapeutic target in this disease. Ironically, both nonsteroidal agonists and antagonists for the AR are undergoing clinical trials, making AR a complicated target to understand in breast cancer. This review provides a detailed account of AR's therapeutic role in breast cancer.

Keywords: androgen receptor; breast cancer; selective androgen receptor modulator (SARM); estrogen receptor; triple-negative breast cancer (TNBC)

---

1. Introduction

Over 240,000 women will develop breast cancer and ~40,000 will die from the disease in the United States in 2016 [1]. Globally, about 1.7 million women were diagnosed with breast cancer in 2012, emphasizing the urgent need for effective and safe therapeutic approaches [2]. Although the majority of breast cancers are slow growing or indolent [3], a subset acquires an aggressive phenotype due to a variety of reasons. Molecular, genotypic, and phenotypic studies clearly provide evidence for the heterogeneity of breast cancer with multiple subtypes and classifications [4,5].

2. Breast Cancer Classification

For therapeutic purposes, breast cancer has been historically classified based on the expression or lack of expression of estrogen receptor (ER), progesterone receptor (PR), and human epidermal growth factor receptor (HER2) [6]. Breast cancers expressing these three targets are classified as triple-positive, while those that lack their expression are classified as triple-negative (TNBC).

In 2000, Perou et al. completed a genome-wide molecular analysis of patient specimens to classify breast cancer based on cell-type and molecular signature [4]. Breast cancer specimens that expressed keratin 8/18, markers of luminal epithelial cells, were classified as luminal breast cancers, while those that expressed keratin 5/6, markers of basal epithelial cells, were classified as basal breast cancer. Further, using gene expression signatures, breast cancers were classified into luminal A, luminal B, HER2-enriched, and basal-like (BLBC).

The luminal A subtype is characterized by the expression of ER, lack of HER2, and a lower expression of the proliferative marker, Ki67 (ER+/HER2-/Ki67 low). The luminal A subtype is an indolent disease that is typically treated with hormonal therapies that either antagonize or degrade ER or inhibit aromatase, an enzyme critically involved in biosynthesis of estradiol.

The luminal B subtype is characterized by the expression of ER, lack of HER2, and high Ki67 (ER+/HER2-/Ki67 high). Although luminal B is predominantly HER2-negative, a subset of it expresses HER2 while still retaining other characteristics of HER2-negative luminal B. Markers of proliferation such as cyclin B1 (CCNB1), Ki67 (MKI67), and Myb proto-oncogene like 2 (MYBL2) [7,8] and proliferative growth factor signaling [9,10] are highly expressed in the luminal B subtype. The luminal B subtype is associated with high recurrence, poor disease-free survival [7] with much lower five- and ten- year survival rates than the luminal A subtype [7,11,12], and failure to respond consistently to any existing treatments [13].

The HER2 subtype is comprised of tumors that are ER-negative and HER2-positive [4]. This subtype is treated with HER2 inhibitors such as traztuzumab. The HER2 subtype frequently metastasizes to brain [14], escaping further inhibition by HER2-targeting antibodies that seldom cross the blood-brain barrier due to their large size.

The BLBC subtype is the most aggressive subtype of breast cancer and is associated with high mortality in women. While 75%–80% of the basal subtype is TNBC, the remaining 20%–25% express ER and/or HER2 [15]. It is still regarded as TNBC for therapeutic purposes and treated with a cocktail of chemotherapeutic agents that provide a pCR of about 40%–45% [16]. The cancer genome atlas (TCGA) studies indicate that the basal subtype has several features, including a high percentage of p53 mutations that confer an ovarian cancer phenotype rather than breast cancer [17].

3. TNBC Sub-Classification

Genome-wide studies to understand the underlying mechanisms for the aggressive phenotype of TNBC and to identify new therapeutic targets led to the classification of TNBC into six subtypes [5], including: Basal-like (BL1 and BL2) subtypes that are enriched in genes representing cell cycle, cell division, and DNA damage response. These two subtypes also express high levels of Ki67 at about 70% compared to 42% for other subtypes. Immunomodulatory (IM) subtype that is enriched in genes representing immune cell signaling. Mesenchymal (M) and mesenchymal stem cell like (MSL) subtypes that are enriched in pathways involved in cell motility, kinases, and differentiation. Luminal Androgen Receptor (LAR) subtype with high expression of Androgen Receptor (AR) mRNA and enrichment of hormonal signaling.

This subtyping provides an opportunity to develop focused therapeutics and conduct clinical trials in which the subjects belong to a particular subtype.

4. Androgen Receptor

The AR is a member of the nuclear hormone receptor family of ligand-activated transcription factors that is activated by androgen (i.e., testosterone or its locally synthesized and more potent metabolite, dihydrotestosterone (DHT). The AR gene is located on the X chromosome at q11 and contains eight exons encoding for an N terminus domain (NTD), a DNA binding domain (DBD), a hinge region, and a ligand binding domain (LBD). The NTD contains the activation function 1 domain (AF-1) that retains most of the AR activity [18]. The DBD contains two zinc finger motifs that recognize consensus androgen response elements (AREs) and anchoring of the AR to recognized sequences [19]. The hinge region is responsible for nucleo-cytoplasmic shuttling of the AR and the LBD that contains the ligand binding pocket is important for ligand recognition. The LBD of the AR contains 11 helices (unlike other receptors that contain 12 helices as the AR lacks helix 2) and the AF-2 domain [20].

The unliganded AR is maintained in an inactive complex by heat shock proteins, HSP-70 and HSP-90. Upon ligand binding, the HSPs dissociate from the AR enabling it to translocate into the nucleus and bind to DNA elements that are located both proximal and distal to the transcription start site [21]. Once bound to DNA, the AR recruits coactivators and general transcription factors to alter the transcription and translation of the target genes. While agonists recruit coactivators to augment transcription and translation of target genes, antagonists either recruit corepressors, prevent coactivators from associating with the AR, or retain the AR in the cytoplasm resulting in inactive AR.

5. Prognostic Value of the AR in Breast Cancer

Perhaps surprisingly, the AR is the most widely expressed nuclear hormone receptor in breast cancer with about 85%–95% of the ER-positive and 15%–70% of the ER-negative breast cancers expressing AR. In a study conducted with 2171 patient specimens, AR was found to be expressed in 77% of invasive breast carcinomas [22]. About 91% of the luminal A subtype tumors were positive for the AR, while 68% of the luminal B and 59% of the HER2 subtypes were positive for the AR. In addition, 32% of BLBCs expressed the AR in this cohort of 2171 patient specimens [22]. Interestingly, the study found an inverse correlation between the AR expression and tumor size, lymph node status, and histological grade. A higher proportion of the AR-positive tumors had smaller size compared to AR-negative tumors (24.6% vs. 15.8% for tumors less than 1 cm). Similarly, the majority of the AR-negative tumors were histological grade 3 tumors, while AR-positive tumors typically were histological grades 1 and 2 [22].

A review of a database containing data from 19 studies with a total of 7693 women demonstrated that the AR is expressed in 61% of the patients [23]. While 75% of the ER-positive tumors expressed AR, only 32% of the ER-negative breast cancers expressed the AR [23]. Tumors that expressed the AR were associated with improved overall survival (OS) and disease-free survival (DFS) compared to AR-negative tumors [23]. Considering the significance in this finding, the authors recommended that the AR be considered as one of three prognostic markers to classify breast cancers as triple-positive (ER, HER2, and AR-expressing) or triple-negative (ER, HER2, and AR-negative). Since *PR* is an ER-target gene, *PR* is most likely to align with ER expression pattern and hence was logical to exclude from the list of prognostic markers. These results were reproduced in other studies conducted in different patient cohorts around the world [24–29], including one clearly showing that expression of the AR was associated with reduced recurrence of the disease and reduced incidence of death in TNBC [28].

Noh et al. included 334 ER-negative HER2-positive or -negative breast cancers in a study to evaluate the expression of AR and clinical outcome [30]. Most of the AR-negative breast cancer patients were younger and had higher Ki67 compared to AR-positive breast cancer patients. While 27% of the TNBC patients were AR-positive, 53% of the ER-negative HER2-positive patients were AR-positive. Metabolic markers such as carbonic anhydrase (CAIX), which are associated with shorter DFS and OS, were significantly lower in AR-positive TNBC and ER-negative tumors [30].

One of the breast cancer subtypes where AR's prognostic value was debated is the molecular apocrine type [31]. Molecular apocrine breast cancers, which constitute about 5%–10% of the breast cancers, are ER- and PR- negative [31,32]. The lack of these hormone receptors makes them unresponsive to associated hormonal therapies. One of the unique features of the molecular apocrine breast cancers is that they express AR, potentially making AR a valuable prognostic and therapeutic target [5]. Since AR and androgens increase the proliferation of a molecular apocrine breast cancer cell line, MDA-MB-453, it is widely perceived, albeit falsely, that AR is an unfavorable therapeutic target and prognostic marker in molecular apocrine subtype [33,34]. However, a study compared 20 molecular apocrine cancers with 26 non-apocrine cancers for AR expression and other clinical features [35]. All apocrine carcinomas were AR-positive, while all non-apocrine tumors were AR-negative. While apocrine tumors had grades between G1 and G3 and low T stage (TNM classification where T corresponds to tumor size), all non-apocrine tumors were G3 and high T stage. In addition, 80% of the apocrine tumor patients showed no disease-related mortality. These results present additional evidence to support the idea that the AR is a good prognostic marker with potentially favorable function in breast cancer.

In addition to measuring AR expression, some studies measured the expression of androgen-synthesizing enzymes such as 17βHSD5 (also known as AKR1C3) and 5α-reductase. 17βHSD5 converts the weaker androgen, androstenedione, to a more potent testosterone, while 5α-reductase further amplifies the activity by converting testosterone to the more highly potent DHT [36]. McNamara et al. evaluated 203 TNBC specimens from Thailand and Japan in a study to measure the expression of the AR and androgen-synthesizing enzymes [37]. While 25% of the patients were AR-positive, 72% were 5α-reductase-positive and 70% were 17βHSD5-positive. AR expression inversely correlated with Ki67 staining. Co-expression of the AR and androgen-synthesizing enzymes negatively correlated with Ki67 staining. Although no significant improvement in OS and DFS was observed in the AR- and 5α-reductase- positive cohort, the AR-negative 5α-reductase-positive cohort had worse survival in an 80 month follow-up.

A recent study evaluated the expression of AR and other genes in 1141 patient specimens [38]. Nuclear AR expression, which is an indirect measure of activated AR, was associated with favorable prognosis such as smaller tumor size, lower grade, and overall survival, suggesting that AR activation is favorable in breast cancer [38]. These observations were more pronounced in the luminal breast cancer subtypes [38].

An overwhelming number of publications demonstrate that the AR is a favorable prognostic marker (i.e., that the AR is a protective protein), regardless of the tumor subtype, and suggest that in most, if not all, cases AR expression is inversely proportional to tumor size, aggressiveness, pathological grade, and directly proportional to DFS, progression-free survival (PFS), and OS. However, a few reports have identified a subset of cancers where AR expression is directly proportional to Ki67 staining and correlates with poorer OS and DFS [39,40]. For example, a study conducted in a Chinese cohort of 450 breast cancer patients [40] showed that AR expression correlated with an increase in DFS in luminal breast cancer patients but a decrease in DFS in patients with TNBC. These results further illustrate the complex role of the AR in breast cancer. This information is summarized in Table 1.

Table 1. Summary of studies showing the prognostic value of androgen receptor (AR) expression in breast cancer.

Reference	Ref	Summary
Pistelli et al., 2014	[29]	• AR expression in TNBC (n = 81) was inversely correlated with Ki67 ($p < 0.0001$).
Vera-Badillo et al., 2014	[23]	• A review of data from 19 studies that included 7693 women. • AR expression was associated with improved OS and DFS (both in ER + ve and TNBC) at both 3 and 5 years $p < 0.001$).
Noh et al., 2014	[30]	• 334 ER − ve (HER2 + ve or −ve) cases were included in this study. • AR − ve Her2 − ve patients were younger and had higher ki67 than AR + ve patients. • Metabolic markers such as CAIX, which are associated with shorter DFS and OS, were lower in AR + ve Her2 − ve cancers
Sultana et al., 2014	[24]	• Patients (in a study that included 200 women) with AR + ve tumors had higher OS. • AR + ve ER-ve women had a trend for longer OS and encountered only 2 deaths (n = 16). On the other hand, AR − ve ER − ve women had shorter OS and had 10 deaths (n = 37).
McNamara et al., 2014	[25]	• AR expression was associated with lower ki67, mostly TNBCs. • AR was the only correlative marker for ki67 staining (lower)
McNamara et al., 2013	[37]	• 25% (51 samples) of 203 TNBC patients were AR + ve, 72% for 5-α reductase and 70% for 17βHSD5. • AR negatively correlated with ki67. • Co-expression of AR and androgenic enzymes negatively correlated with ki67 staining. • AR − ve 5αR group had worse survival in an 80 month follow up.
Luo et al., 2010	[26]	• Of 137 TNBC patients 38 were AR + ve. Of 132 non-TNBC patients 110 were AR + ve. • AR + ve correlated with 5 year survival in TNBC, but not in non-TNBC.

Table 1. *Cont.*

Reference	Ref	Summary
Agoff et al., 2003	[28]	• 89% of ER + ve (n = 19) and 49% of ER − ve (n = 69) tumors were AR + ve. • Patients with ER − ve and AR + ve tumors were older than AR − ve patients. AR − ve tumors had higher ki67 staining. • ER − ve AR + ve tumors were lower grade, smaller and Her-2/neu over-expression. • In ER + ve tumors AR positivity correlates with PR positivity. • 84% of ER − ve, AR + ve patients were disease free after treatment, while only 53% of ER − ve, AR − ve patients were disease free after treatment. • None of the ER-negative, AR-positive patients died, while 4 of ER-negative, AR-negative patients died.
Qu et al., 2013	[27]	• 109 breast cancer (ER + ve, ER − ve, TNBC) were included in this study. • AR + ve breast cancers (all types) had better OS and DFS. • AR was also associated with lower risk of recurrence.

6. AR as Predictor of Therapeutic Response

While the above studies strongly suggest that AR expression predicts favorable prognosis, AR expression also provides information on the treatment response. In a study evaluating 913 patients, AR expression was associated with a favorable outcome to treatment [41]. Patients with tumors that expressed ER, but not AR, failed aromatase inhibitor (AI) therapy earlier. Since aromatase converts testosterone to estradiol, inhibiting the enzyme will potentially increase intracellular testosterone, an AR agonist. This observation suggests that activation of the AR is an important factor for sustained therapeutic outcome with AI. In addition to the above study, an interesting observation [42] indicated that patients with AR-positive tumors benefited from tamoxifen treatment, whereas patients with AR-negative tumors had worse outcome.

Loibl et al. evaluated 673 core primary breast cancer biopsies from patients who have received neoadjuvant chemotherapy [43]. AR was detected in 53% of the entire cohort with 67% in luminal A and 21% in TNBC. Similar to several other studies, AR expression correlated with better DFS and OS in both luminal breast cancer and TNBC. However, the pathological complete response (pCR) in the AR-positive group was only 13%, which is similar to rates observed for the luminal A subtype, compared to 25% in the AR-negative cohort, which is similar to rates observed in the luminal B or TNBC subtype. This data indicates that the AR-negative cohort had a better chance of attaining pCR and provides evidence that, regardless of the breast cancer subtype and ER/PR/HER2 expression, AR-expressing tumors appear to retain the characteristics of the luminal A subtype when responding to chemotherapeutic agents. This hypothesis was corroborated by other studies. Lehmann et al. in their TNBC sub-classification study found that the LAR subtype of the TNBC expressed a luminal gene expression pattern including luminal markers such as FOXA1, KRT18, and XBP1 [5]. Indolent AR-positive luminal A subtype has a pCR of only 10% in response to chemotherapeutic agents, while the BLBC or TNBC tumors have approximately 50% pCR [16,44]. In addition, out of the six molecular subtypes in TNBC, basal-like is the only subtype that provided a significant association between pCR and survival after chemotherapy [45].

7. Role of Intracrine Androgen Synthesis in Breast Cancer

Intracrine hormone synthesis in breast and prostate cancers has been recognized in the recent years as a vital but previously unrecognized driver of continued tumor growth [46–48]. Fernand Labrie's elegant work in this area for over two decades shed light on how, why, when, and the extent to which intracrine hormone synthesis occurs [46,47,49,50]. Studies have shown that estradiol concentrations were significantly higher intra-tumorally compared to serum and that the levels did not differ between pre- and post- menopausal women [51]. Also, estradiol concentration was >2 fold higher in breast carcinoma tissues than in surrounding normal tissues [52]. Recchione et al. determined the serum and tumor levels of estradiol, testosterone, and DHT in 34 patient specimens [53]. While the levels of testosterone were comparable between serum and tumor tissues, the concentration of estradiol and DHT was much higher in the tumor tissues than in blood [53]. In addition, cancers of the breast and prostate overcome pharmacological inhibition by synthesizing hormones through unconventional pathways [54–58]. These data support the importance of intracrine hormone synthesis in breast cancer.

The activation and inactivation of steroid hormones are influenced by a class of enzymes called hydroxysteroid dehydrogenases (HSD), which catalyze the NAD(P)(H)-dependent oxidoreduction of the hydroxyl/keto groups of androgens, estrogens and their precursors [59,60] and thereby regulate the intracellular availability of steroid hormone ligands to their receptors [61]. HSDs modify the 3, 5, 11, 17, or 20 positions of the steroid backbone [61–63]. Fourteen of these enzymes are classified as mammalian 17β-HSDs [59]. Between 75% and 100% of circulating estradiol in pre- and post- menopausal women, respectively, is synthesized from adrenal precursors by steroidogenic enzymes (i.e., the 17-βHSD family and aromatase) [46,64]. One of the fourteen 17-βHSDs important for the activation of adrenal precursors is aldo keto reductase 1C3 (17-βHSD5 or AKR1C3). AKR1C3 converts estrone to estradiol, androstenedione (A′dione) to testosterone, and progesterone to 20α-hydroxy progesterone [65–67] (Figure 1).

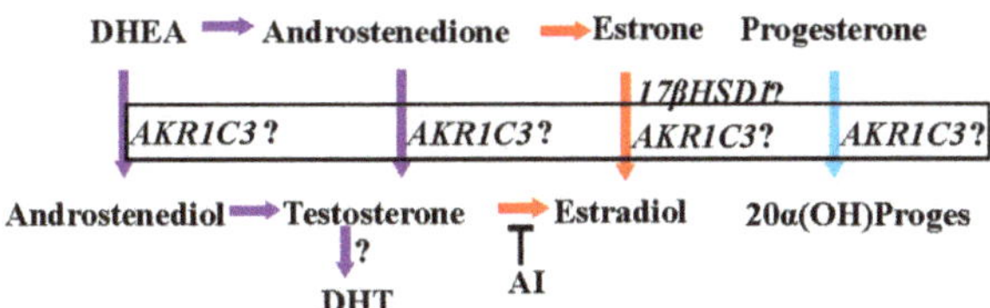

Figure 1. Intracrine synthesis of androgens, estrogens, and progesterone. AI: aromatase inhibitor; ?: functional importance in clinical breast cancer is not clear.

Estrogens in pre-menopausal and post-menopausal women are synthesized from their adrenal androgen precursors, dihydroepiandrosterone sulphate (DHEAS) and dihydroepiandrosterone (DHEA) [46]. DHEAS and DHEA are converted to androstenedione (4′dione) and then to highly active androgens and estrogens in peripheral tissues. Tumor protective functions have been attributed to these adrenal androgen precursors. On one hand, low circulating levels of DHEA and DHEAS have been found in patients with breast cancer [68]. On the other hand, administration of DHEA and maintenance of serum DHEA levels similar to that of healthy pre-menopausal women resulted in significant inhibition of mammary carcinogenesis in rats [69]. Further, DHT was detected at higher concentrations in breast cancer tissues [53], supporting the hypothesis that a combination of AR expression and higher DHT levels are associated with a favorable prognosis in AR-expressing breast cancer tissues.

Together, these lines of evidence suggest that intracrine androgen synthesis, higher androgen concentrations, and AR expression are strongly associated with a better prognosis, favorable therapeutic outcome, and a reduction in tumor in patients with AR-positive breast cancers.

8. AR as Therapeutic Target for Breast Cancer

Steroidal androgens were the mainstay of clinical treatment for breast cancer before the discovery of tamoxifen or other ER antagonists and AIs [70,71]. Early preclinical evidence for the anti-proliferative effects was generated in 1950s when Huggins and colleagues showed shrinkage of chemically-induced mammary tumors by ovariectomy or by the administration of DHT, long before either the ER or AR had been cloned [72–74]. However, the use of androgens was discontinued after the discovery of ER antagonists or selective estrogen receptor modulators (SERMs) and AIs, owing largely to the undesirable masculinizing effects of steroidal androgens and the commercial promise of the newer therapies.

Despite or perhaps because of plentiful historical evidence, a controversy remains with respect to whether an AR agonist such as an androgen or an AR antagonist will be effective in treating breast cancer. The conflict is primarily due to the skewed outcome of experiments performed with preclinical immortalized cell line models. Below we summarize the clinical and preclinical evidence supporting the use of both AR agonists and antagonists as treatment options for breast cancer.

9. Preclinical Evidence Supporting the Beneficial Effects of AR agonists in Breast Cancer

Preclinical models to evaluate the role of the AR in breast cancer are highly variable. ZR-75-1 is an ER-positive luminal A breast cancer cell line that expresses high levels of the AR. Treatment of this cell line with DHT resulted in significant growth inhibition [75]. DHT inhibited both estradiol-dependent and estradiol–independent growth completely [75]. Unlike other cell lines, ZR-75-1 responds to physiologically relevant concentrations of DHT. These anti-proliferative effects were reversed by hydroxyflutamide, an AR antagonist. These in vitro results were extended in vivo in ovariectomized, estradiol-supplemented, nude mice bearing ZR-75-1 tumors [76]. In this study, DHT completely inhibited the tumor growth and even regressed the tumors. Due to very slow growth properties of ZR-75-1 cells, which is characteristic of ER-positive luminal A tumors, it is difficult to conduct xenograft studies in this model.

Tilley and colleagues using MCF-7 and T47D ER- and AR- positive luminal breast cancer cell lines demonstrated that two steroidal androgens (DHT and mibolerone) inhibited the cell proliferation [77]. Although the inhibition of proliferation was not as robust as that obtained in ZR-75-1 cells, the inhibition was also reversed by AR antagonists [77]. The differences in the magnitude of effects between cell lines could be due to the level of AR expression. MCF-7 cells have relatively lower AR expression compared to ZR-75-1 cells. Studies have also shown that androgens induce apoptosis in MCF-7 cells. On the other hand, some studies have also reported growth-stimulatory effects of androgens in modified MCF-7 cells [78]. Although these results define the variability in cell-based models, predominantly anti-proliferative effects were observed with androgens in ER- and AR-positive cells.

More convincing results evolved from the dimethylbenzanthracene (DMBA)-induced mammary carcinogenesis rat model [76]. Rats bearing DMBA-induced mammary tumors regressed significantly when treated with either strong androgens such as DHT or with weak androgen precursors such as DHEA, DHEAS, or 4′dione [69,76]. All these in vitro and in vivo results in multiple models unequivocally prove that AR agonists are inhibitors of ER-positive luminal breast cancers.

When analyzing the preclinical data in TNBC or BLBC models, the landscape is complex and inconclusive. Most of the data were generated in one ER-negative apocrine breast cancer cell line, MDA-MB-453. The proliferation of MDA-MB-453 cells or growth of MDA-MB-453 xenografts are stimulated by androgens and inhibited by AR antagonists [33,79]. It is yet unclear if the mutation in the AR LBD, p53, and PTEN, and constitutive activation of PIK3CA contribute to this phenotype of the cells [34,80]. However, ectopic expression of wildtype AR in MDA-MB-231 ER-negative cells restored the growth inhibitory effects of steroidal androgens and selective androgen receptor modulators (SARMs), which could be partially reversed by AR antagonists [79].

Barton et al. used TNBC cell lines to evaluate the effect of DHT [81]. Treatment of SUM159PT, HCC1806, BT549, and MDA-MB-231 cells with 10 nM DHT increased the proliferation of only SUM159PT, but not the other cell lines, while the proliferation of all cell lines was inhibited by enzalutamide, a nonsteroidal AR antagonist. The induction of proliferation by DHT in SUM159PT cells was modest. For unknown reasons, the proliferation of BT549 cells, which express AR at a level comparable to that of SUM159PT, was not induced by DHT. Growth of all cell lines was inhibited by AR antagonist enzalutamide or AR siRNA.

Ince and colleagues evaluated the effect of DHT in various ER-negative and TNBC cell lines [82,83]. While 10 nM DHT inhibited the proliferation of AR-positive CAL-148, MFM-223, and BT-474 in 8–10 days, DHT failed to inhibit the proliferation of AR-negative MDA-MB-468, SUM-159PT, or BT-20 cells. This group also evaluated the AR antagonist enzalutamide in these cell lines; some of which express the AR and some of which do not express the AR [82]. While enzalutamide inhibited the proliferation of prostate cancer cell lines with a 5-fold difference in IC_{50} values between AR-positive and -negative prostate cancer cell lines, it inhibited TNBC cell lines at comparable concentrations regardless of the AR expression. These results suggest that the effect of AR antagonist enzalutamide in TNBC cell lines could be AR independent.

Multiple lines of evidence suggest that the AR is a favorable prognostic indicator in breast cancer and that AR agonists would be the preferred approach for choice of androgenic treatment for ER-positive breast cancer. However, data is conflicting in TNBC. With multiple players involved in TNBC, the action of the AR in TNBC appears to be influenced by cross-talk with other pathways that differ between cell types and cancer subtypes.

10. Clinical Evidence Supporting the Use of AR Ligands in Hormone-Receptor-Positive Breast Cancer

Clinical evidence supporting the use of steroidal androgens for breast cancer dates back to the 1940s when testosterone and DHT were used to treat women with breast cancer [71,84]. Several studies using natural androgens demonstrated that the breast cancers regressed by 30%–50% in pre- and in post-menopausal women and that these effects were predominant in breast cancers expressing the AR [85–88]. Tumor growth regression with androgens was also observed after the removal of the pituitary, establishing that the effect of androgens is mediated directly through the AR expressed in the breast cancer tissue rather than through an effect on the hypothalamus pituitary hypogonadal axis [85].

Initial evidence of synthetic steroidal androgens showing growth inhibitory effects in breast cancer came from the use of fluoxymesterone (Halotestin™) and medroxyprogesterone acetate [89–91]. These synthetic androgens were not only effective in eliciting breast cancer regression, but were also effective in providing additive effects in combination with tamoxifen, providing a survival advantage to patients [92]. Although medroxyprogesterone has PR activity, it was effective in TNBCs that do not express PR, suggesting that the effects were achieved by through the ability of medroxyprogesterone to activate the AR [93].

Despite the historic and positive clinical results achieved with androgens in breast cancer, there have been few controlled clinical trials. As such, it remains unclear which subtypes respond best to androgens and the magnitude of response that can be expected. Ongoing clinical trials with newer nonsteroidal SARMs and nonsteroidal antiandrogens are poised to fill this knowledge gap. DHT, testosterone, and fluoxymesterone are steroidal androgens that have androgenic effects not only in breast, but also in other tissues including uterus, ovaries, skin, and hair follicles. SARMs were first reported in the late 1990s and subsequently shown to tissue selectively activate the AR in breast, muscle, and bone, without side effects associated with steroidal androgens [94–98]. Clinical trials with enobosarm (a nonsteroidal SARM being developed by GTx, Inc., Memphis, TN, USA) are ongoing to evaluate its efficacy and safety in breast cancer [94,95]. A phase II proof-of-concept clinical trial in 18 ER- and AR-positive breast cancer demonstrated a favorable response of stable disease in 42% of the evaluable patients. Since all the patients had bone-only disease, partial response or complete response could not be achieved. These results were presented at the San Antonio Breast Cancer Conference in 2015. Currently, enobosarm is being tested in Phase II clinical trials in subjects with ER-positive breast cancer and TNBC (NCT02463032 and NCT02368691, respectively). These early clinical results corroborate the clinical utility of androgens in breast cancer and suggest that nonsteroidal SARMs without the side effects commonly associated with steroidal androgens could provide a new avenue of hormonal therapy for certain subtypes of breast cancer.

Abiraterone acetate is an inhibitor of Cyp17A1 enzyme, an enzyme upstream in the steroidogenesis pathway. An intriguing result was obtained in a clinical trial with abiraterone in ER-positive breast cancer patients [99]. The central hypothesis for the study was that a complete inhibition of androgen and estrogen signaling would provide a better response in breast cancer. In this trial, 297 patients were stratified into three arms; with one arm receiving 1000 mg abiraterone plus 5 mg prednisone, one arm receiving 25 mg exemestane alone and one arm receiving exemestane and abiraterone [99]. The primary end-point was PFS. No significant difference in PFS was observed when abiraterone was combined with exemestane. The investigators found an increase in serum progesterone levels, which they believe could have contributed to the lack of clinical activity with abiraterone. However, recently a publication reported a protective effect of progesterone in breast cancer [100]. This has to be mechanistically further evaluated to understand why abiraterone did not provide a better outcome in both ER-positive breast cancer and in TNBC, while enzalutamide did in a TNBC clinical trial.

11. Clinical Evidences Supporting the Use of AR Ligands in ER-Negative Breast Cancer

The results obtained in MDA-MB-453 cells provided an impetus to evaluate antagonists in breast cancer, TNBC in particular. Two AR antagonists, bicalutamide and enzalutamide, and a CYP17A1 inhibitor, abiraterone, are currently used in the clinical treatment of prostate cancer. Repurposing these drugs to treat TNBC should prove straightforward if they are found to be effective in the clinic. An investigator-initiated clinical trial was conducted to evaluate the efficacy and safety of bicalutamide [101]. Out of the 424 patients with TNBC screened to determine the AR expression, only 51 were found to express AR. The trial treated 26 subjects with 150 mg bicalutamide daily. Although there were no partial or complete responses in the study, stable disease was observed in two patients for up to 6 months and five patients for greater than 6 months with a clinical benefit rate (CBR) of 19%. Although a modestly favorable response to bicalutamide was observed, it was interesting that subjects with tumor specimens that stained strongly for the AR were the least responsive to the drug while subjects with tumor specimens that stained very weakly for AR demonstrated the most durable responses.

A follow-up case report of one patient with AR-positive TNBC who relapsed after chemotherapy and progressed after multiple treatments and surgery and responded to treatment with 150 mg bicalutamide has also been published [102]. The patient achieved a complete response according to RECIST 1.1 criteria after 4 months of treatment and responded as long as 12 months when the report was published.

Based partially on the modest success achieved with bicalutamide, clinical trials in TNBC and ER-positive breast cancer were initiated with a second generation AR antagonist, enzalutamide. Enzalutamide has a unique mechanism of action where it blocks AR nuclear translocation and is more potent than bicalutamide [103]. Although no publications have come out on the trial, data presented in San Antonio breast cancer conference in 2014 and 2015 and in American Society for Clinical oncology (ASCO) 2015 annual meeting indicated a favorable response, including partial and complete responses, in approximately 40% of the patients. Details will emerge when the data are published.

Abiraterone, the CYP17A1 inhibitor, was tested in 34 AR-positive TNBC patients [104]. Patients were treated with 1000 mg abiraterone combined with 5 mg prednisone. At 6 months a CBR of 20% was achieved, which included one complete response and five subjects with stable disease of greater than 6 months. The overall response rate was 6.7% with median PFS of 2.8 months, which was far less than that observed with enzalutamide. Table 2 has a summary of clinical data.

Table 2. Summary of clinical data on AR agonists and antagonists in breast cancer.

Reference	Ref	Summary
Hermann and Adair, 1947, 1946	[71,84]	• Treatment of patients with breast cancer with testosterone propionate showed significant regression of cancer and disappearance of metastases. • Four out of 11 breast cancer patients treated with testosterone propionate exhibited favorable response.
Bines et al., 2014	[88]	• Clinical trial with Megesterol acetate, a synthetic progestin that also has AR agonistic activity was conducted in ER-positive breast cancer patients. • Clinical benefit rate of 40% was achieved with a duration of clinical benefit of 10 months.

Table 2. *Cont.*

Reference	Ref	Summary
Hermann and Adair, 1947, 1946	[71,84]	• Treatment of patients with breast cancer with testosterone propionate showed significant regression of cancer and disappearance of metastases. • Four out of 11 breast cancer patients treated with testosterone propionate exhibited favorable response.
Bines et al., 2014	[88]	• Clinical trial with Megesterol acetate, a synthetic progestin that also has AR agonistic activity was conducted in ER-positive breast cancer patients. • Clinical benefit rate of 40% was achieved with a duration of clinical benefit of 10 months.
Tormey et al.,1983	[90]	• Combination of halotestin and tamoxifen was tested in a clinical trial conducted in ER-positive breast cancer patients. • Combination was more effective with 38% partial and complete remission rates, while tamoxifen had only 15%. • The duration of response was also longer in the combination group than in the tamoxifen group.
Gucalp et al., 2013	[101]	• Clinical trial with an AR antagonist, bicalutamide, was performed in ER-negative breast cancer patients. • The 6 month clinical benefit rate was 19% and the median PFS was 12 weeks. The drug was well tolerated.
Arce-Salinas et al., 2016	[102]	• Case report of a patient with ER-negative breast cancer treated with bicalutamide. • The patient showed a complete response and the response was also durable for over a year.
Bonnefoi et al., 2016	[104]	• A clinical trial with abiraterone+prednisone in 30 AR-positive TNBC patients was performed. • A clinical benefit rate of 20% was observed in this trial with an overall response rate of 6.7%.
O'Shaughnessy et al., 2016	[99]	• Abiraterone acetate was tested alone or in combination with exemestane in patients with ER-positive breast cancer. • There was no significant difference in the PFS in the combination arm compared to the exemestane arm.

12. Mechanisms of Action of the AR in Breast Cancer

Studies from several groups support the concept that AR elicits anti-proliferative effects in ER-positive breast cancers by antagonizing ER action. Data also suggests that the AR in the presence of agonists binds to estrogen response elements (EREs) by competing for common binding regions [105] (Figure 2). Likewise, gonist-activated AR may compete for the limited coactivator pool, thereby inhibiting ER function by sequestering coactivators from the ER.

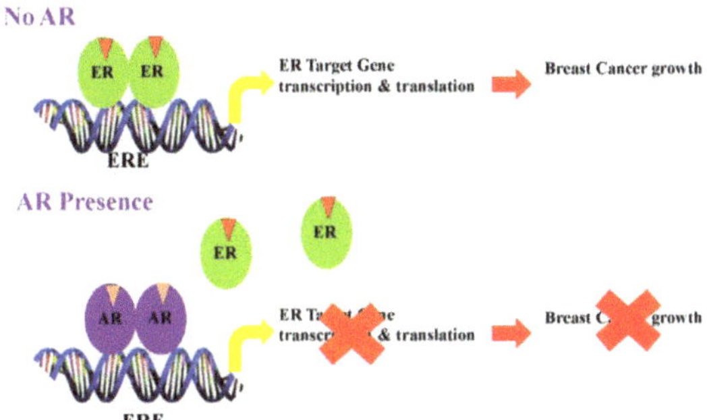

Figure 2. Mechanism for inhibition of estrogen receptor (ER)-positive breast cancer by the Androgen receptor (AR). (**A**) ER, in the presence of estrogens, binds to estrogen response elements (ERE) and activates the transcription and translation of target genes. AR, when activated by androgens, displaces ER and binds to EREs to form an inactive transcriptional complex, leading to inhibition of ER-target genes; (**B**) On the other hand, the AR, when activated by androgens, competes with ER for a limited pool of coactivators. This competition inhibits ER target genes and activates AR target genes. (Modified version of the figure published by McNamara et al. [25]).

While the mechanism is, safe to say, modestly clear in an ER-positive setting, it is still ambiguous in TNBC, especially considering that only one cell line MDA-MB-453 was used for mechanistic studies. The AR has been shown to cross-talk with several proteins in MDA-MB-453 cells. FOXA1 regulates AR and ER DNA binding and has significant overlapping binding regions in MDA-MB-453 [106]. Similarly, androgens were shown to increase extracellular signal-regulated kinase (ERK) and HER2 signaling in TNBC. Evaluation of PIK3CA kinase mutation in TNBC specimens showed that 40% of the AR-positive and 4% of the AR-negative specimens had mutations and concurrent amplifications [107,108]. Considering that the MDA-MB-453 cell line also contains a PIK3CA mutation, combination of the AR antagonist and PI3K/mTOR inhibitors provided additional effects [108]. Androgens in the presence of the AR have also been shown to abrogate the interaction between epithelial cells and mesenchymal stem cells to inhibit the paracrine metastatic factors [79].

13. Conclusions

The AR is a favorable prognostic marker and a promising therapeutic target in breast cancer. In ER-positive breast cancer, the landscape is clear suggesting that androgens and in particular nonsteroidal AR agonists may provide beneficial effects. On the other hand, data on TNBC is conflicting with historical data favoring the use of agonists, data from enzalutamide clinical trials supporting antagonists, and data from abiraterone clinical trials suggesting that inhibition of AR signaling is not beneficial. This is likely to come down to the subtypes in TNBC where a subtype might respond to agonists, while another subtype might respond to antagonists. A clear picture can be obtained only with new preclinical translational models such as the patient-derived xenografts (PDXs) that will provide clarity. Even in this case, the outcome and mechanisms might vary between patient specimens and exposure to prior treatments. In addition, the evolving AR splice variants (AR-SVs) have to be taken into consideration while planning a strategy [109]. Considering that splice variants lack the LBD, neither agonists nor antagonists that bind to the LBD are likely to provide a meaningful outcome. Similar to prostate cancer, prolonged treatment of patient's specimen with enzalutamide resulted in an increase in the AR-SVs [109]. The AR-SVs in breast cancer is a nascent field requiring additional data before any direction could be chartered.

Overall the next few years, when results from clinical trials with enobosarm and enzalutamide will be available, are critical to provide greater clarity on the role of the AR in ER-positive and –negative breast cancers. Considering that new agonists and antagonists for the AR are available, the emergence of nonsteroidal drugs targeting the AR as a new hormonal treatment for breast cancer is almost certainly on the horizon.

Conflicts of Interest: R.N. is a consultant to GTx, Inc.

References

1. Siegel, R.L.; Miller, K.D.; Jemal, A. Cancer statistics, 2016. *CA Cancer J. Clin.* **2016**, *66*, 7–30. [CrossRef] [PubMed]
2. Torre, L.A.; Bray, F.; Siegel, R.L.; Ferlay, J.; Lortet-Tieulent, J.; Jemal, A. Global cancer statistics, 2012. *CA Cancer J. Clin.* **2015**, *65*, 87–108. [CrossRef] [PubMed]
3. Sherry, M.M.; Greco, F.A.; Johnson, D.H.; Hainsworth, J.D. Metastatic breast cancer confined to the skeletal system. An indolent disease. *Am. J. Med.* **1986**, *81*, 381–386. [CrossRef]
4. Perou, C.M.; Sorlie, T.; Eisen, M.B.; van de Rijn, M.; Jeffrey, S.S.; Rees, C.A.; Pollack, J.R.; Ross, D.T.; Johnsen, H.; Akslen, L.A.; et al. Molecular portraits of human breast tumours. *Nature* **2000**, *406*, 747–752. [CrossRef] [PubMed]
5. Lehmann, B.D.; Bauer, J.A.; Chen, X.; Sanders, M.E.; Chakravarthy, A.B.; Shyr, Y.; Pietenpol, J.A. Identification of human triple-negative breast cancer subtypes and preclinical models for selection of targeted therapies. *J. Clin. Investig.* **2011**, *121*, 2750–2767. [CrossRef] [PubMed]

6. Onitilo, A.A.; Engel, J.M.; Greenlee, R.T.; Mukesh, B.N. Breast cancer subtypes based on ER/PR and HER2 expression: Comparison of clinicopathologic features and survival. *Clin. Med. Res.* **2009**, *7*, 4–13. [CrossRef] [PubMed]
7. Cheang, M.C.; Chia, S.K.; Voduc, D.; Gao, D.; Leung, S.; Snider, J.; Watson, M.; Davies, S.; Bernard, P.S.; Parker, J.S.; et al. Ki67 index, HER2 status, and prognosis of patients with luminal B breast cancer. *J. Natl. Cancer Inst.* **2009**, *101*, 736–750. [CrossRef] [PubMed]
8. Sotiriou, C.; Pusztai, L. Gene-expression signatures in breast cancer. *N. Engl. J. Med.* **2009**, *360*, 790–800. [CrossRef] [PubMed]
9. Loi, S.; Sotiriou, C.; Haibe-Kains, B.; Lallemand, F.; Conus, N.M.; Piccart, M.J.; Speed, T.P.; McArthur, G.A. Gene expression profiling identifies activated growth factor signaling in poor prognosis (Luminal-B) estrogen receptor positive breast cancer. *BMC Med. Genom.* **2009**. [CrossRef] [PubMed]
10. Wirapati, P.; Sotiriou, C.; Kunkel, S.; Farmer, P.; Pradervand, S.; Haibe-Kains, B.; Desmedt, C.; Ignatiadis, M.; Sengstag, T.; Schutz, F.; et al. Meta-analysis of gene expression profiles in breast cancer: Toward a unified understanding of breast cancer subtyping and prognosis signatures. *Breast Cancer Res.* **2008**. [CrossRef] [PubMed]
11. Nguyen, P.L.; Taghian, A.G.; Katz, M.S.; Niemierko, A.; Abi Raad, R.F.; Boon, W.L.; Bellon, J.R.; Wong, J.S.; Smith, B.L.; Harris, J.R. Breast cancer subtype approximated by estrogen receptor, progesterone receptor, and HER-2 is associated with local and distant recurrence after breast-conserving therapy. *J. Clin. Oncol.* **2008**, *26*, 2373–2378. [CrossRef] [PubMed]
12. Nam, B.H.; Kim, S.Y.; Han, H.S.; Kwon, Y.; Lee, K.S.; Kim, T.H.; Ro, J. Breast cancer subtypes and survival in patients with brain metastases. *Breast Cancer Res.* **2008**. [CrossRef] [PubMed]
13. Tran, B.; Bedard, P.L. Luminal-B breast cancer and novel therapeutic targets. *Breast Cancer Res.* **2011**. [CrossRef] [PubMed]
14. Leyland-Jones, B. Human epidermal growth factor receptor 2-positive breast cancer and central nervous system metastases. *J. Clin. Oncol.* **2009**, *27*, 5278–5286. [CrossRef] [PubMed]
15. Prat, A.; Adamo, B.; Cheang, M.C.; Anders, C.K.; Carey, L.A.; Perou, C.M. Molecular characterization of basal-like and non-basal-like triple-negative breast cancer. *Oncologist* **2013**, *18*, 123–133. [CrossRef] [PubMed]
16. Prat, A.; Ellis, M.J.; Perou, C.M. Practical implications of gene-expression-based assays for breast oncologists. *Nat. Rev. Clin. Oncol.* **2012**, *9*, 48–57. [CrossRef] [PubMed]
17. Cancer Genome Atlas Network. Comprehensive molecular portraits of human breast tumours. *Nature* **2012**, *490*, 61–70.
18. Jenster, G.; van der Korput, H.A.; Trapman, J.; Brinkmann, A.O. Identification of two transcription activation units in the N-terminal domain of the human androgen receptor. *J. Biol. Chem.* **1995**, *270*, 7341–7346. [PubMed]
19. Verrijdt, G.; Tanner, T.; Moehren, U.; Callewaert, L.; Haelens, A.; Claessens, F. The androgen receptor DNA-binding domain determines androgen selectivity of transcriptional response. *Biochem. Soc. Trans.* **2006**, *34*, 1089–1094. [CrossRef] [PubMed]
20. Matias, P.M.; Donner, P.; Coelho, R.; Thomaz, M.; Peixoto, C.; Macedo, S.; Otto, N.; Joschko, S.; Scholz, P.; Wegg, A.; et al. Structural evidence for ligand specificity in the binding domain of the human androgen receptor. Implications for pathogenic gene mutations. *J. Biol. Chem.* **2000**, *275*, 26164–26171. [CrossRef] [PubMed]
21. Wang, Q.; Li, W.; Zhang, Y.; Yuan, X.; Xu, K.; Yu, J.; Chen, Z.; Beroukhim, R.; Wang, H.; Lupien, M.; et al. Androgen receptor regulates a distinct transcription program in androgen-independent prostate cancer. *Cell* **2009**, *138*, 245–256. [CrossRef] [PubMed]
22. Collins, L.C.; Cole, K.S.; Marotti, J.D.; Hu, R.; Schnitt, S.J.; Tamimi, R.M. Androgen receptor expression in breast cancer in relation to molecular phenotype: Results from the Nurses' Health Study. *Mod. Pathol.* **2011**, *24*, 924–931. [CrossRef] [PubMed]
23. Vera-Badillo, F.E.; Templeton, A.J.; de Gouveia, P.; Diaz-Padilla, I.; Bedard, P.L.; Al-Mubarak, M.; Seruga, B.; Tannock, I.F.; Ocana, A.; Amir, E. Androgen receptor expression and outcomes in early breast cancer: A systematic review and meta-analysis. *J. Natl. Cancer Inst.* **2014**. [CrossRef] [PubMed]
24. Sultana, A.; Idress, R.; Naqvi, Z.A.; Azam, I.; Khan, S.; Siddiqui, A.A.; Lalani, E.N. Expression of the Androgen Receptor, pAkt, and pPTEN in Breast Cancer and Their Potential in Prognostication. *Transl. Oncol.* **2014**, *7*, 355–362. [CrossRef] [PubMed]

25. McNamara, K.M.; Yoda, T.; Nurani, A.M.; Shibahara, Y.; Miki, Y.; Wang, L.; Nakamura, Y.; Suzuki, K.; Yang, Y.; Abe, E.; et al. Androgenic pathways in the progression of triple-negative breast carcinoma: A comparison between aggressive and non-aggressive subtypes. *Breast Cancer Res. Treat.* **2014**, *145*, 281–293. [CrossRef] [PubMed]
26. Luo, X.; Shi, Y.X.; Li, Z.M.; Jiang, W.Q. Expression and clinical significance of androgen receptor in triple negative breast cancer. *Chin. J. Cancer* **2010**, *29*, 585–590. [CrossRef] [PubMed]
27. Qu, Q.; Mao, Y.; Fei, X.C.; Shen, K.W. The impact of androgen receptor expression on breast cancer survival: A retrospective study and meta-analysis. *PLoS ONE* **2013**, *8*, e82650. [CrossRef] [PubMed]
28. Agoff, S.N.; Swanson, P.E.; Linden, H.; Hawes, S.E.; Lawton, T.J. Androgen receptor expression in estrogen receptor-negative breast cancer. Immunohistochemical, clinical, and prognostic associations. *Am. J. Clin. Pathol.* **2003**, *120*, 725–731. [CrossRef] [PubMed]
29. Pistelli, M.; Caramanti, M.; Biscotti, T.; Santinelli, A.; Pagliacci, A.; De Lisa, M.; Ballatore, Z.; Ridolfi, F.; Maccaroni, E.; Bracci, R.; et al. Androgen receptor expression in early triple-negative breast cancer: Clinical significance and prognostic associations. *Cancers* **2014**, *6*, 1351–1362. [CrossRef] [PubMed]
30. Noh, S.; Kim, J.Y.; Koo, J.S. Metabolic differences in estrogen receptor-negative breast cancer based on androgen receptor status. *Tumour Biol.* **2014**, *35*, 8179–8192. [CrossRef] [PubMed]
31. Doane, A.S.; Danso, M.; Lal, P.; Donaton, M.; Zhang, L.; Hudis, C.; Gerald, W.L. An estrogen receptor-negative breast cancer subset characterized by a hormonally regulated transcriptional program and response to androgen. *Oncogene* **2006**, *25*, 3994–4008. [CrossRef] [PubMed]
32. Cha, Y.J.; Jung, W.H.; Koo, J.S. The clinicopathologic features of molecular apocrine breast cancer. *Korean J. Pathol.* **2012**, *46*, 169–176. [CrossRef] [PubMed]
33. Cochrane, D.R.; Bernales, S.; Jacobsen, B.M.; Cittelly, D.M.; Howe, E.N.; D'Amato, N.C.; Spoelstra, N.S.; Edgerton, S.M.; Jean, A.; Guerrero, J.; et al. Role of the Androgen Receptor in Breast Cancer and Preclinical Analysis of Enzalutamide. *Breast Cancer Res.* **2014**. [CrossRef] [PubMed]
34. Moore, N.L.; Buchanan, G.; Harris, J.M.; Selth, L.A.; Bianco-Miotto, T.; Hanson, A.R.; Birrell, S.N.; Butler, L.M.; Hickey, T.E.; Tilley, W.D. An androgen receptor mutation in the MDA-MB-453 cell line model of molecular apocrine breast cancer compromises receptor activity. *Endocr. Relat. Cancer* **2012**, *19*, 599–613. [CrossRef] [PubMed]
35. Mills, A.M.; Chelsea, E.G.; Scott, M.W.; Christiana, M.B.; Atkins, K.A. Pure Apocrine Carcinomas Represent a Clinicopathologically Distinct Androgen Receptor-Positive Subset of Triple-Negative Breast Cancers. *Am. J. Surg. Pathol.* **2016**, *40*, 1109–1116. [CrossRef] [PubMed]
36. Yepuru, M.; Wu, Z.; Kulkarni, A.; Yin, F.; Barrett, C.M.; Kim, J.; Steiner, M.S.; Miller, D.D.; Dalton, J.T.; Narayanan, R. Steroidogenic enzyme AKR1C3 is a novel androgen receptor-selective coactivator that promotes prostate cancer growth. *Clin. Cancer Res.* **2013**, *19*, 5613–5625. [CrossRef] [PubMed]
37. McNamara, K.M.; Yoda, T.; Miki, Y.; Chanplakorn, N.; Wongwaisayawan, S.; Incharoen, P.; Kongdan, Y.; Wang, L.; Takagi, K.; Mayu, T.; et al. Androgenic pathway in triple negative invasive ductal tumors: Its correlation with tumor cell proliferation. *Cancer Sci.* **2013**, *104*, 639–646. [CrossRef] [PubMed]
38. Aleskandarany, M.A.; Abduljabbar, R.; Ashankyty, I.; Elmouna, A.; Jerjees, D.; Ali, S.; Buluwela, L.; Diez-Rodriguez, M.; Caldas, C.; Green, A.R.; et al. Prognostic significance of androgen receptor expression in invasive breast cancer: Transcriptomic and protein expression analysis. *Breast Cancer Res. Treat.* **2016**, *159*, 215–227. [CrossRef] [PubMed]
39. Safarpour, D.; Pakneshan, S.; Tavassoli, F.A. Androgen receptor (AR) expression in 400 breast carcinomas: Is routine AR assessment justified? *Am. J. Cancer Res.* **2014**, *4*, 353–368. [PubMed]
40. Choi, J.E.; Kang, S.H.; Lee, S.J.; Bae, Y.K. Androgen receptor expression predicts decreased survival in early stage triple-negative breast cancer. *Ann. Surg. Oncol.* **2015**, *22*, 82–89. [CrossRef] [PubMed]
41. Elebro, K.; Borgquist, S.; Simonsson, M.; Markkula, A.; Jirstrom, K.; Ingvar, C.; Rose, C.; Jernstrom, H. Combined Androgen and Estrogen Receptor Status in Breast Cancer: Treatment Prediction and Prognosis in a Population-Based Prospective Cohort. *Clin. Cancer Res.* **2015**, *21*, 3640–3650. [CrossRef] [PubMed]
42. Hilborn, E.; Gacic, J.; Fornander, T.; Nordenskjold, B.; Stal, O.; Jansson, A. Androgen receptor expression predicts beneficial tamoxifen response in oestrogen receptor-alpha-negative breast cancer. *Br. J. Cancer* **2016**, *114*, 248–255. [CrossRef] [PubMed]

43. Loibl, S.; Muller, B.M.; von Minckwitz, G.; Schwabe, M.; Roller, M.; Darb-Esfahani, S.; Ataseven, B.; du Bois, A.; Fissler-Eckhoff, A.; Gerber, B.; et al. Androgen receptor expression in primary breast cancer and its predictive and prognostic value in patients treated with neoadjuvant chemotherapy. *Breast Cancer Res. Treat.* **2011**, *130*, 477–487. [CrossRef] [PubMed]
44. Parker, J.S.; Mullins, M.; Cheang, M.C.; Leung, S.; Voduc, D.; Vickery, T.; Davies, S.; Fauron, C.; He, X.; Hu, Z.; et al. Supervised risk predictor of breast cancer based on intrinsic subtypes. *J. Clin. Oncol.* **2009**, *27*, 1160–1167. [CrossRef] [PubMed]
45. Prat, A.; Lluch, A.; Albanell, J.; Barry, W.T.; Fan, C.; Chacon, J.I.; Parker, J.S.; Calvo, L.; Plazaola, A.; Arcusa, A.; et al. Predicting response and survival in chemotherapy-treated triple-negative breast cancer. *Br. J. Cancer* **2014**, *111*, 1532–1541. [CrossRef] [PubMed]
46. Labrie, F. Intracrinology. *Mol. Cell Endocrinol.* **1991**, *78*, C113–C118. [CrossRef]
47. Labrie, F. All sex steroids are made intracellularly in peripheral tissues by the mechanisms of intracrinology after menopause. *J. Steroid Biochem. Mol. Biol.* **2015**, *145*, 133–138. [CrossRef] [PubMed]
48. Labrie, F.; Luu-The, V.; Labrie, C.; Belanger, A.; Simard, J.; Lin, S.X.; Pelletier, G. Endocrine and intracrine sources of androgens in women: Inhibition of breast cancer and other roles of androgens and their precursor dehydroepiandrosterone. *Endocr. Rev.* **2003**, *24*, 152–182. [CrossRef] [PubMed]
49. Labrie, F.; Belanger, A.; Luu-The, V.; Labrie, C.; Simard, J.; Cusan, L.; Gomez, J.L.; Candas, B. DHEA and the intracrine formation of androgens and estrogens in peripheral target tissues: Its role during aging. *Steroids* **1998**, *63*, 322–328. [CrossRef]
50. Luu-The, V.; Labrie, F. The intracrine sex steroid biosynthesis pathways. *Prog. Brain Res.* **2010**, *181*, 177–192. [PubMed]
51. Miyoshi, Y.; Ando, A.; Shiba, E.; Taguchi, T.; Tamaki, Y.; Noguchi, S. Involvement of up-regulation of 17beta-hydroxysteroid dehydrogenase type 1 in maintenance of intratumoral high estradiol levels in postmenopausal breast cancers. *Int. J. Cancer* **2001**, *94*, 685–689. [CrossRef] [PubMed]
52. Chetrite, G.S.; Cortes-Prieto, J.; Philippe, J.C.; Wright, F.; Pasqualini, J.R. Comparison of estrogen concentrations, estrone sulfatase and aromatase activities in normal, and in cancerous, human breast tissues. *J. Steroid Biochem. Mol. Biol.* **2000**, *72*, 23–27. [CrossRef]
53. Recchione, C.; Venturelli, E.; Manzari, A.; Cavalleri, A.; Martinetti, A.; Secreto, G. Testosterone, dihydrotestosterone and oestradiol levels in postmenopausal breast cancer tissues. *J. Steroid Biochem. Mol. Biol.* **1995**, *52*, 541–546. [CrossRef]
54. Sharifi, N. Minireview: Androgen metabolism in castration-resistant prostate cancer. *Mol. Endocrinol.* **2013**, *27*, 708–714. [CrossRef] [PubMed]
55. Fukami, M.; Homma, K.; Hasegawa, T.; Ogata, T. Backdoor pathway for dihydrotestosterone biosynthesis: Implications for normal and abnormal human sex development. *Dev. Dyn.* **2013**, *242*, 320–329. [CrossRef] [PubMed]
56. Kamrath, C.; Hochberg, Z.; Hartmann, M.F.; Remer, T.; Wudy, S.A. Increased activation of the alternative "backdoor" pathway in patients with 21-hydroxylase deficiency: Evidence from urinary steroid hormone analysis. *J. Clin. Endocrinol. Metab.* **2012**, *97*, E367–E375. [CrossRef] [PubMed]
57. Mohler, J.L.; Titus, M.A.; Bai, S.; Kennerley, B.J.; Lih, F.B.; Tomer, K.B.; Wilson, E.M. Activation of the androgen receptor by intratumoral bioconversion of androstanediol to dihydrotestosterone in prostate cancer. *Cancer Res.* **2011**, *71*, 1486–1496. [PubMed]
58. Mohler, J.L.; Titus, M.A.; Wilson, E.M. Potential prostate cancer drug target: Bioactivation of androstanediol by conversion to dihydrotestosterone. *Clin. Cancer Res.* **2011**, *17*, 5844–5849. [CrossRef] [PubMed]
59. Lukacik, P.; Kavanagh, K.L.; Oppermann, U. Structure and function of human 17beta-hydroxysteroid dehydrogenases. *Mol. Cell. Endocrinol.* **2006**, *248*, 61–71. [CrossRef] [PubMed]
60. Moeller, G.; Adamski, J. Multifunctionality of human 17beta-hydroxysteroid dehydrogenases. *Mol. Cell. Endocrinol.* **2006**, *248*, 47–55. [CrossRef] [PubMed]
61. Penning, T.M. Hydroxysteroid dehydrogenases and pre-receptor regulation of steroid hormone action. *Hum. Reprod. Update* **2003**, *9*, 193–205. [CrossRef] [PubMed]
62. Walker, E.A.; Stewart, P.M. 11beta-hydroxysteroid dehydrogenase: Unexpected connections. *Trends Endocrinol. Metab.* **2003**, *14*, 334–339. [CrossRef]
63. Nobel, S.; Abrahmsen, L.; Oppermann, U. Metabolic conversion as a pre-receptor control mechanism for lipophilic hormones. *Eur. J. Biochem.* **2001**, *268*, 4113–4125. [CrossRef] [PubMed]

64. Nagasaki, S.; Miki, Y.; Akahira, J.; Suzuki, T.; Sasano, H. 17beta-hydroxysteroid dehydrogenases in human breast cancer. *Ann. N. Y. Acad. Sci.* **2009**, *1155*, 25–32. [CrossRef] [PubMed]
65. Lin, H.K.; Steckelbroeck, S.; Fung, K.M.; Jones, A.N.; Penning, T.M. Characterization of a monoclonal antibody for human aldo-keto reductase AKR1C3 (type 2 3alpha-hydroxysteroid dehydrogenase/type 5 17beta-hydroxysteroid dehydrogenase); immunohistochemical detection in breast and prostate. *Steroids* **2004**, *69*, 795–801. [CrossRef] [PubMed]
66. Penning, T.M.; Burczynski, M.E.; Jez, J.M.; Lin, H.K.; Ma, H.; Moore, M.; Ratnam, K.; Palackal, N. Structure-function aspects and inhibitor design of type 5 17beta-hydroxysteroid dehydrogenase (AKR1C3). *Mol. Cell. Endocrinol.* **2001**, *171*, 137–149. [CrossRef]
67. Penning, T.M.; Byrns, M.C. Steroid hormone transforming aldo-keto reductases and cancer. *Ann. N. Y. Acad. Sci.* **2009**, *1155*, 33–42. [CrossRef] [PubMed]
68. Zumoff, B.; Levin, J.; Rosenfeld, R.S.; Markham, M.; Strain, G.W.; Fukushima, D.K. Abnormal 24-hr mean plasma concentrations of dehydroisoandrosterone and dehydroisoandrosterone sulfate in women with primary operable breast cancer. *Cancer Res.* **1981**, *41*, 3360–3363. [PubMed]
69. Li, S.; Yan, X.; Belanger, A.; Labrie, F. Prevention by dehydroepiandrosterone of the development of mammary carcinoma induced by 7,12-dimethylbenz(a)anthracene (DMBA) in the rat. *Breast Cancer Res. Treat.* **1994**, *29*, 203–217. [CrossRef] [PubMed]
70. Adair, F.E.; Herrmann, J.B. The Use of Testosterone Propionate in the Treatment of Advanced Carcinoma of the Breast. *Ann. Surg.* **1946**, *123*, 1023–1035. [CrossRef] [PubMed]
71. Herrmann, J.B.; Adair, F.E. The effect of testosterone propionate on carcinoma of the female breast with soft tissue metastases. *J. Clin. Endocrinol. Metab.* **1946**, *6*, 769–775. [CrossRef] [PubMed]
72. Huggins, C.; Briziarelli, G.; Sutton, H., Jr. Rapid induction of mammary carcinoma in the rat and the influence of hormones on the tumors. *J. Exp. Med.* **1959**, *109*, 25–42. [CrossRef] [PubMed]
73. Lubahn, D.B.; Joseph, D.R.; Sullivan, P.M.; Willard, H.F.; French, F.S.; Wilson, E.M. Cloning of human androgen receptor complementary DNA and localization to the X chromosome. *Science* **1988**, *240*, 327–330. [CrossRef] [PubMed]
74. Chang, C.S.; Kokontis, J.; Liao, S.T. Molecular cloning of human and rat complementary DNA encoding androgen receptors. *Science* **1988**, *240*, 324–326. [CrossRef] [PubMed]
75. Poulin, R.; Baker, D.; Labrie, F. Androgens inhibit basal and estrogen-induced cell proliferation in the ZR-75-1 human breast cancer cell line. *Breast Cancer Res. Treat.* **1988**, *12*, 213–225. [CrossRef] [PubMed]
76. Dauvois, S.; Geng, C.S.; Levesque, C.; Merand, Y.; Labrie, F. Additive inhibitory effects of an androgen and the antiestrogen EM-170 on estradiol-stimulated growth of human ZR-75-1 breast tumors in athymic mice. *Cancer Res.* **1991**, *51*, 3131–3135. [PubMed]
77. Cops, E.J.; Bianco-Miotto, T.; Moore, N.L.; Clarke, C.L.; Birrell, S.N.; Butler, L.M.; Tilley, W.D. Antiproliferative actions of the synthetic androgen, mibolerone, in breast cancer cells are mediated by both androgen and progesterone receptors. *J. Steroid Biochem. Mol. Biol.* **2008**, *110*, 236–243. [CrossRef] [PubMed]
78. Macedo, L.F.; Guo, Z.; Tilghman, S.L.; Sabnis, G.J.; Qiu, Y.; Brodie, A. Role of androgens on MCF-7 breast cancer cell growth and on the inhibitory effect of letrozole. *Cancer Res.* **2006**, *66*, 7775–7782. [CrossRef] [PubMed]
79. Narayanan, R.; Ahn, S.; Cheney, M.D.; Yepuru, M.; Miller, D.D.; Steiner, M.S.; Dalton, J.T. Selective androgen receptor modulators (SARMs) negatively regulate triple-negative breast cancer growth and epithelial:mesenchymal stem cell signaling. *PLoS ONE* **2014**, *9*, e103202. [CrossRef] [PubMed]
80. Hall, R.E.; Birrell, S.N.; Tilley, W.D.; Sutherland, R.L. MDA-MB-453, an androgen-responsive human breast carcinoma cell line with high level androgen receptor expression. *Eur. J. Cancer* **1994**, *30A*, 484–490. [CrossRef]
81. Barton, V.N.; D'Amato, N.C.; Gordon, M.A.; Lind, H.T.; Spoelstra, N.S.; Babbs, B.L.; Heinz, R.E.; Elias, A.; Jedlicka, P.; Jacobsen, B.M.; et al. Multiple molecular subtypes of triple-negative breast cancer critically rely on androgen receptor and respond to enzalutamide in vivo. *Mol. Cancer Ther.* **2015**, *14*, 769–778. [CrossRef] [PubMed]
82. Thakkar, A.; Wang, B.; Picon-Ruiz, M.; Buchwald, P.; Ince, T.A. Vitamin D and androgen receptor-targeted therapy for triple-negative breast cancer. *Breast Cancer Res. Treat.* **2016**, *157*, 77–90. [CrossRef] [PubMed]
83. Santagata, S.; Thakkar, A.; Ergonul, A.; Wang, B.; Woo, T.; Hu, R.; Harrell, J.C.; McNamara, G.; Schwede, M.; Culhane, A.C.; et al. Taxonomy of breast cancer based on normal cell phenotype predicts outcome. *J. Clin. Investig.* **2014**, *124*, 859–870. [CrossRef] [PubMed]

84. Adair, F.E.; Herrmann, J.B. The use of testosterone propionate in the treatment of advanced carcinoma of the breast. *Ann Surg* **1946**, *123*, 1023–1035. [CrossRef] [PubMed]
85. Trams, G.; Maass, H. Specific binding of estradiol and dihydrotestosterone in human mammary cancers. *Cancer Res.* **1977**, *37*, 258–261. [PubMed]
86. Bryan, R.M.; Mercer, R.J.; Bennett, R.C.; Rennie, G.C.; Lie, T.H.; Morgan, F.J. Androgen receptors in breast cancer. *Cancer* **1984**, *54*, 2436–2440. [CrossRef]
87. Gordon, G. *Anabolic-Androgenic Steroids*; Springer-Verlag: New York, NY, USA, 1976.
88. Bines, J.; Dienstmann, R.; Obadia, R.M.; Branco, L.G.; Quintella, D.C.; Castro, T.M.; Camacho, P.G.; Soares, F.A.; Costa, M.E. Activity of megestrol acetate in postmenopausal women with advanced breast cancer after nonsteroidal aromatase inhibitor failure: A phase II trial. *Ann. Oncol.* **2014**, *25*, 831–836. [CrossRef] [PubMed]
89. Kennedy, B.J. Fluoxymesterone therapy in advanced breast cancer. *N. Engl. J. Med.* **1958**, *259*, 673–675. [CrossRef] [PubMed]
90. Tormey, D.C.; Lippman, M.E.; Edwards, B.K.; Cassidy, J.G. Evaluation of tamoxifen doses with and without fluoxymesterone in advanced breast cancer. *Ann. Intern. Med.* **1983**, *98*, 139–144. [CrossRef] [PubMed]
91. Muggia, F.M.; Cassieth, P.A.; Ochoa, M., Jr.; Flatow, F.A.; Gellhorn, A.; Hyman, G.A. Treatment of breast cancer with medroxyprogesterone acetate. *Ann. Intern. Med.* **1968**, *68*, 328–337. [CrossRef] [PubMed]
92. Ingle, J.N.; Twito, D.I.; Schaid, D.J.; Cullinan, S.A.; Krook, J.E.; Mailliard, J.A.; Tschetter, L.K.; Long, H.J.; Gerstner, J.G.; Windschitl, H.E.; et al. Combination hormonal therapy with tamoxifen plus fluoxymesterone versus tamoxifen alone in postmenopausal women with metastatic breast cancer. An updated analysis. *Cancer* **1991**, *67*, 886–891. [CrossRef]
93. Birrell, S.N.; Roder, D.M.; Horsfall, D.J.; Bentel, J.M.; Tilley, W.D. Medroxyprogesterone acetate therapy in advanced breast cancer: The predictive value of androgen receptor expression. *J. Clin. Oncol.* **1995**, *13*, 1572–1577. [PubMed]
94. Dalton, J.T.; Mukherjee, A.; Zhu, Z.; Kirkovsky, L.; Miller, D.D. Discovery of nonsteroidal androgens. *Biochem. Biophys. Res. Commun.* **1998**, *244*, 1–4. [CrossRef] [PubMed]
95. Dalton, J.T.; Barnette, K.G.; Bohl, C.E.; Hancock, M.L.; Rodriguez, D.; Dodson, S.T.; Morton, R.A.; Steiner, M.S. The selective androgen receptor modulator GTx-024 (enobosarm) improves lean body mass and physical function in healthy elderly men and postmenopausal women: Results of a double-blind, placebo-controlled phase II trial. *J. Cachexia Sarcopenia Muscle* **2011**, *2*, 153–161. [CrossRef] [PubMed]
96. Jones, A.; Hwang, D.J.; Narayanan, R.; Miller, D.D.; Dalton, J.T. Effects of a novel selective androgen receptor modulator on dexamethasone-induced and hypogonadism-induced muscle atrophy. *Endocrinology* **2010**, *151*, 3706–3719. [CrossRef] [PubMed]
97. Kearbey, J.D.; Gao, W.; Narayanan, R.; Fisher, S.J.; Wu, D.; Miller, D.D.; Dalton, J.T. Selective Androgen Receptor Modulator (SARM) treatment prevents bone loss and reduces body fat in ovariectomized rats. *Pharm. Res.* **2007**, *24*, 328–335. [CrossRef] [PubMed]
98. Narayanan, R.; Coss, C.C.; Yepuru, M.; Kearbey, J.D.; Miller, D.D.; Dalton, J.T. Steroidal androgens and nonsteroidal, tissue-selective androgen receptor modulator, S-22, regulate androgen receptor function through distinct genomic and nongenomic signaling pathways. *Mol. Endocrinol.* **2008**, *22*, 2448–2465. [CrossRef] [PubMed]
99. O'Shaughnessy, J.; Campone, M.; Brain, E.; Neven, P.; Hayes, D.; Bondarenko, I.; Griffin, T.W.; Martin, J.; De Porre, P.; Kheoh, T.; et al. Abiraterone acetate, exemestane or the combination in postmenopausal patients with estrogen receptor-positive metastatic breast cancer. *Ann. Oncol.* **2016**, *27*, 106–113. [CrossRef] [PubMed]
100. Mohammed, H.; Russell, I.A.; Stark, R.; Rueda, O.M.; Hickey, T.E.; Tarulli, G.A.; Serandour, A.A.; Birrell, S.N.; Bruna, A.; Saadi, A.; et al. Progesterone receptor modulates ERalpha action in breast cancer. *Nature* **2015**, *523*, 313–317. [CrossRef] [PubMed]
101. Gucalp, A.; Tolaney, S.; Isakoff, S.J.; Ingle, J.N.; Liu, M.C.; Carey, L.A.; Blackwell, K.; Rugo, H.; Nabell, L.; Forero, A.; et al. Phase II Trial of Bicalutamide in Patients with Androgen Receptor-Positive, Estrogen Receptor-Negative Metastatic Breast Cancer. *Clin. Cancer Res.* **2013**, *19*, 5505–5512. [CrossRef] [PubMed]
102. Arce-Salinas, C.; Riesco-Martinez, M.C.; Hanna, W.; Bedard, P.; Warner, E. Complete Response of Metastatic Androgen Receptor-Positive Breast Cancer to Bicalutamide: Case Report and Review of the Literature. *J. Clin. Oncol.* **2016**, *34*, e21–e24. [CrossRef] [PubMed]

103. Tran, C.; Ouk, S.; Clegg, N.J.; Chen, Y.; Watson, P.A.; Arora, V.; Wongvipat, J.; Smith-Jones, P.M.; Yoo, D.; Kwon, A.; et al. Development of a second-generation antiandrogen for treatment of advanced prostate cancer. *Science* **2009**, *324*, 787–790. [CrossRef] [PubMed]
104. Bonnefoi, H.; Grellety, T.; Tredan, O.; Saghatchian, M.; Dalenc, F.; Mailliez, A.; L'Haridon, T.; Cottu, P.; Abadie-Lacourtoisie, S.; You, B.; et al. A phase II trial of abiraterone acetate plus prednisone in patients with triple-negative androgen receptor positive locally advanced or metastatic breast cancer (UCBG 12–1). *Ann. Oncol.* **2016**, *27*, 812–818. [CrossRef] [PubMed]
105. Peters, A.A.; Buchanan, G.; Ricciardelli, C.; Bianco-Miotto, T.; Centenera, M.M.; Harris, J.M.; Jindal, S.; Segara, D.; Jia, L.; Moore, N.L.; et al. Androgen receptor inhibits estrogen receptor-alpha activity and is prognostic in breast cancer. *Cancer Res.* **2009**, *69*, 6131–6140. [CrossRef] [PubMed]
106. Robinson, J.L.; Macarthur, S.; Ross-Innes, C.S.; Tilley, W.D.; Neal, D.E.; Mills, I.G.; Carroll, J.S. Androgen receptor driven transcription in molecular apocrine breast cancer is mediated by FoxA1. *EMBO J.* **2011**, *30*, 3019–3027. [CrossRef] [PubMed]
107. Adamczyk, A.; Niemiec, J.; Janecka, A.; Harazin-Lechowska, A.; Ambicka, A.; Grela-Wojewoda, A.; Domagala-Haduch, M.; Cedrych, I.; Majchrzyk, K.; Kruczak, A.; et al. Prognostic value of PIK3CA mutation status, PTEN and androgen receptor expression for metastasis-free survival in HER2-positive breast cancer patients treated with trastuzumab in adjuvant setting. *Pol. J. Pathol.* **2015**, *66*, 133–141. [CrossRef] [PubMed]
108. Lehmann, B.D.; Bauer, J.A.; Schafer, J.M.; Pendleton, C.S.; Tang, L.; Johnson, K.C.; Chen, X.; Balko, J.M.; Gomez, H.; Arteaga, C.L.; et al. PIK3CA mutations in androgen receptor-positive triple negative breast cancer confer sensitivity to the combination of PI3K and androgen receptor inhibitors. *Breast Cancer Res.* **2014**. [CrossRef] [PubMed]
109. Hickey, T.E.; Irvine, C.M.; Dvinge, H.; Tarulli, G.A.; Hanson, A.R.; Ryan, N.K.; Pickering, M.A.; Birrell, S.N.; Hu, D.G.; Mackenzie, P.I.; et al. Expression of androgen receptor splice variants in clinical breast cancers. *Oncotarget* **2015**, *6*, 44728–44744. [PubMed]

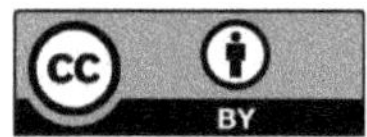

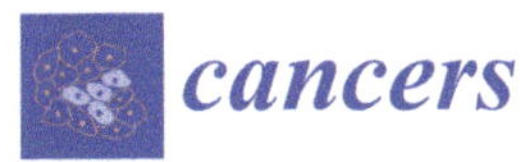

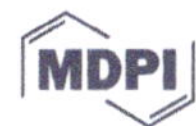

Article

Expression and Clinical Significance of Androgen Receptor in Triple-Negative Breast Cancer

Yuka Asano [1], Shinichiro Kashiwagi [1,*], Wataru Goto [1], Sayaka Tanaka [2], Tamami Morisaki [1], Tsutomu Takashima [1], Satoru Noda [1], Naoyoshi Onoda [1], Masahiko Ohsawa [2], Kosei Hirakawa [1] and Masaichi Ohira [1]

1 Department of Surgical Oncology, Osaka City University Graduate School of Medicine, 1-4-3 Asahi-machi, Abeno-ku, Osaka 545-8585, Japan; asnyk0325@yahoo.co.jp (Y.A.); saraikazemaru@gmail.com (W.G.); spitz4_5@yahoo.co.jp (T.M.); tsutomu-@rd5.so-net.ne.jp (T.T.); s-noda@med.osaka-cu.ac.jp (S.N.); nonoda@med.osaka-cu.ac.jp (N.O.); hirakawa@med.osaka-cu.ac.jp (K.H.); masaichi@med.osaka-cu.ac.jp (M.O.)

2 Department of Diagnostic Pathology, Osaka City University Graduate School of Medicine, 1-4-3 Asahi-machi, Abeno-ku, Osaka 545-8585, Japan; m1153321@med.osaka-cu.ac.jp (S.T.); m-ohsawa@med.osaka-cu.ac.jp (M.O.)

* Correspondence: spqv9ke9@view.ocn.ne.jp; Tel.: +81-6-6645-3838; Fax: +81-6-6646-6450

Academic Editor: Emmanuel S. Antonarakis
Received: 10 November 2016; Accepted: 4 January 2017; Published: 6 January 2017

Abstract: Background: Triple-negative breast cancer (TNBC) has a poor prognosis because of frequent recurrence. Androgen receptor (AR) is involved in the pathogenesis of breast cancer, but its role is not clearly defined. The aim of this study was to explore the expression of AR and its relationship with clinicopathologic features in TNBC. Methods: This study investigated 1036 cases of sporadic invasive breast carcinoma. Immunohistochemical assays were performed to determine the expression of AR in 190 TNBC samples. The relationships between AR expression and clinicopathologic data and prognosis were analyzed. Results: In 190 TNBC cases, the prognosis of AR-positive patients was significantly better ($p = 0.019$, log-rank) than AR-negative patients, and in multivariate analysis, AR expression was an independent indicator of good prognosis ($p = 0.039$, hazard ratio = 0.36). In patients with disease relapse, AR positivity was significantly correlated with better prognosis ($p = 0.034$, log-rank). Conclusions: AR expression may be useful as a subclassification marker for prognosis in TNBC.

Keywords: triple-negative breast cancer; androgen receptor; prognostic marker; individualized treatment; intrinsic subtype

1. Introduction

Breast cancer is a highly diverse disease that can be classified into subtypes comprising different clinical or cellular characteristics. It is commonly subclassified into five subtypes including luminal A, luminal B, human epidermal growth factor receptor 2 (HER2)-enriched, basal-like, and normal-like, according to the mRNA expression profile; these breast cancer types are frequently referred to as the "intrinsic subtype" [1–4]. The basal-like subtype almost always coincides with estrogen receptor (ER)-negative, progesterone receptor (PR)-negative, and HER2-negative triple-negative breast cancer (TNBC) [3,5,6]. However, compared to the basal-like classification that is based on a molecular approach, classifying a tumor as a TNBC is based on an immunohistochemical approach that is easy to use in actual clinical practice. TNBC is an intractable breast cancer because of its highly malignant biological potential, including aggressive tumor growth and rapid dissemination to important organs [7–9]. Patients with TNBC often require systemic anti-cancer therapy to manage the progression of the disease. Endocrine and anti-HER2 therapies are ineffective against TNBC as they lack the molecular targets (ER and HER2, respectively), and chemotherapy is considered the only remedy for TNBCs [10,11].

However, recent research indicates that TNBC can be further classified according to its genetic profile. Androgen receptor (AR)-positive TNBC is one of these subtypes [12]. AR-positive TNBC shows preserved androgenic signaling that could be a possible therapeutic molecular target similar to ER-positive breast cancer [10,13]. Additionally, AR expression has been identified in 70%–90% of breast tumors, similar to the frequency of ER expression in breast tumors [14]. Although previous reports indicated that androgens inhibit the progression of breast cancer [15–17], the precise mechanisms and clinical significance of AR in breast cancer remain unclear. International phase II studies aiming to develop a novel individualized treatment strategy against TNBC are currently underway in AR-positive TNBC [13]. There have been several reports investigating the clinical features of AR-positive TNBC [10,18–22]; most have found non-aggressive characteristics with a favorable prognosis compared with AR-negative TNBCs [18,22,23]. However, some reports have suggested positive correlations between AR positivity and progressive disease or poor prognosis [19]. Thus, controversies still exist concerning the clinical significance of AR expression in TNBC [24].

In this study, we classified 190 cases of breast cancer with the triple-negative phenotype from 1036 breast carcinomas. We addressed the significance of clinicopathologic features and AR expression in order to identify additional prognostic markers that can help identify tumors with more aggressive behavior.

2. Materials and Methods

2.1. Patient Background

This study investigated a consecutive series of 1036 patients with primary infiltrating breast cancer who underwent operations at the Osaka City University Hospital from 2000 to 2006. Additionally, 190 patients with TNBC treated at the Osaka City General Hospital were included. All of the patients who had undergone conservative breast surgery received postoperative radiotherapy to the residual breast. TNBC patients received adjuvant chemotherapy by either an anthracycline-based regimen (doxorubicin or epirubicin) or a 5-fluorouracil (5-FU)-based regimen, depending on the stage or risk of recurrence, in accordance with the National Comprehensive Cancer Network guidelines or the guidelines for breast cancer in Japan. The median follow-up time was 6.6 years (range, 0.2–8.0 years). Relapse-free survival (RFS) was defined as the interval between the date of surgical removal of the primary tumor and the date at which relapse was confirmed or the date of the last follow-up (for censored patients). Cancer-specific survival (CSS) was the time, in years, from the date of the primary surgery to the time of breast cancer-related death. Tumors were confirmed histopathologically and staged according to the TNM classification. This research conformed to the provisions of the Declaration of Helsinki in 1995. All patients were informed of the investigational nature of this study and provided their written, informed consent. The study protocol was approved by the Ethics Committee of Osaka City University (#926).

2.2. Immunohistochemistry

Immunohistochemical studies were performed as previously described [25]. The tumor specimens were fixed in a 10% formaldehyde solution and embedded in paraffin, after which they were cut into 4-μm thick sections and mounted on glass slides. The slides were deparaffinized in xylene and heated in an autoclave for 20 min at 105 °C and 0.4 kg/m^2 in Target Retrieval Solution (Dako, Carpinteria, CA, USA). The specimens were then incubated with 3% hydrogen peroxide in methanol for 15 min to block endogenous peroxidase activity, and then incubated in 10% normal goat or rabbit serum to block nonspecific reactions.

Primary monoclonal antibodies directed against ER (clone 1D5, dilution 1:80; Dako), PR (clone PgR636, dilution 1:100; Dako), HER2 (HercepTest™; Dako, Carpinteria, CA, USA), Ki67 (clone MIB-1, dilution 1:100; Dako), and AR (clone AR441, dilution 1:100; Dako) were used. The tissue sections were incubated with antibody for 70 min at room temperature or overnight at 4 °C (HER2: 70 min; ER, PgR, Ki67, AR: overnight), and were then incubated with horseradish peroxidase-conjugated anti-rabbit or anti-mouse Ig polymer as a secondary antibody (HISTOFINE (PO)™ kit; Nichirei, Tokyo, Japan). The slides were subsequently treated with streptavidin–peroxidase reagent and incubated in phosphate-buffered saline-diaminobenzidine and 1% hydrogen peroxide (*v*/*v*), followed by counterstaining with Mayer's hematoxylin. Positive and negative controls for each marker were used according to the supplier's data sheet.

2.3. Immunohistochemical Scoring

Immunohistochemical scoring was performed by two pathologists who specialized in mammary gland pathology using the blind method to confirm the objectivity and reproducibility of the diagnosis. In line with previous studies, the cut-off value for ER and PR positivity was set at ≥1%, and the same cut-off was adopted for AR positivity. HER2 expression was graded according to the accepted grading system as 0, 1+, 2+, or 3+. The following criteria were used for scoring: 0, no reactivity or membranous reactivity in <10% of cells; 1+, faint/barely perceptible membranous reactivity in ≥10% of cells or reactivity in only part of the cell membrane; 2+, weak to moderate complete or basolateral membranous reactivity in ≥10% of tumor cells; 3+, strong complete or basolateral membranous reactivity in ≥10% of tumor cells. HER2 was considered positive if the grade of immunostaining was 3+, or 2+ with gene amplification via fluorescent in situ hybridization (FISH). In the FISH analysis, each copy of the HER2 gene and a reference gene (centromere 17; CEP17) was counted. The interpretation followed the criteria of the American Society of Clinical Oncology (ASCO)/College of American Pathologists (CAP) guidelines for HER2 immunohistochemistry classification for positive breast cancer if the HER2/CEP17 ratio was higher than 2.0 [26]. A Ki67-labeling index of ≥14% was classified as positive [27]. Immunohistochemical scoring of AR expression was evaluated as previously described [28–30]. AR expression was semi-quantitatively analyzed according to the percentage of cells showing nuclear positivity: 0, 0%; 1+, 1%–29%; 2+, 30%–69%; 3+, ≥70%. Scores ≥1 were considered positive, and a score of 0 was negative (Figure 1) [28–30].

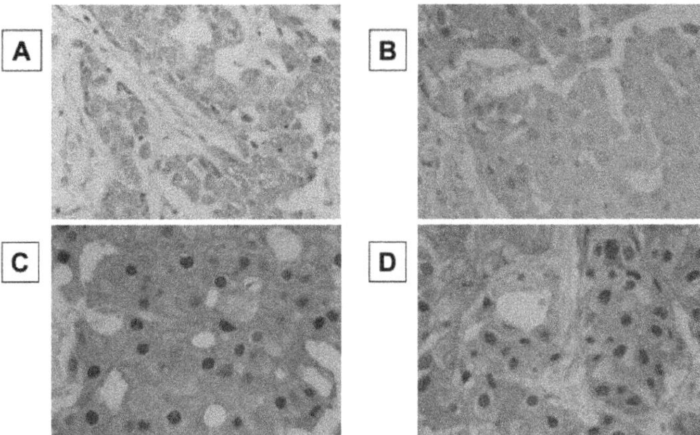

Figure 1. Immunohistochemical determination of androgen receptor. Androgen receptor (AR) expression was semi-quantitatively analyzed according to the percentage of cells showing nucleus tipositivity: 0, 0% (**A**); 1+, 1%–29% (**B**); 2+, 30%–69% (**C**); 3+, ≥70% (**D**). AR expression was considered positive when scores were ≥1, and negative when scores were 0. (×400).

2.4. Statistical Analysis

Statistical analysis was performed using the SPSS® version 19.0 statistical software package (IBM, Armonk, New York, NY, USA). Categorical data are reported with numbers and percentage, and continuous data as median and range. The association between TNBC and other clinicopathologic variables and the significance of different prognostic markers were analyzed using the chi-squared test (or Fisher's exact test when necessary). Association with survival was analyzed by the Kaplan-Meier plot and log-rank test. The Cox proportional hazards model was used to compute univariate and multivariate hazard ratios (HRs) for the study parameters with 95% confidence intervals (95% CIs). In all of the tests, a p-value of less than 0.05 was considered statistically significant. Cutoff values for different biomarkers included in this study were chosen before statistical analysis.

3. Results

The prognoses of 1036 patients with breast cancer who underwent surgery were analyzed retrospectively according to pathological subclassification. Among these, 190 (18.3%) were diagnosed with TNBC, and 846 (81.7%) with non-TNBC. Adjuvant chemotherapy was provided to 138/190 (72.6%) TNBC patients; 60 patients received an anthracycline-based regimen and 78 received a 5-FU-based regimen. Patients with TNBC had a significantly higher relapse rate compared to those with non-TNBC ($p < 0.001$, log-rank) (Supplemental Figure S1A). Furthermore, patients with TNBC also had a significantly poorer CSS rate than those with non-TNBC ($p < 0.001$, log-rank) (Supplemental Figure S1B).

Fifty-six of 190 (29.5%) TNBC tumors expressed AR. No correlation was found between clinicopathologic characteristics and AR expression (Table 1). Additionally, no significant difference was observed in RFS rates between patients with AR-positive and -negative TNBC ($p = 0.348$, log-rank) (Figure 2A). However, the patients with AR-expressing tumors had significantly better prognoses than those with non-AR-expressing tumors ($p < 0.001$, log-rank) (Figure 2B). A statistical analysis of clinical factors demonstrated that advanced disease stage, tumor diameter $\geq$2 cm, positive axillary lymph node metastasis, higher histological grade, and negative tumor AR expression correlated significantly with poorer RFS. A multivariate analysis demonstrated that positive axillary lymph node metastasis was an independent and the strongest factor indicating higher risk of recurrence in patients with TNBC ($p = 0.011$, HR = 3.30). In addition, AR expression was found to be an independent factor indicating favorable prognosis in patients with TNBC ($p = 0.039$, HR = 0.36) (Table 2).

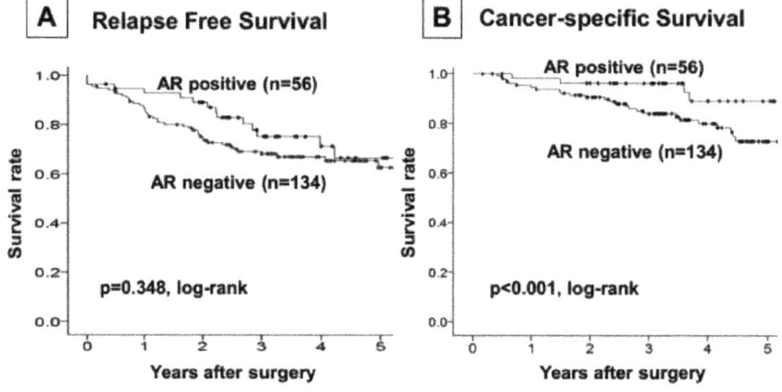

Figure 2. Cancer specific and relapse-free survival of patients based on AR expression in triple-negative breast cancers. AR expression cases had significantly good prognosis compared to the non-expression cases (**A**), but no significant difference in relapse-free survival rate was observed between AR-positive and negative triple-negative breast caluncer (TNBC) cases (**B**).

Table 1. Correlation between clinicopathological features and androgen receptor expression in 190 triple-negative breast cancer.

Parameters	Androgen Receptor		p Value
	Positive (n = 56)	Negative (n = 134)	
Age at operation			
≤55	27 (48.2%)	57 (42.5%)	
>55	29 (51.8%)	77 (57.5%)	0.473
Stage			
1	16 (28.6%)	43 (32.1%)	
2–4	40 (71.4%)	91 (67.9%)	0.633
Tumor size (cm)			
≤2	21 (37.5%)	54 (40.3%)	
>2	35 (62.5%)	80 (59.7%)	0.719
Lymph node status			
Negative	34 (60.7%)	81 (60.4%)	
Positive	22 (39.3%)	53 (39.6%)	0.973
Lymphatic invasion			
Negative	44 (78.6%)	91 (67.9%)	
Positive	12 (21.4%)	43 (32.1%)	0.140
Vascular invasion			
Negative	56 (100.0%)	129 (96.3%)	
Positive	0 (0%)	5 (3.7%)	0.171
Histologic type			
IDC	48 (85.6%)	116 (86.6%)	
Special type	8 (14.3%)	18 (13.4%)	0.876
Histological grade			
1–2	28 (50.0%)	55 (41.0%)	
3	28 (50.0%)	79 (59.0%)	0.257
Ki67			
Negative	24 (42.9%)	57 (42.5%)	
Positive	32 (57.1%)	77 (57.5%)	0.968

IDC, invasive ductal carcinoma.

Table 2. Univariate and multivariate analysis with respect to progression free survival in 190 triple-negative breast cancers.

Parameters	Univarite Analysis			Multivariate Analysis		
	Hazard Ratio	95% CI	p Value	Hazard Ratio	95% CI	p Value
Androgen receptor Positive vs. Negative	0.34	0.13–0.87	0.025	0.36	0.14–0.95	0.039
Pathological stage I vs. II and III	2.54	1.04–6.22	0.041	0.40	0.62–2.54	0.329
Tumor size (cm) ≤2 vs. >2	2.46	1.11–5.45	0.027	2.71	0.63–11.77	0.183
Lymph node status n0 vs. n1, n2, n3	3.39	1.67–6.88	0.001	3.30	1.32–8.25	0.011
Lymphatic invasion ly0 vs. ly1, ly2, ly3	1.94	0.99–3.75	0.054	1.23	0.65–2.66	0.565
Histological grade 1, 2 vs. 3	2.36	1.01–5.21	0.034	1.78	0.79–4.01	0.162

Among 43 patients who suffered from disease relapse, 10 (23.3%) had AR-positive TNBC. When CSS after the relapse was investigated, patients with AR-positive TNBC had a significantly better prognosis than those with AR-negative TNBC (p = 0.034, log-rank) (Figure 3). However, there were no clinical features or pathological characteristics observed that may have influenced the increased survival rate in patients with AR-positive TNBC in comparison with those with AR-negative TNBC (Table 3).

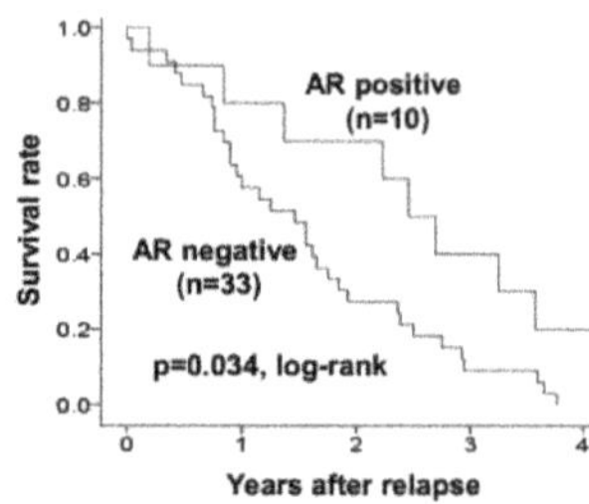

Figure 3. In relapse cases of TNBC. AR-positive TNBC had significantly good prognosis compared to negative cases.

Table 3. Correlation between clinicopathological features and androgen receptor expression among 43 relapsed cases in 190 triple-negative breast cancer.

Parameters	Androgen Receptor		p Value
	Positive (n = 10)	Negative (n = 33)	
Age at operation			
≤55	5 (50.0%)	20 (60.6%)	
>55	5 (50.0%)	13 (39.4%)	0.551
Stage			
1	2 (20.0%)	8 (24.2%)	
2–4	8 (80.0%)	25 (75.8%)	0.575
Tumor size (cm)			
≤2	3 (30.0%)	9 (27.3%)	
>2	7 (70.0%)	24 (72.3%)	0.579
Lymph node status			
Negative	5 (50.0%)	14 (42.4%)	
Positive	5 (50.0%)	19 (57.6%)	0.673
Lymphatic invasion			
Negative	6 (60.0%)	14 (42.4%)	
Positive	4 (40.0%)	19 (57.6%)	0.269
Vascular invasion			
Negative	10 (100.0%)	31 (93.9%)	
Positive	0 (0%)	2 (6.1%)	0.585
Histologic type			
IDC	10 (100.0%)	28 (84.8%)	
Special type	0 (0.0%)	5 (15.2%)	0.247
Histological grade			
1–2	3 (30.0%)	8 (24.2%)	
3	7 (70.0%)	25 (75.8%)	0.504
Ki67			
Negative	1 (10.0%)	11 (33.3%)	
Positive	9 (90.0%)	22 (66.7%)	0.149
Relapse and metastases			
Locoregional	6 (60.0%)	19 (57.6%)	
Distant	4 (40.0%)	14 (42.4%)	0.594

IDC, invasive ductal carcinoma.

4. Discussion

In recent studies, it has been determined that TNBC may further be classified into seven subtypes according to its gene expression profile [10,11], and the subtypes may respond differently to standardized therapeutic efforts [31]. According to previous studies, AR expression is commonly found in tumors that also express ER, and the prevalence of AR expression in TNBCs is reported less frequently, ranging from 13.7% to 64.3% (total 317/1227; 25.8%) [8,30,32–34]. This variability may be caused by differences in the techniques or criteria used to define AR positivity [8,29,30,32–34]. For AR positivity, many studies have adopted the standardized criteria for determining ER and PR positivity in breast cancer, defined as >1% positive cancer cells, which was also used in our study [29,30]. We found 30% of TNBCs expressed AR, which was in line with previous reports. Our study included as many as 190 TNBCs, although we did not examine the genetic profiles of each AR-positive tumor to determine which of these tumors could be classified into the luminal androgen receptor (LAR) subtype [30]. However, we did demonstrate that AR-positive TNBCs had different characteristics than AR-negative TNBCs. Thus, we believe that most of the AR-positive TNBCs could be categorized as the LAR subtype, and the population of the LAR subtype in TNBC would not be rare, as has been described by Lehmann et al. [10]. As with the luminal A and B (ER+) subtypes, overexpression of FOXA1 is observed as in LAR subtype TNBCs [10]. Breast tumors with FOXA1 overexpression have been reported to have a good prognosis, and we expect that the expression of FOXA1 will be tested in AR-positive TNBCs in the future.

As has been suggested in previous reports, we observed a significant difference in disease-free survival between patients with AR-positive and -negative TNBC [30,32,34]. Patients with AR-positive TNBC had disease recurrence later, by approximately 2 years, compared with those with AR-negative TNBC. Previous studies have shown that AR-positive tumors are associated with lower Ki-67 index [33], postmenopausal status, positive nodal status [30], higher tumor grade, and development of distant metastasis [8]. However, in our samples, the profiles of the patient or the initial disease did not differ between AR-positive and -negative TNBC. We also observed no difference in the site of recurrence (loco-regional or distant). These observations suggested that AR-positive TNBC has similar clinical characteristics to AR-negative TNBC. There have been consistent results concerning the difference in the population of TNBC and AR positivity according to race. AR-positive TNBCs in Japanese women may have unknown characteristics distinct from TNBCs as a whole that could contribute to the longer time to disease relapse. Signals generated by AR expression have been confirmed to display adverse effects on cellular proliferation in some breast cancer cell lines treated with 5-alpha-dihydrotestosterone [35]. These molecular mechanisms could be involved in delaying disease relapse.

AR expression also had a significant effect on CSS. Patients with AR-positive TNBCs survived longer after recurrence than those with AR-negative TNBCs. This clearly suggests a difference in malignant potential between AR-positive and -negative TNBC. However, we could not identify any specific factor responsible for this increase in survival. This was a retrospective study, and thus we could not alter the treatment strategies as the result of AR expression for any patient. Therefore, the difference in survival might be caused by differences in sensitivity to conventional treatments or by the innate nature of the AR-positive TNBC phenotype. Further investigation is required to identify the precise characteristics of AR-positive TNBCs. We have previously reported that TNBCs that are positive for AR expression have a significantly lower rate of pathological complete response (pCR) in neoadjuvant chemotherapy (NAC) and are chemotherapy-resistant [28].

A study examining treatment with AR antagonists in AR-expressing breast cancers is currently underway for clinical application [36]. There have been several agents that have been shown to have adverse effects on AR-positive cancer cells, and two clinical studies have already been conducted using targeted agents in AR-positive breast cancer [13]. The administration of bicalutamide to patients with metastatic AR-positive TNBC resulted in stable disease for 24 months in 19% of patients. These agents could become important treatment options for AR-positive TNBC in the near future [37].

In this study, we carried out protein expression analysis on TNBCs using immunohistochemical staining and investigated the clinical significance of AR expression. Although we observed no significant difference in the RFS rate between AR-positive and -negative TNBC cases, many late relapse cases (4 or more years to recurrence) showed luminal type relapse. Thus, we believe that AR-positive TNBC has biological properties different from those of the basal-like TNBCs that display a high degree of malignancy, and that are more similar to the hormone receptor-positive luminal subtypes. We believe that among the TNBC subtypes, the biological malignancy of AR-positive TNBC is lower than other subtypes.

5. Conclusions

We conclude that AR expression may be useful as a subclassification marker for good prognosis in TNBC, and that AR-positive TNBCs may be responsive to anti-androgen endocrine therapy.

Supplementary Materials: The following are available online at http://www.mdpi.com/2072-6694/9/1/4/s1. Figure S1: Correlation between the triple-negative phenotype and cancer specific survival and relapse-free survival. The patients with triple-negative breast cancers had a significantly poorer outcome in all breast cancers (A,B).

Acknowledgments: This study was supported in part by Grants-in Aid for Scientific Research (KAKENHI 25461992 and 26461957) from the Ministry of Education, Science, Sports, Culture and Technology of Japan. We thank Yayoi Matsukiyo and Tomomi Ohkawa (Department of Surgical Oncology, Osaka City University Graduate School of Medicine) for helpful advice regarding data management.

Author Contributions: Y.A. participated in the design of the study and drafted the manuscript. S.K. helped with study data collection and manuscript preparation. W.G., T.M., and T.T. helped with study data collection and participated in its design. S.N. and N.O. helped with data collection and manuscript preparation. S.T. and M. Ohsawa were responsible for the pathological diagnosis. K.H. and M. Ohira conceived the study, and participated in its design and coordination and helped to draft the manuscript. All authors have read and approved the final manuscript.

Conflicts of Interest: The authors declare no conflict of interest.

References

1. Abd El-Rehim, D.M.; Ball, G.; Pinder, S.E.; Rakha, E.; Paish, C.; Robertson, J.F.; Macmillan, D.; Blamey, R.W.; Ellis, I.O. High-throughput protein expression analysis using tissue microarray technology of a large well-characterised series identifies biologically distinct classes of breast cancer confirming recent cDNA expression analyses. *Int. J. Cancer* **2005**, *116*, 340–350. [CrossRef] [PubMed]
2. Mattie, M.D.; Benz, C.C.; Bowers, J.; Sensinger, K.; Wong, L.; Scott, G.K.; Fedele, V.; Ginzinger, D.; Getts, R.; Haqq, C. Optimized high-throughput microRNA expression profiling provides novel biomarker assessment of clinical prostate and breast cancer biopsies. *Mol. Cancer* **2006**, *5*, 24. [CrossRef] [PubMed]
3. Perou, C.M.; Sorlie, T.; Eisen, M.B.; van de Rijn, M.; Jeffrey, S.S.; Rees, C.A.; Pollack, J.R.; Ross, D.T.; Johnsen, H.; Akslen, L.A.; et al. Molecular portraits of human breast tumours. *Nature* **2000**, *406*, 747–752. [CrossRef] [PubMed]
4. Sorlie, T.; Perou, C.M.; Tibshirani, R.; Aas, T.; Geisler, S.; Johnsen, H.; Hastie, T.; Eisen, M.B.; van de Rijn, M.; Jeffrey, S.S.; et al. Gene expression patterns of breast carcinomas distinguish tumor subclasses with clinical implications. *Proc. Natl. Acad. Sci. USA* **2001**, *98*, 10869–10874. [CrossRef] [PubMed]
5. Nielsen, T.O.; Hsu, F.D.; Jensen, K.; Cheang, M.; Karaca, G.; Hu, Z.; Hernandez-Boussard, T.; Livasy, C.; Cowan, D.; Dressler, L.; et al. Immunohistochemical and clinical characterization of the basal-like subtype of invasive breast carcinoma. *Clin. Cancer Res.* **2004**, *10*, 5367–5374. [CrossRef] [PubMed]
6. Perou, C.M. Molecular stratification of triple-negative breast cancers. *Oncologist* **2011**, *16*, S61–S70. [CrossRef] [PubMed]
7. Bauer, C.; Peigne, V.; Gisselbrecht, M. Unusual presentation of myeloma in an elderly woman: Breast and cutaneous involvement. *Eur. J. Intern. Med.* **2008**, *19*, 150–151. [CrossRef] [PubMed]
8. Rakha, E.A.; El-Sayed, M.E.; Green, A.R.; Lee, A.H.; Robertson, J.F.; Ellis, I.O. Prognostic markers in triple-negative breast cancer. *Cancer* **2007**, *109*, 25–32. [CrossRef] [PubMed]

9. Sorlie, T.; Tibshirani, R.; Parker, J.; Hastie, T.; Marron, J.S.; Nobel, A.; Deng, S.; Johnsen, H.; Pesich, R.; Geisler, S.; et al. Repeated observation of breast tumor subtypes in independent gene expression data sets. *Proc. Natl. Acad. Sci. USA* **2003**, *100*, 8418–8423. [CrossRef] [PubMed]
10. Lehmann, B.D.; Bauer, J.A.; Chen, X.; Sanders, M.E.; Chakravarthy, A.B.; Shyr, Y.; Pietenpol, J.A. Identification of human triple-negative breast cancer subtypes and preclinical models for selection of targeted therapies. *J. Clin. Investig.* **2011**, *121*, 2750–2767. [CrossRef] [PubMed]
11. Metzger-Filho, O.; Tutt, A.; de Azambuja, E.; Saini, K.S.; Viale, G.; Loi, S.; Bradbury, I.; Bliss, J.M.; Azim, H.A., Jr.; Ellis, P.; et al. Dissecting the heterogeneity of triple-negative breast cancer. *J. Clin. Oncol.* **2012**, *30*, 1879–1887. [CrossRef] [PubMed]
12. Gucalp, A.; Traina, T.A. Triple-negative breast cancer: Role of the androgen receptor. *Cancer J.* **2010**, *16*, 62–65. [CrossRef] [PubMed]
13. Gucalp, A.; Tolaney, S.; Isakoff, S.J.; Ingle, J.N.; Liu, M.C.; Carey, L.A.; Blackwell, K.; Rugo, H.; Nabell, L.; Forero, A.; et al. Phase II trial of bicalutamide in patients with androgen receptor-positive, estrogen receptor-negative metastatic Breast Cancer. *Clin. Cancer Res.* **2013**, *19*, 5505–5512. [CrossRef] [PubMed]
14. Kuenen-Boumeester, V.; Van der Kwast, T.H.; Claassen, C.C.; Look, M.P.; Liem, G.S.; Klijn, J.G.; Henzen-Logmans, S.C. The clinical significance of androgen receptors in breast cancer and their relation to histological and cell biological parameters. *Eur. J. Cancer* **1996**, *32A*, 1560–1565. [CrossRef]
15. Ando, S.; De Amicis, F.; Rago, V.; Carpino, A.; Maggiolini, M.; Panno, M.L.; Lanzino, M. Breast cancer: From estrogen to androgen receptor. *Mol. Cell. Endocrinol.* **2002**, *193*, 121–128. [CrossRef]
16. De Launoit, Y.; Veilleux, R.; Dufour, M.; Simard, J.; Labrie, F. Characteristics of the biphasic action of androgens and of the potent antiproliferative effects of the new pure antiestrogen EM-139 on cell cycle kinetic parameters in LNCaP human prostatic cancer cells. *Cancer Res.* **1991**, *51*, 5165–5170. [PubMed]
17. Poulin, R.; Baker, D.; Labrie, F. Androgens inhibit basal and estrogen-induced cell proliferation in the ZR-75-1 human breast cancer cell line. *Breast Cancer Res. Treat.* **1988**, *12*, 213–225. [CrossRef] [PubMed]
18. He, J.; Peng, R.; Yuan, Z.; Wang, S.; Peng, J.; Lin, G.; Jiang, X.; Qin, T. Prognostic value of androgen receptor expression in operable triple-negative breast cancer: A retrospective analysis based on a tissue microarray. *Med. Oncol.* **2012**, *29*, 406–410. [CrossRef] [PubMed]
19. Hu, R.; Dawood, S.; Holmes, M.D.; Collins, L.C.; Schnitt, S.J.; Cole, K.; Marotti, J.D.; Hankinson, S.E.; Colditz, G.A.; Tamimi, R.M. Androgen receptor expression and breast cancer survival in postmenopausal women. *Clin. Cancer Res.* **2011**, *17*, 1867–1874. [CrossRef] [PubMed]
20. McGhan, L.J.; McCullough, A.E.; Protheroe, C.A.; Dueck, A.C.; Lee, J.J.; Nunez-Nateras, R.; Castle, E.P.; Gray, R.J.; Wasif, N.; Goetz, M.P.; et al. Androgen receptor-positive triple negative breast cancer: A unique breast cancer subtype. *Ann. Surg. Oncol.* **2014**, *21*, 361–367. [CrossRef] [PubMed]
21. Mrklic, I.; Pogorelic, Z.; Capkun, V.; Tomic, S. Expression of androgen receptors in triple negative breast carcinomas. *Acta Histochem.* **2013**, *115*, 344–348. [CrossRef] [PubMed]
22. Robinson, J.L.; Macarthur, S.; Ross-Innes, C.S.; Tilley, W.D.; Neal, D.E.; Mills, I.G.; Carroll, J.S. Androgen receptor driven transcription in molecular apocrine breast cancer is mediated by FoxA1. *EMBO J.* **2011**, *30*, 3019–3027. [CrossRef] [PubMed]
23. Sutton, L.M.; Cao, D.; Sarode, V.; Molberg, K.H.; Torgbe, K.; Haley, B.; Peng, Y. Decreased androgen receptor expression is associated with distant metastases in patients with androgen receptor-expressing triple-negative breast carcinoma. *Am. J. Clin. Pathol.* **2012**, *138*, 511–516. [CrossRef] [PubMed]
24. Fioretti, F.M.; Sita-Lumsden, A.; Bevan, C.L.; Brooke, G.N. Revising the role of the androgen receptor in breast cancer. *J. Mol. Endocrinol.* **2014**, *52*, R257–R265. [CrossRef] [PubMed]
25. Kashiwagi, S.; Yashiro, M.; Takashima, T.; Aomatsu, N.; Kawajiri, H.; Ogawa, Y.; Onoda, N.; Ishikawa, T.; Wakasa, K.; Hirakawa, K. c-Kit expression as a prognostic molecular marker in patients with basal-like breast cancer. *Br. J. Surg.* **2013**, *100*, 490–496. [CrossRef] [PubMed]
26. Wolff, A.C.; Hammond, M.E.; Hicks, D.G.; Dowsett, M.; McShane, L.M.; Allison, K.H.; Allred, D.C.; Bartlett, J.M.; Bilous, M.; Fitzgibbons, P.; et al. Recommendations for human epidermal growth factor receptor 2 testing in breast cancer: American Society of Clinical Oncology/College of American Pathologists clinical practice guideline update. *J. Clin. Oncol.* **2013**, *31*, 3997–4013. [CrossRef] [PubMed]

27. Goldhirsch, A.; Wood, W.C.; Coates, A.S.; Gelber, R.D.; Thurlimann, B.; Senn, H.J. Panel members. Strategies for subtypes—Dealing with the diversity of breast cancer: Highlights of the St. Gallen International Expert Consensus on the Primary Therapy of Early Breast Cancer 2011. *Ann. Oncol.* **2011**, *22*, 1736–1747. [CrossRef] [PubMed]
28. Asano, Y.; Kashiwagi, S.; Onoda, N.; Kurata, K.; Morisaki, T.; Noda, S.; Takashima, T.; Ohsawa, M.; Kitagawa, S.; Hirakawa, K. Clinical verification of sensitivity to preoperative chemotherapy in cases of androgen receptor-expressing positive breast cancer. *Br. J. Cancer* **2016**, *114*, 14–20. [CrossRef] [PubMed]
29. Castellano, I.; Allia, E.; Accortanzo, V.; Vandone, A.M.; Chiusa, L.; Arisio, R.; Durando, A.; Donadio, M.; Bussolati, G.; Coates, A.S.; et al. Androgen receptor expression is a significant prognostic factor in estrogen receptor positive breast cancers. *Breast Cancer Res. Treat.* **2010**, *124*, 607–617. [CrossRef] [PubMed]
30. Luo, X.; Shi, Y.X.; Li, Z.M.; Jiang, W.Q. Expression and clinical significance of androgen receptor in triple negative breast cancer. *Chin. J. Cancer* **2010**, *29*, 585–590. [CrossRef] [PubMed]
31. Masuda, H.; Baggerly, K.A.; Wang, Y.; Zhang, Y.; Gonzalez-Angulo, A.M.; Meric-Bernstam, F.; Valero, V.; Lehmann, B.D.; Pietenpol, J.A.; Hortobagyi, G.N.; et al. Differential response to neoadjuvant chemotherapy among 7 triple-negative breast cancer molecular subtypes. *Clin. Cancer Res.* **2013**, *19*, 5533–5540. [CrossRef] [PubMed]
32. Gasparini, P.; Fassan, M.; Cascione, L.; Guler, G.; Balci, S.; Irkkan, C.; Paisie, C.; Lovat, F.; Morrison, C.; Zhang, J.; et al. Androgen receptor status is a prognostic marker in non-basal triple negative breast cancers and determines novel therapeutic options. *PLoS ONE* **2014**, *9*, e88525. [CrossRef] [PubMed]
33. McNamara, K.M.; Yoda, T.; Miki, Y.; Chanplakorn, N.; Wongwaisayawan, S.; Incharoen, P.; Kongdan, Y.; Wang, L.; Takagi, K.; Mayu, T.; et al. Androgenic pathway in triple negative invasive ductal tumors: Its correlation with tumor cell proliferation. *Cancer Sci.* **2013**, *104*, 639–646. [CrossRef] [PubMed]
34. Mohammadizadeh, F.; Sajadieh, S.; Sajjadieh, H.; Kasaei, Z. Androgen receptor expression and its relationship with clinicopathological parameters in an Iranian population with invasive breast carcinoma. *Adv. Biomed. Res.* **2014**, *3*, 132. [PubMed]
35. Greeve, M.A.; Allan, R.K.; Harvey, J.M.; Bentel, J.M. Inhibition of MCF-7 breast cancer cell proliferation by 5alpha-dihydrotestosterone; a role for p21(Cip1/Waf1). *J. Mol. Endocrinol.* **2004**, *32*, 793–810. [CrossRef] [PubMed]
36. Narayanan, R.; Dalton, J.T. Androgen receptor: A complex therapeutic target for breast cancer. *Cancers* **2016**, *8*, 108. [CrossRef] [PubMed]
37. Cochrane, D.R.; Bernales, S.; Jacobsen, B.M.; Cittelly, D.M.; Howe, E.N.; D'Amato, N.C.; Spoelstra, N.S.; Edgerton, S.M.; Jean, A.; Guerrero, J.; et al. Role of the androgen receptor in breast cancer and preclinical analysis of enzalutamide. *Breast Cancer Res.* **2014**, *16*, R7. [CrossRef] [PubMed]

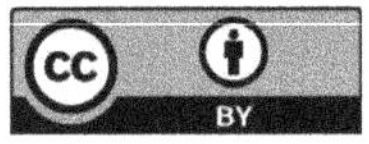

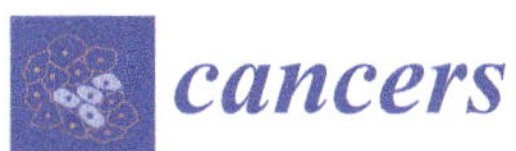

MDPI

Review

Androgen Receptor Signaling in Bladder Cancer

Peng Li [1,2,3], Jinbo Chen [4,5,6] and Hiroshi Miyamoto [1,2,4,5,7,*]

1. Department of Pathology, Johns Hopkins University School of Medicine, Baltimore, MD 21287, USA; 001lipeng@163.com
2. Department of Urology, Johns Hopkins University School of Medicine, Baltimore, MD 21287, USA
3. Minimally Invasive Urology Center, Shandong Provincial Hospital Affiliated to Shandong University, Jinan 250021, China
4. Department of Pathology & Laboratory Medicine, University of Rochester Medical Center, Rochester, NY 14642, USA; jinbo_chen@urmc.rochester.edu
5. James P. Wilmot Cancer Center, University of Rochester Medical Center, Rochester, NY 14642, USA
6. Department of Urology, Xiangya Hospital of Central South University, Changsha 410008, China
7. Department of Urology, University of Rochester Medical Center, Rochester, NY 14642, USA

* Correspondence: hiroshi_miyamoto@urmc.rochester.edu

Academic Editor: Emmanuel S. Antonarakis
Received: 1 December 2016; Accepted: 16 February 2017; Published: 22 February 2017

Abstract: Emerging preclinical findings have indicated that steroid hormone receptor signaling plays an important role in bladder cancer outgrowth. In particular, androgen-mediated androgen receptor signals have been shown to correlate with the promotion of tumor development and progression, which may clearly explain some sex-specific differences in bladder cancer. This review summarizes and discusses the available data, suggesting the involvement of androgens and/or the androgen receptor pathways in urothelial carcinogenesis as well as tumor growth. While the precise mechanisms of the functions of the androgen receptor in urothelial cells remain far from being fully understood, current evidence may offer chemopreventive or therapeutic options, using androgen deprivation therapy, in patients with bladder cancer.

Keywords: androgen; androgen receptor; anti-androgen; carcinogenesis; tumor progression; urothelial cancer

---

1. Introduction

Urinary bladder cancer, mostly urothelial carcinoma, is the second most common genitourinary malignancy, with an estimate of 429,800 new cases and 165,100 deaths in 2012 worldwide [1]. Despite significant advances in diagnostic technologies as well as surgical techniques and adjuvant/neoadjuvant treatment strategies, the prognosis of patients with bladder cancer has remained largely unchanged over the last few decades. Thus, patients with a non-muscle-invasive bladder tumor still carry a life-long risk of recurrence with occasional progression to muscle invasion following transurethral surgery, while those with a muscle-invasive tumor are at a high risk of metastasis following radical cystectomy. Indeed, current non-surgical conventional treatments, such as intravesical pharmacotherapy and systemic chemotherapy, do not result in complete prevention of tumor recurrence or significant reduction in mortality [2,3]. Of note, mainly due to the life-long need for monitoring for recurrence, bladder cancer has been reported to have the highest lifetime costs per patient among all malignancies [4,5]. As a result, further studies are urgently needed to better understand the molecular mechanisms for bladder cancer development and progression, which may not only provide effective targeted therapy but also contribute to the reduction of treatment costs.

Men are at a significantly higher risk of bladder cancer than women in the US as well as virtually all countries/regions, while there is an approximately 10-fold variation in its incidence internationally [1,6]. Cigarette smoke and exposure to industrial work-related chemicals—well-established risk factors for bladder cancer—were thought to contribute to the sex-disparity. However, men are still 3–4 times more likely to develop bladder cancer than women even after controlling these environmental or lifestyle factors [1,6–8]. Accordingly, intrinsic factors are likely to play a critical role in urothelial carcinogenesis. Meanwhile, preclinical evidence has strongly suggested the involvement of androgen receptor (AR) signaling in bladder tumorigenesis and cancer progression.

Previous studies have thus demonstrated that AR activation generally correlates with the promotion of the development and growth of urothelial cancer. In this article, we review these available data and highlight underlying molecular mechanisms.

2. Androgens, AR Signaling, and Their Physiological Functions in the Bladder

Androgens, first discovered in 1936, are a class of steroid hormones, mainly secreted by the testis, ovary, and adrenal cortex. These include testosterone and its metabolite via 5α-reductase in certain tissues, dihydrotestosterone (DHT), as well as adrenal androgens, dehydroepiandrosterone, androstenediol, and androstenedione. In males, androgens can stimulate the differentiation and maturation of the sex organs and the development of secondary sex characteristics as well as maintain sexual activity and reproductive function [9,10]. The physiological functions of androgens are mainly dependent on their binding to AR in target cells to stimulate a series of post-receptor biochemical changes [9–12].

The AR, a 110 kD protein composed of 919 amino acids, is a member of the nuclear receptor superfamily that functions as a ligand-inducible transcription factor and mediates the biological effects of androgens in a wide range of physiological and pathological processes [11–13]. The human *AR* gene locates on the X chromosome (Xq11–12) and contains eight exons and seven introns with the total length exceeding 90 kb. The AR encodes four distinct functional domains: the N-terminal transactivation domain, the DNA-binding domain (DBD), a hinge region, and the C-terminal ligand-binding domain (LBD) [13]. It usually locates in the cytoplasm coupling with heat shock proteins. Upon binding of androgens at the LBD, AR is released from heat shock proteins and is translocated into the nucleus in the form of a phosphorylated homodimer. Then, AR binds to androgen response elements (AREs) in the genome as well as to a variety of co-regulators, leading to a series of specific activation or repression of gene transcription [13,14]. An alternative mechanism of AR activation independent of androgen binding includes its phosphorylation via kinases [e.g., epidermal growth factor receptor (EGFR)] in, for instance, prostate cancer cells [15–17]. Truncated AR isoforms that lack the LBD have also been found and are constitutively active in the absence of androgens [18].

Male internal genitalia, including the prostate and bulbourethral gland as well as urothelium, are derived from the urogenital sinus endoderm. Simultaneously, it is well known that the differentiation of the prostate and its development require the induction of AR signaling [19]. Thus, we can infer that AR signaling also contributes to bladder development. Meanwhile, AR expression has been documented in a variety of human or rodent tissues [20,21]. AR has also been found to be present in urothelium as well as bladder submucosa, such as smooth muscle cells and neurons [20–24]. However, physiological functions of AR in some of the organs, including the bladder, remain far from being fully understood. Animal studies have shown that AR is involved in the regulation of urine storage and urinary tract functions. Castration in male animals resulted in significant decreases in the activity and expression of tissue enzymes closely related to cholinergic and non-cholinergic nerve functions [25,26]. Androgen supplementation in castrated male rats also re-augmented the thickness of urothelium, the quantity of smooth muscle fibers, and the number of vessels in their bladders [27]. In addition, androgen deficiency was found to induce bladder fibrosis and reduce the bladder capacity and compliance in male rats [28]. Thus, androgens appear to contribute to improving/maintaining bladder functions. It has indeed been shown in a few clinical studies that testosterone treatment is beneficial to men with lower urinary tract symptoms [29,30]. Conversely, testosterone was shown to inhibit neurogenic and chemogenic responses in the rat bladder, resulting in the reduction of detrusor muscle contraction [31].

To the best of our knowledge, there are no recent clinical studies further assessing the efficacy of androgen treatment in those with lower urinary tract symptoms.

3. Alterations of AR in Bladder Cancer

Prior to its cloning, a binding assay suggested higher levels of AR content in bladder tumor (49.5 Fm/mg) than in normal bladder mucosa (17.2 Fm/mg), as well as in male (68.0 Fm/mg) or low-grade (43.8 (male)/27.7 (female) Fm/mg) tumors than in female (27.7 Fm/mg) or high-grade (32.4 Fm/mg) tumors, respectively [32]. Thereafter, immunohistochemical studies in surgical specimens have assessed the expression status of AR in different grades/stages of bladder tumors, in comparison with normal/non-neoplastic urothelial tissues in some of them [33–44] (Table 1). Of note, a PCR-based method could detect the *AR* gene in all 33 superficial bladder cancer specimens examined [45].

Table 1. Immunohistochemical studies showing correlations between androgen receptor (AR) expression in bladder cancer and clinicopathological features.

Study [Reference]	N	AR Positivity							
		Non-tumor vs. Tumor		Patient Gender		Tumor Grade		Tumor Stage	
		Non-tumor	Tumor	Male	Female	Low	High	NMI	MI
Zhuang et al., 1997 [33]	9	NA	44.4%	50.0%	33.3%	NA	NA	20.0%	75.0%
Boorjian et al., 2004 [34]	49	86.5%	53.1%	61.1%	30.1%	88.9%	48.5%	75.0%	21.4%
Boorjian et al., 2009 [35]	55	NA	43.6%	NA	NA	NA	NA	59.1%	33.3%
Mir et al., 2011 [37]	472	NA	12.9%	14.0%	8.1%	12.2%	13.1%	9.0%	15.1%
Tuygun et al., 2011 [38]	139	0%	51.1%	66.7%	61.5%	63.9%	37.3%	60.4%	21.2%
Zheng et al., 2011 [39]	24	NA	33.3%	NA	NA	40.0%	31.6%	NA	NA
Miyamoto et al., 2012 [40]	188	80.1%	42.0%	41.9%	42.5%	55.4%	36.4%	50.5%	33.0%
Jing et al., 2014 [41]	58	NA	53.4%	56.8%	42.9%	55.0%	50.0%	48.9%	69.2%
Mashhadi et al., 2014 [42]	120	0%	21.7%	NA	NA	NA	NA	NA	NA
Nam et al., 2014 [43]	169	NA	37.3%	38.5%	30.8%	39.2%	32.7%	NA	NA
Williams et al., 2015 [44]	297	NA	24.6%	NA	NA	NA	NA	33.6%	19.5%

N: number of cases; NMI: non-muscle-invasive; MI: muscle-invasive; NA: not applicable.

The positive rates of AR expression immunohistochemically detected in bladder tumor tissues involving more than 40 cases range from 13% to 55%, which are significantly lower than those in non-neoplastic urothelial samples in some studies [34,36,40]. In contrast, at least two studies have demonstrated no detectable AR in normal urothelial tissues examined [38,42]. These conflicting findings may have resulted from differences in tissue preservation (e.g., formalin fixation), staining protocol (e.g., antibody), and/or signal scoring. In addition, the so-called cancer field effect may have affected the immunoreactivity because normal-appearing tissues from patients with bladder cancer were used in most of these studies. Nonetheless, these immunohistochemical studies have failed to reveal significant sex-related differences in AR expression in male versus female tissues (normal, tumor). A significant decrease in the AR positive rate was also reported in urothelial carcinomas of the upper urinary tract, compared with corresponding non-neoplastic urothelial tissues [46].

Some of these studies have compared the rates of AR positivity in low-grade or non-muscle-invasive tumors versus high-grade or muscle-invasive tumors. Similar to the AR positivity in bladder tumors compared with non-neoplastic bladders, its significant or insignificant down-regulation is observed in high-grade and/or muscle-invasive tumors [34–36,38,40,43]. Similar findings were observed in upper urinary tract tumors [46–48]. Thus, AR expression appears to be down-regulated or lost during steps of tumorigenesis and tumor progression in spite of the promoting effects of AR signals as described below. In contrast, a few other studies showed slight increases in AR positivity in high-grade and/or muscle-invasive bladder tumors [37,41].

Prognostic values of AR expression in bladder cancer patients have also been assessed, and the findings remain controversial. Two studies indicated a correlation between AR positivity and a lower risk of tumor recurrence [38,43]. Meanwhile, AR expression was shown to correlate with the risk of tumor progression [40,42]. Other studies have failed to show prognostic significance of AR expression in bladder or upper urinary tract tumors [36,37,46,47]. It has also been suggested that muscle-invasive bladder cancers are initially androgen-sensitive for their growth, which is eventually lost due to the activation of certain genes possessing an ARE in their promoter region in an androgen-independent manner—as seen in prostate cancer—and induces metastatic potential of tumor cells [49]. Thus, AR expression may not necessarily serve as a prognosticator in patients with bladder cancer.

In addition to the differential expression of AR protein, genetic alterations involving the *AR* gene have been documented in bladder cancer. Loss of heterozygosity at the AR locus was identified in muscle-invasive tumors and concurrent lesions of carcinoma in situ from female patients [50]. In addition, several studies have demonstrated differences in the number of polyglutamine (CAG) repeats within exon 1 of the *AR* gene, which in general is inversely correlated with its transcriptional activity, between bladder tumors and controls or different grades/stages of bladder tumors. Men and women who had 23 (odds ratio = 2.09) and 44 (cumulative; odds ratio = 4.95) CAG repeats were found to have a significantly elevated risk of urothelial carcinoma, compared to those with longer CAG [51]. A significantly shorter CAG repeat length was also identified in 95 male patients with bladder cancer (mean: 19.8), compared with 94 control males (mean: 21.1) [52]. Moreover, there appeared to be a link between shorter CAG repeat length and more aggressive features of bladder cancer in a relatively small number of cases [53]. Short CAG repeat lengths (20 in UMUC3 and 22 in TCCSUP) were also identified in two AR-positive human bladder cancer cell lines [35]. Meanwhile, although no somatic mutations in the *AR* gene were found in 99 cases of bladder cancer [54], a molecular profiling data search [55,56] identified them in up to 4% (2 of 50) of urothelial carcinomas of the bladder as well as in 6.1% (2 of 33) of plasmacytoid urothelial carcinomas. AR isoforms (i.e., 90 kDa, 60 kDa) were also detected in some of tumor specimens [33], suggesting the presence of its splice variants in bladder cancer.

4. Role of AR Signaling in Urothelial Carcinogenesis

The gender-specific difference in the incidence of bladder cancer as well as AR expression in benign and cancerous urothelium suggests the involvement of AR signaling in urothelial tumorigenesis. High incidence of high-grade prostatic intraepithelial neoplasia and prostatic adenocarcinoma—in the development of both of which, AR plays a critical role—in cystoprostatectomy specimens undergone for bladder urothelial carcinoma (e.g., 24.4% for the latter in a meta-analysis involving 13,140 patients [57]) may also support the presence of common tumorigenesis signals between these two malignancies. Based on these observations, previous studies using various approaches have assessed the role of androgens and/or AR in urothelial carcinogenesis.

A chemical carcinogen, *N*-butyl-*N*-4-hydroxybutyl nitrosamine (BBN), which is known to induce a bladder tumor effectively in experimental rodents and more rapidly in male animals than in females [58], has been used to assess the effects of androgens, AR, and anti-AR treatment on bladder carcinogenesis. In 1975, it was shown that testosterone treatment in female rats increased the incidence of BBN-induced bladder tumors while a synthetic estrogen diethylstilbestrol in males decreased it [59]. In 1997, hormonal treatment with a gonadotropin-releasing hormone analogue as chemical castration or an anti-androgen flutamide was shown to prevent the development of BBN-mediated tumors in male rats [60]. Subsequently, BBN was found to fail to induce bladder cancer in male or female AR knockout (ARKO) mice [45]. Testosterone treatment and surgical orchiectomy were also shown to increase and decrease, respectively, the incidence of bladder tumors in male rats with administration of another carcinogen *N*-nitrosobis(2-oxopropyl)amine [61]. Thus, androgen-mediated AR signals appeared to play a critical role in bladder carcinogenesis induced by chemical carcinogens. However, a subset of male ARKO mice treated with BBN and supplemented with DHT developed bladder tumors [45], suggesting the involvement of androgen-mediated non-AR pathways in bladder tumorigenesis. Otherwise, because only DBD in exon 2 of the *AR* gene was disrupted in the ARKO mice [62], the androgen effect on bladder tumorigenesis might be mediated through the truncated AR protein that is unable to bind to DNA. An additional possibility was that the second zinc finger of the DBD in exon 3 had residual DNA binding activity. More recently, BBN was also found to fail to induce bladder tumors in male mice having normal levels of testosterone yet lacking AR specifically in the urothelium [63]. Similarly, the incidence of a BBN-induced bladder tumor in a transgenic mouse model where AR is conditionally expressed in the bladder urothelium was higher than that in age and sex matched controls [64]. In addition, castration inhibited the development of bladder tumors in another transgenic mouse model in which constitutive active β-catenin in the urothelial basal cells spontaneously induced high-grade urothelial cancer [65]. These observations further suggest a critical role of urothelial AR, but not ARs in other organs, in bladder carcinogenesis.

Several recent retrospective cohort studies have supported these findings in animals indicating that AR activation correlates with the induction of bladder tumorigenesis. First, men undergoing androgen deprivation therapy (ADT) for their prostate cancer were shown to have a considerably lower risk of subsequent development of bladder cancer (0/266 (0%)), compared with those undergoing surgery alone (5/437 (1.1%)) or radiotherapy (14/631 (2.2%)) [66]; second, in 162 men with a history of prostate and bladder cancers, ADT used for the treatment of the former strongly prevented the recurrence of the latter, compared with those without ADT [67]. In this cohort, AR expression in their bladder tumors was also found to be an independent predictor of the preventive effects of ADT on tumor recurrence [68]; third, in 228 men with a history of bladder cancer, ADT (for their prostate cancer) or a 5α-reductase inhibitor dutasteride treatment (for their benign prostatic hyperplasia) resulted in significant reduction in the rate of bladder tumor recurrence, compared with 196 control patients without hormonal treatment [69]; finally, in a prospective cohort study involving 72,370 men, treatment with a 5α-reductase inhibitor finasteride primarily prescribed for their symptomatic benign prostatic hyperplasia significantly reduced the risk of bladder cancer development (hazard ratio = 0.634; $p = 0.0004$) [70], although a preclinical study failed to show a significant inhibitory effect of finasteride on a BBN-induced bladder tumor [60].

Androgens have been shown to modulate the activity and/or expression of certain enzymes via the AR pathway. These enzymes include cytochrome P450 (e.g., CYP4B1) and UDP-glucuronosyltransferase (e.g., UGT1A subtypes) that are known to involve the activation and detoxification, respectively, of bladder carcinogens, such as aromatic amines. The levels of *CYP4B1* gene expression in male mouse bladders were found to be higher than those in female mouse bladders, and castration in males resulted in a decrease in its expression [71]. Similarly, the expression levels of mouse Ugt1a subtypes were elevated in the bladders from intact female or ARKO male mice, compared with those from intact/control male mice [72]. In addition, orchiectomy [72] or ovariectomy [73] up- or down-regulated, respectively, the expression of some Ugt1a subtypes in the mouse bladders. Meanwhile, in SVHUC human normal urothelial cells stably expressing wild-type full-length AR, DHT treatment resulted in considerable decreases in the expression of all UGT1A subtypes, and an anti-androgen hydroxyflutamide blocked the DHT effects [72]. Moreover, in a mouse model, castration was shown to reduce bladder susceptibility to a carcinogen 4-aminobiphenyl via modulating UGT1A3 in the liver [74].

GATA3 is a zinc-finger transcription factor and is highly expressed in urothelial cells. Loss of GATA3 expression in a subset of bladder cancers, especially high-grade and/or muscle-invasive tumors [75], as well as its correlation with the induction of tumor cell migration and invasion in vitro [76], suggests the role of GATA3 as a tumor suppressor. Indeed, in an in vitro transformation model using SVHUC cells, GATA3 silencing resulted in the induction of malignant transformation as well as down- or up-regulation of the expression of tumor suppressors (e.g., p53, p21, p27, PTEN, UGT1A) or oncogenic molecules (e.g., c-myc, cyclin D1/D3/E, FGFR3), respectively [77]. In SVHUC sublines with or without undergoing neoplastic transformation induced by carcinogen challenge, AR overexpression or androgen treatment considerably reduced GATA3 expression [77]. In addition, orchiectomy increased and ovariectomy decreased the levels of GATA3 expression in the mouse bladders [77]. Thus, in non-neoplastic urothelial cells, AR activation appears to correlate with the down-regulation of the expression of GATA3 that prevents neoplastic transformation.

5. Role of AR Signaling in Urothelial Cancer Progression

In addition to its involvement in urothelial carcinogenesis, there have been a variety of studies suggesting that androgens and/or AR promote bladder cancer progression. As seen in prostate cancer cells, androgens could induce AR expression and its nuclear translocation as well as ARE promoter activity in bladder cancer cells [39,41,45,78–83]. In some of these studies, AR antagonists, such as flutamide, bicalutamide, and enzalutamide, were shown to block the effects of androgens on AR expression or transcription.

Using cell viability or colony formation assays, androgens have been shown to induce the growth of AR-positive bladder cancer cells [39,45,79,80,82–89]. Accordingly, AR knockdown as well as treatment with AR antagonists inhibited the cell proliferation of bladder cancer lines cultured with androgens. In an earlier study using the R198 transplantable bladder cancer line, tumor growth in male mice was facilitated by DHT administration [90]. Subsequent studies using mouse xenograft models for bladder cancer demonstrated that orchiectomy or treatment with anti-AR compounds could considerably inhibit tumor growth [41,45,84,86–88,91]. In a transgenic mouse model expressing SV40 large T antigen specifically in urothelium (via uroplakin II) and spontaneously developing bladder cancer, castration after tumor formation retarded its growth, which was restored by DHT supplement [92]. Similarly, in vitro assays have demonstrated that androgen-mediated AR signals promote the migration and invasion of bladder cancer cells [41,82,83,88]. Then, AR knockdown or anti-androgen treatment was shown to inhibit them [41,83,86–88]. Additionally, in the uroplakin II-SV40T transgenic model, castration reduced microvessel density in bladder tumors and increased the expression of an anti-angiogenic factor TSP-1 [92], indicating the promotion of angiogenesis by AR activation in bladder cancer.

In AR-positive bladder cancer cells, androgens are able to modulate the expression or activity of various molecules/pathways. Those known to involve bladder cancer cell proliferation/ migration/invasion as well as angiogenesis/metastasis include β-catenin/Wnt signaling and its downstream targets c-myc/cyclin D1 [65,81,84,86], CD24 [80,88], EGFR family and its downstream AKT/ERK [39,79], ELK1 [82], matrix metalloproteinases (MMPs) [45,65,83,86,88,93], and vascular endothelial growth factor [45,88]. Androgen-mediated AR signals were also shown to induce epithelial-to-mesenchymal transition via modulating the expression of Slug and the activity of β-catenin/Wnt signaling in bladder cancer cells [41,87]. More recently, in vitro assays demonstrated that bladder cancer cells could recruit B cells [94], T cells [95], and neutrophils [93], leading to the induction of cell invasion as well as the expression of AR and MMPs. These observations may represent underlying molecular mechanisms for the promoting effects of androgens on bladder cancer progression.

As seen in prostate cancer cells, non-androgens, such as epidermal growth factor (EGF), could increase AR transcriptional activity in bladder cancer cells, which was blocked by AR antagonists [79]. EGF could also induce AR-positive bladder cancer cell proliferation in the absence of androgens [79,85]. More interestingly, EGF and DHT appeared to show synergistic effects on the proliferation as well as phosphorylation of EGFR, AKT, and ERK in bladder cancer cells [39,79].

Recent in vitro studies have suggested a correlation between AR activity in bladder cancer cells and chemosensitivity. AR-positive cell lines were more resistant to cisplatin than control AR-negative or AR knockdown cells cultured in the presence of androgens [96]. Furthermore, androgen or anti-androgen treatment resulted in a decrease or an increase, respectively, in sensitivity to cisplatin in AR-positive bladder cancer cells, presumably via modulating the activity of a key factor of cisplatin resistance NF-κB [96]. Similarly, bladder cancer cells overexpressing AR or those treated with DHT were found to be more resistant to doxorubicin, an anti-cancer agent often used for intravesical pharmacotherapy, than respective control cells [84]. However, there were no significant differences in sensitivity to 5-fluorouracil [84] or gemcitabine [96] between AR-positive versus AR-negative bladder cancer cells or between AR-positive cells with versus without androgen treatment. In addition, enzalutamide treatment or AR knockdown was shown to inhibit the growth of gemcitabine-resistant bladder cancer cells, while whether it could increase chemosensitivity was not tested [89]. Of note, in these studies, AR expression was shown to be considerably elevated in "resistant" cell lines after long-term culture with cisplatin [96], doxorubicin [84], or gemcitabine [89], compared with control lines.

6. AR Co-Regulators in Bladder Cancer

As aforementioned, androgen-mediated AR transcriptional activity can be further enhanced by co-activators. Indeed, several AR co-regulators have been implicated in the modulation of bladder cancer cell growth. A cross-talk between AR-co-regulators and other signaling pathways in bladder cancer cells may further promote urothelial tumorigenesis and tumor progression.

Immunohistochemistry in tissue samples showed the expression of NCOA1, NCOA2, NCOA3, CREBBP, and EP300, in 85%–100% of bladder tumors—some of which even lacked AR expression [35]. Furthermore, of these AR co-activators, only NCOA1 expression was significantly down-regulated in tumors, compared with non-neoplastic urothelial tissues. Meanwhile, knockdown of each co-activator led to significant reduction in cell proliferation of AR-positive bladder cancer lines, although, inconsistent with the findings in prostate cancer cells, androgen treatment failed to up-regulate the expression levels of these co-activators in these cells [35]. Therefore, distinct mechanisms may underlie co-regulator functions in bladder cancer versus other AR-positive malignancies such as prostate cancer.

Immunohistochemistry in radical cystectomy specimens also showed strong correlations of the expression of JMJD2A and LSD1, both of which were shown to mediate AR transactivation via histone-lysine demethylation mechanisms, with that of AR [36]. Moreover, significant down- and up-regulation of JMJD2A and LSD1, respectively, were found in bladder cancer specimens, compared with benign urothelial tissues. Loss of JMJD2A was also associated with lymphovascular invasion or worse overall survival, but not cancer-specific mortality. Remarkably, pharmacological inhibition of LSD1 resulted in significant decreases in the growth and androgen-induced AR transcription in bladder cancer cells [36].

Altered expression of β-catenin is well known to correlate with the progression of bladder cancer and poor patient outcomes [41,81,97]. Additionally, as described above, constitutive active β-catenin in mouse bladder cells could induce urothelial tumorigenesis [65]. In AR-positive bladder cancer cells, androgens have also been shown to activate β-catenin/Wnt signaling [65,81]. Moreover, AR and β-catenin co-express at the nuclei of bladder cancer cells and form a complex with T-cell factor, a co-factor of β-catenin and a downstream component of Wnt signaling, in the presence of androgens [81]. Thus, androgen-mediated AR signals appear to synergize with β-catenin in bladder cancer cells and may thereby promote tumor growth.

7. Concluding Remarks

Current evidence indicating correlations of AR activation with the promotion of urothelial tumorigenesis and tumor progression supports that bladder cancer is a member of endocrine-related tumors. It is thus likely that at least AR and its associated signaling pathways, as depicted in Figure 1, play an important role in the pathogenesis of bladder cancer, which also helps explain the sex disparities, especially its incidence between men and women. However, underlying mechanisms of how AR and related signals regulate bladder cancer outgrowth still need to be elucidated. It also remains unclear whether androgen-mediated AR signals are the central pathway in modulating bladder carcinogenesis. Accordingly, further mechanistic studies are required to determine the precise functional role of AR signaling in the development and progression of bladder cancer.

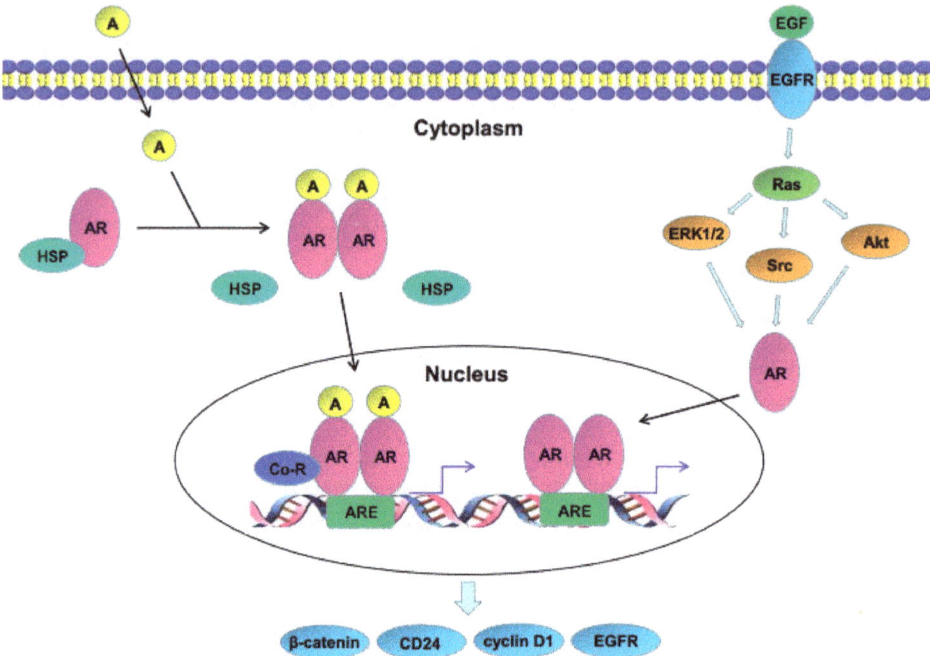

Figure 1. AR signaling in bladder cancer. A, androgen; AR, androgen receptor; ARE, androgen response element; Co-R, co-regulator; EGF, epidermal growth factor; EGFR, epidermal growth factor receptor; HSP, heat shock protein.

Again, current non-surgical conventional treatments, such as intravesical pharmacotherapy and systemic chemotherapy, often fail to completely prevent the recurrence of superficial bladder tumors or significantly reduce the mortality rate in patients with advanced bladder cancer. Moreover, no approved targeted therapy for bladder cancer is available. As aforementioned, AR signals likely promote the development and progression of urothelial cancer. We therefore anticipate that AR inactivation—even via available options clinically used for the treatment of, for instance, prostate cancer—offers an effective chemopreventive or therapeutic approach for urothelial cancer. Indeed, two phase II clinical trials are being conducted to assess the preventive effects of enzalutamide on tumor recurrence in patients with non-muscle-invasive bladder cancer (NCT02605863) and the therapeutic effects of abiraterone—an androgen biosynthesis inhibitor prescribed in men with castration-resistant prostate cancer—in patients with advanced bladder cancer (NCT02788201). In addition, a phase I trial (NCT02300610) assessing the combination effects of enzalutamide with gemcitabine and cisplatin in patients with urothelial cancer is recruiting participants. Further prospective cohort studies of anti-AR treatment in patients with bladder cancer are thus encouraged.

Conflicts of Interest: The authors declare no conflict of interest.

References

1. Torre, L.A.; Bray, F.; Siegel, R.L.; Ferlay, J.; Lortet-Tieulent, J.; Jemal, A. Global cancer statistics, 2012. *Cancer J. Clin.* **2015**, *65*, 87–108. [CrossRef] [PubMed]
2. Carneiro, B.A.; Meeks, J.J.; Kuzel, T.M.; Scaranti, M.; Abdulkadir, S.A.; Giles, F.J. Emerging therapeutic targets in bladder cancer. *Cancer Treat. Rev.* **2015**, *41*, 170–178. [CrossRef] [PubMed]

3. Knowles, M.A.; Hurst, C.D. Molecular biology of bladder cancer: New insights into pathogenesis and clinical diversity. *Nat. Rev. Cancer* **2015**, *15*, 25–41. [CrossRef] [PubMed]
4. Sievert, K.D.; Amend, B.; Nagele, U.; Schilling, D.; Bedke, J.; Horstmann, M.; Hennenlotter, J.; Kruck, S.; Stenzl, A. Economic aspects of bladder cancer: What are the benefits and costs? *World J. Urol.* **2009**, *27*, 295–300. [CrossRef] [PubMed]
5. Norm, D.; Sandip, M.; Amit, R.; Adam, B.; Joseph, J.; Aria, R.; Chieko, M.; Todd, S.; Brandon, P.; Gary, D. Bladder cancer mortality in the United States: A geographic and temporal analysis of socioeconomic and environmental factors. *J. Urol.* **2016**, *195*, 290–296.
6. Siegel, R.L.; Miller, K.D.; Jemal, A. Cancer statistics, 2016. *Cancer J. Clin.* **2016**, *66*, 7–30. [CrossRef] [PubMed]
7. Hartge, P.; Harvey, E.B.; Linehan, W.M.; Silverman, D.T.; Sullivan, J.W.; Hoover, R.N.; Fraumeni, J.F., Jr. Unexplained excess risk of bladder cancer in men. *J. Natl. Cancer Inst.* **1990**, *82*, 1636–1640. [CrossRef]
8. Hemelt, M.; Yamamoto, H.; Cheng, K.K.; Zeegers, M.P. The effect of smoking on the male excess of bladder cancer: A meta-analysis and geographical analyses. *Int. J. Cancer* **2009**, *124*, 412–419. [CrossRef] [PubMed]
9. Mowszowicz, I.; Stamatiadis, D.; Wright, F.; Kuttenn, F.; Mauvais-Jarvis, P. Androgen receptor in sexual differentiation. *J. Steroid Biochem.* **1989**, *32*, 157–162. [CrossRef]
10. Khera, M. Male hormones and men's quality of life. *Curr. Opin. Urol.* **2016**, *26*, 152–157. [CrossRef] [PubMed]
11. Boonyaratanakornkit, V.; Edwards, D.P. Receptor mechanisms mediating non-genomic actions of sex steroids. *Semin. Reprod. Med.* **2007**, *25*, 139–153. [CrossRef] [PubMed]
12. Torres, V.; Carreño, D.V.; San Francisco, I.F.; Sotomayor, P.; Godoy, A.S.; Smith, G.J. Androgen receptor in human endothelial cells. *J. Endocrinol.* **2015**, *224*, 131–137. [CrossRef] [PubMed]
13. Heinlein, C.A.; Chang, C. Androgen receptor in prostate cancer. *Endocr. Rev.* **2004**, *25*, 276–308. [CrossRef] [PubMed]
14. Mudryj, M.; Tepper, C.G. On the origins of the androgen receptor low molecular weight species. *Horm. Cancer* **2013**, *4*, 259–269. [CrossRef] [PubMed]
15. Singer, E.A.; Golijanin, D.J.; Miyamoto, H.; Messing, E.M. Androgen deprivation therapy for prostate cancer. *Expert Opin. Pharmacother.* **2008**, *9*, 211–228. [CrossRef] [PubMed]
16. Devlin, H.L.; Mudryj, M. Progression of prostate cancer: Multiple pathways to androgen independence. *Cancer Lett.* **2009**, *274*, 177–186. [CrossRef] [PubMed]
17. Lamont, K.R.; Tindall, D.J. Minireview: Alternative activation pathways for the androgen receptor in prostate cancer. *Mol. Endocrinol.* **2011**, *25*, 897–907. [CrossRef] [PubMed]
18. Antonarakis, E.S.; Armstrong, A.J.; Dehm, S.M.; Luo, J. Androgen receptor variant-driven prostate cancer: clinical implications and therapeutic targeting. *Prostate Cancer Prostatic Dis.* **2016**, *19*, 231–241. [CrossRef] [PubMed]
19. Thomas, J.C.; Oottamasathien, S.; Makari, J.H.; Honea, L.; Sharif-Afshar, A.R.; Wang, Y.; Adams, C.; Wills, M.L.; Bhowmick, N.A.; Adams, M.C. Temporal-spatial protein expression in bladder tissue derived from embryonic stem cells. *J. Urol.* **2008**, *180*, 1784–1789. [CrossRef] [PubMed]
20. Wilson, C.M.; McPhaul, M.J. A and B forms of the androgen receptor are expressed in a variety of human tissues. *Mol. Cell. Endocrinol.* **1996**, *120*, 51–57. [CrossRef]
21. Pelletier, G. Localization of androgen and estrogen receptors in rat and primate tissues. *Histol. Histopathol.* **2000**, *15*, 1261–1270. [PubMed]
22. Rosenzweig, B.A.; Bolina, P.S.; Birch, L.; Moran, C.; Marcovici, I.; Prins, G.S. Location and concentration of estrogen, progesterone, and androgen receptors in the bladder and urethra of the rabbit. *Neurourol. Urodyn.* **1995**, *14*, 87–96. [CrossRef] [PubMed]
23. Salmi, S.; Santti, R.; Gustafsson, J.A.; Makela, S. Co-localization of androgen receptor with estrogen receptor beta in the lower urinary tract of the male rat. *J. Urol.* **2001**, *166*, 674–677. [CrossRef]
24. Celayir, S.; Ilce, Z.; Dervisoglu, S. The sex hormone receptors in the bladder in childhood-I: Preliminary report in male subjects. *Eur. J. Pediatr. Surg.* **2002**, *12*, 312–317. [CrossRef] [PubMed]
25. Filippi, S.; Morelli, A.; Sandner, P.; Fibbi, B.; Mancina, R.; Marini, M.; Gacci, M.; Vignozzi, L.; Vannelli, G.B.; Carini, M.; et al. Characterization and functional role of androgen-dependent PDE5 activity in the bladder. *Endocrinology* **2007**, *148*, 1019–1029. [CrossRef] [PubMed]
26. Juan, Y.S.; Onal, B.; Broadaway, S.; Cosgrove, J.; Leggett, R.E.; Whietbeck, C.; De, E.; Sokol, R.; Levin, R.M. Effect of castration on male rabbit lower urinary tract tissue enzymes. *Mol. Cell. Biochem.* **2007**, *301*, 227–233. [CrossRef] [PubMed]

27. Madeiro, A.; Girão, M.; Sartori, M.; Acquaroli, R.; Baracat, E.; Rodrigues De Lima, G. Effects of the association of androgen/estrogen on the bladder and urethra of castrated rats. *Clin. Exp. Obstet. Gynecol.* **2002**, *29*, 117–120. [PubMed]
28. Zhang, Y.; Chen, J.; Hu, L.; Chen, Z. Androgen deprivation induces bladder histological abnormalities and dysfunction via TGF-β in orchiectomized mature rats. *Tohoku J. Exp. Med.* **2012**, *226*, 121–128. [CrossRef] [PubMed]
29. Holmäng, S.; Mårin, P.; Lindstedt, G.; Hedelin, H. Effect of long-term oral testosterone undecanoate treatment on prostate volume and serum prostate-specific antigen concentration in eugonadal middle-aged men. *Prostate* **1993**, *23*, 99–106. [CrossRef] [PubMed]
30. Yassin, A.A.; El-Sakka, A.I.; Saad, F.; Gooren, L.J. Lower urinary-tract symptoms and testosterone in elderly men. *World J. Urol.* **2008**, *26*, 359–364. [CrossRef]
31. Hall, R.; Andrews, P.L.; Hoyle, C.H. Effects of testosterone on neuromuscular transmission in rat isolated urinary bladder. *Eur. J. Pharmacol.* **2002**, *449*, 301–309. [CrossRef]
32. Laor, E.; Schiffman, Z.J.; Braunstein, J.D.; Reid, R.E.; Tolia, B.M.; Koss, L.G.; Freed, S.Z. Androgen receptors in bladder tumors. *Urology* **1985**, *25*, 161–163. [CrossRef]
33. Zhuang, Y.H.; Bläuer, M.; Tammela, T.; Tuohimaa, P. Immunodetection of androgen receptor in human urinary bladder cancer. *Histopathology* **1997**, *30*, 556–562. [CrossRef] [PubMed]
34. Boorjian, S.; Ugras, S.; Mongan, N.P.; Gudas, L.J.; You, X.; Tickoo, S.K.; Scherr, D.S. Androgen receptor expression is inversely correlated with pathologic tumor stage in bladder cancer. *Urology* **2004**, *64*, 383–388. [CrossRef] [PubMed]
35. Boorjian, S.A.; Heemers, H.V.; Frank, I.; Farmer, S.A.; Schmidt, L.J.; Sebo, T.J.; Tindall, D.J. Expression and significance of androgen receptor coactivators in urothelial carcinoma of the bladder. *Endocr. Relat. Cancer* **2009**, *16*, 123–137. [CrossRef] [PubMed]
36. Kauffman, E.C.; Robinson, B.D.; Downes, M.J.; Powell, L.G.; Lee, M.M.; Scherr, D.S.; Gudas, L.J.; Mongan, N.P. Role of androgen receptor and associated lysine-demethylase coregulators, LSD1 and MJD2A, in localized and advanced human bladder cancer. *Mol. Carcinog.* **2011**, *50*, 931–944. [CrossRef] [PubMed]
37. Mir, C.; Shariat, S.F.; van der Kwast, T.H.; Ashfaq, R.; Lotan, Y.; Evans, A.; Skeldon, S.; Hanna, S.; Vajpeyi, R.; Kuk, C.; et al. Loss of androgen receptor expression is not associated with pathological stage, grade, gender or outcome in bladder cancer: A large multi-institutional study. *BJU Int.* **2011**, *108*, 24–30. [CrossRef] [PubMed]
38. Tuygun, C.; Kankaya, D.; Imamoglu, A.; Sertcelik, A.; Zengin, K.; Oktay, M.; Sertcelik, N. Sex-specific hormone receptors in urothelial carcinomas of the human urinary bladder: A comparative analysis of clinicopathological features and survival outcomes according to receptor expression. *Urol. Oncol.* **2011**, *29*, 43–51. [CrossRef] [PubMed]
39. Zheng, Y.; Izumi, K.; Yao, J.L.; Miyamoto, H. Dihydrotestosterone upregulates the expression of epidermal growth factor receptor and ERBB2 in androgen receptor-positive bladder cancer cells. *Endocr. Relat. Cancer* **2011**, *18*, 451–464. [CrossRef]
40. Miyamoto, H.; Yao, J.L.; Chaux, A.; Zheng, Y.; Hsu, I.; Izumi, K.; Chang, C.; Messing, E.M.; Netto, G.J.; Yeh, S. Expression of androgen and oestrogen receptors and its prognostic significance in urothelial neoplasm of the urinary bladder. *BJU Int.* **2012**, *109*, 1716–1726. [CrossRef]
41. Jing, Y.; Cui, D.; Guo, W.; Jiang, J.; Jiang, B.; Lu, Y.; Zhao, W.; Wang, X.; Jiang, Q.; Han, B. Activated androgen receptor promotes bladder cancer metastasis via Slug mediated epithelial-mesenchymal transition. *Cancer Lett.* **2014**, *348*, 135–145. [CrossRef] [PubMed]
42. Mashhadi, R.; Pourmand, G.; Kosari, F.; Mehrsai, A.; Salem, S.; Pourmand, M.R.; Alatab, S.; Khonsari, M.; Heydari, F.; Beladi, L.; et al. Role of steroid hormone receptors in formation and progression of bladder carcinoma: A case-control study. *Urol. J.* **2014**, *11*, 1968–1973. [PubMed]
43. Nam, J.K.; Park, S.W.; Lee, S.D.; Chung, M.K. Prognostic value of sex-hormone receptor expression in non-muscle-invasive bladder cancer. *Yonsei Med. J.* **2014**, *55*, 1214–1221. [CrossRef] [PubMed]
44. Williams, E.M.; Higgins, J.P.; Sangoi, A.R.; McKenney, J.K.; Troxell, M.L. Androgen receptor immunohistochemistry in genitourinary neoplasms. *Int. Urol. Nephrol.* **2015**, *47*, 81–85. [CrossRef] [PubMed]
45. Miyamoto, H.; Yang, Z.; Chen, Y.T.; Ishiguro, H.; Uemura, H.; Kubota, Y.; Nagashima, Y.; Chang, Y.J.; Hu, Y.C.; Tsai, M.Y.; et al. Promotion of bladder cancer development and progression by androgen receptor signals. *J. Natl. Cancer Inst.* **2007**, *99*, 558–568. [CrossRef] [PubMed]

46. Kashiwagi, E.; Fujita, K.; Yamaguchi, S.; Fushimi, H.; Ide, H.; Inoue, S.; Mizushima, T.; Reis, L.O.; Sharma, R.; Netto, G.J.; et al. Expression of steroid hormone receptors and its prognostic significance in urothelial carcinoma of the upper urinary tract. *Cancer Biol. Ther.* **2016**, *17*, 1188–1196. [CrossRef] [PubMed]
47. Rau, K.M.; Chen, Y.J.; Sun, M.T.; Kang, H.Y. Prognostic effects and regulation of activin A, maspin, and the androgen receptor in upper urinary tract urothelial carcinoma. *Anticancer Res.* **2011**, *31*, 1713–1720. [PubMed]
48. Shyr, C.R.; Chen, C.C.; Hsieh, T.F.; Chang, C.H.; Ma, W.L.; Yeh, S.; Messing, E.; Li, T.H.; Chang, C. The expression and actions of androgen receptor in upper urinary tract urothelial carcinoma (UUTUC) tissues and the primary cultured cells. *Endocrine* **2013**, *43*, 191–199. [CrossRef] [PubMed]
49. Gakis, G.; Stenzl, A. Gender-specific differences in muscle-invasive bladder cancer: The concept of sex steroid sensitivity. *World J. Urol.* **2013**, *31*, 1059–1064. [CrossRef] [PubMed]
50. Cheng, L.; MacLennan, G.T.; Pan, C.X.; Jones, T.D.; Moore, C.R.; Zhang, S.; Gu, J.; Patel, N.B.; Kao, C.; Gardner, T.A. Allelic loss of the active X chromosome during bladder carcinogenesis. *Arch. Pathol. Lab. Med.* **2004**, *128*, 187–190. [PubMed]
51. Liu, C.H.; Huang, J.D.; Huang, S.W.; Hour, T.C.; Huang, Y.K.; Hsueh, Y.M.; Chiou, H.Y.; Lee, T.C.; Jan, K.Y.; Chen, C.J.; et al. Androgen recpetor gene polymorphism may affect the risk of urothelial carcinoma. *J. Biomed. Sci.* **2008**, *15*, 261–269. [CrossRef] [PubMed]
52. Teng, X.Y.; Liu, G.Q.; Diao, X.L.; Wu, Z.Y.; Li, L.; Zhang, W.; Zhang, X.; Su, Q. CAG repeats in the androgen receptor gene are shorter in patients with pulmonary, esophageal or bladder carcinoma and longer in women with uterine leiomyoma. *Oncol. Rep.* **2010**, *23*, 811–818. [PubMed]
53. Gonzalez-Zulueta, M.; Ruppert, J.M.; Tokino, K.; Tsai, Y.C.; Spruck, C.H., III; Miyao, N.; Nichols, P.W.; Hermann, G.G.; Horn, T.; Steven, K.; et al. Microsatellite instability in bladder cancer. *Cancer Res.* **1993**, *53*, 5620–5623. [PubMed]
54. Wu, S.; Lv, Z.; Zhu, J.; Dong, P.; Zhou, F.; Li, X.; Cai, Z. Somatic mutation of the androgen receptor gene is not associated with transitional cell carcinoma: A "negative" study by whole-exome sequencing analysis. *Eur. Urol.* **2013**, *64*, 1018–1019. [CrossRef] [PubMed]
55. Cerami, E.; Gao, J.; Dogrusoz, U.; Gross, B.E.; Sumer, S.O.; Aksoy, B.A.; Jacobsen, A.; Byrne, C.J.; Heuer, M.L.; Larsson, E.; et al. The cBio cancer genomics portal: An open platform for exploring multidimensional cancer genomics data. *Cancer Discov.* **2012**, *2*, 401–404. [CrossRef] [PubMed]
56. Gao, J.; Aksoy, B.A.; Dogrusoz, U.; Dresdner, G.; Gross, B.; Sumer, S.O.; Sun, Y.; Jacobsen, A.; Sinha, R.; Larsson, E.; et al. Integrative analysis of complex cancer genomics and clinical profiles using the cBioPortal. *Sci. Signal.* **2013**. [CrossRef] [PubMed]
57. Fahmy, O.; Khairul-Asri, M.G.; Schubert, T.; Renninger, M.; Stenzl, A.; Gakis, G. Clinicopathological features and prognostic value of incidental prostatic adenocarcinoma in radical cystoprostatectomy specimens: A systematic review and meta-analysis of 13,140 patients. *J. Urol.* **2017**, *197*, 385–390. [CrossRef] [PubMed]
58. Bertram, J.S.; Craig, A.W. Specific induction of bladder cancer in mice by butyl-(4-hydroxybutyl)-nitrosamine and the effects of hormonal modifications on the sex difference in response. *Eur. J. Cancer* **1972**, *8*, 587–594. [CrossRef]
59. Okajima, E.; Hiramatsu, T.; Iriya, K.; Ijuin, M.; Matsushima, S. Effects of sex hormones on development of urinary bladder tumours in rats induced by *N*-butyl-*N*-(4-hydroxybutyl) nitrosamine. *Urol. Res.* **1975**, *3*, 73–79. [CrossRef] [PubMed]
60. Imada, S.; Akaza, H.; Ami, Y.; Koiso, K.; Ideyama, Y.; Takenaka, T. Promoting effects and mechanisms of action of androgen in bladder carcinogenesis in male rats. *Eur. Urol.* **1997**, *31*, 360–364. [PubMed]
61. Pour, P.M.; Stepan, K. Induction of prostatic carcinomas and lower urinary tract neoplasms by combined treatment of intact and castrated rats with testosterone propionate and *N*-nitrosobis(2-oxopropyl)amine. *Cancer Res.* **1987**, *47*, 5699–5706. [PubMed]
62. Yeh, S.; Tsai, M.Y.; Xu, Q.; Mu, X.M.; Lardy, H.; Huang, K.E.; Lin, H.; Yeh, S.D.; Altuwaijri, S.; Zhou, X.; et al. Generation and characterization of androgen receptor knockout (ARKO) mice: An in vivo model for the study of androgen functions in selective tissues. *Proc. Natl. Acad. Sci. USA* **2002**, *99*, 13498–13503. [CrossRef] [PubMed]
63. Hsu, J.W.; Hsu, I.; Xu, D.; Miyamoto, H.; Liang, L.; Wu, X.R.; Shyr, C.R.; Chang, C. Decreased tumorigenesis and mortality from bladder cancer in mice lacking urothelial androgen receptor. *Am. J. Pathol.* **2013**, *182*, 1811–1820. [CrossRef] [PubMed]

64. Johnson, D.T.; Hooker, E.; Luong, R.; Yu, E.J.; He, Y.; Gonzalgo, M.L.; Sun, Z. Conditional expression of the androgen receptor increases susceptibility of bladder cancer in mice. *PLoS ONE* **2016**, *11*, e0148851. [CrossRef] [PubMed]
65. Lin, C.; Yin, Y.; Stemler, K.; Humphrey, P.; Kibel, A.S.; Mysorekar, I.U.; Ma, L. Constitutive β-catenin activation induces male-specific tumorigenesis in the bladder urothelium. *Cancer Res.* **2013**, *73*, 5914–5925. [CrossRef] [PubMed]
66. Shiota, M.; Yokomizo, A.; Takeuchi, A.; Imada, K.; Kiyoshima, K.; Inokuchi, J.; Tatsugami, K.; Ohga, S.; Nakamura, K.; Honda, H.; et al. Secondary bladder cancer after anticancer therapy for prostate cancer: Reduced comorbidity after androgen-deprivation therapy. *Oncotarget* **2015**, *6*, 14710–14719. [CrossRef] [PubMed]
67. Izumi, K.; Taguri, M.; Miyamoto, H.; Hara, Y.; Kishida, T.; Chiba, K.; Murai, T.; Hirai, K.; Suzuki, K.; Fujinami, K.; et al. Androgen deprivation therapy prevents bladder cancer recurrence. *Oncotarget* **2014**, *5*, 12665–12674. [CrossRef] [PubMed]
68. Izumi, K.; Ito, Y.; Miyamoto, H.; Miyoshi, Y.; Ota, J.; Moriyama, M.; Murai, T.; Hayashi, H.; Inayama, Y.; Ohashi, K.; et al. Expression of androgen receptor in non-muscle-invasive bladder cancer predicts the preventive effect of androgen deprivation therapy on tumor recurrence. *Oncotarget* **2016**, *7*, 14153–14160. [PubMed]
69. Shiota, M.; Kiyoshima, K.; Yokomizo, A.; Takeuchi, A.; Kashiwagi, E.; Dejima, T.; Takahashi, R.; Inokuchi, J.; Tatsugami, K.; Eto, M. Suppressed recurrent bladder cancer after androgen suppression with androgen-deprivation therapy or 5α-reductase inhibitor. *J. Urol.* **2017**, *197*, 308–313. [CrossRef] [PubMed]
70. Morales, E.E.; Grill, S.; Svatek, R.S.; Kaushik, D.; Thompson, I.M., Jr.; Ankerst, D.P.; Liss, M.A. Finasteride reduces risk of bladder cancer in a large prospective screening study. *Eur. Urol.* **2016**, *69*, 407–410. [CrossRef] [PubMed]
71. Imaoka, S.; Yoneda, Y.; Sugimoto, T.; Ikemoto, S.; Hiroi, T.; Yamamoto, K.; Nakatani, T.; Funae, Y. Androgen regulation of CYP4B1 responsible for mutagenic activation of bladder carcinogens in the rat bladder: Detection of CYP4B1 mRNA by competitive reverse transcription-polymerase chain reaction. *Cancer Lett.* **2001**, *166*, 119–123. [CrossRef]
72. Izumi, K.; Zheng, Y.; Hsu, J.W.; Chang, C.; Miyamoto, H. Androgen receptor signals regulate UDP-glucuronosyltransferases in the urinary bladder: A potential mechanism of androgen-induced bladder carcinogenesis. *Mol. Carcinog.* **2013**, *52*, 94–102. [CrossRef] [PubMed]
73. Izumi, K.; Li, Y.; Ishiguro, H.; Zheng, Y.; Yao, J.L.; Netto, G.J.; Miyamoto, H. Expression of UDP-glucuronosyltransferase 1A in bladder cancer: Association with prognosis and regulation by estrogen. *Mol. Carcinog.* **2014**, *54*, 314–324. [CrossRef] [PubMed]
74. Bhattacharya, A.; Klaene, J.J.; Li, Y.; Paonessa, J.D.; Stablewski, A.B.; Vouros, P.; Zhang, Y. The inverse relationship between bladder and liver in 4-aminobiphenyl-induced DNA damage. *Oncotarget* **2015**, *6*, 836–845. [CrossRef] [PubMed]
75. Miyamoto, H.; Izumi, K.; Yao, J.L.; Li, Y.; Yang, Q.; McMahon, L.A.; Gonzalez-Roibon, N.; Hicks, D.G.; Tacha, D.; Netto, G.J. GATA binding protein 3 is down-regulated in bladder cancer yet strong expression is an independent predictor of poor prognosis in invasive tumor. *Hum. Pathol.* **2012**, *43*, 2033–2040. [CrossRef] [PubMed]
76. Li, Y.; Ishiguro, H.; Kawahara, T.; Kashiwagi, E.; Izumi, K.; Miyamoto, H. Loss of GATA3 in bladder cancer promotes cell migration and invasion. *Cancer Biol. Ther.* **2014**, *15*, 428–435. [CrossRef] [PubMed]
77. Li, Y.; Ishiguro, H.; Kawahara, T.; Miyamoto, Y.; Izumi, K.; Miyamoto, H. GATA3 in the urinary bladder: Suppression of neoplastic transformation and down-regulation by androgens. *Am. J. Cancer Res.* **2014**, *4*, 461–473. [PubMed]
78. Chen, F.; Langenstroer, P.; Zhang, G.; Iwamoto, Y.; See, W. Androgen dependent regulation of BCG induced IL6 expression in human transitional carcinoma cell lines. *J. Urol.* **2003**, *170*, 2009–2013. [CrossRef] [PubMed]
79. Izumi, K.; Zheng, Y.; Li, Y.; Zaengle, J.; Miyamoto, H. Epidermal growth factor induces bladder cancer cell proliferation through activation of the androgen receptor. *Int. J. Oncol.* **2012**, *41*, 1587–1592. [PubMed]
80. Overdevest, J.B.; Knubel, K.H.; Duex, J.E.; Thomas, S.; Nitz, M.D.; Harding, M.A.; Smith, S.C.; Frierson, H.F.; Conaway, M.; Theodorescu, D. CD24 expression is important in male urothelial tumorigenesis and metastasis in mice and is androgen regulated. *Proc. Natl. Acad. Sci. USA* **2012**, *109*, E3588–E3596. [CrossRef] [PubMed]

81. Li, Y.; Zheng, Y.; Izumi, K.; Ishiguro, H.; Ye, B.; Li, F.; Miyamoto, H. Androgen activates β-catenin signaling in bladder cancer cells. *Endocr. Relat. Cancer* **2013**, *20*, 293–304. [CrossRef] [PubMed]
82. Kawahara, T.; Shareef, H.K.; Aljarah, A.K.; Ide, H.; Li, Y.; Kashiwagi, E.; Netto, G.J.; Zheng, Y.; Miyamoto, H. ELK1 is up-regulated by androgen in bladder cancer cells and promotes tumor progression. *Oncotarget* **2015**, *6*, 29860–29876. [PubMed]
83. Kawahara, T.; Ide, H.; Kashiwagi, E.; El-Shishtawy, K.A.; Li, Y.; Reis, L.O.; Zheng, Y.; Miyamoto, H. Enzalutamide inhibits androgen receptor-positive bladder cancer cell growth. *Urol. Oncol.* **2016**, *34*, 432.e15–432.e23. [CrossRef] [PubMed]
84. Shiota, M.; Takeuchi, A.; Yokomizo, A.; Kashiwagi, E.; Tatsugami, K.; Kuroiwa, K.; Naito, S. Androgen receptor signaling regulates cell growth and vulnerability to doxorubicin in bladder cancer. *J. Urol.* **2012**, *188*, 276–286. [CrossRef] [PubMed]
85. Hsieh, T.F.; Chen, C.C.; Ma, W.L.; Chuang, W.M.; Hung, X.F.; Tsai, Y.R.; Lin, M.H.; Zhang, Q.; Zhang, C.; Chang, C.; et al. Epidermal growth factor enhances androgen receptor-mediated bladder cancer progression and invasion via potentiation of AR transactivation. *Oncol. Rep.* **2013**, *30*, 2917–2922. [PubMed]
86. Wu, J.T.; Han, B.M.; Yu, S.Q.; Wang, H.P.; Xia, S.J. Androgen receptor is a potential therapeutic target for bladder cancer. *Urology* **2010**, *75*, 820–827. [CrossRef] [PubMed]
87. Jitao, W.; Jinchen, H.; Qingzuo, L.; Li, C.; Lei, S.; Jianming, W.; Zhenli, G. Androgen receptor inducing bladder cancer progression by promoting an epithelial-mesenchymal transition. *Andrologia* **2014**, *46*, 1128–1133. [CrossRef] [PubMed]
88. Ding, G.; Yu, S.; Cheng, S.; Li, G.; Yu, Y. Androgen receptor (AR) promotes male bladder cancer cell proliferation and migration via regulating CD24 and VEGF. *Am. J. Transl. Res.* **2016**, *8*, 578–587. [PubMed]
89. Kaneyama, K.; Horie, K.; Mizutani, K.; Kato, T.; Fujita, Y.; Kawakami, K.; Kojima, T.; Miyazaki, T.; Deguchi, T.; Ito, M. Enzalutamide inhibits proliferation of gemcitabine-resistant bladder cancer cells with increased androgen receptor expression. *Int. J. Oncol.* **2017**, *50*, 75–84.
90. Reid, L.M.; Leav, I.; Kwan, P.W.L.; Russell, P.; Merk, F.B. Characterization of a human, sex steroid-responsive transitional cell carcinoma maintained as a tumor line (R198) in athymic nude mice. *Cancer Res.* **1984**, *44*, 4560–4573. [PubMed]
91. Zheng, Y.; Ishiguro, H.; Ide, H.; Inoue, S.; Kashiwagi, E.; Kawahara, T.; Jalalizadeh, M.; Reis, L.O.; Miyamoto, H. Compound A inhibits bladder cancer growth predominantly via glucocorticoid receptor transrepression. *Mol. Endocrinol.* **2015**, *29*, 1486–1497. [CrossRef] [PubMed]
92. Johnson, A.M.; O'Connell, M.J.; Miyamoto, H.; Huang, J.; Yao, J.L.; Messing, E.M.; Reeder, J.E. Androgenic dependence of exophytic tumor growth in a transgenic mouse model of bladder cancer: A role for thrombospondin-1. *BMC Urol.* **2008**. [CrossRef] [PubMed]
93. Lin, C.; Lin, W.; Yeh, S.; Li, L.; Chang, C. Infiltrating neutrophils increase bladder cancer cell invasion via modulation of androgen receptor (AR)/MMP13 signals. *Oncotarget* **2015**, *6*, 43081–43089. [PubMed]
94. Ou, Z.; Wang, Y.; Liu, L.; Li, L.; Yeh, S.; Qi, L.; Chang, C. Tumor microenvironment B cells increase bladder cancer metastasis via modulation of the IL-8/androgen receptor (AR)/MMPs signals. *Oncotarget* **2015**, *6*, 26065–26078. [CrossRef] [PubMed]
95. Tao, L.; Qiu, J.; Jiang, M.; Song, W.; Yeh, S.; Yu, H.; Zang, L.; Xia, S.; Chang, C. Infiltrating T cells promote bladder cancer progression via increasing IL1→androgen receptor→HIF1α→VEGFa signals. *Mol. Cancer Ther.* **2016**, *15*, 1943–1951. [CrossRef] [PubMed]
96. Kashiwagi, E.; Ide, H.; Inoue, S.; Kawahara, T.; Zheng, Y.; Reis, L.O.; Baras, A.S.; Miyamoto, H. Androgen receptor activity modulates responses to cisplatin treatment in bladder cancer. *Oncotarget* **2016**, *7*, 49169–49176. [CrossRef] [PubMed]
97. Kastritis, E.; Murray, S.; Kyriakou, F.; Horti, M.; Tamvakis, N.; Kavantzas, N.; Patsouris, E.S.; Noni, A.; Legaki, S.; Dimopoulos, M.A.; et al. Somatic mutations of adenomatous polyposis coli gene and nuclear b-catenin accumulation have prognostic significance in invasive urothelial carcinomas: Evidence for Wnt pathway implication. *Int. J. Cancer* **2009**, *124*, 103–108. [CrossRef] [PubMed]

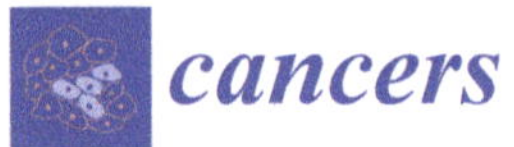 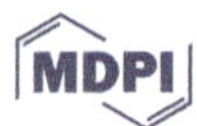

Review

Androgen Receptor Signaling in Salivary Gland Cancer

Martin G. Dalin [1,2,*], Philip A. Watson [1], Alan L. Ho [3] and Luc G. T. Morris [1,4,*]

[1] Human Oncology and Pathogenesis Program, Memorial Sloan Kettering Cancer Center, New York, NY 10065, USA; watsonp@mskcc.org
[2] Department of Pediatrics, Institution for Clinical Sciences, University of Gothenburg, Gothenburg SE-416 86, Sweden
[3] Head and Neck Medical Oncology Service, Department of Medicine, Memorial Sloan Kettering Cancer Center, New York, NY 10065, USA; hoa@mskcc.org
[4] Head and Neck Service, Department of Surgery, Memorial Sloan Kettering Cancer Center, New York, NY 10065, USA
* Correspondence: martin.dalin@gu.se (M.G.D.); morrisl@mskcc.org (L.G.T.M.); Tel.: +46-31-343-8384 (M.G.D.); +1-212-639-3049 (L.G.T.M.)

Academic Editor: Emmanuel S. Antonarakis
Received: 22 December 2016; Accepted: 3 February 2017; Published: 8 February 2017

Abstract: Salivary gland cancers comprise a small subset of human malignancies, and are classified into multiple subtypes that exhibit diverse histology, molecular biology and clinical presentation. Local disease is potentially curable with surgery, which may be combined with adjuvant radiotherapy. However, metastatic or unresectable tumors rarely respond to chemotherapy and carry a poorer prognosis. Recent molecular studies have shown evidence of androgen receptor signaling in several types of salivary gland cancer, mainly salivary duct carcinoma. Successful treatment with anti-androgen therapy in other androgen receptor-positive malignancies such as prostate and breast cancer has inspired researchers to investigate this treatment in salivary gland cancer as well. In this review, we describe the prevalence, biology, and therapeutic implications of androgen receptor signaling in salivary gland cancer.

Keywords: salivary gland cancer; androgen receptor; salivary duct carcinoma; androgen-deprivation therapy (ADT)

---

1. Introduction

Salivary gland cancers (SGCs) are a group of uncommon, heterogeneous tumors that account for 0.3% of all malignancies and 6% of head and neck cancers in the United States [1]. The majority of SGCs are found in the parotid gland (59%–81% of cases), but they also arise in the submandibular gland (6%–21%), or in minor salivary glands (7%–22%) that populate the upper aerodigestive tract [2–4]. The World Health Organization classifies 24 subtypes of SGC, which show significant variation in histological and clinical features [1]. SGC is generally treated with surgery and, in selected cases, adjuvant radiotherapy (RT) [5]. Systemic therapy has not been adequately tested in many SGC subtypes, and cytotoxic chemotherapy has shown a limited effect in SGCs in general. As a consequence, the prognosis of recurrent or metastatic SGC can be poor [2,6,7]. However, recent studies have investigated the molecular landscape of several types of SGCs, such as adenoid cystic carcinoma (ACC), mucoepidermoid carcinoma (MEC), polymorphous low grade adenocarcinoma (PLGA), secretory carcinoma and salivary duct carcinoma (SDC), and uncovered molecular targets of interest in selected patients [8–13].

The androgen receptor (AR) is a nuclear steroid hormone receptor that is physiologically expressed at low levels in many human tissues [14]. Its main ligands are testosterone and 5α-dihydrotestosterone

(DHT). AR regulates the transcription of multiple effector genes through direct DNA binding or interaction with other transcription factors, leading to increased cell growth, differentiation, and survival [15]. Overactive AR signaling is an important oncogenic driver in several tumor types, including prostate cancer and a subset of breast cancers [16,17]. Androgen-deprivation therapy (ADT) has been used in patients with prostate cancer since the 1940s [18], and has more recently gained interest in a growing number of malignancies [17,19–21]. ADT may be achieved by direct inhibition of AR (known as anti-androgen therapy), or by downregulating the gonadotropin-releasing hormone (GnRH) receptor signaling output, which leads to reduced serum testosterone levels (known as chemical castration). These two methods are often combined to achieve what has been termed maximum or complete androgen blockade [22].

2. AR Expression in SGC

Nuclear AR expression based on immunohistochemistry (IHC) is the most widely used marker of active AR signaling, and correlates with the response to ADT in prostate cancer [23]. The prevalence of AR expression varies substantially between different subtypes of SGC (see Table 1 for a summary of published IHC data). AR overexpression is most frequently associated with salivary duct carcinomas (SDC), the majority of which are positive for AR. Several studies have shown AR immunoreactivity in 64%–77% of cases [8,24–30], whereas a recent large report detected AR expression in as many as 98% of SDCs [31]. In that study, several tumors initially diagnosed as AR-negative SDCs were reclassified as other tumor entities after a second evaluation by salivary pathologists. Also, for tumors with conventional SDC morphology and a negative first AR IHC, the staining was repeated and showed AR expression the second time in several cases. This may suggest that the prevalence of AR-positive SDC was previously underestimated due to technical issues or diagnostic difficulties.

Our group recently identified AR positivity by IHC in 75% of SDCs, and RNA sequencing confirmed extremely low but detectable levels of AR mRNA in AR IHC–negative cases, all of which had typical SDC morphology at the time of pathologic re-evaluation [8]. Interestingly, three of four AR IHC-negative cases showed AR signaling activity at levels equivalent to AR IHC-positive cases, as measured by expression of AR-regulated genes. Both AR-negative and AR-positive SDCs showed global gene expression patterns highly similar to AR-positive (also termed molecular apocrine) breast cancers. This raises the possibility that some SDCs with low levels of AR may have acquired alternative mechanisms to activate AR signaling pathways. Furthermore, the remarkable biological similarity between the two cancer types may suggest that treatment results in patients with molecular apocrine breast cancer could be of interest for the design of clinical trials in SDC.

The prognostic relevance of AR expression in SDC is difficult to assess, due to the rarity of the disease and the low number of AR-negative cases. Some investigators have identified a trend suggestive of better disease-free survival in AR-positive compared to AR-negative SDC patients [26,29], but this association has not been identified by other groups [8,24,25]. Similarly, one study detected a higher prevalence of AR expression in men than in women with SDC [30], a finding that has not been replicated in other reports [8,26].

In other subtypes of SGC, nuclear AR expression is found at lower rates. Adenocarcinoma, not otherwise specified (AC NOS) and acinic cell carcinoma (AcCC) are AR-positive in 26% and 15% of the cases, respectively [28,32–35]. On the other hand, only a small subset of MEC and ACC have detectable expression of AR [27,28,32–34,36,37], and some of these cases show weak AR expression (5%–15% stained nuclei) which may not be relevant for the biology of the tumors [32]. Among the rare types of SGC, AR expression has been reported in PLGA and basal cell adenocarcinoma (BCAC) [28,32], whereas all published cases of myoepithelial carcinoma (MECA) have been AR-negative [28,33]. Five cases of AR-positive epithelial-myoepithelial carcinoma (EMC) were reported and suggested to represent a specific variant of the disease, denoted apocrine EMC [38]. However, one study of six unselected EMCs did not detect AR [28], and the prevalence of AR expression in EMC is unknown. Given the challenging nature of salivary gland pathology, it is possible that some of these AR-positive entities in fact represent SDC.

A subset of SGCs result from the malignant transformation of a pre-existing pleomorphic adenoma (PA). PA is the most prevalent salivary gland tumor, and is typically benign and non-metastatic. Around 6% of PAs develop into different types of carcinoma, denoted carcinoma ex-PA [39]. Whereas PAs are AR-positive in 30% of the cases, 90% of carcinoma ex-PAs express AR. This difference may suggest that AR expression is a risk factor for the malignant transformation of PAs. Alternatively, overexpression of AR may act as an oncogenic event in some carcinomas ex-PA [40].

Table 1. Prevalence of positive AR immunoreactivity in different types of SGC.

Histology	AR Positivity [1]	Reported Range [2]	References
SDC	615/713 (86%)	43%–100%	[8,24–31,33,34,41–45]
AC NOS	11/43 (26%)	21%–33%	[28,33,34]
AcCC	6/40 (15%)	0%–31%	[28,32,34,35]
MEC	7/135 (5%)	0%–20%	[27,28,32–34,36]
ACC	7/145 (5%)	0%–20%	[28,32–34,36]
EMC	0/6 (0%)	N/A	[28]
MECA	0/7 (0%)	N/A	[28,33]
BCAC	2/2 (100%)	N/A	[32]
PLGA	1/2 (50%)	N/A	[28]

[1] Number of AR-positive cases/total number of cases, in all studies combined; [2] Range of prevalence detected in the different studies. SDC, salivary duct carcinoma; AC NOS, adenocarcinoma not otherwise specified; AcCC, acinic cell carcinoma; MEC, mucoepodermoid carcinoma; ACC, adenoid cystic carcinoma; EMC, epithelial-myoepithelial carcinoma; MECA, myoepithelial carcinoma; BCAC, basal cell adenocarcinoma; PLGA, polymorphous low grade adenocarcinoma.

3. Expression of AR Splice Variants

The full-length AR (AR-FL) gene consists of eight exons, of which exons 4–8 encode the ligand-binding domain. Expression of alternative AR isoforms lacking the ligand-binding domain (which normally serves as a binding site for anti-androgens, such as enzalutamide) is associated with ADT resistance in prostate cancer [46–50]. AR-V7, a constitutively active AR splice variant that includes only exons 1–3 and a cryptic exon 3, is detected in 37%–50% of SDCs (Figure 1) [8,26]. On average, AR-V7 is expressed at around 5% of AR-FL RNA levels [8], which is similar to the AR-V7/AR-FL ratio seen in prostate cancer [16]. Another AR isoform, AR-V3, including only exons 1, 2 and a cryptic exon 2, is also found in SDC but at lower rates and only in male patients [26]. AR-45, which lacks the majority of exon 1, including the N-terminal domain that mediates ligand-independent transactivation of AR [51], is detected in a minority of SDCs [26]. However, the association between the alternative AR isoforms and response to ADT in SDC, and the prevalence of AR-V7, AR-V3, and AR-45 in other types of SGC, remains unknown.

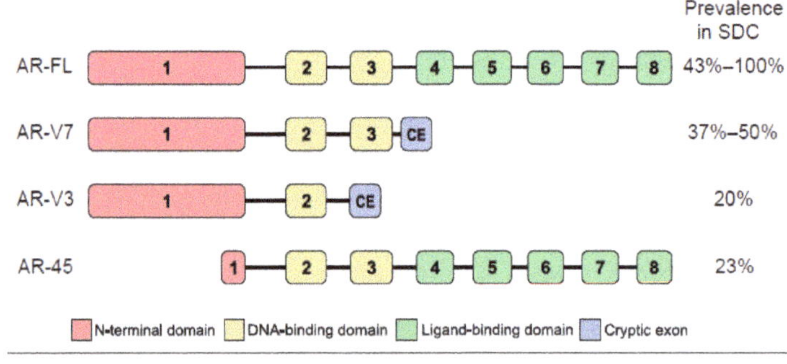

Figure 1. Reported prevalence of AR splice variant expression in SDC. References: For AR-FL, [8,24–31,33,34,41–45]; for AR-V7, [8,26]; for AR-V3 and AR-45, [26].

4. Genetic Alterations Affecting AR Signaling

An extra copy of chromosome X, which includes the AR gene, is found in almost 40% of SDCs. This may contribute to overexpression of AR, although some of the tumors with an extra chromosome X are negative for AR in IHC [26]. Unlike in prostate cancer, focal amplification or protein-altering somatic mutations of AR have not been found in SDC or ACC [8,9,26].

Forkhead box protein A1 (FOXA1) is a transcription factor that mediates the transcription of AR target genes by facilitating the AR/chromatin interaction [52]. *FOXA1* mutations may potentially be associated with ADT resistance in prostate cancer, although this is being actively investigated [53]. In a recent exome sequencing study reported by our group, we identified alteration (either somatic mutations in the DNA-binding domain or high-level amplification) of *FOXA1* in four of 12 AR-positive SDCs. Conversely, no *FOXA1* alterations were found in four AR-negative SDCs [8].

Fatty acid synthase (FASN) is an enzyme that controls fatty acid synthesis and has been shown to promote the growth of prostate cancer as a result of AR signaling. Experimental studies suggest that *FASN* overexpression can mediate resistance to ADT in prostate cancer, although no clinical data are yet available [54]. In our exome study of SDC, alterations (missense mutations, a frameshift insertion, and high-level amplification) of *FASN* were found in four of 12 AR-positive but not in AR-negative tumors [8].

In ACC, which rarely expresses AR, no significant genetic alterations affecting AR signaling have been detected [9]. In other subtypes of SGC, the prevalence of AR-related genetic alterations is unknown.

5. Anti-Androgen Therapy in Patients with SGC

Several ADT drugs have been developed and tested clinically, mainly in patients with prostate cancer. Abiraterone is a CYP17A1 inhibitor which reduces circulating levels of androgen by ultimately blocking the conversion of pregnenolone to DHT. Bicalutamide and flutamide are competitive inhibitors of the AR ligand-binding domain, as is enzalutamide, which was developed more recently and has greater AR affinity compared to the earlier anti-androgens, and may inhibit AR activity via a variety of different mechanisms [55]. Triptorelin and goserelin are GnRH agonists which eventually cause downregulation of luteinizing hormone (LH) and thereby reduced serum testosterone levels [22].

Inspired by results from other cancers [17,56] and functional studies showing AR-dependency in cultured SGC cells [26,57], a number of patients with AR-positive SGC have been treated with different ADT regimens (see Table 2 for a summary of reported cases). In a retrospective analysis of 17 patients with recurrent or metastatic AR-positive SGC, of which the majority had SDC or AC NOS, the overall response rate was 65%. Treatment was generally well tolerated in these patients, both men and women. However, relapse was commonly seen, leading to a three-year progression-free survival (PFS) of 12%, and a five-year overall survival of 19% [58]. Smaller studies of AR-positive SDC patients have reported somewhat less favorable outcomes, with an overall ADT response rate of 25%–50% [8,59]. Several case reports have shown a good effect of ADT alone in patients with AR-positive SDC or AC NOS, including stable disease for several months as well as cases of complete remission [43,60,61]. A few patients with SDC or AC NOS, who initially responded to a combination of bicalutamide and triptorelin but had a relapse, then showed a response to subsequent abiraterone, suggesting resistance mediated by the reactivation of AR signaling during ADT treatment [62,63]. ADT has also been combined with either definitive RT or palliative chemotherapy with robust responses in several single case reports of SGC [64,65].

Patients with AC NOS have been found to respond well to ADT, with partial or complete response in 10 of 11 reported cases, and a median PFS of 20 months. SDC patients appear to have a lower response rate, with partial or complete response in 11 of 26 (42%) reported cases and a median PFS of eight months (Table 2).

Table 2. Reported cases of ADT treatment in patients with AR-positive SGC.

Patient ID [1]	Histology	Sex	Age [2]	ADT Agents	Response	PFS (Months)	Ref.
1	AC NOS	m	73	Bicalutamide + triptorelin	CR	N.K.	[60]
2	AC NOS	m	72	Bicalutamide + triptorelin	CR	2	[58]
3	AC NOS	m	N.K.	Goserelin	PR	N.K.	[61]
4	AC NOS	m	59	Bicalutamide + triptorelin	PR	12	[63]
5	AC NOS	m	44	Bicalutamide + triptorelin	PR	25	[63]
6	AC NOS	m	67	Bicalutamide + triptorelin	PR	22	[58]
7	AC NOS	m	67	Bicalutamide + triptorelin	PR	22	[58]
8	AC NOS	m	46	Bicalutamide + triptorelin	PR	58	[58]
9	AC NOS	m	49	Bicalutamide + triptorelin	PR	7	[58]
10	AC NOS	m	62	Bicalutamide + triptorelin	PR	9	[58]
11	AC NOS	m	69	Bicalutamide + triptorelin	SD	20	[58]
12	Cyst AC	m	79	Bicalutamide + triptorelin	PR	14	[58]
13	Cyst AC	f	68	Triptorelin + cyproterone	PD	0	[58]
14	Poor diff.	m	54	Bicalutamide + triptorelin	PD	0	[58]
15	SDC	f	87	Bicalutamide + leuprolide [3]	CR	24	[64]
16	SDC	m	44	Bicalutamide + triptorelin	CR	39	[58]
17	SDC	m	67	Bicalutamide + triptorelin	CR	11	[58]
18	SDC	m	66	Bicalutamide	PR	14	[43]
19	SDC	m	50	Bicalutamide	PR	8	[59]
20	SDC	f	83	Bicalutamide	PR	26	[59]
21	SDC	m	45	Goserelin	PR	4	[62]
22	SDC	m	45	Bicalutamide + goserelin	PR	10	[62]
23	SDC	m	45	Abiraterone + goserelin	PR	10	[62]
24	SDC	m	51	Bicalutamide + triptorelin	PR	6	[58]
25	SDC	m	67	Bicalutamide + triptorelin	PR	7	[58]
26	SDC	f	68	Bicalutamide + leuprolide	SD	17	[8]
27	SDC	m	57	Bicalutamide	SD	14	[59]
28	SDC	m	56	Bicalutamide + goserelin	SD	12	[59]
29	SDC	m	67	Bicalutamide + goserelin	SD	8	[59]
30	SDC	m	75	Bicalutamide + triptorelin	SD	8	[58]
31	SDC	m	54	Bicalutamide + triptorelin	SD	10	[58]
32	SDC	m	68	Bicalutamide + triptorelin	SD	23	[58]
33	SDC	f	48	Bicalutamide + leuprolide	PD	0	[8]
34	SDC	f	69	Bicalutamide + leuprolide	PD	0	[8]
35	SDC	m	77	Bicalutamide + leuprolide	PD	0	[8]
36	SDC	m	73	Bicalutamide + goserelin	PD	0	[59]
37	SDC	m	68	Bicalutamide + goserelin	PD	0	[59]
38	SDC	f	64	Bicalutamide	PD	0	[59]
39	SDC	m	39	Bicalutamide	PD	0	[59]
40	SDC	m	73	Bicalutamide	PD	0	[59]

[1] Patients are sorted by tumor histology and then best response; [2] At start of ADT; [3] This patient received external beam radiotherapy together with ADT. ADT, androgen deprivation therapy; PFS, progression-free survival; Ref., reference; AC NOS, adenocarcinoma not otherwise specified; Cyst AC, cystadenocarcinoma; Poor diff., poorly differentiated; SDC, salivary duct carcinoma; m, male; f, female; N.K., not known; CR, complete response; PR, partial response; SD, stable disease; PD, progressive disease.

Of note, several dramatic responses to ADT in SGC patients were published only as case reports of extraordinary responders. A recent preliminary study including all SDC patients treated with ADT in the Netherlands showed somewhat more modest results, with partial response in four (13%) cases, stable disease in 10 (32%) cases, and progressive disease in 17 (55%) cases, and a median PFS of 3.8 months [45]. On the other hand, since the majority of SGCs are chemotherapy-resistant, the treatment options for patients with generalized disease are limited and AR is the most promising target for these patients with otherwise incurable disease. Several clinical trials are currently ongoing, investigating the efficacy of ADT in patients with recurrent/metastatic AR-positive SGC, using abiraterone, bicalutamide or enzalutamide in male and female patients (NCT02749903, NCT01969578, NCT02867852). In addition to providing valuable clinical response information, these trials will also collect tumor tissue for correlative research, facilitating further understanding of molecular determinants of response to ADT in AR-positive SGC.

6. Conclusions

AR is expressed in a majority of SDCs and in a minority of other SGCs such as AC NOS, and ADT has emerged as a promising therapy in patients with AR-positive SGC. Several potential mechanisms of resistance to ADT have been described, including the expression of AR splice variants and mutations in *FOXA1* and *FASN*. Ongoing and future clinical trials will likely shed light on the clinical benefit and limitations of ADT in AR-positive SGC.

Acknowledgments: Martin G. Dalin was supported by Sahlgrenska University Hospital, The Swedish Medical Society, and Svensson's Fund for Medical Research. Luc G. T. Morris was supported by NIH K08 DE024774, the Society of MSKCC, the Damon Runyon Cancer Research Foundation, and the Jayme and Peter Flowers Fund.

Author Contributions: Manuscript concept: Martin G. Dalin, Luc G. T. Morris. Literature review: Martin G. Dalin, Philip A. Watson, Alan L. Ho, Luc G. T. Morris. Analysis of data: Martin G. Dalin, Luc G. T. Morris. Interpretation of data: Martin G. Dalin, Philip A. Watson, Alan L. Ho, Luc G. T. Morris. Graphic design: Martin G. Dalin. Preparation of manuscript: Martin G. Dalin, Philip A. Watson, Alan L. Ho, Luc G. T. Morris.

Conflicts of Interest: The authors declare no conflict of interest.

References

1. Eveson, J.W.; Auclair, P.; Gnepp, D.R.; El-Naggar, A.K. Tumors of the salivary glands. In *Pathology and Genetics of Head and Neck Tumours: International Agency for Research on Cancer*; World Health Organization: Geneva, Switzerland, 2005; pp. 210–281.
2. Terhaard, C.H.; Lubsen, H.; van der Tweel, I.; Hilgers, F.J.; Eijkenboom, W.M.; Marres, H.A.; Tjho-Heslinga, R.E.; de Jong, J.M.; Roodenburg, J.L. Salivary gland carcinoma: Independent prognostic factors for locoregional control, distant metastases, and overall survival: Results of the dutch head and neck oncology cooperative group. *Head Neck* **2004**, *26*, 681–693. [CrossRef] [PubMed]
3. Renehan, A.; Gleave, E.N.; Hancock, B.D.; Smith, P.; McGurk, M. Long-term follow-up of over 1000 patients with salivary gland tumours treated in a single centre. *Br. J. Surg.* **1996**, *83*, 1750–1754. [CrossRef] [PubMed]
4. Fitzpatrick, P.J.; Theriault, C. Malignant salivary gland tumors. *Int. J. Radiat. Oncol. Biol. Phys.* **1986**, *12*, 1743–1747. [CrossRef]
5. Panwar, A.; Kozel, J.A.; Lydiatt, W.M. Cancers of major salivary glands. *Surg. Oncol. Clin. N. Am.* **2015**, *24*, 615–633. [CrossRef] [PubMed]
6. Laurie, S.A.; Licitra, L. Systemic therapy in the palliative management of advanced salivary gland cancers. *J. Clin. Oncol.* **2006**, *24*, 2673–2678. [CrossRef] [PubMed]
7. Licitra, L.; Grandi, C.; Prott, F.J.; Schornagel, J.H.; Bruzzi, P.; Molinari, R. Major and minor salivary glands tumours. *Crit. Rev. Oncol. Hematol.* **2003**, *45*, 215–225. [CrossRef]
8. Dalin, M.G.; Desrichard, A.; Katabi, N.; Makarov, V.; Walsh, L.A.; Lee, K.W.; Wang, Q.; Armenia, J.; West, L.; Dogan, S.; et al. Comprehensive molecular characterization of salivary duct carcinoma reveals actionable targets and similarity to apocrine breast cancer. *Clin. Cancer Res.* **2016**, *22*, 4623–4633. [CrossRef] [PubMed]
9. Ho, A.S.; Kannan, K.; Roy, D.M.; Morris, L.G.; Ganly, I.; Katabi, N.; Ramaswami, D.; Walsh, L.A.; Eng, S.; Huse, J.T.; et al. The mutational landscape of adenoid cystic carcinoma. *Nat. Genet.* **2013**, *45*, 791–798. [CrossRef] [PubMed]
10. Ku, B.M.; Jung, H.A.; Sun, J.M.; Ko, Y.H.; Jeong, H.S.; Son, Y.I.; Baek, C.H.; Park, K.; Ahn, M.J. High-throughput profiling identifies clinically actionable mutations in salivary duct carcinoma. *J. Trans. Med.* **2014**. [CrossRef] [PubMed]
11. Weinreb, I.; Piscuoglio, S.; Martelotto, L.G.; Waggott, D.; Ng, C.K.; Perez-Ordonez, B.; Harding, N.J.; Alfaro, J.; Chu, K.C.; Viale, A.; et al. Hotspot activating *PRKD1* somatic mutations in polymorphous low-grade adenocarcinomas of the salivary glands. *Nat. Genet.* **2014**, *46*, 1166–1169. [CrossRef] [PubMed]
12. Kang, H.; Tan, M.; Bishop, J.A.; Jones, S.; Sausen, M.; Ha, P.K.; Agrawal, N. Whole-exome sequencing of salivary gland mucoepidermoid carcinoma. *Clin. Cancer Res.* **2017**, *23*, 283–288. [CrossRef] [PubMed]
13. Skalova, A.; Vanecek, T.; Simpson, R.H.; Laco, J.; Majewska, H.; Baneckova, M.; Steiner, P.; Michal, M. Mammary analogue secretory carcinoma of salivary glands: Molecular analysis of 25 *ETV6* gene rearranged tumors with lack of detection of classical *ETV6-NTRK3* fusion transcript by standard RT-PCR: Report of 4 cases harboring *ETV6-X* gene fusion. *Am. J. Surg. Pathol.* **2016**, *40*, 3–13. [CrossRef] [PubMed]
14. Ruizeveld de Winter, J.A.; Trapman, J.; Vermey, M.; Mulder, E.; Zegers, N.D.; van der Kwast, T.H. Androgen receptor expression in human tissues: An immunohistochemical study. *J. Histochem. Cytochem.* **1991**, *39*, 927–936. [CrossRef] [PubMed]

15. Lu, N.Z.; Wardell, S.E.; Burnstein, K.L.; Defranco, D.; Fuller, P.J.; Giguere, V.; Hochberg, R.B.; McKay, L.; Renoir, J.M.; Weigel, N.L.; et al. International union of pharmacology. Lxv. The pharmacology and classification of the nuclear receptor superfamily: Glucocorticoid, mineralocorticoid, progesterone, and androgen receptors. *Pharmacol. Rev.* **2006**, *58*, 782–797. [CrossRef] [PubMed]
16. Robinson, D.; Van Allen, E.M.; Wu, Y.M.; Schultz, N.; Lonigro, R.J.; Mosquera, J.M.; Montgomery, B.; Taplin, M.E.; Pritchard, C.C.; Attard, G.; et al. Integrative clinical genomics of advanced prostate cancer. *Cell* **2015**, *161*, 1215–1228. [CrossRef] [PubMed]
17. Narayanan, R.; Dalton, J.T. Androgen receptor: A complex therapeutic target for breast cancer. *Cancers* **2016**. [CrossRef] [PubMed]
18. Perlmutter, M.A.; Lepor, H. Androgen deprivation therapy in the treatment of advanced prostate cancer. *Rev. Urol.* **2007**, *9*, S3–S8. [PubMed]
19. Godoy, G.; Gakis, G.; Smith, C.L.; Fahmy, O. Effects of androgen and estrogen receptor signaling pathways on bladder cancer initiation and progression. *Bladder Cancer* **2016**, *2*, 127–137. [CrossRef] [PubMed]
20. Di Lauro, L.; Barba, M.; Pizzuti, L.; Vici, P.; Sergi, D.; Di Benedetto, A.; Mottolese, M.; Speirs, V.; Santini, D.; De Maria, R.; et al. Androgen receptor and antiandrogen therapy in male breast cancer. *Cancer lett.* **2015**, *368*, 20–25. [CrossRef] [PubMed]
21. Kanda, T.; Jiang, X.; Yokosuka, O. Androgen receptor signaling in hepatocellular carcinoma and pancreatic cancers. *World J. Gastroenterol.* **2014**, *20*, 9229–9236. [PubMed]
22. Gomella, L.G. Effective testosterone suppression for prostate cancer: Is there a best castration therapy? *Rev. Urol.* **2009**, *11*, 52–60. [PubMed]
23. Grivas, P.D.; Robins, D.M.; Hussain, M. Predicting response to hormonal therapy and survival in men with hormone sensitive metastatic prostate cancer. *Crit. Rev. Oncol. Hematol.* **2013**, *85*, 82–93. [CrossRef] [PubMed]
24. Luk, P.P.; Weston, J.D.; Yu, B.; Selinger, C.I.; Ekmejian, R.; Eviston, T.J.; Lum, T.; Gao, K.; Boyer, M.; O'Toole, S.A.; et al. Salivary duct carcinoma: Clinicopathologic features, morphologic spectrum, and somatic mutations. *Head Neck* **2016**, *38*, E1838–E1847. [CrossRef] [PubMed]
25. Huang, X.; Hao, J.; Chen, S.; Deng, R. Salivary duct carcinoma: A clinopathological report of 11 cases. *Oncol. Lett.* **2015**, *10*, 337–341. [CrossRef] [PubMed]
26. Mitani, Y.; Rao, P.H.; Maity, S.N.; Lee, Y.C.; Ferrarotto, R.; Post, J.C.; Licitra, L.; Lippman, S.M.; Kies, M.S.; Weber, R.S.; et al. Alterations associated with androgen receptor gene activation in salivary duct carcinoma of both sexes: Potential therapeutic ramifications. *Clin. Cancer Res.* **2014**, *20*, 6570–6581. [CrossRef] [PubMed]
27. Butler, R.T.; Spector, M.E.; Thomas, D.; McDaniel, A.S.; McHugh, J.B. An immunohistochemical panel for reliable differentiation of salivary duct carcinoma and mucoepidermoid carcinoma. *Head Neck Pathol.* **2014**, *8*, 133–140. [CrossRef] [PubMed]
28. Cros, J.; Sbidian, E.; Hans, S.; Roussel, H.; Scotte, F.; Tartour, E.; Brasnu, D.; Laurent-Puig, P.; Bruneval, P.; Blons, H.; et al. Expression and mutational status of treatment-relevant targets and key oncogenes in 123 malignant salivary gland tumours. *Ann. Oncol.* **2013**, *24*, 2624–2629. [CrossRef] [PubMed]
29. Masubuchi, T.; Tada, Y.; Maruya, S.; Osamura, Y.; Kamata, S.E.; Miura, K.; Fushimi, C.; Takahashi, H.; Kawakita, D.; Kishimoto, S.; et al. Clinicopathological significance of androgen receptor, HER2, KI-67 and EGFR expressions in salivary duct carcinoma. *Int. J. Clin. Oncol.* **2015**, *20*, 35–44. [CrossRef] [PubMed]
30. Williams, M.D.; Roberts, D.; Blumenschein, G.R., Jr.; Temam, S.; Kies, M.S.; Rosenthal, D.I.; Weber, R.S.; El-Naggar, A.K. Differential expression of hormonal and growth factor receptors in salivary duct carcinomas: Biologic significance and potential role in therapeutic stratification of patients. *Am. J. Surg. Pathol.* **2007**, *31*, 1645–1652. [CrossRef] [PubMed]
31. Williams, L.; Thompson, L.D.; Seethala, R.R.; Weinreb, I.; Assaad, A.M.; Tuluc, M.; Ud Din, N.; Purgina, B.; Lai, C.; Griffith, C.C.; et al. Salivary duct carcinoma: The predominance of apocrine morphology, prevalence of histologic variants, and androgen receptor expression. *Am. J. Surg. Pathol.* **2015**, *39*, 705–713. [CrossRef] [PubMed]
32. Nasser, S.M.; Faquin, W.C.; Dayal, Y. Expression of androgen, estrogen, and progesterone receptors in salivary gland tumors. Frequent expression of androgen receptor in a subset of malignant salivary gland tumors. *Am. J. Clin. Pathol.* **2003**, *119*, 801–806. [CrossRef] [PubMed]
33. Locati, L.D.; Perrone, F.; Losa, M.; Mela, M.; Casieri, P.; Orsenigo, M.; Cortelazzi, B.; Negri, T.; Tamborini, E.; Quattrone, P.; et al. Treatment relevant target immunophenotyping of 139 salivary gland carcinomas (SGCS). *Oral Oncol.* **2009**, *45*, 986–990. [CrossRef] [PubMed]

34. Sygut, D.; Bien, S.; Ziolkowska, M.; Sporny, S. Immunohistochemical expression of androgen receptor in salivary gland cancers. *Pol. J. Pathol.* **2008**, *59*, 205–210. [PubMed]
35. Thompson, L.D.; Aslam, M.N.; Stall, J.N.; Udager, A.M.; Chiosea, S.; McHugh, J.B. Clinicopathologic and immunophenotypic characterization of 25 cases of acinic cell carcinoma with high-grade transformation. *Head Neck Pathol.* **2016**, *10*, 152–160. [CrossRef] [PubMed]
36. Ito, F.A.; Ito, K.; Coletta, R.D.; Vargas, P.A.; Lopes, M.A. Immunohistochemical study of androgen, estrogen and progesterone receptors in salivary gland tumors. *Braz. Oral Res.* **2009**, *23*, 393–398. [CrossRef] [PubMed]
37. Ishibashi, K.; Ito, Y.; Fujii, K.; Masaki, A.; Beppu, S.; Kawakita, D.; Ijichi, K.; Shimozato, K.; Inagaki, H. Androgen receptor-positive mucoepidermoid carcinoma: Case report and literature review. *Int. J. Surg. Pathol.* **2015**, *23*, 243–247. [CrossRef] [PubMed]
38. Seethala, R.R.; Richmond, J.A.; Hoschar, A.P.; Barnes, E.L. New variants of epithelial-myoepithelial carcinoma: Oncocytic-sebaceous and apocrine. *Arch. Pathol. Lab. Med.* **2009**, *133*, 950–959. [PubMed]
39. Di Palma, S. Carcinoma ex pleomorphic adenoma, with particular emphasis on early lesions. *Head Neck Pathol.* **2013**, *7*, S68–S76. [CrossRef] [PubMed]
40. Nakajima, Y.; Kishimoto, T.; Nagai, Y.; Yamada, M.; Iida, Y.; Okamoto, Y.; Ishida, Y.; Nakatani, Y.; Ichinose, M. Expressions of androgen receptor and its co-regulators in carcinoma ex pleomorphic adenoma of salivary gland. *Pathology* **2009**, *41*, 634–639. [CrossRef] [PubMed]
41. Fan, C.Y.; Melhem, M.F.; Hosal, A.S.; Grandis, J.R.; Barnes, E.L. Expression of androgen receptor, epidermal growth factor receptor, and transforming growth factor alpha in salivary duct carcinoma. *Arch. Otolaryngol. Head Neck Surg.* **2001**, *127*, 1075–1079. [CrossRef] [PubMed]
42. Di Palma, S.; Simpson, R.H.; Marchio, C.; Skalova, A.; Ungari, M.; Sandison, A.; Whitaker, S.; Parry, S.; Reis-Filho, J.S. Salivary duct carcinomas can be classified into luminal androgen receptor-positive, HER2 and basal-like phenotypes. *Histopathology* **2012**, *61*, 629–643. [CrossRef] [PubMed]
43. Yamamoto, N.; Minami, S.; Fujii, M. Clinicopathologic study of salivary duct carcinoma and the efficacy of androgen deprivation therapy. *Am. J. Otolaryngol.* **2014**, *35*, 731–735. [CrossRef] [PubMed]
44. Chiosea, S.I.; Williams, L.; Griffith, C.C.; Thompson, L.D.; Weinreb, I.; Bauman, J.E.; Luvison, A.; Roy, S.; Seethala, R.R.; Nikiforova, M.N. Molecular characterization of apocrine salivary duct carcinoma. *Am. J. Surg. Pathol.* **2015**, *39*, 744–752. [CrossRef] [PubMed]
45. Boon, E.; Bel, M.; van der Graaf, W.T.A.; van Es, R.J.J.; Eerenstein, S.; de Jong, R.B.; van den Brekel, M.; van der Velden, L.-A.; Witjes, M.; Hoeben, A.; et al. Salivary duct carcinoma: Clinical outcomes and prognostic factors in 157 patients and results of androgen deprivation therapy in recurrent disease (n = 31)—Study of the dutch head and neck society (DHNS). *J. Clin. Oncol.* **2016**, *34*, Suppl. abstract 6016.
46. Antonarakis, E.S.; Lu, C.; Wang, H.; Luber, B.; Nakazawa, M.; Roeser, J.C.; Chen, Y.; Mohammad, T.A.; Chen, Y.; Fedor, H.L.; et al. AR-V7 and resistance to enzalutamide and abiraterone in prostate cancer. *N. Engl. J. Med.* **2014**, *371*, 1028–1038. [CrossRef] [PubMed]
47. Dehm, S.M.; Schmidt, L.J.; Heemers, H.V.; Vessella, R.L.; Tindall, D.J. Splicing of a novel androgen receptor exon generates a constitutively active androgen receptor that mediates prostate cancer therapy resistance. *Cancer Res.* **2008**, *68*, 5469–5477. [CrossRef] [PubMed]
48. Guo, Z.; Yang, X.; Sun, F.; Jiang, R.; Linn, D.E.; Chen, H.; Chen, H.; Kong, X.; Melamed, J.; Tepper, C.G.; et al. A novel androgen receptor splice variant is up-regulated during prostate cancer progression and promotes androgen depletion-resistant growth. *Cancer Res.* **2009**, *69*, 2305–2313. [CrossRef] [PubMed]
49. Sun, S.; Sprenger, C.C.; Vessella, R.L.; Haugk, K.; Soriano, K.; Mostaghel, E.A.; Page, S.T.; Coleman, I.M.; Nguyen, H.M.; Sun, H.; et al. Castration resistance in human prostate cancer is conferred by a frequently occurring androgen receptor splice variant. *J. Clin. Investig.* **2010**, *120*, 2715–2730. [CrossRef]
50. Watson, P.A.; Chen, Y.F.; Balbas, M.D.; Wongvipat, J.; Socci, N.D.; Viale, A.; Kim, K.; Sawyers, C.L. Constitutively active androgen receptor splice variants expressed in castration-resistant prostate cancer require full-length androgen receptor. *Proc. Natl. Acad. Sci. USA* **2010**, *107*, 16759–16765. [CrossRef] [PubMed]
51. Metzger, E.; Muller, J.M.; Ferrari, S.; Buettner, R.; Schule, R. A novel inducible transactivation domain in the androgen receptor: Implications for prk in prostate cancer. *EMBO J.* **2003**, *22*, 270–280. [CrossRef] [PubMed]
52. Augello, M.A.; Hickey, T.E.; Knudsen, K.E. Foxa1: Master of steroid receptor function in cancer. *EMBO J.* **2011**, *30*, 3885–3894. [CrossRef] [PubMed]
53. Robinson, J.L.; Holmes, K.A.; Carroll, J.S. *FOXA1* mutations in hormone-dependent cancers. *Front. Oncol.* **2013**. [CrossRef] [PubMed]

54. Wen, S.; Niu, Y.; Lee, S.O.; Yeh, S.; Shang, Z.; Gao, H.; Li, Y.; Chou, F.; Chang, C. Targeting fatty acid synthase with ASC-J9 suppresses proliferation and invasion of prostate cancer cells. *Mol. Carcinog.* **2016**, *55*, 2278–2290. [CrossRef] [PubMed]
55. Armstrong, C.M.; Gao, A.C. Drug resistance in castration resistant prostate cancer: Resistance mechanisms and emerging treatment strategies. *Am. J. Clin. Exp. Urol.* **2015**, *3*, 64–76. [PubMed]
56. Merseburger, A.S.; Alcaraz, A.; von Klot, C.A. Androgen deprivation therapy as backbone therapy in the management of prostate cancer. *OncoTargets Ther.* **2016**, *9*, 7263–7274. [CrossRef] [PubMed]
57. Kamata, Y.U.; Sumida, T.; Murase, R.; Nakano, H.; Yamada, T.; Mori, Y. Blockade of androgen-induced malignant phenotypes by flutamide administration in human salivary duct carcinoma cells. *Anticancer Res.* **2016**, *36*, 6071–6075. [CrossRef] [PubMed]
58. Locati, L.D.; Perrone, F.; Cortelazzi, B.; Lo Vullo, S.; Bossi, P.; Dagrada, G.; Quattrone, P.; Bergamini, C.; Potepan, P.; Civelli, E.; et al. Clinical activity of androgen deprivation therapy in patients with metastatic/relapsed androgen receptor-positive salivary gland cancers. *Head Neck* **2016**, *38*, 724–731. [CrossRef] [PubMed]
59. Jaspers, H.C.; Verbist, B.M.; Schoffelen, R.; Mattijssen, V.; Slootweg, P.J.; van der Graaf, W.T.; van Herpen, C.M. Androgen receptor-positive salivary duct carcinoma: A disease entity with promising new treatment options. *J. Clin. Oncol.* **2011**, *29*, e473–e476. [CrossRef] [PubMed]
60. Locati, L.D.; Quattrone, P.; Bossi, P.; Marchiano, A.V.; Cantu, G.; Licitra, L. A complete remission with androgen-deprivation therapy in a recurrent androgen receptor-expressing adenocarcinoma of the parotid gland. *Ann. Oncol.* **2003**, *14*, 1327–1328. [CrossRef] [PubMed]
61. Van der Hulst, R.W.; van Krieken, J.H.; van der Kwast, T.H.; Gerritsen, J.J.; Baatenburg de Jong, R.J.; Lycklama a Nijeholt, A.A.; Meinders, A.E. Partial remission of parotid gland carcinoma after goserelin. *Lancet* **1994**. [CrossRef]
62. Urban, D.; Rischin, D.; Angel, C.; D'Costa, I.; Solomon, B. Abiraterone in metastatic salivary duct carcinoma. *J. Natl. Compr. Cancer Netw.* **2015**, *13*, 288–290.
63. Locati, L.D.; Perrone, F.; Cortelazzi, B.; Imbimbo, M.; Bossi, P.; Potepan, P.; Civelli, E.; Rinaldi, G.; Quattrone, P.; Licitra, L.; et al. Activity of abiraterone in rechallenging two ar-expressing salivary gland adenocarcinomas, resistant to androgen-deprivation therapy. *Cancer Biol. Ther.* **2014**, *15*, 678–682. [CrossRef] [PubMed]
64. Soper, M.S.; Iganej, S.; Thompson, L.D. Definitive treatment of androgen receptor-positive salivary duct carcinoma with androgen deprivation therapy and external beam radiotherapy. *Head Neck* **2014**, *36*, E4–E7. [CrossRef] [PubMed]
65. Kuroda, H.; Sakurai, T.; Yamada, M.; Uemura, N.; Ono, M.; Abe, T.; Fujii, S.; Maeda, M.; Kohda, K.; Obata, M.; et al. Effective treatment by both anti-androgen therapy and chemotherapy for a patient with advanced salivary duct carcinoma. *Jpn. J. Cancer Chemother.* **2011**, *38*, 627–630.

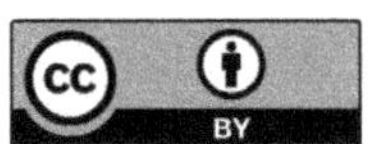

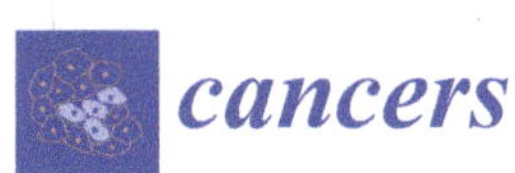

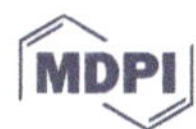

Brief Report

Androgen Receptor Could Be a Potential Therapeutic Target in Patients with Advanced Hepatocellular Carcinoma

Tatsuo Kanda [1,*], Koji Takahashi [1], Masato Nakamura [1], Shingo Nakamoto [1], Shuang Wu [1], Yuki Haga [1], Reina Sasaki [1], Xia Jiang [1,2] and Osamu Yokosuka [1]

1 Department of Gastroenterology and Nephrology, Chiba University, Graduate School of Medicine, 1-8-1 Inohana, Chiba 260-8670, Japan; koji517@gmail.com (K.T.); nkmr.chiba@gmail.com (M.N.); nakamotoer@yahoo.co.jp (S.N.); gosyou100@yahoo.co.jp (S.W.); hagayuki@gmail.com (Y.H.); reina_sasaki_0925@yahoo.co.jp (R.S.); jxia925@yahoo.co.jp (X.J.); yokosukao@faculty.chiba-u.jp (O.Y.)

2 Department of General Surgery, The First Hospital of Hebei Medical University, Donggang Road No. 89, Shijiazhuang 050031, China

* Correspondence: kandat2t@yahoo.co.jp; Tel.: +81-43-226-2086

Academic Editor: Emmanuel S. Antonarakis
Received: 27 February 2017; Accepted: 3 May 2017; Published: 5 May 2017

Abstract: Hepatocellular carcinoma (HCC) is a male-dominant disease with poor prognosis. Sorafenib is the only approved systemic chemotherapeutic drug for patients with advanced HCC. Previous studies have shown that androgen and androgen receptor (AR) are involved in human hepatocarcinogenesis and the development of HCC. Here, we discuss the recent data on AR and HCC, and the combination of sorafenib and inhibitors of AR for advanced-HCC patients. Androgen-dependent and androgen-independent AR activation exist in human hepatocarcinogenesis. AR could directly control hepatocarcinogenesis and regulate the innate immune system to influence HCC progression. Combination of sorafenib with AR inhibitors might represent a potential treatment for patients with advanced HCC.

Keywords: androgen receptor; hepatocellular carcinoma; sorafenib

---

1. Introduction

Hepatocellular carcinoma (HCC) is one of the poor-prognosis cancers [1,2]. In Japan, HCC is the major cancer among primary liver cancers, which have 5- and 10-year survival rates of 34% and 16%, respectively [3]. HCC mostly occurs in patients with cirrhosis. It is not easy to cure HCC by surgical resection other than liver transplantation [4]. In patients with advanced HCC, sorafenib is the only approved systemic chemotherapeutic drug, and new treatment options are eagerly awaited [1].

To surpass the treatment with sorafenib alone for advanced HCC, new treatments have been developed in recent years [2,5,6]. Histone deacetylase inhibitor resminostat plus sorafenib was safe and showed early signs of efficacy for advanced HCC patients progressing on sorafenib-only treatment [5]. Sorafenib plus hepatic arterial infusion chemotherapy with cisplatin achieved favorable overall survival when compared with sorafenib alone for advanced HCC patients [6]. Regorafenib was also shown to provide survival benefit in advanced HCC patients progressing on sorafenib treatment [2].

HCC is one of the male-dominant cancers [7]. We and others have reported that male sex hormone androgen and androgen receptor (AR) are involved in human hepatocarcinogenesis and the development of HCC [8–12]. AR antagonists such as flutamide and bicalutamide have been used for prostate cancer for many decades, and new AR antagonists are also under development [13]. Herein, AR and HCC will be discussed. We also describe the combination treatment of sorafenib and inhibitors of AR for patients with advanced HCC.

2. AR and AR Signaling

Androgens act through AR, a 110-kDa ligand-inducible nuclear receptor (Figure 1A) [14]. The classical steroid receptors such as AR, estrogen receptor, progesterone receptor, glucocorticoid receptor and mineral corticoid receptor are grouped as type 1 nuclear receptors. AR has four functional domains: NH_2-terminal transactivation domain, DNA-binding domain (DBD), hinge region and ligand-binding domain (LBD).

AR regulates the expression of target genes that have androgen response elements (AREs) (Figure 1A) [14,15]. AREs exist in the promoter region of vascular endothelial growth factor (VEGF) [8] and glucose-regulated protein 78 kDa (GRP78) [9], and they play a role in the growth of human hepatocytes. Transforming growth factor, beta 1 (TGF-β1) transcription is also activated by androgen and AR complex in hepatocytes [16,17]. This transcriptional activation function of AR is important in the normal sexual development of the male gender as well as the progression of cancer [8,14,18].

AR co-regulators also influence a number of functional properties of AR, including ligand selectivity and DNA binding capacity [14]. Oncogenes such as erb-b2 receptor tyrosine kinase 2 (ERBB2) and HRas proto-oncogene, GTPase (HRAS) increase mitogen-activated protein kinase signaling, which can cause ligand-independent activation of AR (Figure 1B) [19,20]. There is a cross-talk mechanism between growth factor signaling and androgen in prostate development, physiology, and cancer [20]. Ligand-independent activation of AR pathways also plays a role in human HCC and pancreatic cancer progression [8,21].

The activation of Src kinase is involved in the ligand-independent activation of AR [22]. Two UDP-glucuronosyltransferases (2B15 and 2B7) are also involved in inactivation of androgens, and may have a major role in persons that is null genotype of UGT2B17 [23]. Hepatitis B X (HBx) also augmented AR activity by enhancing the phosphorylation of AR through HBx-mediated activation of the c-Src kinase signaling pathway in human hepatocarcinogenesis [11,24].

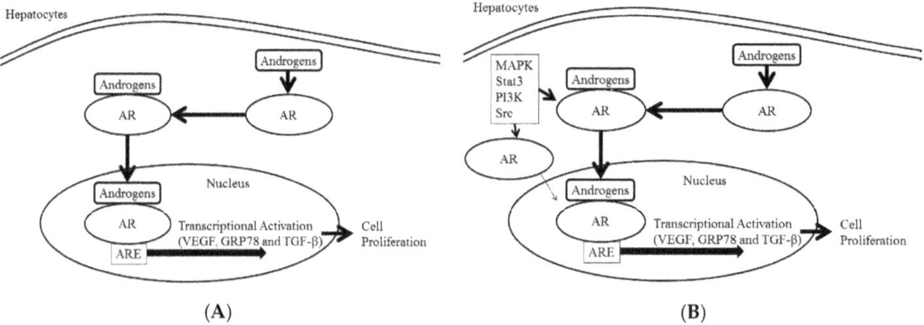

Figure 1. Androgen-dependent and androgen-independent androgen receptor (AR) activation in human hepatocarcinogenesis. (**A**) Androgen-dependent signaling. (**B**) Androgen-independent signaling. Phosphorylation of mitogen-activated protein kinase (MAPK), signal transducer and activator of transcription 3 (Stat3), AKT serine/threonine kinase 1 (Akt) and Proto-oncogene tyrosine-protein kinase (Src) activates AR. VEGF, vascular endothelial growth factor; GRP78, glucose-regulated protein 78 kDa; TGF-β, transforming growth factor, beta 1; PI3K, phosphatidylinositol-4,5-bisphosphate 3-kinase catalytic subunit alpha.

3. AR and HCC

Human HCC and normal liver express AR [7,10,25]. Hepatitis B virus (HBV) and hepatitis C virus (HCV) are two major causes of HCC. AR signaling is involved in human HCC associated with HBV and HCV [26]. AR signaling should be involved in hepatocarcinogenesis to some extent, irrespective of the cause of human and mouse HCC [27]. As androgen and AR-signaling are associated with the development of steatosis [28], AR may be associated with HCC that is related to non-alcoholic steatohepatitis.

Increased expression of variant transcripts from the AR gene (ARVs) has been shown to be involved in the development of castration-resistant prostate cancer [29]. The expression of ARVs was observed in the liver and may be involved in hepatocarcinogenesis [30]. AR variants may also lead to resistance to HCC antiandrogen therapy in the liver.

4. AR and Sorafenib in the Treatment of HCC (Table 1)

At present, sorafenib is the only approved drug for systemic chemotherapy of HCC. We observed that sorafenib-induced apoptosis was enhanced by the inhibition of AR and GRP78 in human hepatoma cell lines [9]. Sorafenib also inhibits AR activation induced by HBx in vitro and in vivo [31]. Of interest, this AR-targeting ability of sorafenib was not mediated by its well-known kinase inhibitory activity; however, this ability of sorafenib was achieved by enhancing the activity of K-box region and MADS-box transcription factor family protein (SHP-1) tyrosine phosphatase [31]. There are contrary opinions concerning hepatic AR and the effect of sorafenib, namely that hepatic AR suppresses HCC metastasis through modulation of cell migration and anoikis [30,32,33]. Natural killer (NK) cells suppress HCC; and interleukin 12 (IL12A), one of the NK cell stimulatory factors, plays a role in the activation of NK cell function [34,35]. In NK cells, AR could suppress IL12A expression at the transcriptional level, resulting in repressing the efficacy of NK cell cytotoxicity against HCC [34]. Sorafenib treatment interacts with AR and enhances IL12A signals [34]. AR could regulate the innate immune system to influence HCC progression [34,36,37]. Although AR suppresses HCC metastasis at late stage [28,32,33,37], androgen and the AR axis maintain and promote cancer cell stemness through activation of Nanog in HCC [38].

Table 1. Molecular targets during anti-cancer drug treatment for hepatocellular carcinoma (HCC) through androgen receptor (AR).

References	Targets	Effects of Anti-Cancer Drugs
Jiang et al. [9]	GRP78	Knockdown of GRP78 and AR enhances apoptosis induced by sorafenib in human hepatoma cells.
Wang et al. [31]	SHP-1	Sorafenib inhibited HBx-enhanced AR activity by activating SHP-1 phosphatase in HBx-transgenic mice.
Shi et al. [34]	IL12A	Sorafenib interacts with AR and enhances IL12A signals.
Shi et al. [36]	ULBP2	By suppressing AR, cisplatin could up-regulate cytotoxicity of NK cells to target HCC.
Ma et al. [28]	p-p38, NFκB, MMP9	Addition of sorafenib improved HCC survival of L-AR$^{-/y}$ mice.
Xu et al. [33]	miR-367	Combining miR-367-3p with Sorafenib showed better efficacy of suppressing HCC cell invasion by altering AR signals in vitro and in vivo.

GRP78, glucose-regulated protein 78 kDa; SHP-1, K-box region and MADS-box transcription factor family protein; HBx, hepatitis B x; IL12A, interleukin 12A; ULBP2, UL16-binding protein 2; p-p38, phosphorylation of p38 kinase; NF-κB, nuclear factor kappa B; MMP9, matrix metalloproteinase 9.

5. Conclusions

We have already reviewed clinical trials targeting androgen in HCC [25]. However, the previous reports demonstrated that anti-androgen therapies did not show any survival benefits in advanced HCC patients [39,40]. That might be considered to be attributed by the lower expression of AR and androgen-independent AR activation mechanism in the advanced HCC. A recent review [13] described phase I/II clinical trials of the androgen antagonist enzalutamide with or without sorafenib for advanced HCC that are currently underway. Enzalutamide binds to the AR with greater relative affinity than the clinically used antiandrogen bicalutamide, reduces the efficiency of its nuclear translocation, and impairs both DNA binding to androgen response elements and recruitment of coactivators [41]. The combination of sorafenib and enzalutamide is a potentially new approach for the treatment of castration-resistant prostate cancer [42]. This combination may present a potential treatment for patients with advanced HCC. In prostatic cancer cells with downregulated AR expression by short interfering RNA, treatment with sorafenib increased apoptosis in an additive manner [43], suggesting that there might be a potential to use inhibitors of AR in HCC as an adjuvant therapy option for sorafenib-resistant HCC patients. Moreover, immune checkpoint inhibitors such as programmed cell death 1 (PD-1), programmed cell death ligand 1 (PD-L1), or cytotoxic T-lymphocyte-associated protein 4 (CTLA-4) are now undergoing clinical trials, and they may open new doors for the treatment of HCC [44]. In this new era, AR could control NK cell function and may be a more attractive target. In conclusion, recent advances regarding AR in HCC have been described. AR is an attractive target with or without anti-cancer drugs in HCC, one of the male dominant diseases.

Acknowledgments: We extended our thanks to Prof. Fumio Imazeki and Prof. Naoya Kato for helpful suggestions. This work was partly supported by grants from the Japan Agency for Medical Research and Development (AMED).

Author Contributions: Tatsuo Kanda, Koji Takahashi, Masato Nakamura, Shingo Nakamoto, Shuang Wu, Yuki Haga, Reina Sasaki, Xia Jiang and Osamu Yokosuka conceived, designed and wrote the paper.

Conflicts of Interest: Tatsuo Kanda received research grants from Merck Sharp and Dohme (MSD), Chugai Pharm and AbbVie. The founding sponsors had no role in the design of the study; in the collection, analyses, or interpretation of data; in the writing of the manuscript, and in the decision to publish the results. The other authors declare no conflict of interest.

References

1. Llovet, J.M.; Ricci, S.; Mazzaferro, V.; Hilgard, P.; Gane, E.; Blanc, J.F.; de Oliveira, A.C.; Santoro, A.; Raoul, J.L.; Forner, A.; et al. SHARP Investigators Study Group. Sorafenib in advanced hepatocellular carcinoma. *N. Engl. J. Med.* **2008**, *359*, 378–390. [CrossRef] [PubMed]
2. Bruix, J.; Qin, S.; Merle, P.; Granito, A.; Huang, Y.H.; Bodoky, G.; Pracht, M.; Yokosuka, O.; Rosmorduc, O.; Breder, V.; et al. RESORCE Investigators. Regorafenib for patients with hepatocellular carcinoma who progressed on sorafenib treatment (RESORCE): A randomised, double-blind, placebo-controlled, phase 3 trial. *Lancet* **2017**, *389*, 56–66. [CrossRef]
3. National Cancer Center. Center for Cancer Control and Information Services. Available online: http://ganjoho.jp/reg_stat/statistics/stat/summary.html (accessed on 23 February 2017).
4. Kanda, T.; Ogasawara, S.; Chiba, T.; Haga, Y.; Omata, M.; Yokosuka, O. Current management of patients with hepatocellular carcinoma. *World J. Hepatol.* **2015**, *7*, 1913–1920. [CrossRef] [PubMed]
5. Bitzer, M.; Horger, M.; Giannini, E.G.; Ganten, T.M.; Wörns, M.A.; Siveke, J.T.; Dollinger, M.M.; Gerken, G.; Scheulen, M.E.; Wege, H.; et al. Resminostat plus sorafenib as second-line therapy of advanced hepatocellular carcinoma—The SHELTER study. *J. Hepatol.* **2016**, *65*, 280–288. [CrossRef] [PubMed]
6. Ikeda, M.; Shimizu, S.; Sato, T.; Morimoto, M.; Kojima, Y.; Inaba, Y.; Hagihara, A.; Kudo, M.; Nakamori, S.; Kaneko, S.; et al. Sorafenib plus hepatic arterial infusion chemotherapy with cisplatin versus sorafenib for advanced hepatocellular carcinoma: Randomized phase II trial. *Ann. Oncol.* **2016**, *27*, 2090–2096. [CrossRef] [PubMed]
7. Nagasue, N.; Yu, L.; Yukaya, H.; Kohno, H.; Nakamura, T. Androgen and oestrogen receptors in hepatocellular carcinoma and surrounding liver parenchyma: Impact on intrahepatic recurrence after hepatic resection. *Br. J. Surg.* **1995**, *82*, 542–547. [CrossRef] [PubMed]
8. Kanda, T.; Steele, R.; Ray, R.; Ray, R.B. Hepatitis C virus core protein augments androgen receptor-mediated signaling. *J. Virol.* **2008**, *82*, 11066–11072. [CrossRef] [PubMed]
9. Jiang, X.; Kanda, T.; Nakamoto, S.; Miyamura, T.; Wu, S.; Yokosuka, O. Involvement of androgen receptor and glucose-regulated protein 78 kDa in human hepatocarcinogenesis. *Exp. Cell Res.* **2014**, *323*, 326–336. [CrossRef] [PubMed]
10. Kanda, T.; Jiang, X.; Yokosuka, O. Androgen receptor signaling in hepatocellular carcinoma and pancreatic cancers. *World J. Gastroenterol.* **2014**, *20*, 9229–9236. [PubMed]

11. Chiu, C.M.; Yeh, S.H.; Chen, P.J.; Kuo, T.J.; Chang, C.J.; Chen, P.J.; Yang, W.J.; Chen, D.S. Hepatitis B virus X protein enhances androgen receptor-responsive gene expression depending on androgen level. *Proc. Natl. Acad. Sci. USA* **2007**, *104*, 2571–2578. [CrossRef] [PubMed]
12. Zheng, Y.; Chen, W.L.; Ma, W.L.; Chang, C.; Ou, J.H. Enhancement of gene transactivation activity of androgen receptor by hepatitis B virus X protein. *Virology* **2007**, *363*, 454–461. [CrossRef] [PubMed]
13. Schweizer, M.T.; Yu, E.Y. AR-Signaling in Human Malignancies: Prostate Cancer and Beyond. *Cancers* **2017**, *9*, 7. [CrossRef] [PubMed]
14. Heinlein, C.A.; Chang, C. Androgen receptor (AR) coregulators: An overview. *Endocr. Rev.* **2002**, *23*, 175–200. [CrossRef] [PubMed]
15. Bolton, E.C.; So, A.Y.; Chaivorapol, C.; Haqq, C.M.; Li, H.; Yamamoto, K.R. Cell- and gene-specific regulation of primary target genes by the androgen receptor. *Genes. Dev.* **2007**, *21*, 2005–2017. [CrossRef] [PubMed]
16. Yoon, G.; Kim, J.Y.; Choi, Y.K.; Won, Y.S.; Lim, I.K. Direct activation of TGF-beta1 transcription by androgen and androgen receptor complex in Huh7 human hepatoma cells and its tumor in nude mice. *J. Cell Biochem.* **2006**, *97*, 393–411. [CrossRef] [PubMed]
17. Koch, D.C.; Jang, H.S.; O'Donnell, E.F.; Punj, S.; Kopparapu, P.R.; Bisson, W.H.; Kerkvliet, N.I.; Kolluri, S.K. Anti-androgen flutamide suppresses hepatocellular carcinoma cell proliferation via the aryl hydrocarbon receptor mediated induction of transforming growth factor-β1. *Oncogene* **2015**, *34*, 6092–6104. [CrossRef] [PubMed]
18. Chen, C.D.; Welsbie, D.S.; Tran, C.; Baek, S.H.; Chen, R.; Vessella, R.; Rosenfeld, M.G.; Sawyers, C.L. Molecular determinants of resistance to antiandrogen therapy. *Nat. Med.* **2004**, *10*, 33–39. [CrossRef] [PubMed]
19. Craft, N.; Shostak, Y.; Carey, M.; Sawyers, C.L. A mechanism for hormone-independent prostate cancer through modulation of androgen receptor signaling by the HER-2/neu tyrosine kinase. *Nat. Med.* **1999**, *5*, 280–285. [CrossRef] [PubMed]
20. Gioeli, D.; Ficarro, S.B.; Kwiek, J.J.; Aaronson, D.; Hancock, M.; Catling, A.D.; White, F.M.; Christian, R.E.; Settlage, R.E.; Shabanowitz, J.; et al. Androgen receptor phosphorylation. Regulation and identification of the phosphorylation sites. *J. Biol. Chem.* **2002**, *277*, 29304–29314. [CrossRef] [PubMed]
21. Okitsu, K.; Kanda, T.; Imazeki, F.; Yonemitsu, Y.; Ray, R.B.; Chang, C.; Yokosuka, O. Involvement of interleukin-6 and androgen receptor signaling in pancreatic cancer. *Genes. Cancer* **2010**, *1*, 859–867. [CrossRef] [PubMed]
22. Szafran, A.T.; Stephan, C.; Bolt, M.; Mancini, M.G.; Marcelli, M.; Mancini, M.A. High-Content Screening Identifies Src Family Kinases as Potential Regulators of AR-V7 Expression and Androgen-Independent Cell Growth. *Prostate* **2017**, *77*, 82–93. [CrossRef] [PubMed]
23. Kuuranne, T.; Kurkela, M.; Thevis, M.; Schänzer, W.; Finel, M.; Kostiainen, R. Glucuronidation of anabolic androgenic steroids by recombinant human UDP-glucuronosyltransferases. *Drug Metab. Dispos.* **2003**, *31*, 1117–1124. [CrossRef] [PubMed]
24. Yang, W.J.; Chang, C.J.; Yeh, S.H.; Lin, W.H.; Wang, S.H.; Tsai, T.F.; Chen, D.S.; Chen, P.J. Hepatitis B virus X protein enhances the transcriptional activity of the androgen receptor through c-Src and glycogen synthase kinase-3beta kinase pathways. *Hepatology* **2009**, *49*, 1515–1524. [CrossRef] [PubMed]
25. Kanda, T.; Yokosuka, O. The androgen receptor as an emerging target in hepatocellular carcinoma. *J. Hepatocell. Carcinoma* **2015**, *2*, 91–99. [CrossRef] [PubMed]
26. Kanda, T.; Yokosuka, O.; Omata, M. Androgen Receptor and Hepatocellular Carcinoma. *J. Gastrointest. Dig. Syst.* **2013**, S12. [CrossRef]
27. Wu, M.H.; Ma, W.L.; Hsu, C.L.; Chen, Y.L.; Ou, J.H.; Ryan, C.K.; Hung, Y.C.; Yeh, S.; Chang, C. Androgen receptor promotes hepatitis B virus-induced hepatocarcinogenesis through modulation of hepatitis B virus RNA transcription. *Sci. Transl. Med.* **2010**, *2*, 32ra35. [CrossRef] [PubMed]
28. Ma, W.L.; Lai, H.C.; Yeh, S.; Cai, X.; Chang, C. Androgen receptor roles in hepatocellular carcinoma, fatty liver, cirrhosis and hepatitis. *Endocr. Relat. Cancer* **2014**, *21*, R165–R182. [CrossRef] [PubMed]
29. Brand, L.J.; Dehm, S.M. Androgen receptor gene rearrangements: New perspectives on prostate cancer progression. *Curr. Drug Targets* **2013**, *14*, 441–449. [CrossRef] [PubMed]
30. Hu, D.G.; Hickey, T.E.; Irvine, C.; Wijayakumara, D.D.; Lu, L.; Tilley, W.D.; Selth, L.A.; Mackenzie, P.I. Identification of androgen receptor splice variant transcripts in breast cancer cell lines and human tissues. *Horm. Cancer* **2014**, *5*, 61–71. [CrossRef] [PubMed]

31. Wang, S.H.; Yeh, S.H.; Shiau, C.W.; Chen, K.F.; Lin, W.H.; Tsai, T.F.; Teng, Y.C.; Chen, D.S.; Chen, P.J. Sorafenib Action in Hepatitis B Virus X-Activated Oncogenic Androgen Pathway in Liver through SHP-1. *J. Natl. Cancer Inst.* **2015**, *107*, pii: djv190. [CrossRef] [PubMed]
32. Ma, W.L.; Hsu, C.L.; Yeh, C.C.; Wu, M.H.; Huang, C.K.; Jeng, L.B.; Hung, Y.C.; Lin, T.Y.; Yeh, S.; Chang, C. Hepatic androgen receptor suppresses hepatocellular carcinoma metastasis through modulation of cell migration and anoikis. *Hepatology* **2012**, *56*, 176–185. [CrossRef] [PubMed]
33. Xu, J.; Lin, H.; Li, G.; Sun, Y.; Chen, J.; Shi, L.; Cai, X.; Chang, C. The miR-367-3p Increases Sorafenib Chemotherapy Efficacy to Suppress Hepatocellular Carcinoma Metastasis through Altering the Androgen Receptor Signals. *EBioMedicine* **2016**, *12*, 55–67. [CrossRef] [PubMed]
34. Shi, L.; Lin, H.; Li, G.; Jin, R.A.; Xu, J.; Sun, Y.; Ma, W.L.; Yeh, S.; Cai, X.; Chang, C. Targeting Androgen Receptor (AR)→IL12A Signal Enhances Efficacy of Sorafenib plus NK Cells Immunotherapy to Better Suppress HCC Progression. *Mol. Cancer Ther.* **2016**, *15*, 731–742. [CrossRef] [PubMed]
35. Manetti, R.; Parronchi, P.; Giudizi, M.G.; Piccinni, M.P.; Maggi, E.; Trinchieri, G.; Romagnani, S. Natural killer cell stimulatory factor (interleukin 12 [IL-12]) induces T helper type 1 (Th1)-specific immune responses and inhibits the development of IL-4-producing Th cells. *J. Exp. Med.* **1993**, *177*, 1199–1204. [CrossRef] [PubMed]
36. Shi, L.; Lin, H.; Li, G.; Sun, Y.; Shen, J.; Xu, J.; Lin, C.; Yeh, S.; Cai, X.; Chang, C. Cisplatin enhances NK cells immunotherapy efficacy to suppress HCC progression via altering the androgen receptor (AR)-ULBP2 signals. *Cancer Lett.* **2016**, *373*, 45–56. [CrossRef] [PubMed]
37. Lai, H.C.; Yeh, C.C.; Jeng, L.B.; Huang, S.F.; Liao, P.Y.; Lei, F.J.; Cheng, W.C.; Hsu, C.L.; Cai, X.; Chang, C.; et al. Androgen receptor mitigates postoperative disease progression of hepatocellular carcinoma by suppressing CD90+ populations and cell migration and by promoting anoikis in circulating tumor cells. *Oncotarget* **2016**, *7*, 46448–46465. [CrossRef] [PubMed]
38. Jiang, L.; Shan, J.; Shen, J.; Wang, Y.; Yan, P.; Liu, L.; Zhao, W.; Xu, Y.; Zhu, W.; Su, L.; et al. Androgen/androgen receptor axis maintains and promotes cancer cell stemness through direct activation of Nanog transcription in hepatocellular carcinoma. *Oncotarget* **2016**, *7*, 36814–36828. [CrossRef] [PubMed]
39. Grimaldi, C.; Bleiberg, H.; Gay, F.; Messner, M.; Rougier, P.; Kok, T.C.; Cirera, L.; Cervantes, A.; De Greve, J.; Paillot, B.; et al. Evaluation of antiandrogen therapy in unresectable hepatocellular carcinoma: Results of a European Organization for Research and Treatment of Cancer multicentric double-blind trial. *J. Clin. Oncol.* **1998**, *16*, 411–417. [CrossRef] [PubMed]
40. Groupe d'Etude et de Traitement du Carcinome Hépatocellulaire. Randomized trial of leuprorelin and flutamide in male patients with hepatocellular carcinoma treated with tamoxifen. *Hepatology* **2004**, *40*, 1361–1369.
41. Tran, C.; Ouk, S.; Clegg, N.J.; Chen, Y.; Watson, P.A.; Arora, V.; Wongvipat, J.; Smith-Jones, P.M.; Yoo, D.; Kwon, A.; et al. Development of a second-generation antiandrogen for treatment of advanced prostate cancer. *Science* **2009**, *324*, 787–790. [CrossRef] [PubMed]
42. Wu, H.; Zhang, L.; Gao, X.; Zhang, X.; Duan, J.; You, L.; Cheng, Y.; Bian, J.; Zhu, Q.; Yang, Y. Combination of sorafenib and enzalutamide as a potential new approach for the treatment of castration-resistant prostate cancer. *Cancer Lett.* **2017**, *385*, 108–116. [CrossRef] [PubMed]
43. Oh, S.J.; Erb, H.H.; Hobisch, A.; Santer, F.R.; Culig, Z. Sorafenib decreases proliferation and induces apoptosis of prostate cancer cells by inhibition of the androgen receptor and Akt signaling pathways. *Endocr. Relat. Cancer.* **2012**, *19*, 305–319. [CrossRef] [PubMed]
44. Kudo, M. Immune Checkpoint Inhibition in Hepatocellular Carcinoma: Basics and Ongoing Clinical Trials. *Oncology* **2017**, *92* (Suppl. 1), 50–62. [CrossRef] [PubMed]

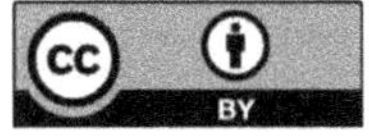

MDPI AG
St. Alban-Anlage 66
4052 Basel, Switzerland
Tel. +41 61 683 77 34
Fax +41 61 302 89 18
http://www.mdpi.com

Cancers Editorial Office
E-mail: cancers@mdpi.com
http://www.mdpi.com/journal/cancers

www.ingramcontent.com/pod-product-compliance
Lightning Source LLC
Chambersburg PA
CBHW051729210326
41597CB00032B/5656

* 9 7 8 3 0 3 8 4 2 7 4 0 7 *